Saunders
Review
of
FAMILY
PRACTICE

Saunders
Review
of
FAMILY
PRACTICE

2nd Edition

EDWARD T. BOPE, MD
Director
Family Practice Residency Program
Family Practice Center
Riverside Methodist Hospitals
Columbus, Ohio

ALVAH R. CASS, MD, ScM
Associate Professor
Department of Family Medicine
University of Texas
Medical Branch—Galveston
Galveston, Texas

MICHAEL D. HAGEN, MD
Nicholas J. Pisacano Professor and
  Associate Chair for Academic Affairs
Department of Family Practice
University of Kentucky
School of Medicine
Attending Physician, University Hospital
Lexington, Kentucky

W.B. SAUNDERS COMPANY
A Division of Harcourt Brace & Company
Philadelphia ● London ● Toronto ● Montreal ● Sydney ● Tokyo

W.B. SAUNDERS COMPANY
A Division of Harcourt Brace & Company

The Curtis Center
Independence Square West
Philadelphia, Pennsylvania 19106

Library of Congress Cataloging-in-Publication Data

Saunders review of family practice /
[edited by] Edward T. Bope, Alvah R. Cass, Michael D. Hagen.—2nd ed.

p. cm.

ISBN 0–7216–5817–2

1. Family medicine. I. Bope, Edward T. II. Cass, Alvah R.
III. Hagen, Michael D. [DNLM: 1. Family Practice—examination
questions. 2. Comprehensive Health Care—examination questions.
WB 18.2 S257 1997]

RC46.S225 1997   610—dc20

DNLM/DLC   96–16715

SAUNDERS REVIEW OF FAMILY PRACTICE   ISBN 0–7216–5817–2

Printed in the United States of America

Last digit is the print number: 9   8   7   6   5   4   3

Contributors

Kent E. Anthony, M.D., M.B.A., B.A.
Assistant Professor, Department of Family Medicine, University of Texas Medical Branch, Galveston, Texas
The Problem-Oriented Medical Record; Managed Health Care; Accounting Systems; Personnel and Time Management

Clyde A. Addison, M.D.
Family Physician, Chenango Memorial Hospital, Norwich, New York
Growth and Development

Gregory H. Blake, M.D., M.P.H.
Associate Professor and Chairman, Department of Family Medicine, University of Tennessee Medical Center, Knoxville, Tennessee
Otolaryngology

Edward T. Bope, B.S., M.D.
Director, Family Practice Residency Program, Family Practice Center, Riverside Methodist Hospitals, Columbus, Ohio
Pulmonary Medicine

Pamela Jelly Boyers, Ph.D.
Director of Medical Education, Riverside Methodist Hospitals at Grant/Riverside, Columbus, Ohio
Establishing Rapport

Alvah R. Cass, M.D., Sc.M.
Associate Professor, Department of Family Medicine, The University of Texas Medical Branch, Galveston, Texas
Assessment of Functional Health Status

Mary Thoesen Coleman, M.D., Ph.D.
Assistant Professor, Department of Family Medicine, The Ohio State University; Rardin Family Practice Center, Columbus, Ohio
Emergency Medicine

Steven A. Crawford, M.D.
Vice-Chair and Clinical Professor, Department of Family Medicine, University of Oklahoma, Oklahoma City, Oklahoma
Endocrinology

Michael Dunaway, M.D.
Faculty Development Fellow, University of Kentucky, Lexington; Medical Staff, (Flemingsburg) Fleming County Hospital, Flemingsburg, Kentucky
Personality Disorders in Office Practice; Dementia

Paul Dusseau, B.A., M.D.
Assistant Instructor, Riverside Methodist Hospital, Family Practice Center, Columbus, Ohio
Neurology in Family Practice

Matthew D. Everett, D.O.
Ohio State University Clinical Faculty, Riverside Methodist Hospital Family Practice Residency, Columbus, Ohio
Care of the Elderly

Carolyn L. Frymoyer, M.D.
Assistant Professor, Health Science Center at Syracuse; Residency Faculty, St. Joseph's Hospital Health Center, Syracuse, New York
Rheumatic Disease

Bill G. Gegas, M.D.
Clinical Assistant Professor, Department of Family Practice, Ohio State University; Associate Program Director, Family Practice Residency Program, Riverside Methodist Hospitals, Columbus, Ohio
Obstetrics

Michael D. Hagen, M.D.
Nicholas J. Pisacano Professor and Associate Chair for Academic Affairs, Department of Family Practice, University of Kentucky School of Medicine; Attending Physician, University Hospital, Lexington, Kentucky
Preventive Health Care; Use of Consultants; Interpretation of the Electrocardiogram; Cardiovascular Disease and Arrhythmias; Orthopedics; Diagnosis and Treatment of Anxiety Disorders; Depression; Crisis Intervention in Office Practice; Alcohol Abuse

Wendy J. Hunter, M.A., B.M. B.Ch., D.Ch., DRCOG, MRCGP
General Practitioner, St. Katherine's Surgery, Herefordshire, England
Care of the Dying Patient

Clarence A. Jernigan, M.D., M.P.H.
Associate Professor, The University of Texas Medical Branch, Galveston, Texas
Computer Applications in Office Practice; Malpractice and Risk Management

Cynda Johnson, M.D.
Professor, Departments of Family Medicine and Obstetrics/Gynecology; Vice Chair, Department of Family Medicine; Residency Program Director, University of Kansas Medical Center, Kansas City, Kansas
Contraception

William Jorgenson, D.O.
Associate Professor, Crouse Irving Memorial Hospital, Syracuse, New York
Allergy

Gary W. Kearl, M.D., M.S.P.H.
Attending Physician, Chandler Medical Center, University of Kentucky College of Medicine, Lexington, Kentucky
Office Surgery; Gynecology

Mitchell S. King, M.D.
Director, Family Practice Residency, St. Francis Hospital of Evanston, Evanston, Illinois
Ophthalmology

Douglas J. Knutson, M.D.
Family Practice Resident, Riverside Methodist Hospitals, Columbus, Ohio
Interpreting Laboratory Tests

Francis P. Kohrs, M.D., M.S.P.H.
Assistant Professor and Director, Predoctoral Education, University of Kentucky College of Medicine; Attending Physician, Chandler Medical Center, University of Kentucky, Lexington, Kentucky
Oncology; Hematology

Andrew Leeman, M.A., B.M. B.Ch., MRCGP
Principal in General Practice, Pendeen Surgery, Ross-on-Wye, England
Ethics in Family Practice

Camille M. Leugers, M.D.
Assistant Professor, Department of Community Medicine, Baylor College of Medicine, Houston, Texas
Care of the Newborn

Thomas G. Maddox, M.D.
Assistant Director, Trinity Lutheran Family Practice Residency, Kansas City, Missouri
Infectious Diseases

Arch G. Mainous III, Ph.D.
Associate Professor and Research Director, University of Kentucky, Lexington, Kentucky
Behavioral Problems in Children and Adolescents; The Somatic Patient

Stephen E. Markovich, M.D.
Family Practice Senior Resident, Riverside Methodist Hospitals, Columbus, Ohio
Interpreting Laboratory Tests

Matthew McHugh, M.D., B.S.(Human Nutrition)
Physician, Riverside Methodist Hospital, Columbus, Ohio
Sports Medicine

Marilyn Mehr, Ph.D.
Professor, Department of Family Practice; Professor and Director, Behavioral Medicine, University of Kentucky Medical School, Lexington, Kentucky
Depression; Crisis Intervention in Office Practice

Peter Nalin, M.D.
Associate Professor, State University of New York Health Science Center, Syracuse, New York
Pulmonary Medicine

Donald E. Nease, Jr., M.D.
Assistant Professor, Department of Family Medicine, University of Texas Medical Branch, Galveston, Texas
Evaluation of Skin Lesions; Nutrition and Family Medicine

Emily R. Nease, M.S., R.D.
Clinical Dietitian, Marriott Management Services at Edgewater Methodist Retirement Community, Galveston, Texas
Nutrition and Family Medicine

Richard Neill, M.D.
Assistant Professor, Residency Director, University of Kentucky, Lexington, Kentucky
Gastroenterology; Clinical Genetics and Genetic Counseling

Dana Nottingham, M.D.
Clinical Instructor, The Ohio State University College of Medicine; Assistant Director, Riverside Family Practice Residency Program, Grant/Riverside Methodist Hospitals, Columbus, Ohio
Patient Compliance; Patient Education

Jeri A. O'Donnell, M.A., LPCC
Director of Behavioral Sciences, Riverside Family Practice Residency, Grant/Riverside Hospitals, Columbus, Ohio
The Family's Influence on Health; Domestic Violence

Juan A. Pérez, M.D.
Assistant Professor, Department of Family Medicine, University of Medicine and Dentistry of New Jersey, Newark; Clinical Associate Professor, Robert Wood Johnson School of Medicine, New Brunswick; Chairman, Family Practice, St. Mary Hospital, Hoboken; Director of Medical Education, Franciscan Health System of New Jersey, New Jersey
Sexual Health Care

Alan R. Roth, D.O.
Clinical Assistant Professor of Family Practice, New York College of Osteopathic Medicine, Old Westbury, and State University of New York Health Science Center at Brooklyn; Director, Family Practice Residency Program, Jamaica Hospital Medical Center, Jamaica, New York
Periodic Health Examination

David R. Rudy, M.D., M.P.H.
Pomerene Professor and Vice Chairman, The Ohio State University College of Medicine, Columbus, Ohio
The Family Physician; Clinical Problem Solving

Victor S. Sierpina, M.D.
Assistant Professor, The University of Texas Medical Branch, Galveston, Texas
Parasitology and Travel Medicine

Janice Kelly Smith, M.D.
Clinical Assistant Professor, Department of Family Medicine, University of Texas Medical Branch, Galveston, Texas
Childhood and Adolescence

Walton Sumner, M.D.
Assistant Professor, Department of Internal Medicine, Division of General Medical Sciences, Washington University School of Medicine, St. Louis, Missouri
Nicotine Addiction

Robert F. Thompson, M.D.
Director of Clinical and Educational Programs, First Choice Community Health Care, Albuquerque, New Mexico
Community-Oriented Primary Care

William A. Verhoff, B.S.N., R.N.
Nurse Manager, Riverside Methodist Hospital, Columbus, Ohio
Psychosocial Influences on Health; Practicing Biopsychosocial Medicine

Betty Walker, Ph.D.
Associate Professor and Director of Education, Department of Family Practice, University of Kentucky Medical School, Lexington, Kentucky
Diagnosis and Treatment of Anxiety Disorders; Alcohol Abuse

Michael B. Weinstock, M.D.
Clinical Assistant Professor, Ohio State University College of Medicine; Faculty Attending, Family Practice Residency Program, Riverside Methodist Hospitals, Columbus, Ohio
Care of the Adult HIV-1–Infected Patient

Betty Young, Dr.P.H.
Assistant Professor, Department of Family Practice, University of Kentucky and Kentucky Clinic, Lexington, Kentucky
Family Genogram; Interviewing Techniques

Roger J. Zoorob, M.D., M.P.H.
Assistant Professor, Family Practice, and Associate Residency Director, University of Kentucky College of Medicine, Lexington, Kentucky
Urinary Tract Disorders; Abuse of Controlled Substances

Foreword

"Curiosity is one of the permanent and certain characteristics of a vigorous intellect."

Samuel Johnson

Inquisitiveness, testing, and retesting are natural to family physicians. We thrive on the varied challenges of medicine and enjoy the variety of problems that confront us daily in practice. We are more comfortable with the unknown than are physicians in other specialties, and we are more willing to let time heal or define the condition more clearly.

Ours was the first specialty to require recertification every six years, so testing and retesting is a way of life for us. We realize how much more we learn from these challenges and recognize how this testing keeps us sharp and up to date. We are eager to learn more and provide the best care possible for our patients. This book helps us do that. It challenges us to be knowledgeable and remain current with recent medical advances.

The authors have captured the essence of the content of *The Textbook of Family Practice* and have designed a variety of questions relating to that material in a manner that is challenging and informative. They also provide a critique of each question, explaining why the answer is correct or incorrect and then reference the source. Everyone, whether experienced physician or second-year medical student, can benefit from this challenging review.

Robert E. Rakel, M.D.

Preface

The family doctor is a student for life, using each patient as a check against the current medical knowledge and as a guide for what we need to learn. The amount of medical literature is vast and is now more accessible through electronic applications. Many offices and homes are now equipped with computers, thus allowing fast, up-to-date referencing. Most clinicians keep a trusted textbook such as Rakel's *Textbook of Family Practice* close at hand. Those who have used this textbook are grateful for both its breadth and depth of information.

The *Saunders Review of Family Practice* is written as a study companion to the Rakel text. It is written by family doctors who have carefully reviewed each chapter and written questions about what they believe to be the most important learning points. In each case, the questions have been edited to be sure that they are accurate and in good form for test-taking practice. To properly use this book, the learner should read the chapter in the *Textbook of Family Practice* and then answer the questions in the corresponding chapter in this textbook. Each of the approximately 1500 questions is followed by a critique that defends both the correct and incorrect answers. There is also a page reference to the *Textbook of Family Practice* to direct the learner if more reading is needed.

This textbook can also be used by itself as a survey of family practice knowledge. The breadth of the material covered by the questions should give the learner some feedback about his or her general knowledge level. If further reading is needed, the *Textbook of Family Practice* should be reviewed.

The *Saunders Review of Family Practice* has been written to help the student of family medicine at any level. The medical student, the resident, and the practicing physician will all find the opportunity to augment their knowledge while assessing their current mastery of the material. Nicholas Pisacano, M.D., late mentor to the editors, said that if we keep in mind what is good for the people, our patients, we will do the right thing. One of the most important ways to do good for our patients is to obtain the best mastery of medical knowledge that we can have. It is hoped that this book will help with this awesome task.

Edward T. Bope, M.D.

Contents

Part I   Principles of Family Practice

1 The Family Physician 3
David R. Rudy

2 Family Genogram 7
Betty Young

3 The Family's Influence on Health 9
Jeri A. O'Donnell

4 Psychosocial Influences on Health 13
William A. Verhoff

5 Practicing Biopsychosocial Medicine 16
William A. Verhoff

6 Domestic Violence 19
Jeri A. O'Donnell

7 Care of the Elderly 23
Matthew D. Everett

8 Care of the Dying Patient 26
Wendy J. Hunter

9 Ethics in Family Practice 29
Andrew Leeman

Part II   Community Medicine

10 Periodic Health Examination 33
Alan R. Roth

11 Preventive Health Care 39
Michael D. Hagen

12 Use of Consultants 49
Michael D. Hagen

13 Community-Oriented Primary Care 53
Robert F. Thompson

14 Assessment of Functional Health Status 56
Alvah R. Cass

Part III   Communication in Family Medicine

15 Establishing Rapport 61
Pamela Jelly Boyers

16 Patient Compliance 66
Dana Nottingham

17 Patient Education.........................69
Dana Nottingham

18 Interviewing Techniques.............73
Betty Young

Part IV   Practice of Family Medicine

19 Clinical Problem Solving 77
David R. Rudy

20 Infectious Diseases 80
Thomas G. Maddox

21 Care of the Adult HIV-1–Infected
Patient 85
Michael B. Weinstock

22 Pulmonary Medicine 89
Edward T. Bope and
Peter Nalin

23 Otolaryngology............................92
Gregory H. Blake

24 Allergy..99
William Jorgenson

25 Parasitology and Travel
Medicine 103
Victor S. Sierpina

26 Obstetrics..................................108
Bill G. Gegas

27 Care of the Newborn.................111
Camille M. Leugers

28 Growth and Development.......117
Clyde A. Addison

29 Childhood and Adolescence ... 122
Janice Kelly Smith

30 Behavioral Problems in Children
and Adolescents 127
Arch G. Mainous III

31 Office Surgery............................131
Gary W. Kearl

32 Gynecology 138
Gary W. Kearl

33 Contraception...........................145
Cynda Johnson

34 Interpretation of the
Electrocardiogram 150
Michael D. Hagen

35 Cardiovascular Disease and
Arrhythmias...............................166
Michael D. Hagen

Cardiovascular Disease 166

Diagnosis and Treatment of
Arrhythmias..............................183

36 Emergency Medicine 190
Mary Thoesen Coleman

37 Sports Medicine 195
Matthew McHugh

38 Orthopedics..............................198
Michael D. Hagen

39 Rheumatic Disease...................213
Carolyn L. Frymoyer

40 Evaluation of Skin Lesions.........218
Donald E. Nease, Jr.

41 Endocrinology 223
Steven A. Crawford

42 Nutrition and Family
Medicine 231
Donald E. Nease, Jr., and
Emily R. Nease

43 Gastroenterology 237
Richard Neill

44 Oncology...................................246
Francis P. Kohrs

45 Hematology 255
Francis P. Kohrs

46 Urinary Tract Disorders...............265
Roger J. Zoorob

47 Ophthalmology 277
    Mitchell S. King

48 Neurology in Family
    Practice 282
    Paul Dusseau

49 Sexual Health Care 286
    Juan A. Pérez

50 Clinical Genetics and Genetic
    Counseling 290
    Richard Neill

51 Diagnosis and Treatment of
    Anxiety Disorders 294
    Michael D. Hagen and
    Betty Walker

52 Depression 299
    Marilyn Mehr and
    Michael D. Hagen

53 Crisis Intervention in Office
    Practice 304
    Marilyn Mehr and
    Michael D. Hagen

54 Personality Disorders in Office
    Practice 307
    Michael Dunaway

55 The Somatic Patient 311
    Arch G. Mainous III

56 Dementia 314
    Michael Dunaway

57 Alcohol Abuse 318
    Michael D. Hagen and
    Betty Walker

58 Nicotine Addiction 324
    Walton Sumner

59 Abuse of Controlled
    Substances 329
    Roger J. Zoorob

60 Interpreting Laboratory
    Tests 332
    Douglas J. Knutson and
    Stephen E. Markovich

Part V   Management of the Practice

61 The Problem-Oriented Medical
    Record 339
    Kent E. Anthony

62 Managed Health Care 342
    Kent E. Anthony

63 Accounting Systems 345
    Kent E. Anthony

64 Personnel and Time
    Management 348
    Kent E. Anthony

65 Computer Applications in
    Office Practice 350
    Clarence A. Jernigan

66 Malpractice and Risk
    Management 352
    Clarence A. Jernigan

Part I

Principles of
Family Practice

1

The Family Physician

David R. Rudy

1. Family Practice, as a new specialty which succeeded general practice, may be said to have been born as a result of reports of the following two studies:

    A. The Hsiao and Willard Reports
    B. The Flexnor and Millis Reports
    C. The Millis and Willard Reports
    D. The Flexnor and Willard Reports
    E. The Millis and GMENAC Reports

Answer: C

Critique: American medicine has undergone a number of significant changes at several junctures in history. The Flexnor Report of 1910 resulted in the scientific revolution that brought medical education into the universities (but set back humanistic medicine), except for a few surviving free-standing schools. In 1966, the "Report of the Citizens' Commission on Graduate Medical Education of the American Medical Association" (Millis Commission Report) and the Ad Hoc Committee on Education for Family Practice of the Council of Medical Education of the American Medical Association (AMA) (the Willard Committee) described and recommended the concept of a new specialty in primary care, which was called family practice. In 1980, the Graduate Medical Education National Advisory Committee (GMENAC) was the body that projected a physician surplus of 150,000 in the United States by the year 2020. The Hsiao Report of 1987 recommended restructuring the Medicare physician fee reimbursement schedule, which tended to elevate fees paid to primary care specialists while reducing those for surgical and other highly paid specialists.

Pages 3–4

2. The American Board of Family Practice (ABFP) came into being in which of the following years?

    A. 1947
    B. 1966
    C. 1776
    D. 1971
    E. 1969

Answer: E

Critique: The ABFP, the examining and certifying body for family practice, was formed in 1969 and took its place beside other specialty boards, such as the American Board of Pediatrics and the American Board of Internal Medicine. The chief protagonist and founder was the late Nicholas Pisicano, M.D., of the University of Kentucky. A lesser-sung hero of those early years was Thomas E. Rardin, M.D., of Columbus, OH, the only general practitioner on the medical staff of the Ohio State University Hospital at the time of the foundation of the ABFP. Dr. Rardin was highly instrumental "behind the scenes" in shepherding legislation through the AMA and other sponsoring organizations providing for the establishment of family practice as a specialty, among others. In 1947, the American Academy of General Practice, forerunner of the ABFP (1971) was founded. The fateful Millis and Willard Reports were published in 1966.

Pages 3–4

3. Rivo and associates in 1994 identified common conditions and diagnoses in primary care and recommended that their training should include at least 90% of them. Which of the following specialties, upon review of their training for the aforementioned purpose, fell short of this goal?

    A. Family practice
    B. Pediatrics
    C. Obstetrics and gynecology
    D. Internal medicine

Answer: C

Critique: The other major primary care specialty that failed to show training of residents in at least 90% of Rivo's primary care group of diseases was emergency medicine.

Page 5

4. The text lists 18 characteristics that, although desirable in all physicians, befit family physicians especially. All of the following are included in that list EXCEPT:

A. Compassion and empathy with a sincere interest in the patient and the family
B. The ability, education, training, and knowledge to deal with all medical problems in both the diagnostic and the therapeutic phase
C. A continuing enthusiasm for learning and for the satisfaction that comes from maintaining current medical knowledge through continuing medical education
D. The ability to deal comfortably with multiple problems occurring in one patient
E. The ability to support children during growth and development and during their adjustment to family and society

Answer: B

Critique: Options A, C, D, and E are all directed toward responsible and respectful patient care with the patient's best interests served. Option B alludes to an unrealistic view of the abilities of any physician in the late 20th century. It appeals to a tendency to aggrandize the doctor as omniscient but not necessarily mindful of the main goal of the practice of medicine, serving the welfare of the patient.

Page 6

5. What percentage of adults consulting a physician one or more times per month is admitted to a hospital (prior to a diagnostic related group [DRG] system of categorizing admissions as a method of determining Medicare reimbursement)?

A. 1%
B. 3.6%
C. 2%
D. 0.4%
E. 25%

Answer: B

Critique: Of 250 adults who consult a physician once per month, nine were admitted to a hospital, as of the tabulation by Greenberg in the *New England Journal of Medicine* (N Engl J Med 265:885, 1961). The percentage today, after 3 decades of a variety of drives toward decreased hospital utilization, would be much smaller.

Page 13, Figure 1–1

6. What percentage of adults *consulting a physician* one or more times per month is admitted to another physician (prior to the growth of health maintenance organizations [HMOs])?

A. 1%
B. 3.6%
C. 2%
D. 0.4%
E. 25%

Answer: C

Critique: This figure would likewise be much smaller today. The growth of HMOs reflects the growing concern during the past 30 years regarding the huge amount of

unnecessary expenses for health care. A great deal of these expenses have been generated by too-ready self-referral by patients and by overly conservative choices by physicians to consult anatomically or systematically defined specialists and subspecialists (see Fig. 1–1, p. 13). At first glance the 5 of 250 (2%) figure may seem to be at odds with the text itself, which states (see p. 15) that 3.3% of *office visits* result in referral to another physician. Apparently, the 2% represents the percentage of *all encounters* with a physician, including telephone conversations.

Page 13, Figure 1–1

7. What percentage of adults consulting a physician one or more times per month is referred to a university medical center (tertiary care facility)?

A. 1%
B. 3.6%
C. 2%
D. 0.4%
E. 25%

Answer: D

Critique: Of 250 adults reporting one or more physician consultations per month, one adult is admitted to a tertiary care facility. This information is taken from Greenberg (N Engl J Med 265:885, 1961) and may be lower in the era of managed care.

Page 13, Figure 1–1

8. From the *patient's* point of view, which of the following symptom complexes is *not* among the top 20 reasons for office visits (to physicians) in the United States, according to the National Center for Health Statistics in 1991?

A. General medical examination
B. Chest pain
C. Earache
D. Abdominal pain, cramps, spasms
E. Head cold and related symptoms

Answer: B

Critique: This point is made to show the huge diversity of problems encountered in family practice, the quintessential primary care field. Although chest pain, with its serious differential diagnoses (e.g., heart disease, reflux esophagitis, pleurisy), is commonly seen in primary care practice, its volume is overshadowed by at least 20 other common fears and complaints.

Page 14, Table 1–1

9. Which of the following is *not* among the top 20 *diagnoses* made in office visits?

A. Essential hypertension
B. Diabetes mellitus
C. Neurotic disorders
D. Breast cancer
E. Asthma

Answer: D

Critique: Although breast cancer has rightfully received much publicity for its increased incidence during the last 10 years, the other diagnoses mentioned (three of which are also potentially lethal) are seen on a daily basis. The top 20 together make up only 35.2% of diagnoses made in office visits.

Page 14, Table 1–2

10. What is the category of the first- and second-most prescribed drugs at office visits in the United States (1991)?

  A. Minor tranquilizers
  B. Thyroid hormones
  C. Antibiotics
  D. Vaccines and serums
  E. Estrogens and progestins

Answer: C

Critique: Amoxicillin alone constitutes 3.3% of all office prescriptions and these, together with cefaclor (Ceclor) and cephalexin (Keflex), comprise 5.1% of prescriptions.

Page 15, Table 1–3

11. The United States has the most expensive health care system in the world. Which of the following figures represents the approximate percentage of the gross national product devoted to health care?

  A. 2%
  B. 10%
  C. 14%
  D. 18%
  E. 20%

Answer: C

Critique: The United States spends 14% of its gross national product on health care. This may be compared with 8% for Canada.

Page 8

12. What is the ratio of internists' referral rate to that of family physicians?

  A. 0.5
  B. 1.0
  C. 1.1
  D. 1.3
  E. 1.7

Answer: D

Critique: Internists refer patients to other physicians 1.3 times as frequently as do family physicians. Option E, 1.7, is the rate at which they refer patients for hospital admission, compared with that of family physicians. The latter, since hospitalization reflects greater degrees of illness, could possibly be influenced by the type of patients seen by internists versus family doctors. The outpatient referral rates would seem to differ based on differing

philosophies and on different training preparation between the two specialties.

Page 8

13. In which of the following testing criteria did family practice residents outperform all other specialties' residents, as reported in 1982 by Gonnella and Veloski?

  A. FLEX examination
  B. Part II National Board scores, compared with those of part I
  C. Specialty board (ABFP) compared with other resident graduates' specialty board examinations
  D. Part III National Board scores compared with part II
  E. State board examinations

Answer: D

Critique: Family practice residents were the only first-year postdoctorate (PD I) residents to improve in National Board Examination part III compared with part II. Part III is taken during the first postdoctoral year of residency.

Page 9

Questions 14–20: (True or False) Regarding office visits or house calls in primary care and their changing profile during the past 3 to 5 years:

14. In the United States, a clear majority of citizens of all ages visit physicians at least once each year.

15. Men live shorter lives and visit physicians more frequently than do women.

16. The average number of visits per person in the United States accelerates at the rate of a little more than one per year per decade of adult life.

17. Visits to family physicians constitute about 50% of all outpatient visits in the United States.

18. House call rates (number per practice and number per patient) by family physicians have increased during the last few years.

19. The number of nursing home beds has been matched by the need for home (and other domiciliary) services.

20. Four times as many family physicians as pediatricians make house calls.

Answers: 14-T, 15-F, 16-T, 17-F, 18-T, 19-F, 20-T

Critique: About 75% of the population of the United States visit physicians at least once per year. Although it is true that men have a shorter average life expectancy than do women, men nevertheless visit doctors at only about two thirds the rate of women. The average number of visits rises with each decade's age group, being 1.8 per year in the 15- to 24-year old group and reaching six per year in the over 74-year-old group. Of all physician visits, 25% are made to family physicians. It is a paradox that the need for outpatient and domiciliary services has increased because of the campaigns of the last decade for shorter and less hospital utilization, in order to reverse the trends of the 1960s and 1970s for fewer home visits by physicians. Although the demand for such services has increased during the last decade at the rate of 20% per year, the number of nursing home beds has risen at only 2% annually. Approximately four times as many family physicians as pediatricians and about 1.33 times as many family physicians as internists make house calls.

2

Family Genogram

Betty Young

1. Which of the following relationships is least likely to be recorded in the index patient's family genogram?

    A. Multiple marriage
    B. Adopted children
    C. Blended family
    D. Heterosexual couple with legal bonds
    E. Same gender couples
    F. Multiple generational households

Answer: E

Critique: Meaningful relationships least likely to be recorded in the index patient's family genogram include individuals living together without legal bonds (either same gender or opposite gender couples). Information about the patient's close relationships is very important when assessing the patient's social support system and also his or her other health risks.

Page 30

2. Which of the demographic variables recorded in the family genogram has predictive value for the patient's increased risk of cardiovascular and renal diseases, diabetes, tuberculosis, cirrhosis of the liver, accidents, and suicides?

    A. Family size
    B. Education level
    C. Ethnicity
    D. Occupation
    E. Geographic locale

Answer: B

Critique: Demographic data recorded in the index patient's family genogram has predictive value for the patient's increased risk for specific health problems. The demographic variable with highest predictive value for increased risk of cardiovascular and renal diseases, diabetes mellitus, tuberculosis, and cirrhosis of the liver is the educational background or level of the patient. The reason why education has such high predictive value is that lower educational achievement (less than high school) is significantly associated with other risk factors, such as low income, poor work environment, less healthy diet, greater exposure to infectious disease due to crowded living arrangements, and family size.

Page 31

3. For purposes of interpreting the family genogram, which of the following theories of human behavior uses all four categories of genogram information (i.e., structure, demographics, events, and problems)?

    A. Life cycle or developmental theory
    B. Family systems theory
    C. Stress-social support theory
    D. Genetic theory
    E. Social learning theory

Answer: C

Critique: The theory of human behavior that is considered most useful when interpreting information obtained in the family genogram is the stress–social support theory because it uses all categories of genogram information (e.g., family structure, demographic data, genetic background, life events, and family relationships or problems). This theory asserts that life events can cause illness unless these events are buffered by social support and that social support may have an independent beneficial effect on health regardless of the absence or presence of stressful events.

Page 31

4. Which of the following is least accurate in describing the advantages of using a family genogram to depict family structure, demographic events, and problems?

    A. Allows the family physician and other health personnel to assess and understand the family
    B. Builds rapport between the physician and the patient by using first names of family members and by knowing who is living in the home
    C. Promotes lifestyle changes and greater emphasis on patient education
    D. Demonstrates that family relationships are a concern of the family physician and are important to the health of the patient

E. Provides a time flow chart that shows significant biomedical and sociomedical events in a troubled family

Answer: E

Critique: There are many advantages in using a family genogram to record the patient's history, including rapport building with the patient, greater understanding of the patient in the context of his or her environment, and promotion of lifestyle changes. The main disadvantage of the genogram is that it does not provide a time flow chart that could demonstrate related events in a troubled family. It is often used as a cross-sectional or one-time study of the patient. If it is kept current by adding appropriate data at subsequent visits, it becomes a much better instrument for gathering data.

Page 29

5. (True or False) The four components of the family genogram are structure, demographics, events, and problems.

Answer: True

Critique: The four components of a family genogram are: structure, demographics, events, and problems. These four types of data are used to assess the patient's health risks based on familial diseases, demographic variables, life events, and current and past problems. The data obtained in the genogram encourage health professionals to apply the biopsychosocial model when interpreting data. Each of the four components of the genogram is seen as a potential risk factor.

Page 29

6. (True or False) Family genograms are not likely to be helpful in identifying significant risk factors for a particular patient.

Answer: False

Critique: Family genograms are very helpful when assessing the patient's risk status. Interpretation of information from a genogram requires that the clinician consider the four types of family information and ask the relevant clinical questions: Does the patient's family structure, demographic profile, life events, or health problems increase or decrease the patient's risk of developing a pre-

ventable condition? Does the information obtained suggest an increase or a decrease in the success rate of a particular management option?

Page 31

7. (True or False) The use of standard genogram symbols is not necessary for interpreting or analyzing the family genogram.

Answer: False

Critique: The use of standard genogram symbols allows other health care providers an opportunity to interpret information that was obtained previously. It also encourages the clinicians who originally obtained the information to use the data and to add to the data in subsequent visits. It is well recognized that information contained in the genogram can help to identify risk factors for the patient.

Page 24

8. (True or False) The model of the family genogram is not readily adaptable to computer-generated programs.

Answer: False

Critique: The model of the family genogram is very adaptable to a computer format. Studies have shown that patients can create a family genogram using a computer program, even when they have had very limited exposure to use of a computer.

Pages 28, 29

9. (True or False) The family genogram is appropriately used to evaluate a somatic complaint by testing biopsychosocial hypotheses.

Answer: True

Critique: The family genogram is used appropriately to evaluate a somatic complaint. Using the basic principles and methods of epidemiology, each of the four components of the genogram (i.e., structure, demographic profile, life events, and problems) is viewed as a potential risk factor that may or may not be related to the biopsychosocial hypothesis or somatic complaint under consideration.

Page 31

3

The Family's Influence on Health

Jeri A. O'Donnell

FAMILY STRESS

1. (True or False) Due to the current technological advances, we are more knowledgeable about why some individuals become ill whereas others remain healthy when exposed to the same pathogens and risk factors.

Answer: False

Critique: Despite significant advances in our understanding of health and illness, little is known about why some people become ill whereas others remain healthy when exposed to the same pathogens and risk factors.

Page 35

2. (True or False) Patients today are more accepting of the diagnosis of too much stress as a reason for their headache or ulcer "acting up."

Answer: True

Critique: Stress has become widely accepted by patients and health care professionals as a factor that influences health. Patients often explain to their physicians that they are under a lot of stress and that their ulcer, back pain, or headache is "acting up."

Page 35

3. (True or False) Census data and cross-sectional studies have consistently shown that widowers have higher death rates from all causes than do married individuals.

Answer: True

Critique: Census data and cross-sectional studies have consistently shown that widowers have much higher death rates from all causes than do married individuals.

Page 35

4. (True or False) Investigators Meyer and Haggerty (1962) noted that chronic stress was associated with higher rates of streptococcal pharyngitis.

Answer: True

Critique: Meyer and Haggerty (1962) found that chronic stress was associated with higher rates of streptococcal pharyngitis and that 30% of the streptococcal infections were preceded by a stressful family event.

Page 35

5. The group with the higher death rate from all diseases is:

    A. Single persons
    B. Married persons
    C. The widowed
    D. Divorcees

Answer: D

Critique: Several cross-sectional studies have shown that divorcees have a higher death rate from all diseases than do single, widowed, or married persons.

Pages 35, 36

6. Social support (e.g., emotional and instrumental) and financial aid that is obtained from one's social network improve health:

    A. Directly
    B. Indirectly

Answer: A

Critique: An extensive body of research has shown that social networks and supports can improve health *directly* and can also buffer the adverse effects of stress (Cohen and Syme, 1985; Rosengren et al., 1993).

Page 36

7. (True or False) Independent of socioeconomic status, Berkman and Syme (1979) showed that social networks were a major predictor of mortality.

Answer: True

Critique: In a seminal study of more than 6000 adults, Berkman and Syme (1979) showed that social networks were a major predictor of mortality over a 9-year period, independent of socioeconomic status, previous health status, or health practices.

Page 36

8. Factors associated with mortality in the elderly are:

   A. One's marital status
   B. The presence of living children
   C. Peer social support
   D. Financial resources
   E. All of the above

Answer: B

Critique: Unlike younger populations, marital status was not associated with mortality in the elderly. The presence and number of living children are the most powerful predictors of survival.

Page 36

IMPACT OF DIVORCE AND REMARRIAGE ON THE FAMILY

1. **(True or False)** It is important for a family physician to remember that a common feature of grief reactions in a family system is that each member may be at a different stage in his or her grief reaction.

Answer: True

Critique: Individuals within a family may have very different experiences of a divorce, and these differences are important for understanding and helping them through this process. The family physician must understand these differences in order to treat individual family members most effectively during these transitions.

Pages 38, 39

2. **(True or False)** Children thrive better overall in a conflictual intact home where both parents are actively involved with them than in a divorced home, even if the divorced home may appear to be more stable.

Answer: False

Critique: Children actually adjust better in a stable divorced home than in an unhappy, highly conflictual intact home (Hetherington et al., 1978).

Page 39

3. **(True or False)** In today's society in which many couples who are divorcing are both employed and have children, the most common method of child custody is joint custody.

Answer: False

Critique: Although much is written about joint custody today, sole custody is by far the most common custodial arrangement following a divorce. In a sole custody arrangement, the custodial parent retains custody of the children and the noncustodial parent has visitation with the children.

Page 39

4. **(True or False)** A noncustodial parent cannot seek medical treatment for a child without the permission of the custodial parent unless there is an emergency situation.

Answer: True

Critique: It is important that family physicians note that usually the custodial parent has the exclusive right to seek medical treatment for the children. This means that, without the permission of the custodial parent, the noncustodial parent can only seek medical treatment in emergency situations.

Page 39

5. The single most powerful sociodemographic predictor of stress-related physical illness is:

   A. Going to jail
   B. Death of a loved one
   C. Loss of a job
   D. Marital disruption
   E. Filing bankruptcy

Answer: D

Critique: Marital disruption is the single most powerful *sociodemographic* predictor of stress-related physical illness (Somers, 1979). Death of a loved one does not indicate whether this individual is in the immediate family. Although all of the aforementioned are stressful, and patients may present to a family physician with stress-related illness, Somers (1979) found that separated individuals have 30% more acute illness and visits to a physician than do married adults. Separated and divorced adults have the highest rates of acute medical problems, chronic medical conditions that interfere with social activity, and disability—even when age, race, and income are controlled (Verbrugge, 1979).

Pages 39, 40

6. Given your knowledge of a normal grief reaction and the length of time that it takes most individuals to adjust and recover; following a divorce, most adults have adjusted to the marital breakup within approximately:

   A. 1 year
   B. 2 years
   C. 3 years
   D. 5 years

Answer: B

Critique: Within approximately 2 years after the divorce, most adults have adjusted to the marital breakup and have developed a new stability in their lives (Bray and Hetherington, 1993).

Page 40

7. The process of divorce has significant effects on children. All of the following are true EXCEPT:

   A. The process is more difficult for boys.
   B. The reaction is age dependent.

C. The postdivorce family relationships affect the child's behavior.

D. Girls tend to manifest academic problems after divorce.

Answer: D

Critique: The effects of divorce vary depending on a number of factors that include the sex of the child, the age of the child, and postdivorce family relationships. It is noted that boys tend to develop more behavioral problems, sex role adjustment problems, and academic problems than do girls.

Page 40

8. (True or False) Most problems exhibited by children after divorce were probably present prior to the marital separation.

Answer: True

Critique: Block and associates (1986) found that many of the problems exhibited by children after divorce may be present prior to the marital separation.

Page 40

9. A common reaction to divorce by children of all ages is:

A. Running away
B. Feeling responsible in some way for the divorce
C. Behavioral problems
D. Anxiety
E. Developmental delays

Answer: C

Critique: Each age group of children has a wide range of reactions, but the most common theme is behavioral problems.

Page 40

10. (True or False) Parenting practices do change after a divorce.

Answer: True

Critique: Parenting practices change, and children respond differently to their parents as the family struggles to find a new equilibrium. Parenting methods that worked prior to the divorce may not be effective after the divorce.

Page 40

Questions 11–14. Match the family physician's advice to the parents of a child with the appropriate age group.

A. Ages 9 to 11
B. Preschool age
C. Adolescents

11. Encourage the parents to be honest.

12. Emphasize that the children are not responsible for the divorce.

13. Encourage peer support.

14. Establish a daily routine.

Answers: 11-A, 12-B, 13-C, 14-B

Critique: Although all of the aforementioned are important parenting practices, the one that most fits the 9- to 11-year-old age group is for the parent to be honest. Options B and D are more relevant for the pre-school age group. Option C is more appropriate for adolescents.

Page 41, Table 3–2

15. (True or False) It is safe for the family physician to assume that the experience of having a divorce is probably a negative one for his or her patient.

Answer: False

Critique: Although it is common to assume that the divorce experience is a negative one, for some individuals it may be quite a positive and welcoming experience.

Page 42

16. Which of the following is most true according to Wallerstein and Kelly (1980)?

A. Less than 25%, but more than 15% of children, had any adult talk to them about the divorce.
B. Less than 50%, but more than 35% of children, had any adult talk to them about the divorce.
C. Less than 10% of children had any adult talk to them about the divorce.
D. Less than 5% of children had any adult talk to them about the divorce.

Answer: C

Critique: Wallerstein and Kelly (1980) noted that less than 10% of children had any adult talk to them about the divorce. Parents may even present unrealistic stories about why one parent has left the household.

Page 42

17. (True or False) Regarding step-parenting, because boys have more trouble adjusting to divorce in general, it follows that they would also take longer to adjust to a step-father than girls do.

Answer: False

Critique: Boys seem to accept a step-father faster and more easily than do girls. Girls often have more conflict with their step-parent and have more negative relationships with their step-fathers.

Page 43

18. (True or False) If a step-family has not adjusted in 2 or 3 years following the second marriage, the family physician should tell the parents that it is normal and time will work it out.

Answer: False

Critique: In the case of severe or long-standing adjustment problems, the family physician may choose to refer the family to a professional counselor. Wood and

Poole (1983) recommended that physicians make a referral if there are multiple problems in the family. It is important to refer to a counselor who has specific experience with the problems encountered by stepfamilies.

Page 44

19. (True or False) After a divorce, it is not uncommon for children to experience grief symptoms because of a new marriage, even if they like their new step-parent.

Answer: True

Critique: Family members, especially children, may experience new grief because the new marriage under-scores the permanence of the divorce (Visher and Visher, 1988).

Page 44

20. (True or False) Marital separation does not seem to affect immune functioning in men or women.

Answer: False

Critique: Marital separation is associated with reduced qualitative and quantitative immune functioning in men and women compared with married controls (Kiecolt-Glaser et al., 1987, 1988), which may explain their increased risk of illness.

Page 40

4

Psychosocial Influences on Health

William A. Verhoff

1. (True or False) In the second half of the 20th century, the sciences of psychoneuroimmunology and psychoneuroendocrinology supported the fact that life stressors generate physiologic responses that alter human homeostasis.

Answer: True

Critique: Life stressors trigger hypothalamic and pituitary mediators, which initiate endocrinologic and immunologic mechanisms. Individuals thus affected are more likely to experience adverse health effects, such as heart disease, infectious disease, cancer, and asthma.

Page 46

2. The clinical application of knowledge of psychosocial influences on health is captured in a model structured on historical and scientific evidence that suggests that every health problem should be assessed on the basis of both:

    A. Environmental and behavioral risks
    B. Psychological and economical risks
    C. Hereditary and geographical risks
    D. Biomedical and psychosocial risks

Answer: D

Critique: Health problems occur for various reasons. Engel (1977, 1980) developed the biopsychosocial model that describes the biomedical and psychosocial influences and their impact on people's health.

Page 46

3. (Matching) The biopsychosocial model describes a variety of forces that influence the relationship between psychosocial risk and health. The following terms and their definitions are taken from the model. Match the correct term with its definition.

    A. Stressors
    B. Crisis
    C. Psychosocial equilibrium
    D. Cognitive appraisal

1. A state of psychological homeostasis in which resources are available to meet the routine challenges of life's stressors

2. A life experience that may disrupt or endanger an individual's personal and social values and relationships

3. The process by which an individual evaluates a life event or role strain in terms of the impact of the experience on his or her emotional and social integrity

4. A state of emotional disequilibrium, usually becoming manifest by anxiety that results from the failure of an individual to identify, or use, resources to resolve a stressor-induced problem

Answers: 1-C, 2-A, 3-D, 4-B

Critique: See Table 4–1 and Figure 4–1 for definitions and their relationship to the various stages on the Cycle of Psychosocial Risk Model.

Pages 47, 48

4. Multiple stressors have an impact on an individual's psyche each day, but not all stressors stimulate an alarm reaction. A response without an alarm reaction usually occurs when past experience with the stressor has been:

    A. Forgotten
    B. Favorable
    C. Misinterpreted
    D. Misunderstood

Answer: B

Critique: Our cognitive appraisal of a stressor allows us to determine whether or not a stressor is a threat. Therefore, a past experience with a stressor that was favorable and had available needed resources would not stimulate an alarm reaction.

Page 47

5. (Choose one) Stressors perceived as threatening can move an individual into a state of psychosocial disequilibrium. As the individual seeks out resources to buffer or neutralize the stressor, the most influential psychosocial support comes from:

    A. Religion
    B. The environment
    C. Friends and family
    D. Cultural background
    E. Educational level

Answer: C

Critique: Social support from family, friends, and work supervisors appears to be the most influential in altering psychosocial risk. If resources are available and remedial coping strategies are employed, the individual usually experiences resolution of the stressor and a return to psychosocial equilibrium.

Page 47

6. (True or False) Crisis is usually associated with anxiety.

Answer: True

Critique: Crisis is usually associated with anxiety. The concept of anxiety as an outcome of crisis is of central importance, because studies have shown that anxiety is the primary emotional mediator of neuroendocrinologic and neuroimmunologic system changes, which alter health outcome.

Pages 47, 48

7. Individuals who demonstrate a low level of illness in the face of high stress have been labeled with the term "hardiness." These individuals have been characterized as having:

    A. A greater sense of control over what occurs in their lives
    B. A feeling of commitment to various activities in which they are engaged
    C. A view of change as a challenge rather than as a threat
    D. A sense of meaningfulness in their lives
    E. All of the above

Answer: E

Critique: It is likely that hardiness reflects past successes in employing resources to overcome life stressors.

Page 48

8. Present medical training and practice place great emphasis on biomedical factors to a point at which a patient's psychosocial symptoms and conditions may be reinforced. This is called:

    A. Physician misinterpretation
    B. Somatic fixation

    C. Psychosocial disequilibrium
    D. Overutilization of health care resources

Answer: B

Critique: This is the process by which a patient becomes locked into a physical problem with the support of a physician who pursues a patient's persistent or exaggerated physical symptoms through an escalation of laboratory tests, office visits, and consultations.

Page 50

9. (True or False) When applying the biopsychosocial model to a patient's condition, the easiest aspect of psychosocial assessment is that of identifying the significance of stressors to the patient.

Answer: False

Critique: This can be the most problematic aspect of the assessment, because physicians and caregivers often assume that they understand the intensity of the patient's stressors based on their own experience. Such an attitude fails to recognize that differences in culture and social backgrounds of physicians and patients results in physicians and patients making different cognitive appraisals of stressors.

Page 52

10. (True or False) Psychosocial intervention begins with a thorough assessment of the patient's stressors and resources. Of these areas of assessment, the identification of the social support resources may be the single most important assessment in the evaluation of psychosocial risk in an individual who is experiencing stress.

Answer: True

Critique: Ruberman and associates (1984) reported that patients who are socially isolated and who have a high degree of life stressors have four times the risk of death as do those with good social support.

Pages 52, 53

11. Even with optimal physician assistance, high-risk patients with poor social support, whose lives are characterized by an accumulation of high-intensity stressors, frequently experience an accentuation of physical and emotional health problems. The most effective treatment for such patients may be long-term supportive therapy. This therapy involves all of the following strategies EXCEPT:

    A. Offering regular appointments at which time positive feedback is given to bolster self-esteem (usually focusing of behavior modification)
    B. Using psychotrophic medications
    C. Addressing stressors as contributions to illness
    D. Searching for new resources at each patient encounter

Answer: B

Critique: Even though medication usage is not prohibited in these patients, the use (when needed) should be specific to the patient's needs. Physicians should recognize that they are major resources in the treatment of patients at psychosocial risk. Remedial coping should be the long-range goal of the physician-patient relationship.

The long-term intervention requires identification of resources that may be directed toward the management of anxiety-producing stressors (e.g., social support person[s], use of counseling, educational programs, social agencies, and psychotherapy).

Page 53

5

Practicing Biopsychosocial Medicine

William A. Verhoff

1. (True or False) American medicine is currently under a second major paradigm shift. This is derived from the notion that the modern-day physician has multiple responsibilities to understand a patient's problems at the micro and macro levels in order to provide the best clinical outcomes.

Answer: True

Critique: On a micro level, the physician deals with the biomedical problems; on a macro level, we deal with the patient and his or her complex relationship with others, the patient's community, and the world community. A failure to comprehend this dualistic role has the potential to flaw fatally any practitioner's best clinical efforts.

Page 56

2. (True or False) The current society is constantly bombarded with startling information that is transmitted instantaneously to the population. This continual transmission of information and visual horrors of the inhumanity perpetrated by humans on each other has decreased the level of stress encountered in our society.

Answer: False

Critique: Regardless of the origin of a patient's dysfunction, stress is the patient's consistent companion during this process. Today, stress is endemic. The information exchange in an instant has worked to produce a level of stress that has heretofore been unencountered in society at large and that has had an unmeasured and untenable impact.

Page 56

3. The physician's social power in our society places him or her in the best position to deal with societal and biomedical problems. The most predominant social powers that are considered to be possessed by physicians are:

A. Reward and legitimate power
B. Referent and expert power
C. Coercive and reward power
D. All the above

Answer: D

Critique: Social scientists have identified an array of social powers; however, five of the most predominant of the powers are possessed by physicians. This power qualifies them, among all the professionals, to influence the behavior of their patients and bring constructive forces to bear at a time when patients are surviving in a destructive environment.

Page 57

4. (Fill in the blank) To restore a patient's power to cope, the physician must employ the five major components of psychotherapy. List three of the five elements:

1. _____
2. _____
3. _____

Answers: 1. The patient has an expectation of receiving help; 2. A therapeutic relationship is established; 3. The patient obtains an external perspective; 4. The physician encourages a corrective experience; and 5. The patient has the opportunity to test reality repeatedly.

Critique: Patients have a unique and distinct view of the world and, although no one can precisely know someone else's view of the world, physicians are in a unique position to enable their patients to cope more effectively. While implementing all of the aforementioned activities, the physician is the supportive listener and occasional commentator as the patient works through the process of problem resolution and self-actualization.

Page 57

5. (True or False) The BATHE technique to obtain the information necessary to assess the patient's psychological situation and react accordingly helps the patient to feel more competent about dealing with his or her situation and about being supported by the physician.

Answer: True

Critique: The BATHE technique is an organized exploration of the patient's problems by first recognizing that stress is contributing to the patient's physical state. Symbolic meaning is then attached and information is obtained on how the patient is handling the situation. Finally, the physician's empathic response provides closure and allows other aspects of the interview to be reviewed.

Page 58

6. (True or False) The BATHE technique is therapeutic because it allows the physician to assume responsibility for the patient's presenting situation.

Answer: False

Critique: The patient continues to own his or her problem, but the physician is better able to assist the patient in the resolution of the problem because the physician has a complete and comprehensive understanding of its derivation.

Page 59

7. (True or False) Patients presenting with psychosocial issues often ask for advice from their physician. The best approach for the physician is to give any necessary advice to his or her patient.

Answer: False

Critique: Although patients ask for advice, treatment is more effective if the patient is made to focus on his or her own resources with some guidance for developing alternatives, rather than the physician giving advice or directly solving the patient's problem, because this action takes away the patient's sense of empowerment. It is better to make the patient aware of his or her own strengths and ability to assess and exercise his or her own options.

Page 59

8. Looking at a trying circumstance or situation as an opportunity to learn a necessary lesson or develop an essential skill is an example of:

    A. Job enhancement
    B. Work re-engineering
    C. Reframing
    D. Restructuring

Answer: C

Critique: Reframing involves finding a way to interpret the situation in positive terms.

Page 59

9. (Fill in the blank) Reframing is one healthy option for handling a bad situation. The other three healthy options are:

    A. _____
    B. _____
    C. _____

Answers: A. Learning it; B. Changing it; and C. Accepting it.

Critique: Option A dictates exploring the best and worst possible outcomes that might result. Option B requires an investigation of what is possible and what additional resources must be brought to bear. Option C recognizes that if it could be different, it would be different.

Page 59

10. When dealing with the difficult patient, the physician needs to arrange appointments that are:

    A. Infrequent, lengthy sessions
    B. Frequent brief sessions
    C. On an as-needed basis
    D. Frequent long sessions

Answer: B

Critique: Except in life-threatening situations, physicians must limit the time that they spend with patients to less than 15 minutes in order to avoid arousing negative emotions. With frequent brief sessions, these patients often feel less rejection and they organize the details of their stories to fit into abbreviated time slots once they are convinced that the physician is listening attentively and is responding appropriately.

Page 60

11. The patient who has multiple complaints, demands to be seen frequently, rarely gets better, and does not appreciate the physician's efforts is a:

    A. Hypochondriacal patient
    B. Chronic complainer
    C. Depressed patient
    D. Schizophrenic patient

Answer: B

Critique: The chronic complainer seems to need his or her disease in order to function and rarely appreciates the physician's efforts. The hypochondriacal patient has numerous somatic complaints and is resistant to reassurance. This patient benefits from frequent visits to the physician.

Page 60

12. (True or False) The psychosocial aspects of medicine can be very challenging, yet gratifying, provided that the physician takes care of himself or herself. Three of the most important rules for survival are:

    1. Exercise right; sleep right; and eat right.
    2. Be helpful to all patients; be courteous to even the most difficult patients; and be kind.

3. Don't take responsibility for things that you cannot control; take care of yourself or you cannot take care of anyone else; and start where the patient is by doing a psychosocial assessment along with the biomedical one.

Answers: 1-T, 2-T, 3-T

Critique: It is essential to apply the aforementioned rules when practicing biopsychosocial medicine. Stuart and Lieberman prescribe 12 rules; however, they rank the aforementioned three as being the most important.

Page 60

6

Domestic Violence

Jeri A. O'Donnell

CHILD ABUSE

1. (True or False) Bodily contact is necessary to define sexual abuse.

Answer: False

Critique: In contrast with physical abuse, tissue damage is not an essential part of the sexual abuse definition; sexual abuse may not involve bodily contact (e.g., sexual conduct intentionally performed in a child's presence).

Page 62

2. Of the abuse cases reported, how many children are victims of more than one type of abuse?

    A. 5%
    B. 10%
    C. 15%
    D. 20%

Answer: B

Critique: In 1992 almost 3 million children were reported to Child Protective Services. Of this total, approximately 800,000 were alleged victims of physical abuse and 500,000 were alleged victims of sexual abuse (McCurdy and Daro, 1993). Over 10% are victims of more than one type of abuse.

Page 62

3. (True or False) The reporting of child abuse has increased primarily because of public awareness.

Answer: True

Critique: The number of child abuse cases continues to increase each year, a fact attributed *primarily* to enhanced public awareness leading to more reporting of cases.

Page 62

4. Finkelhor (1985) described four preconditions necessary for sexual abuse to occur. The precondition that he describes is:

A. A divorce in the family
B. The abuser is abusing substances at the time of the abuse
C. Feeling powerless as an adult
D. Overcoming internal inhibitions

Answer: D

Critique: Finkelhor noted four preconditions necessary for sexual abuse to occur: 1. *motivation,* which includes emotional congruence, sexual arousal by children, and inability to form satisfactory relationships with adults; 2. *overcoming of internal inhibitions,* such as moral and religious beliefs; 3. *removal of external inhibitors, such as parents or witnesses;* and 4. *overcoming resistance in the child.*

Page 63

5. (True or False) Most abusers were abused as children.

Answer: True

Critique: Many abusers were abused as children. This is especially true of physical abuse, because excessive corporal punishment traditionally has been viewed not as child abuse but rather as a parent's undeniable right. Most adolescent sexual offenders were sexually abused as children (Sauzier and Mitkus, 1986).

Page 63

6. (True or False) Most victims of physical abuse are very young, usually younger than 4 years of age.

Answer: True

Critique: In a *clinical* setting, most victims of physical abuse are very young, usually younger than 4 years of age. These young victims tend to require medical attention because they are unable to defend themselves. However, more than 40% of victims of physical abuse are adolescents (U.S. Dept. of Health and Human Services, 1980), many of whom do not actively seek medical assistance.

Page 63

7. The most common cause of death due to child abuse is:

A. Burns
B. Abdominal injuries
C. Fractures
D. Head injuries

Answer: D

Critique: Head injuries are the most common cause of death related to child abuse (Kessler and Hyden, 1991). Abdominal injuries rank second to head injuries as causes of death from abuse (Touloukian, 1968).

Page 64

8. Some long-term psychological consequences of child abuse include:

A. Dropping out of school
B. Overachievement
C. Social isolation
D. Poor problem-solving skills
E. All of the above

Answer: E

Critique: While some children may drop out of school, or on the opposite end of the spectrum become over-achievers, social isolation and poor problem-solving skills are more commonly seen in the victims of child abuse. Many victims suffer from poor self-esteem, a limited ability to relate to others, social isolation with superficial yet dependent and unstable relationships, and poor problem-solving skills (Kempe, 1980b).

Page 65

9. (True or False) When the family physician is confronted with a suspected child abuse situation, the physician should interview the child, using direct statements so as not to confuse the child.

Answer: False

Critique: The physician should interview the child privately, if possible, when abuse is suspected. It is important to use an *indirect* rather than a direct questioning technique, which is less threatening and more likely to elicit disclosure.

Page 65

10. (True or False) Injuries to the skin and subcutaneous tissues are seen in 90% of physically abused children.

Answer: True

Critique: Even though 90% of physically abused children suffer from injuries to the skin and subcutaneous tissue (Kessler and Hyden, 1991), *most soft tissue injuries of childhood are undoubtedly accidental.* However, injuries that occur on the buttocks, abdomen, inner thighs, genitalia, lower back, and sides of the face or head are not typically a result of normal childhood play.

Page 64

11. (True or False) In cases of sexual abuse, vaginal penile penetration results in specific observable evidence.

Answer: False

Critique: Fondling, oral-genital contact, anal penetration, digital vaginal penetration, and vulvar or vestibular penetration are examples of acts that rarely result in specific physical findings. Even vaginal penile penetration may not produce observable evidence.

Page 64

12. In a normal school-aged female (premenstrual age), the size of the opening of the hymen is approximately:

A. One-fourth inch
B. One-half inch
C. Three-quarters inch
D. One inch

Answer: B

Critique: Although many children and adolescent victims may describe penetration of the vagina or anus ("yes, he put it inside"), they may in fact be experiencing vulvar or vestibular penetration, not penetration past the hymen into the vagina. The size of the opening of the hymen in a school-aged child is about *one-half inch,* making vaginal penetration difficult.

Page 64

ELDER ABUSE

1. Although there are many types of elder abuse, the most common form is:

A. Fiscal
B. Physical
C. Material
D. Neglect
E. Psychological

Answer: D

Critique: While our society's most common image of "abuse" is intentional physical violence, several scholars have noted that the most common form of elder abuse is actually neglect (Tayler and Ansello, 1985). Neglect is characterized by inattention to or isolation of the elderly individual; for those who are dependent on others to provide daily necessities, this passive form of abuse can be very serious.

Page 67

2. (True or False) More women in the elderly population are abused than are males.

Answer: False

Critique: Approximately equal numbers of men and women in this population are abused.

Page 67

3. Women are most likely to suffer which of the following consequences of violence?

A. Neglect and financial
B. Physical and psychological
C. Neglect and material

Answer: B

Critique: Pillemer and Finkelhor (1988) reported that abused women suffer more physical and psychological consequences from the violence than do the men.

Page 67

4. (True or False) Adult children caring for their parents tend to be the major perpetrators of elder abuse.

Answer: False

Critique: A predominant image, reinforced by the lay press and media, is that abuse is committed by ungrateful children toward their unreasonable aging parents (Sengstock and Hwalek, 1987). This image has been challenged, however, with findings indicating that the more common perpetrator of elder abuse is the spouse (Pillemer and Finkelhor, 1988; Wolf et al., 1984).

Page 68

5. (True or False) Family physicians should be alert to the fact that signs of fear sounding like paranoia may be a strong indication of abuse.

Answer: True

Critique: Actually, common behavioral indicators of abuse, such as *generalized fear,* may be *misinterpreted as paranoia* related to dementia or a latent psychosis (Council on Scientific Affairs, 1987).

Page 68

6. (True or False) It is difficult to achieve successful identification of abused elders because of unfavorable societal attitudes toward older persons and inconsistent federal, state, and local strategies for reporting abuse of the elderly.

Answer: True

Critique: The successful identification of abused elders and the development of effective prevention plans has been difficult to achieve. Inconsistent federal, state, and local approaches of reporting elder abuse and enforcing legal protection of the abused individual has slowed prevention efforts.

Page 68

SPOUSE ABUSE

1. (True or False) Many married couples report violent behaviors toward each other.

Answer: True

Critique: In two landmark studies of family violence, Straus and Gelles (1986) found that many husbands and wives reported violent behaviors toward each other (see also Cascardi et al., 1992).

Page 69

2. (True or False) Most spousal violence begins at the time of dating.

Answer: False

Critique: Most men do not hit women during courtship; instead, violence begins after both partners have a deep emotional investment in each other. The first violent incident comes as a *complete surprise* to the victim, and is *not* recognized as a precursor to a violent pattern.

Page 69

3. (True or False) In today's society, the costs of men being violent to their family members is quite high.

Answer: False

Critique: A man's violence is rewarded when it stops an emotional argument (and he wins), when he gets his wishes granted, and when he is able to vent his frustrations without fear of retaliation (Browne, 1987). *For men, the cost of being violent to family members is low.*

Page 69

4. (True or False) The consistent risk marker of being an abused wife is:

1. Poor self-esteem
2. Substance abuse
3. Witnessing violence as a child
4. Experiencing violence as a child

Answers: 1-F, 2-F, 3-T, 4-T

Critique: Hotaling and Sugarman (1986), in a systematic review of 52 students, found that the *only* consistent risk marker of being an abused wife was witnessing violence as a child, which was significant in 11 out of 15 studies. A second variable was worth noting: Experience of violence as a child was significantly related to being an abused wife in 9 of 13 studies.

Page 70

5. (True or False) It is easier for a family physician to identify a woman at risk for victimization than to identify a man at risk for abusive behavior.

Answer: False

Critique: It may be easier to identify a man at risk for abusive behavior than a woman at risk for victimization.

Page 70

6. Victimized women demonstrate higher health care utilization, increasing health care costs by:

A. 1.5 times
B. 2.5 times
C. 3.5 times
D. 4.5 times

Answer: B

Critique: Victimized women demonstrate higher health care utilization than do other women. Visits to a physician are twice as frequent, and health care costs are *2.5* times higher (Koss et al., 1991).

Page 70

ADULT VICTIMS OF SEXUAL ASSAULT

1. (True or False) All 50 states now have laws against sex without consent between spouses who live together.

Answer: False

Critique: It is noteworthy that in Texas, sexual assault between spouses who live together is undefined; thus, a cohabiting husband is *legally* allowed to force his wife to have sex.

Page 72

2. (True or False) When a male spouse rapes his wife, the consequences to the wife are not as severe as they probably would be with a stranger.

Answer: False

Critique: Some husbands rape their wives, with consequences to their victims that are *parallel to those who are raped by a stranger.*

Page 72

3. (True or False) Women often perpetrate sexual assault against men.

Answer: False

Critique: Men can be sexually assaulted too, but their perpetrators are almost always other men. The prevalence of victimization is less clear, because most men who are assaulted do not report it.

Page 73

4. (True or False) According to feminists, rape functions as a social control for women's behavior, which is an advantage to all men.

Answer: True

Critique: Feminists note that rape functions as a social control for women's behavior. Fear of rape limits women's freedom and keeps them dependent on men for protection. All men can claim this advantage (Epstein, 1988).

Page 73

5. (True or False) Almost 50% of all rapists who are arrested are younger than 25 years of age.

Answer: True

Critique: Perpetrators of sexual assault tend to be young men; *47%* of all rapists who are arrested are younger than 25 years of age (Koss, 1988); however, most sexual aggressors are not arrested.

Page 73

6. (True or False) When comparing stranger and acquaintance rape, the main difference in the abuse is that strangers are likely to be more aggressive and more willing to use weapons than is someone who the woman knows.

Answer: True

Critique: Strangers were more aggressive and were more likely to use threats, hitting and slapping, and weapons. Both strangers and acquaintances were equally likely to use arm twisting, holding down, or *beating.*

Page 73

7. (True or False) Women who have been sexually assaulted may seek acute medical care from their family physician rather than from an emergency room.

Answer: True

Critique: The more likely scenario is that the victim will refuse to report the assault to the police and will present acutely to her family physician for the purpose of treating injuries or preventing sexually transmitted diseases.

Page 74

7

Care of the Elderly

Matthew D. Everett

1. Regarding the elderly population, only one of the following is correct:

A. Older individuals account for two thirds of all patient stays in hospital.
B. Older women are 10 times more likely to be widowed than are men, and older women are five times more likely to be living alone.
C. The average health care expenditure for older individuals is approximately four times that spent on younger persons. Hospital costs account for the major portion of this expense.
D. Persons older than 65 years of age represent the fastest growing segment of the population.
E. By the year 2030, it is projected that 10% of the population will be older than 65 years of age.

Answer: C

Critique: Older individuals account for one third of all patient stays in hospital. Older women are five times more likely to be widowed than are men, and older women are three times more likely to be living alone. Persons older than 85 years of age represent the fastest growing segment of the population. Of the population, 22% will be older than 65 years of age by the year 2030.

Page 78

2. (True or False) There is no way to prevent the fact that total body fat composition will double between the ages of 25 and 75 years.

Answer: False

Critique: Doubling of total body fat composition has been reported to occur between 25 and 75 years of age; however, in less developed societies with different diets and physical activities, this does not occur.

Pages 78, 79

3. (True or False) Geriatric evaluation and management units (GEMUS) have been demonstrated to be effective by significantly reducing mortality rates, by increasing an elderly person's chances to return to home after discharge from the hospital, and by reducing rates of readmission to the hospital.

Answer: True

Critique: Mortality rates have been shown to decrease by 35%, and odds of a patient returning to his or her own home after discharge from the hospital have doubled with the advent of GEMUS.

Page 86

4. (True or False) Following a stroke, one determinant of functional prognosis is the patient's functional status prior to the stroke.

Answer: True

Critique: The degree of early recovery, the presence of a supportive caregiver and environment, the patient's ability to learn, and his or her motivation are also important determinants of the prognosis.

Page 87

5. (True or False) Of patients with unilateral below-the-knee amputations, 20% become ambulatory.

Answer: False

Critique: About two thirds of patients with unilateral below-the-knee amputations become ambulatory, whereas only 20% of patients with unilateral above-the-knee amputations become ambulatory.

Page 88

6. (True or False) By making house calls, a family physician may gain important additional information about a patient, including safety issues and possible barriers to compliance.

Answer: True

Critique: Information about patient hygiene and other sources where a patient may be obtaining additional medications can be better understood by the physician.

Page 89

7. (True or False) When assessing a patient for nursing home placement, one important factor to be considered carefully is the availability of support systems.

Answer: True

Critique: The physician must also consider the patient's level of functional and physiologic impairment, the presence of chronic illnesses, and the patient's personal preferences.

Page 91

8. (True or False) Thirst, dryness of the skin, changes in skin turgor, postural pulse and blood pressure changes, and low-grade fever are reliable methods of assessing hydration status in older nursing home patients.

Answer: False

Critique: These methods are not helpful in the case of older nursing home patients. The clinician must assess for tongue dryness, longitudinal tongue furrows, dryness of mucous membranes of the mouth, upper body muscular weakness, confusion, slurred speech, and sunken eyes, and the physician must also calculate the patient's water deficit.

Page 92

9. (True or False) The most common noninfectious cause of fever in the elderly nursing home patient is mechanical blockage of a hollow viscus, causing a local inflammatory response.

Answer: True

Critique: Common examples include atelectasis or mucous plugs in a bronchus, repeated microaspiration, fecal impaction, and blockage of a urinary catheter.

Page 93

10. (True or False) In an elderly patient, when fever is associated with an altered mental status, malaise, lethargy, or coma, it is suggestive of bacteremia.

Answer: True

Critique: By itself, fever is a sensitive indicator of illness, but not necessarily of bacteremia.

Page 95

11. (True or False) In the nursing home patient, incontinence alone is an indication for prolonged catheterization via a Foley catheter.

Answer: False

Critique: Foley catheters should be maintained in only several well-defined circumstances, which include chronic outlet obstruction due to strictures or benign prostatic hypertrophy, the need for strict measurement of fluid intake and output, and possibly in patients with pelvic girdle pressure ulcers or other disruptions of skin integrity.

Page 97

12. (True or False) The cardinal signs of illness in the elderly relate predominantly to changes in mentation, functional status, and a failure to thrive.

Answer: True

Critique: Among the elderly, the signs of illness common to the younger population, such as pain, fever, thirst, and breathlessness, are less reliable and less consistent.

Page 98

13. (True or False) Illnesses rarely seen in patients younger than 60 years of age include polymyalgia rheumatica, temporal arteritis, osteoporosis, Paget's disease, macular degeneration, and pseudogout.

Answer: True

Critique: These conditions occur almost entirely in older patients.

Page 98

14. (True or False) Giant cell arteritis occurs in approximately 50% of patients with polymyalgia rheumatica.

Answer: False

Critique: About 20% of patients with polymyalgia rheumatica develop giant cell arteritis.

Page 99

15. (True or False) When an older patient presents with acute or subacute abdominal pain and has an underlying arrhythmia, the possibility of a mesentric embolus must be a high consideration.

Answer: True

Critique: Acute mesenteric vascular insufficiency is a catastrophic abdominal disorder characterized by severe abdominal pain, accompanied by nausea and bloody diarrhea. The mortality rate is high in acute phases of the illnesses.

Page 101

16. Common causes of syncope in the elderly are:

    A. Metabolic disorders
    B. Intracranial pathology
    C. Drug toxicities
    D. Poor cerebral circulation
    E. All of the above

Answer: E

Critique: All of these are common causes of syncope in the elderly and must be considered in the complete evaluation.

Page 101

17. (True or False) A serum ferritin level of less than 75 μg/l, combined with a transferrin saturation of less than 8%, is virtually diagnostic of anemia in chronic disease.

Answer: False

Critique: In iron deficiency anemia, the serum iron level, the ferritin level, and the transferrin level are usually very low, whereas iron-binding capacity is high. In anemia of chronic disease, serum ferritin levels are elevated and iron-binding capacity is decreased.

Page 107

18. (True or False) The risk of heart disease triples in obese patients who are 20% or more above their ideal weight.

Answer: False

Critique: The risk of heart disease doubles in these obese patients. It is also thought that fat distribution is important when assessing the risk of myocardial infarction. Abdominal obesity is thought to pose a much higher risk than does fat deposition in the hips or thighs.

Page 109

19. Historical features suggestive of Alzheimer's disease include which of the following:

    A. A slow, insidious course with an indistinct onset
    B. A progression over months to years
    C. Initial symptoms of memory loss, impaired judgment, and disturbed social functioning
    D. All of the above

Answer: D

Critique: The historical features of Alzheimer's disease include all of the above.

Page 117

8

Care of the
Dying Patient
Wendy J. Hunter

1. (True or False) When discussing the prognosis of the terminal illness the patient will:

1. Indicate his or her wish to discuss the prognosis
2. Always need a full explanation of the likely course of the disease
3. Use denial as a means of coping with the illness
4. Gain comfort from nonverbal contact
5. Often need to repeat the conversation many times

Answers: 1-T, 2-F, 3-F, 4-T, 5-T

Critique: Patients will often indicate that they need to discuss their prognosis either verbally or often by nonverbal cues. They may, however, feel unable to accept bad news all at once, and many doctors reveal the nature of a terminal illness gradually or in stages. This process may need to be repeated many times. It is important to remain alert to nonverbal cues and not to force such a discussion on an unwilling individual. Even when patients are fully aware of their prognosis, they will often continue to employ denial as a means of fighting their disease. Eye contact and gentle touch will help to reassure the patient that the doctor will support the patient throughout his or her last illness. It is a very powerful way of reinforcing the patient-doctor relationship.

Page 135

2. For patients who are dying, all of the following are true EXCEPT:

A. They usually give up hope as death approaches.
B. They need to feel in control.
C. They need to talk to their families and friends.
D. They may focus on completion of a certain project.

Answer: A

Critique: While the physician should not raise false hopes in the patient's mind, anticipation of an achievable goal (e.g., a final phase of life that has dignity) becomes particularly important. The terminally ill need to believe that they are still in control of their lives and their affairs, which they may wish to put in order. Many will focus on a special event, such as an anniversary or a visit from a relative. Close communication with family and friends becomes particularly important as death approaches, and avoidance and withdrawal may well replace this hope with despair.

Pages 138, 139

3. Perception of chronic pain may be altered by:

A. Past experience
B. Fear
C. Boredom
D. Fatigue
E. All of the above

Answer: E

Critique: All these factors may worsen the patient. Analgesia alone is less likely to be effective unless the patient's fears about his or her illness are addressed when he or she is tired, bored, or lonely.

Page 140

4. Which of the following statements is correct?

A. Opiates are the most effective analgesic for all forms of cancer pain.
B. Analgesia should only be taken if necessary.
C. Patients receiving opiates for chronic or severe cancer pain are likely to become dependent on their analgesia.
D. Opiates may be given rectally, parenterally, orally, or subcutaneously.
E. All oral opiates are equally suitable for use in terminal care.

Answer: D

Critique: Some painful cancer-related problems may respond to simple measures (e.g., oral candidiasis, constipation, infected wounds). Opiates may be inappropriate in these circumstances. Other painful problems may respond well to coanalgesics. As pain control is influenced by anxiety and anticipation of pain, regular and adequate dosage is necessary and may result in a lower requirement for analgesia as the cycle of fear is broken. When medication is given regularly and prior to the onset of pain, craving for the medication does not occur. Two opiate agents that are available orally are not recommended for cancer pain: (1) meperidine has a very low oral potency with short duration of action and produces toxic metabolites that can cause tremors or even seizures, and (2) pentazocine is an agonist-antagonist that is not particularly powerful and often causes hallucinations or confusion in terminally ill patients.

Pages 140–142

5. All of the following agents may be used as coanalgesics in terminal care patients EXCEPT:

    A. Nonsteroidal anti-inflammatory drugs (NSAIDs)
    B. Amitriptyline
    C. Carbamazepine
    D. Steroids
    E. Methotrimeprazine

Answer: D

Critique: All the aforementioned drugs may be helpful when caring for certain terminally ill patients, although steroids are not strictly regarded as coanalgesics. Bony lesions or those in the skeletal muscle may benefit from the addition of NSAIDs. Pain caused by nerve damage may respond well to low-dose amitriptyline or to anticonvulsants. Anxiety may affect a patient's perception of any sort of pain. Methotrimeprazine is a potent sedative and antiemetic as well as having analgesic activity.

Page 142

6. When considering opiate use for terminally ill patients, after careful titration, which of the following side effects poses a significant problem?

    A. Sedation
    B. Respiratory depression
    C. Constipation
    D. Nausea
    E. Hypotension

Answer: C

Critique: When opiate use is titrated sensitively to the needs of the patient sedation, hypotension and respiratory depression are rarely a problem, although opiates may often be effective in controlling dyspnea in terminal disease. Nausea associated with opiate use usually settles after a few days and may be controlled effectively with an appropriate antiemetic. Constipation, however, may be a persistent problem with regular opiate use, and patients should always be encouraged to use a regular daily dose of laxative.

Page 140

7. Once causes such as anemia, bronchospasm, or congestive heart failure have been excluded, dyspnea in the

terminally ill patient may be managed by using: (1) opiates, (2) oxygen, and (3) antibiotics. Which in your opinion would be the most appropriate therapy?

    A. Opiates alone
    B. Oxygen alone
    C. Antibiotics alone
    D. Opiates and oxygen
    E. All of the above

Answer: A

Critique: Opiates are the most effective means of relieving dyspnea in the terminally ill patient. Oxygen may give a little extra benefit. The use of antibiotics will not improve control of dyspnea itself, and their use should be considered carefully so that both the physician and the patient are clear as to whether antibiotics will improve the quality of life or prolong the dying phase.

Page 144

8. Which of the following situations best describes a "conspiracy of silence"?

    A. A physician provides a patient with an overoptimistic prognosis.
    B. A physician agrees to give an unrealistic picture of the prognosis either to the patient or to his or her family.
    C. The physician refuses to tell the family the prognosis.
    D. The physician refuses to tell the patient the diagnosis.

Answer: B

Critique: A conspiracy of silence arises when either the patient or the relatives may, at the request of the other party, be given an unrealistic picture of the patient's illness and prognosis. This almost always creates tension between the two parties and results in isolation of the patient or the relatives. The doctor becomes entangled in the deception, a position that may be extremely uncomfortable.

Page 137

9. Arrange the following analgesics in ascending order of potency:

    A. Hydromorphone 2 mg
    B. Fentanyl patches, 50 μg/hr
    C. Codeine 30 mg + acetaminophen 300 mg (Tylenol no. 3)
    D. Oxycodone 5 mg + aspirin 325 mg (Percodan)
    E. Morphine 30 mg

Answers: (from least to most potent) C, D, A, B, E

Critique: Understanding the relative potency of analgesics allows the physician to best meet the patient's needs for pain control.

Page 140, Table 8–1

10. (True or False) Which of the following measures are effective in managing the nutritional status of patients with terminal disease?

1. High-calorie food supplements
2. Gastrostomy feeds
3. Oral steroids
4. Total parenteral nutrition
5. Alleviation of guilt in relatives

Answers: 3-T, 5-T

Critique: There is little evidence that forced supplementary feeding, whether given orally, via a nasogastric tube, or parenterally, improves the prognosis. Indeed, in some cases it may hasten death. The most important measure may well be to alleviate the guilt of relatives who may struggle to feed the patient in the belief that it will be helpful. Oral steroids may stimulate the appetite and, in addition, attention to analgesia, control of nausea, and constipation may all be effective in encouraging the patient to eat a little.

Page 145

11. (True or False) Which of the following statements about hospice care are true?

1. Hospice care focuses only on the needs of the patient.
2. Hospice care can only be administered in an inpatient setting.
3. Patients wanting admission to the hospice care program must have an inevitably fatal illness.
4. The hospice is staffed exclusively by professional health care workers.
5. Medical supervision is available to patients at all times.

Answers: 3-T, 5-T

Critique: Hospice care focuses not only on the patient but also on the family and may continue to follow the family in the year following their bereavement. Family members are encouraged to participate in the program, and volunteers provide the hospice's many extra services. Hospice care may take place in an inpatient or home setting, and medical advice is available at all times. All patients who are admitted to a hospice care program should have an incurable and inevitably fatal disease with a prognosis of weeks or months.

Pages 146, 147

12. Which of the following statements about subcutaneous infusions is correct?

A. Up to 10 ml of medication may be infused daily.
B. Subcutaneous infusions should only be managed in an inpatient setting.

C. Different drugs should be given by way of separate subcutaneous pumps.
D. The pump may give booster doses of medication when needed.
E. The butterfly needle used to deliver the medication may be placed anywhere on the body.

Answer: D

Critique: Up to 50 ml of volume may be infused by a subcutaneous pump daily. Although the infusion may be started in the inpatient unit, with appropriate supervision most families will usually manage to maintain the pump at home. Various medications (e.g., antiemetics and opiates) may be combined within the same syringe, although it is important to check their compatibility first. Most pumps can deliver a booster dose of medication when required. It is important that the infusion site is located in an area where there is adequate subcutaneous tissue. The areas that are used most often are the abdomen, the chest wall, or the thigh.

Page 144

13. (True or False) Which of the following statements apply to advanced directives or "living wills"?

1. More than 50% of Americans have written a "living will."
2. Federal law requires that all patients entering a hospice program must be offered the chance to make a "living will."
3. A living will should allow for witnesses appointed by the patient to act as guardians of the individual's wishes and the specific circumstances in which the will may be used.
4. A living will will provide a substitute for informed discussion with the family practitioner.

Answer: 2-T, 3-T

Critique: Although approximately 90% of Americans say that they would not wish for extraordinary means to be taken if they were dying, only 20% have made "living wills." All patients entering a hospital or hospice program must be offered the chance to make an advanced directive, which is a legal requirement. To cover any given circumstance, it is advisable for witnesses (usually two) to be appointed to act on the patient's behalf. Although useful, it seems unlikely that a living will will provide any substitute for the lasting nature of the doctor-patient relationship and the trust that this relationship may engender.

Page 149

9

Ethics in Family Practice

Andrew Leeman

1. (True or False) A physician's respect for the patient's autonomy must come before all other obligations.

Answer: False

Critique: The physician must balance respect for the patient's autonomy with his or her own professional moral and religious convictions. This should result in a spirit of co-operation between the physician and the patient.

Page 153

2. (True or False) The physician who performs a pre-employment physical examination:

1. Owes a duty to existing workers in the business
2. Should have access to a job description and any physical or psychological requirements or dangers
3. Should not discuss the results with the patient
4. Should not release any medical records to the employer

Answers: 1-T, 2-T, 3-F, 4-T

Critique: The physician should inform the employee of any problems found at the examination and warn the employee of any health risks of the occupation.

Page 153

3. (True or False) Under which circumstances may a physician pass on medical information without consent?

1. When certifying absence from work
2. To any relatives of the patient
3. When treating venereal or communicable diseases
4. To any other physician
5. Gunshot wounds

Answers: 1-F, 2-F, 3-T, 4-F, 5-T

Critique: An employer should only be supplied with a statement on whether or not the patient is fit to work. The patient may not want medical information divulged to relatives, and this should always be clarified before disclosure. Confidential information should only be shared with another physician when he or she is involved with the patient's care.

Page 155

4. Informed consent is:

A. Written about in the works of Hippocrates
B. Only strictly necessary when discussing potentially life-threatening interventions
C. Only valid in written and signed form
D. Not necessary if it could cause psychological harm

Answer: D

Critique: Informed consent is a relatively recent concept, which first appeared as a phrase in 1957. Consent should be sought for all treatments, whether minor or life-endangering. Written and signed consent only serves to provide evidence of the discussions that have already taken place. Informed consent is not needed if it could cause psychological harm to the patient.

Page 155

5. (True or False) In which of the following circumstances will most states allow a teenager to give consent to an intervention in the absence of a parent?

1. Contraception
2. If the teenager has good grades at college
3. If the teenager lives away from home and manages his or her own affairs
4. In an emergency medical situation
5. If the teenager wants an abortion

Answers: 1-T, 2-F, 3-T, 4-T, 5-F

Critique: Informed consent requires the patient to be able to receive, remember, assess, and decide upon information given. This does not require advanced education. Consent for abortion for teenagers is a difficult subject, and it cannot be assumed that the patient's consent alone is always valid.

Page 156

Questions 6–9. Match the following types of noncompliance and the appropriate clinical response.

    A. Involve other physicians.
    B. Respect the patient's wishes.
    C. Treat the patient's psychological problems.
    D. Reinform the patient about the need for treatment.

6. An informed elderly patient who withholds consent for surgery for bowel cancer

7. A patient with whom a physician has had a disagreement over a previous illness, who is now refusing treatment for severe hypertension

8. A patient who keeps forgetting what he or she is told

9. A bereaved and tearful patient who cannot decide whether to undergo joint replacement surgery for osteoarthritis

Answers: 6-B, 7-A, 8-D, 9-C

Critique: The questions in turn relate to issues of value conflict (question 6), failure of trust (question 7), problems of communication (question 8), and psychological factors (question 9). The patient who keeps forgetting what he or she is told may be helped by reviewing how the information is given and the type of information given.

Page 157, Table 9–2

10. Which of the following statements, concerning referral to subspecialists, is or are correct?

    A. A low referral rate is an indication of good practice.
    B. Responsibility of the overall care of the patient always rests with the family practice physician.
    C. The patient should be encouraged to make his or her own arrangements for a subspecialist's opinion.
    D. A referring physician must include all details of a patient's medical history to a subspecialist.
    E. The referral process is complete once an initial appointment has been made.

Answer: B

Critique: A physician must be aware of his or her own limitations, and a low referral rate may reflect a lack of such an awareness. The patient must be guided to a suitable choice of subspecialty and specialist. Not all details of a patient's past history need be included in a referral. Some disclosures may inadvertently break a patient's con-

fidentiality. The referral process is complete only when the full result of the referral has been discussed, understood, and acted upon as necessary.

Page 158

11. (True or False) Physicians have high rates of:

    1. Alcoholism
    2. Suicide
    3. Divorce
    4. Burn-out
    5. Substance abuse

Answers: 1-T, 2-T, 3-T, 4-T, 5-T

Critique: There are many reasons for physicians not caring for their own health. Acceptance of one's own humanity and emotions and making time for one's own needs and family needs are important factors in one's ability to cope.

Page 159

12. (True or False) The criteria for physician-endorsed euthanasia in the Netherlands include which of the following?

    1. Intolerable suffering despite all attempts at relief
    2. An unacceptable social, psychological, financial burden on the patient's family
    3. The written consent of the family attorney
    4. The agreement of two physicians
    5. A rational and informed patient

Answers: 1-T, 2-F, 3-F, 4-T, 5-T

Critique: The family's suffering is not taken into direct consideration when acceding to a request for euthanasia. The family's attorney need not be involved in the decision-making process.

Page 160

13. (True or False) The American Medical Association opposes euthanasia because it would:

    1. Tarnish medicine's image as a healing profession
    2. Confuse patients
    3. Violate the Hippocratic oath
    4. Slow the introduction of new treatments for terminal disease
    5. Oppose the expressed desire of the majority of Americans

Answers: 1-T, 2-T, 3-T, 4-F, 5-F

Critique: Euthanasia would not affect the development of treatments for terminal diseases. In November 1993, 73% of Americans responded "Yes" to this question: "Do you think the law should allow doctors to comply with the wishes of a dying patient in severe distress who asks to have his or her life ended, or not?"

Part II

Community Medicine

10

Periodic Health Examination

Alan R. Roth

1. The periodic health examination was designed to help integrate prevention into clinical care. It is best described by which of the following:

    A. Defines the annual physical examination
    B. Lists appropriate screening procedures
    C. Creates a lifetime health care plan
    D. Determines the efficacy of routine tests
    E. Decreases the amount of time needed for preventive services in family medicine

Answer: C

Critique: The changes in primary care medicine are showing a shift toward the prevention of disease rather than the treatment of illness, thus family physicians are now spending more time on preventive services. The periodic health examination is a health protection package whose aim is to create a lifetime health care plan for the individual patient. The periodic health examination is based on a series of age- and sex-related preventive interventions. The examination consists of a group of tasks that have been formulated by the Canadian Task Force (CTF) on the periodic health examination (1979) and the United States Preventive Services Task Force (USPSTF) (1989).

The purpose of the periodic health examination is to determine the risk of disease or to identify diseases as early as possible in their symptomless state. The historical complete physical examination as well as many screening tests and procedures have not proved to be efficacious or effective. The future of preventive medicine lies in the periodic health examination and its health protection packages.

Page 165

2. Which of the following is an example of a *primary* preventive intervention?

    A. Tetanus prophylaxis
    B. Screening sigmoidoscopy
    C. Papanicolaou smear

    D. Blood pressure screening
    E. Mantoux skin test for tuberculosis

Answer: A

Critique: Primary prevention is a technique aimed at avoiding diseases before they begin. This is accomplished by modifying exposure to disease states or modifying ill health behaviors or risk factors. The goal of primary prevention is to prevent the occurrence of disease. The goal of secondary prevention is to identify diseases in their early state and initiate measures to modify the disease process. Tetanus prophylaxis is the only example of primary prevention given. Other examples of primary prevention include fluoridation of water, accident prevention through patient education, and most immunizations. Screening sigmoidoscopy, Papanicolaou testing, blood pressure screening, and the Mantoux test for tuberculosis are all examples of secondary prevention.

Page 165

3. The best method to evaluate the efficacy and effectiveness of preventive interventions is which of the following.

    A. Cohort study
    B. Randomized controlled trial
    C. Case control study
    D. Descriptive studies
    E. Case reports

Answer: B

Critique: The decline of the conventional annual checkup is based on the fact that most of the tests and procedures included in the comprehensive annual examination have not been found to be effective or efficacious. In the past, practice recommendations have been based on evidence as simple as the opinions of respected authorities or on clinical experience. The randomized controlled trial is the preferred technique used to evelute the efficacy and effectiveness of preventive interventions. The goal is to evaluate each preventive intervention on clinical outcomes, such as mortality, morbidity or improved quality of life. The ideal preventive intervention should be accurate, safe, simple, and inexpensive.

Pages 165–167

4. The proportion of individuals who have a positive test result and who are actually affected by the disease in question is known as:

    A. Positive predictive value
    B. Negative predictive value
    C. Sensitivity of test
    D. Specificity of test
    E. Effectivenss of a test

Answer: A

Critique: The positive predictive value is the proportion of individuals who are actually affected by the disease tested and who have a positive test result. In the screening of asymptomatic individuals, high performance is crucial to the early detection of disease states. The positive predictive value of a test is of utmost importance when determining the test's effectiveness. The negative predictive value is the number of individuals who are free of the disease and who have a negative test result.

The sensitivity is the proportion of diseased individuals correctly identified by the procedure. The specificity is the proportion of healthy individuals who are not affected by the disease and are classified as being disease free by the procedure. The effectiveness of a test is that it results in more good than harm to those whom the procedure is offered.

The inclusion of clinical procedures in the periodic health examination is based on rules of evidence that show that there is good information that a recommendation should be included. These rules of evidence include randomized controlled trials, well-designed controlled trials without randomization, and cohort or case-controlled analytic studies. The clinical procedure in question is then graded based on current scientific certainty as to whether or not it should be included as a preventive intervention.

Pages 166, 167

5. A 40-year-old man presents to your office with symptoms of seasonal allergic rhinitis. On physical examination his blood pressure is noted to be 160/100. Which of the following *best* describes this clinical situation?

    A. Case finding
    B. Screening
    C. Secondary prevention
    D. Early detection procedure
    E. None of the above

Answer: A

Critique: Detection of disease, risk factors for disease, or even pertinent history or physical findings in patients who present to a physician for unrelated conditions is known as case finding. Primary preventive intervention in the course of management of an acute medical illness or intercurrent health problems is increasing in importance and popularity. Most of the activities of the periodic

health examination can be done as part of a patient-triggered encounter for an acute problem or follow-up of a medical condition. Screening is the use of a clinical procedure to a population in order to classify individuals into groups of high or low probability of being affected with a particular condition. Secondary prevention uses a screening test followed by a primary preventive intervention. An early detection procedure is often used synonymously with secondary prevention and can be a history question, physical examination, or laboratory test.

Pages 165–167, 170

6. Which of the following clinical procedures is recommended at the first prenatal visit in a 28-year-old woman with a 12-week intrauterine pregnancy. The woman has had only one sexual partner and has no significant past medical history.

    A. Routine ultrasound
    B. Screening for herpes simplex
    C. Serologic testing for toxoplasmosis
    D. Fasting blood sugar
    E. Serologic screening for syphilis

Answer: E

Critique: Serologic testing for syphilis using the Venereal Disease Research Laboratory (VDRL) or rapid plasma reagin (RPR) blood test is still recommended on all prenatal patients. The test should be performed at the first prenatal visit and at delivery. In those patients who are at high risk for a sexually transmitted disease (STD), an additional test at 28 weeks is recommended. Routine ultrasound is recommended only for women at high risk for intrauterine growth retardation. Ultrasonography has not been shown to significantly affect perinatal morbidity and mortality. Screening for herpes simplex is not recommended, except in individuals at high risk for exposure to sexually transmitted diseases. Toxoplasmosis screening may be indicated for women who have a cat at home. These individuals should be counseled to avoid cat litter and raw meat. The effectiveness of screening for gestational diabetes remains controversial and has not been thoroughly investigated. Screening with an oral glucose challenge test may result in a decreased incidence of macrosomia and birth trauma.

Pages 168–170, 186

7. Screening for neural tube defects and Down syndrome with the maternal serum alpha-fetoprotein (MSAFP) is most appropriately performed at what gestational age?

    A. 8–10 weeks
    B. 12–14 weeks
    C. 16–18 weeks
    D. 20–24 weeks
    E. Screening is recommended only for high-risk individuals.

Answer: C

Critique: Measurement of MSAFP is recommended for the screening of the asymptomatic general population for neural tube defects. MSAFP should be measured on all prenatal patients between 16 and 18 weeks' gestation. The test should be accompanied by adequate counseling as well as follow-up by ultrasonography and amniocentesis if necessary. The high-risk population for developing Down syndrome may also be screened using MSAFP. This test, however, does not replace amniocentesis for karyotyping, which should be offered to all pregnant women aged 35 years and older. Elevated MSAFP levels correlate with an increased risk of neural tube defects. Low MSAFP levels are associated with an increased risk of fetal Down syndrome. Tests done at a gestational age other than 16 to 18 weeks are not considered as reliable. Determination of the correct gestational age is essential when evaluating the accuracy of any MSAFP.

Page 169

8. Routine preventive interventions at birth in a healthy full-term infant should include which of the following clinical procedures?

  A. VDRL of cord blood
  B. Hemoglobin electrophoresis
  C. Sweat test for cystic fibrosis
  D. Screening for coagulation defects
  E. Screening T4 from heel prick for neonatal hypothyroidism

Answer: E

Critique: The periodic health examination includes a series of preventive interventions that should be done at birth, such as screening for neonatal hypothyroidism by T4 testing from a heel prick. These routine screening tests have proved to be effective and are best performed 3 to 6 days after birth.

Screening for congenital syphilis is only indicated when the mother is positive for syphilis and should include weekly quantitative reagin tests during the first month. Hemoglobin electrophoresis is recommended only when the prevalence of sickle cell disease or thalassemia is high. The sweat test for cystic fibrosis may be used to screen for cystic fibrosis in those with affected siblings. Screening for hemorrhagic disease of the newborn is not recommended. To prevent vitamin K–dependent hemorrhagic disease and coagulation disorders, every neonate should receive a single intramuscular dose of vitamin K, 1 mg within 1 hour of birth.

Pages 171, 174

9. The USPSTF recommendation for prophylaxis against ophthalmia neonatorum is which of the following:

  A. Routine eye culture in the nursery
  B. Saline irrigation of eyes
  C. Silver nitrate prophylaxis
  D. Erythromycin 0.5% ophthalmic ointment
  E. None of the above

Answer: D

Critique: Preventive intervention at birth in the asymptomatic general population is indicated for the prevention of ophthalmia neonatorum. The USPSTF recommends

that erythromycin 0.5% ophthalmic ointment should be applied to the eyes of all newborns as soon as possible after birth and no later than 1 hour of age. Silver nitrate has limited efficacy in preventing chlamydial infections and has increased side effects, such as irritation and chemical conjunctivitis. Routine culture and sensitivity of the eyes is not indicated. Saline irrigation has no prophylactic effect, and its use should be avoided especially after the administration of prophylactic antibiotics.

Page 171

10. Which of the following is the USPSTF recommendation for routine visual screening in asymptomatic children and adolescents?

  A. Annual routine screening for refractive errors in all school children
  B. Annual testing for refractive error, strabismus, and amblyopia
  C. Comprehensive examination by an ophthalmologist prior to school entry
  D. Testing for amblyopia and strabismus for all children at 3 or 4 years of age
  E. Annual vision screening of all adolescents

Answer: D

Critique: Screening for refractive defects, strabismus, and amblyopia has usually been part of the routine comprehensive examination. Visual acuity testing, stereotesting, and the cover-uncover test are simple office procedures that can be done by any family physician. The USPSTF only recommends that children be tested once prior to entering school at 3 to 4 years of age for strabismus and amblyopia. Routine testing for refractive errors by visual acuity testing is not recommended for school children or asymptomatic adolescents. The CTF recommends routine screening (including visual acuity testing) in preschool years to decrease the prevalence of uncorrected disorders. The American Academy of Ophthalmology differs from the aforementioned recommendations and states that eye and vision screening should be performed at birth, 6 months, 3 years, and 5 years of age.

Page 175

11. Routine voluntary human immunodeficiency virus (HIV) screening tests are recommended in which of the following groups?

  A. All newborns
  B. All prenatal patients
  C. All adolescents
  D. Premarital examinations
  E. Only those individuals with risk factors for HIV disease

Answer: E

Critique: Routine screening for HIV is recommended for those individuals at high risk for the disease. All physicians should take a complete history from the patient, including sexual activity and drug use. Sexually active patients should be advised that abstaining from sex and maintaining a mutually faithful monogamous sexual relationship with a partner known to be uninfected are the most effective strategies to prevent infection with HIV and other STDs. Counseling should be given to patients about safe sexual practices, including the proper use of condoms and spermicides. High-risk groups include homosexual and bisexual men, prostitutes, past or present intravenous drug abusers, individuals with a history of multiple sexual partners, patients with STDs, sexual contacts of HIV-positive people, patients with a history of blood transfusion between 1978 and 1985, and people from a country with a high prevalence rate of HIV infections. Retesting every 6 to 12 months should be recommended to high-risk patients, particularly if they continue to engage in high-risk behavior. Voluntary HIV testing should be performed only after obtaining informed consent and adequate pre- and post-test counseling.

Pages 175, 183

12. A 30-year-old man presents to your office for a routine examination. His blood pressure is 120/80. You should recommend that the patient have his blood pressure checked again in:

    A. 6 months
    B. 1 year
    C. 2 years
    D. 5 years
    E. 10 years

Answer: C

Critique: The screening for hypertension in the asymptomatic general population is part of the periodic health examination of all adults. The CTF recommends that an individual's blood pressure measurement should be taken at every visit. The USPSTF recommends that patients whose initial screening is normal (systolic <140 mm Hg, diastolic <85 mm Hg) should receive a blood pressure measurement at least once every 2 years. Persons with borderline elevations (systolic >140 mm Hg or diastolic 85 to 89 mm Hg) should have their blood pressures checked annually. The American Academy of Family Physicians recommends that an individual's blood pressure be measured at every visit, with a minimum frequency of every 2 years.

Page 179

13. In which of the following groups should routine total serum cholesterol (nonfasting) be measured at an interval of every 5 years?

    A. Asymptomatic children and adolescents
    B. All adults 20 to 64 years of age
    C. All adults with a total blood cholesterol level higher than 6.2 mmol/l on routine examination
    D. Only those adults with a family history of premature coronary artery disease or hyperlipidemia
    E. Individuals with risk factors for coronary artery disease

Answer: B

Critique: Periodic measurement of total serum cholesterol (nonfasting) has been found to be effective as part of the periodic health examination of healthy adults. To date there is no recommendation to do screening on healthy children or adolescents. Children who have a parent with an elevated total cholesterol level or those with a family history of premature cardiovascular disease should be screened for lipoprotein levels. Routine screening should be performed on all adults at an interval of every 5 years. All abnormal results (total cholesterol >6.2 mmol/l) should be confirmed with repeat blood tests. Those individuals with abnormal or borderline (5.15 to 6.15 mmol/l) results and risk factors for coronary artery disease should be followed more closely. Risk factors include male gender, family history of premature coronary heart disease, smoking tobacco, hypertension, high-density lipoprotein C (<0.90 mmol/l), diabetes mellitus, previous stroke, peripheral vascular disease, or obesity. All individuals with abnormal results or two or more risk factors should receive counseling on nutrition, exercise, and risk reduction. Routine follow-up at 6 months should be recommended.

Page 179

14. Which of the following clinical procedures has proved to be effective for the detection of colorectal carcinoma in asymptomatic adult patients?

    A. An annual hemoccult test for occult blood in stool in adults older than 40 years of age
    B. An annual sigmoidoscopy in persons older than 50 years of age
    C. A colonoscopy every 3 years after 50 years of age
    D. An annual colonoscopy
    E. None of the above

Answer: E

Critique: Despite the fact that digital rectal examination, hemoccult testing, sigmoidoscopy, and colonoscopy may be useful in the early detection of colorectal carcinoma, there has been no clinical procedure that has proved to be efficacious. The USPSTF is currently reviewing this issue. Occult fecal blood testing has shown benefits in mortality after screening patients for more than 10 years. The test has a high false positivity combined with a poor sensitivity on annual testing. Screening sigmoidoscopy will miss all right-sided colon carcinomas. Colonoscopy is an excellent test for the detection of colon carcinoma; however, it is expensive and the yield is low in asymptomatic individuals, making this a poorly effective screening procedure. The American Cancer Society recommends that an annual digital rectal examination should be performed for all patients, starting at 40 years of age. Annual fecal occult blood testing should be done for all asymptomatic individuals without known risk factors beginning at 50 years of age. Those patients at normal risk should be screened with sigmoidoscopy every 3 to 5 years, beginning at 50 years of age.

Pages 183, 186

15. The routine use of fasting blood glucose tests is least controversial in which of the following?

A. All prenatal patients
B. All newborns
C. One baseline test in early childhood or adolescence
D. Annually for elderly patients (>65 years of age)
E. Periodic measurements in persons at high risk for diabetes mellitus

Answer: E

Critique: The use of periodic fasting blood glucose measurements has been shown to be most appropriate in persons at high risk for diabetes mellitus. The American Diabetes Association recommends screening for diabetes mellitus every 3 years in adults with any risk factors for the disease. High-risk groups include the markedly obese, persons with a family history of diabetes, persons of Hispanic or African-American heritage, persons with hypertension, persons with hyperlipidemia, or women with a history of gestational diabetes. Routine periodic fasting blood glucose measurements have not been effective in asymptomatic infants, children, adolescents, or even the elderly. The effectiveness of screening for gestational diabetes has not been properly evaluated in the general population.

Page 183

16. (True or False) Routine screening tests for the early detection of disease in asymptomatic persons has been effective in the following conditions and should, therefore, be included in the periodic health examination:

1. Cervical cancer
2. Lung cancer
3. Endometrial cancer
4. Osteoporosis

Answers: 1-T, 2-F, 3-F, 4-F

Critique: The Papanicolaou smear to screen for cervical cancer has been shown to be a safe and effective screening test. Annual screening is recommended for all sexually active women or beginning at age 18, whichever occurs first. After a woman has had three or more consecutive satisfactory normal annual examinations, the Papanicolaou test may be performed every 1 to 3 years at the discretion of the physician and patient. Increased frequency of testing is recommended for those women with risk factors for cervical carcinoma (e.g., age of first sexual intercourse <18 years, multiple sexual partners, smoking, or low socioeconomic groups). Testing may stop at age 65 if previous smears have been normal. Screening for lung cancer with chest radiographic studies or sputum cytology is not recommended as a preventive intervention, even for cigarette smokers. Evidence exists that neither procedure is valid for the early detection of a lesion or significant changes in the mortality rate. Screening for endometrial cancer by endometrial biopsy or cytologic examination of the endometrium is not recommended as part of the periodic health examination. Early detection procedures for evaluating hyperplasia are unreliable, and there are no controlled studies that show the effectiveness of early treatment. Screening for osteoporosis by bone densitometry is not recommended. The procedure is expensive, and it has not been shown that bone mass is an accurate predictor of fractures.

Pages 179, 188

17. (True or False) The following clinical procedures are considered controversial as to whether or not they should be included or excluded from the periodic health examination:

1. Scoliosis screening by physical examination
2. Digital rectal examination and prostate-specific antigen for prostate cancer
3. Hearing evaluation in the elderly (>65 years old)
4. Electronic fetal monitoring during labor

Answers: 1-T, 2-T, 3-F, 4-T

Critique: Screening for scoliosis by physical examination is a controversial clinical procedure. Screening leads to a high rate of overreferral, and there is controversy about the efficacy of treatment even when scoliosis is detected at an earlier stage. Screening for prostate cancer by digital rectal examination and prostate-specific antigen is a controversial issue. There is no conclusive evidence to support that either clinical procedure is beneficial in the early detection of disease. In addition, the benefits of treatment at these stages is also inconclusive. The American Cancer Society recommends that annual digital rectal examination should be performed on patients at 40 years of age, and annual prostate-specific antigen testing beginning at age 50. The testing of the elderly population (>65 years of age) for hearing impairment by history and audiometry is recommended as part of the periodic health examination. All elderly patients should be evaluated, and appropriate counseling should be given for the use of hearing aids. The routine use of electronic fetal monitoring during labor for the detection of intrapartum asphyxia is an extremely controversial preventive intervention. Although its use is widespread, there is no definite evidence that neonatal morbidity or mortality rates have been reduced. In addition, the use of electronic fetal monitoring has been associated with an increased rate of cesarean section.

Pages 185, 186

18. (True or False) True statements relating to current immunization practices include which of the following?

1. Diphtheria, tetanus, and pertussis (DTP) and *Haemophilus influenzae* type b (HIB) at 2, 4, 6, and 15 months of age
2. Measles, mumps, and rubella (MMR) at 15 months and booster at 4 to 6 years of age
3. Tetanus and diphtheria booster at age 14 to 16 years of age
4. Tetanus and diphtheria booster every 10 years until age 60

Answers: 1-T, 2-T, 3-T, 4-F

Critique: Current recommendations for immunizations include the following: The DTP should be given at 2, 4, 6, and 15 months and at 4 to 6 years. The acellular pertussis vaccine (DTaP) may be substituted at 15 months and 4 to 6 years of age. The trivalent oral polio vaccine (OPV) at 2, 4, and 15 months and at 4 to 6 years. The HIB conjugate vaccine should be given at 2, 4, 6, and 15 months. This vaccine may be combined with DTP vaccine as the DTP/HIB. The MMR vaccine should be administered at 15 months and 4 to 6 years. In areas with measles epidemics, the monovalent measles vaccine should be administered as early as 9 months of age. The MMR vaccine should also be given to all nonpregnant persons born after 1956 who lack evidence of immunity to measles or rubella. Women should be counseled not to become pregnant for 3 months after immunization. The tetanus and diphtheria (Td) booster should be administered at age 14 to 16 years and *every 10 years* thereafter. There is no recommendation to stop giving Td boosters at any age.

Pages 172, 175, 180

19. (True or False) The USPSTF recommendation for breast cancer prevention includes which of the following?

1. Annual clinical breast examination starting at 20 years of age
2. Baseline mammogram at 35 years of age
3. Mammography every 1 to 2 years for women aged 50 to 75
4. Regular screening for women with a strong family history, beginning at 35 years of age

Answers: 1-F, 2-F, 3-T, 4-T

Critique: The USPSTF recommendations for breast cancer prevention are the following: (1) All women older than 40 years of age should receive an annual clinical breast examination; (2) Mammography is recommended every 1 to 2 years for women aged 50 to 75; and (3) For women with a family history of breast cancer in first-degree relatives, regular screening should begin at 35 years of age. Of note is the fact that the teaching of breast self-examination is considered controversial as to its inclusion as a preventive intervention. Breast self-examination may produce anxiety and cause the performance of unnecessary procedures. In addition, there is little evidence that breast self-examination reduces mortality.

The American Cancer Society's recommendations for breast cancer prevention include the following: (1) Women should have clinical breast examinations every 3 years from ages 20 to 39; (2) An annual clinical breast examination should be performed on women 40 years of age and older; (3) Women should be encouraged to examine their breasts every month; (4) Women 40 to 49 years of age should receive screening mammograms every 1 to 2 years; and (5) Women 50 years of age and older should have routine annual screening mammography

Pages 179, 186

20. (True or False) Which of the following individuals should receive prophylaxis with the pneumococcal vaccination?

1. All persons older than 50 years of age
2. Patients with chronic cardiac or pulmonary disease
3. Sickle cell disease
4. Renal disease or nephrotic syndrome
5. Alcoholics

Answers: 1-F, 2-T, 3-T, 4-T, 5-T

Critique: Recommendations for the prevention of pneumococcal pneumonia using the pneumococcal vaccine include the following: (1) All persons 65 years of age or older; (2) Those with medical conditions that increase the risk of pneumococcal infection (e.g., chronic cardiac or pulmonary disease, sickle cell disease, Hodgkin's disease, asplenia, diabetes mellitus, alcoholism, cirrhosis, multiple myeloma, renal disease, and conditions associated with immunosuppression), and (3) Patients living in environments (institutions) with an increased risk of pneumococcal disease. Revaccination should be strongly considered for patients who received the 14-valent vaccine or for those in high-risk groups who received the 23-valent vaccine 6 or more years ago.

Page 184

11

Preventive Health Care

Michael D. Hagen

1. A proposed procedure should meet several criteria before use in primary or secondary screening activities. Of the following, which *one* is *not* a criterion for accepting a screening procedure in practice?

A. The disease or condition for which screening is conducted must have a significant impact on the quantity or quality of life.

B. If the procedure can detect the disorder before clinical manifestations develop, treatment in the asymptomatic state must yield better results than are possible after the disorder becomes apparent.

C. As long as a test is available, clinicians should apply the procedure regardless of the test's cost or morbidity.

D. Interventions for disorders identified at an early stage must demonstrate acceptable effectiveness, risk, patient acceptability, and cost.

Answer: C

Critique: Before clinicians accept a screening procedure for general use, the technique must meet several criteria: (1) the disease or disorder in question must demonstrate a significant burden of suffering (impact on quantity or quality of life, significant prevalence in the population) for the screened population; (2) a procedure must be available to detect individuals at risk in the presymptomatic phase or before they develop the condition; (3) the procedure should demonstrate acceptable accuracy, morbidity, and cost; (4) if the procedure can detect the disorder at an early stage, treatment must be available that yields better results than those obtained by waiting until the disease becomes clinically apparent; (5) the treatment for the disorder must demonstrate acceptable effectiveness, risk, morbidity, cost, and acceptance by the patient.

Further Reading

Morse RM, Heffron WA: Preventive health care. *In* Rakel RE: *Textbook of Family Practice.* Philadelphia, WB Saunders, 1995, p 192.

2. The incidence rate for a particular disorder or condition is described as:

A. The percentage of a population afflicted with the condition at a point in time

B. The number of deaths per 100,000 persons per year

C. The annual number of deaths in 40 year olds in a defined population

D. The number of new cases of a disorder occurring annually in a defined population

Answer: D

Critique: The incidence rate reflects the number of new cases of a disorder occurring annually in a defined population. The number of deaths per 100,000 per year represents the mortality rate for a population. The percentage of people afflicted at a certain point in time constitutes the condition's prevalence. The annual number of deaths among 40 year olds in a population represents an age-specific mortality rate.

Further Reading

Morse RM, Heffron WA: Preventive health care. *In* Rakel RE: *Textbook of Family Practice.* Philadelphia, WB Saunders, 1995, p 192.

3. The sensitivity of a diagnostic or screening test is best described as:

A. The likelihood that a normal person will have a negative screening test result

B. The likelihood that a person with a positive test result has the disease in question

C. The likelihood that an afflicted person will have a positive test result

D. The likelihood that a person with a negative test result is indeed normal

Answer: C

Critique: The sensitivity of a test represents the likelihood that an afflicted individual will have a positive or abnormal test result. The likelihood that a person with a positive test result has the disease in question represents the positive predictive value for that test. Specificity represents the likelihood that a normal person will have a negative or normal test result. The likelihood that a person with a negative test result is indeed normal represents the negative predictive value for the test.

Further Reading

Morse RM, Heffron WA: Preventive health care. *In* Rakel RE: *Textbook of Family Practice.* Philadelphia, WB Saunders, 1995, pp 192–193.

4. Assume that you are evaluating a new screening test in a population of 1000 people, 75 of whom have the disorder for which you are screening. Of the 75 afflicted persons, 50 yield positive test results; 75 of the normal people also have positive test results.

From this information, the *sensitivity* for the test is:

A. 85%
B. 67%
C. 58%
D. 92%

From this information, the *specificity* for the test is:

E. 9%
F. 33%
G. 40%
H. 87%
I. 92%

From this information, the *positive predictive value* for the test is:

J. 60%
K. 40%
L. 20%
M. 10%

From this information, the *negative predictive value* for the test is:

N. 50%
O. 88%
P. 97%
Q. 33%

Answers: B, I, K, P

Critique: The operating characteristics for a diagnostic test can be calculated from a 2 × 2 (or "four-square") table. Such a table for the hypothetical data presented here looks like this:

Disease	Test Positive	Test Negative	Total
Present	50	25	75
Absent	75	850	925
	125	875	1000

The test's sensitivity represents the number of diseased persons (75) who have a positive test result (50):

$$\text{Sensitivity} = \frac{50}{75} = 67\%$$

The test's specificity represents the number of normal persons (925) who have a negative test result (850):

$$\text{Specificity} = \frac{850}{925} = 92\%$$

The test's positive predictive value represents the likelihood that a person with a positive test result (125) actually has the disease (50):

$$\text{Positive predictive value} = \frac{50}{125} = 40\%$$

The test's negative predictive value represents the likelihood that a person with a negative test result (875) is indeed normal (850):

$$\text{Negative predictive value} = \frac{850}{875} = 97\%.$$

Further Reading

Morse RM, Heffron WA: Preventive health care. *In* Rakel RE: *Textbook of Family Practice.* Philadelphia, WB Saunders, 1995, pp 192–194.

5. Assume that you have available to you a screening test that operates with 80% sensitivity and specificity. You apply this test to a population of 1000 people, in which the prevalence of the disorder for which you are testing is 10%. What is the positive predictive value of a positive result in this population?

A. 44%
B. 97%
C. 80%
D. 31%

If the prevalence in this population were 20%, what positive predictive value would a positive test result yield?

E. 25%
F. 6%
G. 20%
H. 50%

Answers: D, H

Critique: The positive predictive value for a test result depends not only on the test's sensitivity and specificity but also on the prevalence of the condition in the population being tested. In the 10% prevalence example, the 2 × 2 table looks like this:

Disease	Test Positive	Test Negative	Total
Present	80	20	100
Absent	180	720	900
	260	740	1000

In this scenario, the positive predictive value is:

$$\frac{80}{260} = 31\%.$$

In the 20% prevalence situation, the 2×2 table looks like this:

Disease	Test Positive	Test Negative	Total
Present	160	40	200
Absent	160	640	800
	320	680	1000

In this population, operating with the same sensitivity and specificity, a positive test result yields:

$$\text{Positive predictive value} = \frac{160}{320} = 50\%.$$

The same test, operating with the same sensitivity and specificity, yields quite different positive predictive values in the two populations. This demonstrates how the positive predictive value depends on the population prevalence. A positive test result in a population with a low prevalence will have a quite different meaning from the same result in the context of a higher prevalence.

Further Reading

Morse RM, Heffron WA: Preventive health care. *In* Rakel RE: *Textbook of Family Practice.* Philadelphia, WB Saunders, 1995, pp 192–194.

6. (True or False) Risk factors for coronary heart disease (CHD) include which of the following?

1. Family history of premature CHD
2. Elevated high-density lipoprotein (HDL) levels
3. Elevated total cholesterol (TC):HDL cholesterol ratio
4. Elevated low-density lipoprotein (LDL) cholesterol

Answers: 1-T, 2-F, 3-T, 4-T

Critique: A family history of CHD confers increased risk independent of lipid levels. An elevated HDL level actually lowers the risk for CHD. Elevated TC:HDL ratios predict risk independently of the LDL cholesterol level. An elevated LDL level is a recognized risk factor for CHD.

Suggested Reading

Kinosian B, Glick H, Preiss L, Puder KL: Cholesterol and coronary heart disease: predicting risks in men by changes in levels and ratios. J Invest Med 43:443–450, 1995.
Morse RM, Heffron WA: Preventive health care. *In* Rakel RE: *Textbook of Family Practice.* Philadelphia, WB Saunders, 1995, pp 194–195.

Roncaglioni MC (for the GISSI-EFRIM Investigators): Role of family history in patients with myocardial infarction: An Italian case-control study. Circulation 85:2065–2072, 1992.

7. Nonpharmacologic measures that physicians should recommend to improve lipid profiles include all of the following EXCEPT:

A. Increased proportion of dietary fat consumed as monounsaturated fats
B. Increased soluble dietary fiber
C. Dietary fat limited to 50% of total calories
D. Weight control and exercise

Answer: C

Critique: Weight control and exercise and increased soluble dietary fiber can improve lipid profiles. Additionally, an increase in the proportion of dietary fat consumed as monounsaturated fat lowers the LDL cholesterol level. Total dietary fat should be limited to 30% of total calories, rather than 50%.

Further Reading

Morse RM, Heffron WA: Preventive health care. *In* Rakel RE: *Textbook of Family Practice.* Philadelphia, WB Saunders, 1995, pp 194–195.

8. According to the National Cholesterol Education Program (NCEP), which of the following conditions call for pharmacologic intervention?

1. Documented CHD with LDL cholesterol greater than 100 mg/dl (2.6 mmol/l) and less than 130 mg/dl (3.4 mmol/l)
2. Two or more CHD risk factors without documented CHD and LDL greater than 130 mg/dl (3.4 mmol/l) and less than 160 mg/l (4.1 mmol/l)
3. Fewer than two CHD risk factors without documented CHD and LDL greater than 190 mg/dl (4.9 mmol/l)
4. Two or more CHD risk factors without documented CHD and LDL greater than 160 mg/dl (4.1 mmol/l)

Answers: 1-F, 2-F, 3-T, 4-T

Critique: The NCEP has provided guidelines for initiating dietary and drug treatment of hypercholesterolemia. A person with CHD whose LDL is between 100 mg/dl (2.6 mmol/l) and 130 mg/dl (3.4 mmol/l) should be treated initially with dietary management. The CHD-free individual who has two risk factors or more and an LDL level between 130 mg/dl (3.4 mmol/l) and 160 mg/dl (4.1 mmol/l) should also receive dietary therapy. The situations described in options C and D both require drug therapy.

Further Reading

Blake GH, Triplett LC: Management of hypercholesterolemia. Am Fam Physician 51:1157–1166, 1995.
Morse RM, Heffron WA: Preventive health care. *In* Rakel RE: *Textbook of Family Practice.* Philadelphia, WB Saunders, 1995, pp 195–196.

9. Lifestyle modifications that physicians should recommend to reduce the risk of CHD include all of the following EXCEPT:

    A. Maintenance of ideal body weight
    B. Smoking cessation
    C. Moderation of alcohol intake
    D. Avoidance of moderately strenuous exercise

Answer: D

Critique: A number of lifestyle modifications can lower the risks for developing CHD. Maintenance of ideal body weight, control of alcohol intake, and discontinuation of tobacco use all diminish the risk for CHD. Physical activity actually confers protection against CHD, and physicians should recommend moderate exercise to patients who are able to undertake such a program.

Futher Reading

Berlin JA, Colditz GA: A meta-analysis of physical activity in the prevention of coronary heart disease. Am J Epidemiol 132:612–628, 1990.

Morse, RM, Heffron WA: Preventive health care. *In* Rakel RE: *Textbook of Family Practice.* Philadelphia, WB Saunders, 1995, pp 195–196.

10. Of the following potential risk factors, which one confers the highest risk for ischemic stroke?

    A. Smoking
    B. Noninsulin-dependent diabetes mellitus
    C. Hypercholesterolemia
    D. Obesity
    E. Systolic or diastolic hypertension

Answer: E

Critique: Of the many risk factors for ischemic stroke, hypertension confers the highest risk. Hypertension contributes to stroke in approximately 70% of the cases. The risk for stroke increases 10 to 12-fold for patients whose diastolic blood pressures lie in the highest (average of 105 mm Hg) versus lowest (average of 76 mm Hg) categories. Conversely, when a person's blood pressure is lowered, this has been shown to decrease the risk of a stroke. Noninsulin-dependent diabetes confers a relative risk of 1.8 to 3.0. Smoking is associated with a relative risk of about 1.5. Obesity increases the risk factor by 1.5 to 2.0 times. Hypercholesterolemia appears to affect the risk of having a stroke in a complex fashion, by demonstrating a U-shaped risk curve. This behavior might reflect differential effects on hemorrhagic and ischemic stroke.

Further Reading

Bronner LL, Kanter DS, Manson JE: Primary prevention of stroke. N Engl J Med 333:1392–1400, 1995.

Morse RM, Heffron WA: Preventive health care. *In* Rakel RE: *Textbook of Family Practice.* Philadelphia, WB Saunders, 1995, p. 197.

11. (True or False) Carotid bruits appear to confer risk for stroke ipsilateral to the affected vessel. True statements regarding the approach to asymptomatic carotid bruits include:

    1. Carotid endarterectomy must be performed to decrease the risk of having a stroke.
    2. Affected patients should be encouraged to modify their behavior to reduce risk factors such as smoking and hypercholesterolemia.
    3. Prophylaxis with aspirin should be instituted due to proven effectiveness in preventing a stroke in patients with asymptomatic carotid bruits.
    4. Clinicians should examine the neck for carotid bruits approximately every 5 years in patients older than 40 years of age.

Answers: 1-F, 2-T, 3-F, 4-T

Critique: Asymptomatic carotid bruits represent a vexing primary care management problem. Although the presence of bruits appears to increase the risk for subsequent ipsilateral stroke, the evidence supporting active intervention for the associated carotid stenoses is mixed. Endarterectomy should be recommended only for carotid stenoses greater than 60% and only in circumstances in which the combined surgical and angiographic mortality rates are equal to or less than 3%. Patients should be encouraged to modify behaviors that constitute risk factors for CHD, because carotid bruits serve as a marker for atherosclerotic disease. Aspirin has not been demonstrated to yield significant benefit in the *asymptomatic* patient. Clinicians should listen to the carotids every 5 years in patients older than 40 years of age (the reader should note that the U.S. Preventive Services Task Force [USPSTF] made no recommendation for or against carotid bruit screening).

Further Reading

Brott T, Toole JF: Medical compared with surgical treatment of asymptomatic carotid artery stenosis. Ann Intern Med 123:720–722, 1995.

Coté R, Battista RN, Abrahamowicz M, et al: Lack of effect of aspirin in asymptomatic patients with carotid bruits and substantial carotid narrowing. Ann Intern Med 123:649–655, 1995.

Morse RM, Heffron WA: Preventive health care. *In* Rakel RE: *Textbook of Family Practice.* Philadelphia, WB Saunders, 1995, p 197.

12. (True or False) True statements regarding techniques available for screening for alcohol abuse include which of the following?

    1. Two questions, "Have you ever had a health, legal, or personal problem as a result of drinking?" and "When was your last drink?" perform poorly in identifying alcohol abuse.
    2. Two or more affirmative answers on the CAGE questionnaire suggest highly that the responder abuses alcohol.
    3. Family history of alcoholism has no predictive value for alcoholism in a first-degree relative.
    4. The addition of the open-ended question "Please tell me about your drinking" improves the yield of information from the CAGE questionnaire.

Answers: 1-F, 2-T, 3-F, 4-T

Critique: Several techniques exist to facilitate the clinician's identification of alcohol abusers in his or her practice. The two questions noted in item A perform with quite good sensitivity and specificity. Two or more affirmative answers on the CAGE questionnaire also perform with good sensitivity (74%) and specificity (91%). The yield from the CAGE can be improved by starting the questioning with "Please tell me about your drinking." A history of alcoholism in a first-degree relative has predictive value for alcohol abuse.

Further Reading

Buchsbaum DG, Buchanan RG, Centor RG, et al: Screening for alcohol abuse using CAGE scores and likelihood ratios. Ann Intern Med 115:774–777, 1991.
Morse RM, Heffron WA: Preventive health care. *In* Rakel RE: *Textbook of Family Practice.* Philadelphia, WB Saunders, 1995, pp 198–199.
Steinweg Dl, Worth H: Alcoholism: The keys to the CAGE. Am J Med 94:520–523, 1993.

13. The top five sites for cancer incidence include all of the following EXCEPT:

    A. Breast
    B. Colon/rectum
    C. Lung
    D. Prostate
    E. Ovary

Answer: E

Critique: The top five sites for cancer incidence include breast, colon/rectum, prostate, lung, and urinary tract.

Further Reading

Morse RM, Heffron WA: Preventive health care. *In* Rakel RE: *Textbook of Family Practice.* Philadelphia, WB Saunders, 1995, pp 198–199.

14. (True or False) True statements regarding the association of diet with cancer include which of the following?

    1. Obesity increases the risk for colon and breast cancers.
    2. Antioxidant-containing foods appear to increase the likelihood for cancer.
    3. Smoked and nitrite-cured foods increase the risk for gastrointestinal cancer.
    4. High-fat diets increase the risk of prostate cancer.

Answers: 1-T, 2-F, 3-T, 4-T

Critique: Dietary factors are thought to account for approximately 35% of deaths from cancer. Obesity increases the risk for colon, breast, and uterine cancers. Antioxidants appear to have a protective effect against some cancers. Smoked and nitrite-cured foods appear to increase the risk for upper gastrointestinal cancer. High-fat diets appear to confer an increased risk for prostate cancer.

Further Reading

Morse RM, Heffron WA: Preventive health care. *In* Rakel RE: *Textbook of Family Practice.* Philadelphia, WB Saunders, 1995, p 199.

15. Which one of the following represents a valid statement regarding colorectal cancer in the United States?

    A. Mortality from colorectal cancer has increased during the last 30 years.
    B. Regular use of aspirin increases the risk for colorectal cancer.
    C. The likelihood for cancer in an adenomatous polyp increases directly with the polyp's size.
    D. Most colonic polyps are adenomas.

Answer: C

Critique: Mortality from colorectal cancer has declined somewhat during the past 30 years. Regular use of aspirin has actually demonstrated decreased risk of colorectal cancer. The probability of cancer in an adenomatous polyp increases directly with the polyp's size, from 1 to 2% for adenomas less than 1 cm to 60% for those greater than 4 cm in size. Adenomata constitute only 20 to 30% of colonic polyps.

Further Reading

Morse RM, Heffron WA: Preventive health care. *In* Rakel RE: *Textbook of Family Practice.* Philadelphia, WB Saunders, 1995, pp 199–200.

16. (True or False) Screening for and prevention of colorectal cancer should include which of the following?

    1. A high-fat, low-fiber diet
    2. Flexible sigmoidoscopy every 5 years after 50 years of age
    3. An assessment of the family history for colorectal cancer or polyps
    4. A rectal examination and fecal occult blood testing starting at 30 years of age

Answers: 1-F, 2-T, 3-T, 4-F

Critique: Patients should be encouraged to consume a high-fiber, low-fat diet to minimize the risk of colorectal cancer. The recommendations for flexible sigmoidoscopy have generated some controversy. The USPSTF found insufficient evidence to recommend for or against flexible sigmoidoscopic screening. Studies published since their 1989 report have provided evidence to support this approach, although long-term mortality data are not yet available. The family history regarding colorectal cancer should be assessed, because such history confers an increased risk. Similar to the sigmoidoscopy case, the USPSTF declined to recommend fecal occult blood testing. Recent evidence suggests that this procedure may be beneficial, but testing should begin at 40 years of age rather than at 30 years of age.

Further Reading

Mandel JS, Bond JH, Church TR, et al: Reducing mortality from colorectal cancer by screening for fecal occult blood. N Engl J Med 328:1365–1371, 1993.
Morse RM, Heffron WA: Preventive health care. *In* Rakel RE: *Textbook of Family Practice.* Philadelphia, WB Saunders, 1995, pp 199–200.
Selby JV, Friedman GD, Quesenberry CP, et al: A case-control study of screening sigmoidoscopy and mortality from colorectal cancer. N Engl J Med 326:653–657, 1992.

17. Factors that appear to increase the risk for breast cancer in women include all of the following EXCEPT:

A. Family history of premenopausal bilateral breast cancer
B. First pregnancy before age 35
C. History of atypical hyperplasia
D. Advancing age

Answer: B

Critique: A first pregnancy after 35 years of age constitutes a risk factor for breast cancer. The other options all identify established risk factors for breast cancer.

Further Reading

Morse RM, Heffron WA: Preventive health care. *In* Rakel RE: *Textbook of Family Practice.* Philadelphia, WB Saunders, 1995, pp 200–201.

18. Of the following available techniques, which one demonstrates the highest sensitivity for detecting breast cancer?

A. Breast self-examination (BSE)
B. Clinical breast examination (CBE) (by a health professional)
C. Mammography
D. Mammography plus CBE

Answer: D

Critique: Mammography plus a CBE performs with the highest sensitivity (75%). A BSE unfortunately demonstrates only 26% sensitivity. The CBE performs with about 45% sensitivity, and mammography alone exhibits 71% sensitivity.

Further Reading

Morse RM, Heffron WA: Preventive health care. *In* Rakel RE: *Textbook of Family Practice.* Philadelphia, WB Saunders, 1995, p 200.

19. The American Cancer Society (ACS) and the USPSTF have promoted different recommendations for breast cancer screening in women who are at average risk. For which of the following options do these two organizations agree?

A. Monthly BSE and CBE every 3 years from 20 to 34 years of age
B. Monthly BSE and CBE every 3 years from 35 to 39 years of age
C. Monthly BSE, CBE, and mammography every year from 40 to 49 years of age
D. CBE and mammography yearly from 50 to 59 years of age

Answer: D

Critique: The USPSTF and the ACS have promoted quite different recommendations for young age groups but converge for people 50 years of age and older. The USPSTF and ACS recommend an annual CBE and mammography in persons older than 50 years of age.

Further Reading

Morse RM, Heffron WA: Preventive health care. *In* Rakel RE: *Textbook of Family Practice.* Philadelphia, WB Saunders, 1995, pp 200–202.

20. (True or False) The effects of smoking on the smoker and his or her family unit include which of the following?

1. Smoking represents the single largest risk factor for lung cancer.
2. Secondary smoke presents an increased risk for lung cancer in exposed family members.
3. Children exposed to secondary tobacco smoke exhibit higher school absenteeism.
4. Secondary smoke increases the risk for heart disease in exposed family members.

Answers: 1-T, 2-T, 3-T, 4-T

Critique: Tobacco use represents the single most important risk factor for lung cancer. Smokers represent a risk to others as well as to themselves. Exposure to secondary smoke increases the risk of lung cancer and heart disease in family members. Such exposure also increases the risk for upper respiratory infection and school absenteeism in children. The only effective preventive measure is to stop smoking, and clinicians should recommend smoking cessation at every opportunity.

Further Reading

Morse RM, Heffron WA: Preventive health care. *In* Rakel RE: *Textbook of Family Practice.* Philadelphia, WB Saunders, 1995, pp 202–203.

21. Risk factors for cervical cancer include all of the following EXCEPT:

A. Multiple sexual partners
B. Smoking
C. History of human papilloma virus (HPV) infection
D. Late age for first intercourse

Answer: D

Critique: Multiple sexual partners, smoking, and HPV infection all represent risk factors for cervical cancer. Initiating intercourse at early, rather than late, age confers increased risk.

Further Reading

Morse RM, Heffron WA: Preventive health care. *In* Rakel RE: *Textbook of Family Practice.* Philadelphia, WB Saunders, 1995, pp 203–204.

22. (True or False) True statements regarding Papanicolaou (Pap) smear screening for cervical cancer include which of the following?

1. Pap smear screening should begin when sexual activity begins.
2. Pap smear screening should begin no later than age 18.
3. Pap smear screening should be performed annually in all women.
4. Pap smear screening performs with 95% sensitivity in identifying cervical neoplasia.

Answers: 1-T, 2-T, 3-F, 4-F

Critique: Pap smear screening should begin when women become sexually active, and no later than age 18 (according to the ACS and the American College of Obstetricians and Gynecologists). Pap smear frequency can be decreased to every 3 years when a woman has had three negative annual examinations. Pap smears perform with 55 to 80% sensitivity. Note that Eddy has demonstrated that the most cost-effective strategy for cervical cancer screening is Pap testing every 3 to 4 years in women who are 20 to 75 years of age: Screening every 4 years in this age group yields a cost-effectiveness ratio of $10,000 per year of life saved (a very acceptable cost-effectiveness ratio), whereas screening every 3 years costs about $185,000 per year of life saved. However, in considering the frequency of Pap smears, the clinician should remember that other issues such as birth control and breast cancer screening require visits more frequently than every 3 years, depending on the woman's age.

Further Reading

Eddy DM: Screening for cervical cancer. Ann Intern Med 113:214–226, 1990.
Morse RM, Heffron WA: Preventive health care. *In* Rakel RE: *Textbook of Family Practice.* Philadelphia, WB Saunders, 1995, pp 203–204.
U.S. Preventive Services Task Force: Screening for cervical cancer. Am Fam Physician 41:853–857, 1990.

23. Measures that clinicians should recommend for the prevention of skin cancer include all of the following EXCEPT:

    A. Use of sunscreens with a high sun-protective factor (SPF) number (≥SPF 15)
    B. Use of protective clothing
    C. Self-examination of the skin
    D. Tanning at least once yearly for skin protection

Answer: D

Critique: Exposure to ultraviolet (UV) light constitutes a major risk factor for skin cancer. Patients should be counseled to use high SPF number sunscreens and protective clothing when exposed to UV light. Patients should be encouraged to practice periodic skin self-examination. Tanning requires UV exposure and should be discouraged just as any exposure to UV light.

Further Reading

Morse RM, Heffron WA: Preventive health care. *In* Rakel RE: *Textbook of Family Practice.* Philadelphia, WB Saunders, 1995, p 204.

24. (True or False) Risk factors for prostate cancer include which of the following?

    1. African-American race
    2. Low-fat diet
    3. Advancing age

Answers: 1-T, 2-F, 3-T

Critique: African-American race confers substantial risk of prostate cancer. Evidence also suggests that a high-fat diet imposes increased risk. Advancing age also confers

increased risk: as many as 30% of men older than 50 years of age might harbor microscopic evidence of prostate cancer. The prevalence clearly increases with age: about 22% in men aged 50 to 59, 36% in men aged 60 to 69, about 38% in men between the ages of 70 and 79, and 54% in men older than 80 years of age.

Further Reading

Morse RM, Heffron WA: Preventive health care. *In* Rakel RE: *Textbook of Family Practice.* Philadelphia, WB Saunders, 1995, p 204.
U.S. Public Health Service: Cancer detection in adults by physical examination. Am Fam Physician 51:871–885, 1995.
Woolf SH: Screening for prostate cancer with prostate-specific antigen: An examination of the evidence. N Engl J Med 333:1401–1405, 1995.

25. Which one of the following statements regarding prostate-specific antigen (PSA) testing as a screen for prostate cancer is valid?

    A. The USPSTF strongly recommends annual PSA testing for men older than 40 years of age.
    B. PSA testing appears to perform with high sensitivity and specificity (i.e., >90%).
    C. PSA testing performs with at least 75% positive predictive value in screening for prostate cancer.
    D. A combination of the PSA with a digital rectal examination improves the positive predictive value for prostate cancer.

Answer: D

Critique: PSA screening to detect asymptomatic prostate cancer remains quite controversial. Although the ACS recommends annual testing in men older than 50 years of age, the USPSTF, the Canadian Task Force on the Periodic Health Examination, and the Canadian Urological Association have recommended against PSA screening. PSA testing appears to perform with sensitivity about 80%; the test performs with much lower specificity due to false-positive results associated with benign prostatic hypertrophy. PSA testing functions with positive predictive value of 28 to 35% in published studies; however, these results reflect performance in selected populations. The test probably performs more poorly in the undifferentiated populations seen in primary care practices. A combination of the PSA with a digital rectal examination appears to improve positive predictive value.

Further Reading

Morse RM, Heffron WA: Preventive health care. *In* Rakel RE: *Textbook of Family Practice.* Philadelphia, WB Saunders, 1995, p 204.
Woolf SH: Screening for prostate cancer with prostate-specific antigen: An examination of the evidence. N Engl J Med 333:1401–1405, 1995.

26. (True or False) True statements regarding osteoporosis include which of the following?

    1. Bone mass peaks during linear skeletal growth.
    2. After age 30, women lose 3 to 5% of their bone mass annually until menopause.
    3. Cortical bone loss rate exceeds that of trabecular bone in menopausal women.

4. Estrogen replacement therapy (ERT) greatly diminishes bone loss after menopause.

Answers: 1-F, 2-F, 3-F, 4-T

Critique: Bone mass peaks shortly after linear skeletal growth ceases. After age 30, women lose 0.3 to 0.5% of their bone mass annually until menopause, at which time the rate accelerates. The trabecular bone loss exceeds that of cortical bone in menopausal women. ERT represents the most effective intervention for preventing bone loss in menopausal women.

Further Reading

Morse RM, Heffron WA: Preventive health care. *In* Rakel RE: *Textbook of Family Practice*. Philadelphia, WB Saunders, 1995, pp 205–206.

27. Risk factors for osteoporosis include all of the following EXCEPT:

A. Positive family history for osteoporosis
B. Active lifestyle
C. Cigarette smoking
D. Caucasian race
E. Inadequate dietary calcium intake

Answer: B

Critique: An active lifestyle actually provides some protection against osteoporosis. Weight-bearing exercise can actually increase bone density. The other options denote recognized risk factors.

Further Reading

Morse RM, Heffron WA: Preventive health care. *In* Rakel RE: *Textbook of Family Practice*. Philadelphia, WB Saunders, 1995, pp 205–206.

28. (True or False) Recommendations for the prevention of osteoporosis include:

1. Estrogen replacement therapy in menopausal women
2. Calcium supplementation
3. Aerobic weight-bearing exercise
4. Counseling regarding smoking cessation

Answers: 1-T, 2-T, 3-T, 4-T

Critique: Estrogen replacement therapy clearly benefits menopausal women who do not have contraindications to such treatment. Calcium supplementation and aerobic weight-bearing exercise also impede the development of osteoporosis. Cigarette smoking is a risk factor for osteoporosis; smokers should be counseled to discontinue tobacco use. Parenthetically, recent studies indicate that biphosphonates can actually reverse established osteoporosis.

Further Reading

Liberman UA, Weiss SR, Bröll J, et al: Effect of oral alendronate on bone mineral density and the incidence of fractures in postmenopausal women. N Engl J Med 333:1437–1443, 1995.

Morse RM, Heffron WA: Preventive health care. *In* Rakel RE: *Textbook of Family Practice*. Philadelphia, WB Saunders, 1995, pp 205–206.

29. Among the following sexually transmitted diseases (STDs), which one occurs with the highest overall annual incidence?

A. Syphilis
B. Gonorrhea
C. Herpes genitalis
D. Chlamydia

Answer: D

Critique: Among the listed STDs, chlamydia demonstrates the highest annual incidence: 3 to 4 million cases. The number of cases of gonorrhea is approximately 2 million per year, and herpes generates approximately 270,000 new cases annually. Syphilis accounts for about 35,000 cases each year.

Further Reading

Morse RM, Heffron WA: Preventive health care. *In* Rakel RE: *Textbook of Family Practice*. Philadelphia, WB Saunders, 1995, p 206.

30. (True or False) Screening for gonorrhea and chlamydia should be considered in which of the following groups?

1. As part of the annual female examination in women at average risk
2. As part of the prenatal evaluation of pregnant women
3. In patients who have multiple sexual partners

Answers: 1-F, 2-T, 3-T

Critique: Screening for gonorrhea and chlamydia should be considered in patients at high risk (e.g., those who have multiple sexual partners) and in pregnant women because of the risk of transmission to the fetus.

Further Reading

Morse RM, Heffron WA: Preventive health care. *In* Rakel RE: *Textbook of Family Practice*. Philadelphia, WB Saunders, 1995, p 206.

31. (True or False) Patient characteristics that indicate increased risk for human immunodeficiency virus (HIV) infection include:

1. Intravenous drug use
2. History of multiple sexual partners
3. History of blood transfusions between 1977 and 1985
4. Hemophilia

Answers: 1-T, 2-T, 3-T, 4-T

Critique: All of the options describe risk factors for acquiring HIV. Counseling to prevent HIV infection should include patient education regarding risky behaviors. This counseling should include education regarding safer sex practices (e.g., monogramy, condom and spermicide use, avoidance of anal intercourse). The prevalence of HIV in asymptomatic family practice office populations appears to be about 0.5%. Although low, this number emphasizes that physicians and their office staff should practice universal precautions in their interactions with patients.

Further Reading

Kurata J, Ounanian L, Chetkovich D, et al: Seroprevalence of human immunodeficiency virus among family practice outpatients. J Am Board Fam Pract 6:347–352, 1993.
Morse RM, Heffron WA: Preventive health care. *In* Rakel RE: *Textbook of Family Practice.* Philadelphia, WB Saunders, 1995, pp 207–208.

32. True statements regarding immunizations in adults include all of the following EXCEPT:

    A. Booster doses of diphtheria toxoid should be administered every 10 years.
    B. Patients older than 65 years of age should receive annual trivalent influenza vaccine.
    C. Previously un-immunized adults should receive inactivated polio vaccine rather than oral polio vaccine.
    D. Patients older than 65 years of age should receive pneumococcal vaccine every 3 years.

Answer: D

Critique: Booster doses of diphtheria vaccine should be administered every 10 years to counter waning immunity. Patients older than 65 years of age should receive annual influenza vaccination. Adults who have not undergone previous polio immunization should receive inactivated polio vaccine rather than the live attenuated virus oral polio vaccine. Patients older than 65 years of age should receive pneumococcal vaccine once. Some evidence suggests that a subset of patients might benefit from re-vaccination after 6 years. Patients with nephrotic syndrome, renal failure, or asplenia are candidates for re-vaccination. Additionally, patients who received the 14-valent vaccine should be re-immunized with the current 23-valent product.

Further Reading

Morse RM, Heffron WA: Preventive health care. *In* Rakel RE: *Textbook of Family Practice.* Philadelphia, WB Saunders, 1995, pp 208–209.
Zimmerman RK, Clover RD: Adult immunizations—a practical approach for clinicians: Part I. Am Fam Physician 51:859–867, 1995.

33. (True or False) Hepatitis B vaccination for adults not previously immunized should be considered for which of the following groups?

    1. Heterosexuals who have multiple sexual partners
    2. Health care workers
    3. Patients receiving hemodialysis
    4. Intravenous drug users

Answers: 1-T, 2-T, 3-T, 4-T

Critique: All of the noted groups should receive hepatitis B vaccine. The Advisory Committee for Immunization Practices (ACIP) has also published specific recommendations for postexposure prophylaxis against hepatitis B (MMWR 40:22,1991).

Further Reading

Morse RM, Heffron WA: Preventive health care. *In* Rakel RE: *Textbook of Family Practice.* Philadelphia, WB Saunders, 1995, pp 208–209.
Zimmerman RK, Clover RD: Adult immunizations—a practical approach for clinicians: Part II. Am Fam Physician 51:1139–1148, 1995.

34. Risk factors for increased risk for glaucoma include all of the following EXCEPT:

    A. Diabetes mellitus
    B. White race
    C. Advancing age
    D. Family history of glaucoma

Answer: B

Critique: Diabetes mellitus, advancing age, and a positive family history all confer increased risk for glaucoma. African-American race confers a fourfold increased risk.

Further Reading

Morse RM, Heffron WA: Preventive health care. *In* Rakel RE: *Textbook of Family Practice.* Philadelphia, WB Saunders, 1995, pp 209–210.

35. (True or False) True statements regarding Schiøtz tonometry include:

    1. Schiøtz tonometry should be performed annually starting at 40 years of age.
    2. Schiøtz tonometry performs with high sensitivity and specificity in glaucoma screening.
    3. Schiøtz tonometry combined with funduscopy performs better than does tonometry alone in glaucoma screening.

Answers: 1-F, 2-F, 3-T

Critique: Schiøtz tonometry performs poorly as a glaucoma screening procedure: The test exhibits low sensitivity and specificity. Insufficient evidence exists to support tonometry screening in family practice; however, if the clinician chooses to offer this procedure, screening of the patient should begin at 40 years of age and occur every 5 years until 60 years of age. The screening interval should be decreased to every 2 to 3 years beginning at 60 years of age. Concomitant funduscopy appears to improve the performance of tonometry.

Further Reading

Morse RM, Heffron WA: Preventive health care. *In* Rakel RE: *Textbook of Family Practice.* Philadelphia, WB Saunders, 1995, pp 209–210.

36. Which one of the following statements regarding scoliosis screening is valid?

    A. Most cases detected at screening will require treatment.
    B. The physical examination of the back operates with high predictive value for scoliosis in typical screening environments.
    C. Brace therapy initiated on the basis of screening does not appear to yield significant benefit in long-term outcomes.

D. The USPSTF recommends annual scoliosis screening in asymptomatic adolescents.

Answer: C

Critique: Several organizations, including the Scoliosis Research Society, the American Academy of Pediatrics, and the American Academy of Orthopedic Surgeons, have recommended screening for scoliosis. However, a systematic review by the USPSTF found insufficient evidence to support this recommendation. They noted that most cases identified by screening require no treatment and that the back examination performs with poor positive predictive value in the usual screening setting. Their review of the evidence indicated that treatment with a brace provides no significant benefit in long-term outcomes.

Further Reading

U.S. Preventive Services Task Force: Screening for adolescent idiopathic scoliosis: Policy statement. JAMA 269:2664–2666, 1993.
U.S. Preventive Services Task Force: Screening for adolescent idiopathic scoliosis: Review article. JAMA 269:2667–2672, 1993.

12

Use of Consultants

Michael D. Hagen

Questions 1–4. Match the following characteristics with the appropriate concept:

    A. Consultations
    B. Referrals
    C. Both A and B
    D. Neither A nor B

1. The process of one physician asking another for an opinion or assistance

2. The transfer of responsibility for a patient's care from one physician to another

3. Represents the majority of exchanges between family physicians and other specialists

4. Usually involves requesting a particular service for a limited time (e.g., surgical procedure)

Answers: 1-A, 2-B, 3-B, 4-B

Critique: A consultation consists of one physician asking another specialist colleague for his/her opinion and/or assistance in managing a particular patient's problem. Referral connotes transfer of responsibility for the patient's care from one physician to another. Referrals comprise the majority of exchanges between family physicians and other specialists. Additionally, referrals are usually made for a particular service (e.g., a surgical procedure) for a limited time.

Further Reading

Rakel RE: Use of consultants. *In* Rakel RE: *Textbook of Family Practice.* Philadelphia, WB Saunders, 1995, p 214.

5. Family physicians refer approximately what percentage of patients they see?

    A. 5%
    B. 10%
    C. 15%
    D. 20%

Answer: A

Critique: On the basis of studies done in the United States and elsewhere, family physicians refer only about 5% of their patients to other specialists. Additionally, approximately half of these referrals represent elective transfers to another physician.

Further Reading

Rakel RE: Use of consultants. *In* Rakel RE: *Textbook of Family Practice.* Philadelphia, WB Saunders, 1995, p 215.

6. Dixon has identified five fundamental reasons for referrals. These reasons include all of the following EXCEPT:

    A. Assistance in diagnosis
    B. Assistance in managing the patient's problem
    C. The patient's request
    D. Physician ownership of the referral facility

Answer: D

Critique: Dixon identified five fundamental reasons for referrals: (1) assistance with diagnosis; (2) assistance with management; (3) assistance with both diagnosis and management; (4) the patient's request; and (5) to reinforce or confirm the referring physician's diagnosis or management plan. Although physician ownership might influence selection of a referral physician, such ownership should not itself serve as the impetus for referral.

Further Reading

Rakel RE: Use of consultants. *In* Rakel RE: *Textbook of Family Practice.* Philadelphia, WB Saunders, 1995, pp 214, 222.

7. In requesting, conducting, and concluding a consultation, the family physician should include all of the following considerations EXCEPT:

    A. The family physician should consider the patient's emotional, socioeconomic, medical, and cultural characteristics.
    B. The family physician should inform the patient and family regarding expectations and indications for the consultation.

C. The family physician should not evaluate the appropriateness of the consultant's recommendations but should rather follow the expert's advice without question.

D. The family physician should provide feedback to the consultant regarding the patient's progress.

Answer: C

Critique: When initiating a consultation, the family physician should consider those demographic and medical patient characteristics that might affect the process. Additionally, the family physician should educate the patient and family regarding the indications for, and the mechanics of, the consultation. The family physician should evaluate the consultant's recommendations in the context of the patient's overall circumstances. The family physician might consider obtaining a consultation with a different consultant if the first specialist's recommendations do not appear appropriate for the patient. The family physician should provide feedback to the consultant regarding the patient's progress.

Further Reading

Rakel RE: Use of consultants. *In* Rakel RE: *Textbook of Family Practice.* Philadelphia, WB Saunders, 1995, pp 215–220.

8. (True or False) Characteristics a family physician should consider in selecting a consultant include which of the following?

1. The consultant's knowledge and skills should be appropriate for the patient's problem.
2. The consultant need not be available to see the patient within a reasonable time interval.
3. The consultant should have maintained his or her skills as demonstrated by frequent use of the necessary techniques.
4. The consultant's personality should not be a factor in the selection process.

Answers: 1-T, 2-F, 3-T, 4-F

Critique: When selecting a consultant, the family physician should consider multiple factors in the decision. The consultant should possess appropriate knowledge and skill and should have demonstrated continued competence in areas germane to the patient's clinical situation. The consultant should be available in a reasonable time frame. Lastly, the consultant's personality should be appropriate to the patient's expectations for the physician-patient interaction.

Further Reading

Rakel RE: Use of consultants. *In* Rakel RE: *Textbook of Family Practice.* Philadelphia, WB Saunders, 1995, p 216.

9. (True or False) Items that the family physician should include in a consultation or referral request include which of the following?

1. A note stating the reason for the consultation or referral (e.g., help with the diagnosis or a referral for a specific procedure)

2. Copies of pertinent progress notes from the patient's medical record
3. Laboratory reports pertaining to the patient's problem
4. Radiographic information that relates to the patient's problem

Answers: 1-T, 2-T, 3-T, 4-T

Critique: To optimize the likelihood of a successful and meaningful consultation, the referring family physician should provide information regarding the patient's progress to date. Additionally, the referring doctor should state explicitly his or her expectations for the consultation or referral (e.g., help with a diagnosis or performance of a specific procedure). The referring doctor should provide copies of pertinent progress notes, laboratory data, and the results of related diagnostic investigations, such as x-rays.

Further Reading

Rakel RE: Use of consultants. *In* Rakel RE: *Textbook of Family Practice.* Philadelphia, WB Saunders, 1995, p 216.

10. Approximately 10 to 20% of patients do not keep a consultation appointment. Techniques that the family physician can use to increase the patient's compliance with the consultation process include all of the following EXCEPT:

A. The family physician should fully inform the patient regarding the need for, and expectations of, the consultation.
B. The family physician should obtain the patient's consent to proceed with the consultation request.
C. The family physician should reassure the patient that he or she will maintain responsibility for the patient's care during and after the consultation.
D. The family physician should select the consultant without regard for the patient's preferences.

Answer: D

Critique: The family physician can use several approaches to increase the likelihood that his or her patient will keep an appointment with a consultant. The patient should be informed fully regarding the reasons for, and expected outcomes of, the consultation or referral. The referring doctor should seek the patient's consent to proceed with the consultation or referral request. Additionally, the referring doctor should attempt to reassure the patient that he or she will maintain responsibility for the patient's care during the consultation process. The family physician should involve the patient in selecting the consultant. Ideally, several appropriate consultants with whom the family physician is familiar will be available; the family physician can then describe these physicians to the patient and allow the patient to collaborate in the selection process.

Further Reading

Rakel RE: Use of consultants. *In* Rakel RE: *Textbook of Family Practice.* Philadelphia, WB Saunders, 1995, pp 217–218.

11. Patient factors that appear related to compliance with consultation include which one of the following?

    A. The nature of the clinical problem
    B. The severity of the clinical problem
    C. The duration of the clinical problem
    D. The adequate discussion of the clinical problem with the family physician

Answer: D

Critique: Lloyd and colleagues have demonstrated that the duration, nature, and severity of the patient's clinical problem do not relate significantly to patient compliance with the referral process. On the other hand, they also demonstrated that patients were less likely to keep their consultation or referral appointments if they had not discussed the problem adequately with the referring physician.

Further Reading

Lloyd M, Bradford C, Webb S: Non-attendance at outpatient clinics: Is it related to the referral process? Fam Pract 10:11, 1993.
Rakel RE: Use of consultants. *In* Rakel RE: *Textbook of Family Practice.* Philadelphia, WB Saunders, 1995, p 218.

12. (True or False) True statements regarding the role of consultants in the care of hospitalized patients include which of the following?

    1. The consultant should see the patient promptly.
    2. The consultant should write orders.
    3. The consultant should provide therapeutic suggestions in the patient's record.
    4. The consultant should call in additional specialists prior to discussions with the family physician.

Answers: 1-T, 2-F, 3-T, 4-F

Critique: When consulted to see a hospitalized patient, the consultant should see the patient promptly and render a note in the patient's chart detailing his or her opinion and management recommendations. The consultant should not write orders unless specifically directed by the attending family physician to do so. The consultant should not consult additional specialists without first discussing this with the attending family physician.

Further Reading

Rakel RE: Use of consultants. *In* Rakel RE: *Textbook of Family Practice.* Philadelphia, WB Saunders, 1995, p 219.

13. Among the following specialties in the United States, which specialty is consulted most by family physicians?

    A. Obstetrics-gynecology
    B. Dermatology
    C. Otolaryngology
    D. General surgery
    E. Cardiology

Answer: D

Critique: On the basis of results from several studies, family physicians consult general surgeons most often among the listed specialties.

Further Reading

Rakel RE: Use of consultants. *In* Rakel RE: *Textbook of Family Practice.* Philadelphia, WB Saunders, 1995, pp 210, 221.

14. (True or False) True statements regarding physician self-referral (e.g., referring a patient to a facility in which the physician has a financial interest) include which of the following?

    1. The most common types of self-referral consist of sending a patient to a laboratory or medical equipment supplier in which the referring doctor has a financial interest.
    2. Professional "kickbacks" from a consultant to a referring physician are considered appropriate if they do not influence the consultation process and do not involve a Medicare patient.
    3. Professional kickbacks involving a Medicare patient constitute a felony.

Answers: 1-T, 2-F, 3-T

Critique: Referrals to laboratories and medical equipment suppliers constitute the most common forms of physician self-referral. Professional kickbacks from a consultant to a referring physician constitute unethical behavior under any circumstance. Kickbacks involving Medicare patients constitute a felony under current law.

Further Reading

Rakel RE: Use of consultants. *In* Rakel RE: *Textbook of Family Practice.* Philadelphia, WB Saunders, 1995, p 222.

15. The referring physician-consultant relationship should be characterized by all of the following EXCEPT:

    A. The consultant should confirm the referring physician's findings, even if this provides no new information.
    B. The consultant should perform additional testing and procedures because this is expected in consultation.
    C. The referring physician should use and interpret the consultant's report in a manner similar to evaluating laboratory results.
    D. The consultant should admit when he or she has nothing further to offer in evaluating the patient's case.

Answer: B

Critique: The good consultant will admit when he or she has nothing to offer beyond the referring physician's opinions and evaluation. Additionally, if the consultant generates no new information, he or she should confirm the referring physician's clinical evaluation and impressions. The consultant should not perform additional testing unless the patient's clinical context warrants further investigation. The referring physician should interpret the consultant's report in the same manner as a new piece of laboratory information, rather than accept without reflection the consultant's opinions and recommendations.

Further Reading

Rakel RE: Use of consultants. *In* Rakel RE: *Textbook of Family Practice.* Philadelphia, WB Saunders, 1995, p 222.

16. (True or False) Which of the following represent common reasons for referrals to family physicians?

1. For a procedure such as flexible sigmoidoscopy or vasectomy
2. For the family physician to serve as coordinator of a patient's care
3. To establish care with a family physician for patients who have not previously had a family physician

Answers: 1-T, 2-T, 3-T

Critique: Family physicians receive referrals from other specialists and generalist colleagues for a variety of reasons. Generalists commonly refer patients to a family physician colleague who can provide a service (e.g., fiberoptic sigmoidoscopy) that the referring physician is unable to offer. Additionally, family physicians frequently receive referrals to establish care with a family physician. Coordination of care represents another common reason for referrals to family physicians. The family physician's broad, comprehensive background facilitates such coordination when multiple specialists are involved in the patient's care.

Further Reading

Rakel RE: Use of consultants. *In* Rakel RE: *Textbook of Family Practice.* Philadelphia, WB Saunders, 1995, p 223.

13

Community-Oriented Primary Care

Robert F. Thompson

1. Of the following concepts, identify the one most applicable to community-oriented primary care (COPC).

    A. Ratio
    B. Probability
    C. Denominator
    D. Average
    E. Numerator

Answer: C

Critique: The numerator concept is applied to an individual patient or the most active patients in a practice. Focusing on the numerator can lead to erroneous assumptions about the population. COPC is most interested in the denominator. The denominator refers to the population being cared for, or the population at risk. This permits broadening of the physician's perspective from the patient(s) with whom he or she is confronted to that of a much broader population or community to which the patient belongs. Focusing on the denominator helps to avoid numerator bias. Probabilities, averages, and ratios are epidemiologic concepts that are useful in expressing information about a population.

Page 227

2. "Practice population" in COPC terminology refers to:

    A. Active patients (i.e., patients seen in the last 2 years)
    B. Registered patients in a practice plus their household members
    C. Active patients plus all their family members within an arbitrary radius or distance
    D. The population living in the geographical area serviced by the practice

Answer: B

Critique: In COPC terminology, the practice population consists of active patients, inactive but registered patients, and household members who have not been patients.

Sometimes patients living in the geographical area served by the practice may be surveyed; however, they are not included in the definition of practice population.

Pages 229–231

3. Basic elements or components of COPC include all of the following EXCEPT:

    A. A practice with a broad spectrum of services
    B. A primary care practice
    C. A defined population
    D. A process by which health problems of the population are addressed

Answer: A

Critique: The basic elements or components of COPC are: (1) a primary care practice or program, (2) a defined population that the practitioner wishes to serve, and (3) a process by which the major health problems of the target population are addressed. COPC is not directly related to a defined spectrum of services, although it may be included in any COPC program.

Page 226

4. Which of the following "communities" would be *least* appropriate for developing a COPC activity?

    A. Members of a Rotary Club
    B. Active patients in an office practice
    C. Persons ticketed for driving while intoxicated during a 1-month time interval
    D. A housing project

Answer: C

Critique: The term "community" may be difficult to define. In general, one seeks a community or group that has something in common, a group with which one might plan a health-related activity. Commonly, communities are chosen on the basis of shared interest or "turf." A community has the potential for being drawn together to meet and plan an activity. Of these four examples, the group least likely to be organized together around the issues of a health problem would be those ticketed for driving while intoxicated.

Pages 226, 227

5. The process through which COPC works includes all of the following EXCEPT:

    A. Choosing a group or site in which to work
    B. Identification of the health problems
    C. Modification of services or practice patterns
    D. Monitoring the way in which services are used
    E. Surveying of the community's perceptions of problems

Answer: D

Critique: The COPC process includes identifying and characterizing the community, identifying and prioritizing health problems, planning interventions or modifying practice patterns in response to selected health problems or concerns, and monitoring the impact of program modifications on behaviors or health outcomes. The options offered are restatements of the recognized steps in the COPC process, except for monitoring the way services are used. Although monitoring of services currently being used might be useful information, it is not a recognized step in the COPC process.

Pages 227, 228

6. Obstacles to putting COPC into practice include all of the following EXCEPT:

    A. Lack of financial incentives
    B. Limited applicability to most common problems
    C. Lack of training of health professionals
    D. Difficulty in managing data

Answer: B

Critique: COPC has been difficult to put into practice. Lack of financial incentives is widely recognized in that this is a significant variation from the traditional "curative" focus. Primary care physicians and other health professionals generally lack specific training in COPC methodology. An important part of the COPC process is that of managing data, especially epidemiologic information; tools are being developed to manage data, although, to date, they have not been well developed. One of the most important selling points of the value of COPC is its impressive applicability to the more common problems for which people seek medical help; this is NOT an obstacle. Examples are abundant.

Pages 228, 229

7. Individuals specifically identified with the historical development and promotion of COPC include all of the following EXCEPT:

    A. Gayle Stephens
    B. David Garr

    C. Paul Nutting
    D. Sidney Kark

Answer: A

Critique: To appreciate COPC, its historical development should be recognized to some degree. Sidney Kark, in South Africa and Israel, has written about community approaches to health care for more than 30 years and defined the concept of COPC in 1981. Paul Nutting, a family practitioner for many years in a small Colorado community, has been a prolific writer on the subject of COPC for more than 10 years. David Garr, a faculty member in family medicine in South Carolina, is another contributor to the COPC literature. Although Gayle Stephens is a widely appreciated leader in family medicine from its conception here in the United States, he has had no involvement in the evolution of COPC.

Pages 225–234

Questions 8–11 (True or False). In planning a COPC activity or project, information about the community and its problems should come from:

8. Subjective data from individuals in the community and health professionals

9. Secondary or existing data (i.e., published or public sources of information)

10. Data collected by the practice

11. Medical histories of patients during their visits to the clinic

Answers: 8-T, 9-T, 10-T, 11-F

Critique: To carry out COPC, information is needed, especially regarding the epidemiology of problems and populations at risk. This information should be systematically collected. In general, data come from two sources; (1) printed or existing data, and (2) information from the community itself. Information from a practice may also be useful to define and manage problems. Information from individuals during clinic visits, acquired in a nonsystematic fashion, is not likely to be helpful.

Page 232

Questions 12–15 (True or False). Community-oriented primary care is:

12. The reunion of traditions of public health and clinical services

13. The modification of traditional health care delivery to better assess disease management outcomes

14. Tailored to the health needs of specific communities

15. A modification of the traditional health care model to deal with health problems of a defined population

Answers: 12-T, 13-F, 14-T, 15-T

Critique: COPC systematically identifies and addresses health problems of a defined or specific population or community. It is often characterized as a "marriage" between public health and traditional curative medicine. Characteristically, it is tailored to specific health problems and the needs of communities. It is not meant to focus on specific diseases but to merely monitor outcomes.

Page 225

14

Assessment of Functional Health Status

Alvah R. Cass

1. A comprehensive functional assessment (CFA) is most suited for:

 A. Recognizing early signs of impaired social function in caregivers for the frail elderly
 B. Identifying functional deficits in patients with chronic illnesses
 C. Documenting disease-specific limitations in functional status
 D. Generating a detailed evaluation of instrumental activities of daily living
 E. Constructing a functional problem list for individuals identified by screening to have a significant functional impairment

Answer: E

Critique: A CFA can be used for individuals identified by screening to have a significant functional impairment. The physician can construct a functional problem list based on the CFA. Office-based screening is the best method to identify functional impairment in at-risk groups, including the elderly, chronically ill, and caregivers of the elderly and chronically ill. Numerous multidimensional instruments are available for measuring disease-specific changes in functional status. An evaluation of instrumental activities of daily living is best accomplished with the Instrumental Activities of Daily Living Index.

Pages 237, 239, 243

2. Which one of the following is the most widely used and best studied global functional health status instrument?

 A. Duke Health Profile
 B. Dartmouth Cooperative Charts
 C. Rand 36-Item Health Survey (SF-36)
 D. Functional Status Index
 E. Activities of Daily Living Index

Answer: C

Critique: The Rand 36-Item Health Survey (SF-36) is the most widely used and best studied global functional health status measure. The Duke Health Profile and the Dartmouth Cooperative Charts are the other commonly used measures of global functional health status; however, they are limited in some respects by psychometric properties. They have not enjoyed equally widespread use and evaluation in multiple settings compared with the SF-36 instrument. The Functional Status Index is limited, because it addresses only physical, emotional, and mental dimensions and is sensitive only to direction not to magnitude of change in functional status. The Activities of Daily Living Index is widely used but does not measure global functional health status.

Pages 239–243

Questions 3–8. Match the following indicators with the corresponding component of functional status. Each option may be used once, more than once, or not at all.

 A. Physical function
 B. Social function
 C. Emotional function
 D. Cognitive function

3. Bathing and toileting

4. Ability to cope with change and stress

5. Sexual performance

6. Managing personal financial affairs

7. Extent to which a person maintains interpersonal contacts

8. Ability to comply with medication schedules

Answers: 3-A, 4-C, 5-B, 6-D, 7-B, 8-D

Critique: Functional status is a multidimensional construct of which physical, social, emotional, and cognitive functions are critical elements. Physical function is the ability to perform certain activities, including bathing, toileting, cooking, exercising, and dressing. Emotional function may include measures of self-esteem and the ability to cope with stress, anxiety, and depression. Social function is a measure of an individual's ability to maintain his or her role and may include maintenance of interpersonal relationships and sexual performance. Cognitive function includes measures of orientation, memory, judgment, communication, and reasoning.

Page 236

Questions 9–14. Match each of the numbered items with the best response from the following lettered options. Each option may be used once, more than once, or not at all.

    A. Activities of Daily Living Index
    B. Instrumental Activities of Daily Living Index
    C. Both A and B
    D. Neither A nor B

9. Useful for screening for impairment in various elements of functional status

10. Assesses the need for assistance with getting into and out of bed or a chair

11. Developed to detect unsuspected or subtle forms of functional impairment

12. Measures a person's ability to manage money

13. Possesses exceptional psychometric properties

14. Evaluates a person's ability to do routine household chores

Answers: 9-C, 10-A, 11-B, 12-B, 13-D, 14-B

Critique: The Activities of Daily Living Index and the Instrumental Activities of Daily Living Index are both excellent screening tools for identifying impairment in various components of functional status. Because these measures do not fall into neat conceptual categories, their psychometric properties are difficult to quantify. The Activities of Daily Living Index measures the need for assistance with toileting, bathing, dressing, eating, and getting into and out of bed or a chair. The Instrumental Activities of Daily Living Index measures a person's ability to prepare meals, manage money, take medications, do routine household chores, shop for groceries, and get to places out of walking distance.

Page 243

Questions 15–19 (True or False). Systematic screening of the functional status of elderly patients in a primary care setting can be used to:

15. Aid in diagnosis of problems

16. Anticipate needed social interventions

17. Develop treatment plans

18. Facilitate communications between specialists or disciplines involved in the care of elderly patients

19. Approach patients and families about institutional placement and care

Answers: 15-T, 16-T, 17-T, 18-T, 19-T

Critique: As many as 50% of elderly living at home may have some form of physical impairment that interferes with the performance of activities of daily living. Systematic screening of the functional status in the elderly can be applied usefully in a primary care setting as an aid in diagnosis, a method to anticipate needed social interventions, and a guide when developing plans for treatment and approaching the possible institutionalization of elderly patients. Systematic screening of functional status in the elderly can also enhance communication between specialties and disciplines involved in their health care.

Page 238

Questions 20–23 (True or False). Caregivers, spouses, and family members of the elderly or chronically ill have been identified as "hidden" patients because they frequently experience a decline in functional status. Components for which they are at the highest risk of impairment include:

20. Physical function

21. Emotional function

22. Cognitive function

23. Social function

Answers: 20-F, 21-T, 22-F, 23-T

Critique: Caregivers, spouses, and family members of the elderly or chronically ill are often at high risk of emotional (e.g., depression, anxiety, exhaustion) and social impairment (e.g., sleep deprivation, absences from work, inability to leave the home) related to their dedication to debilitated family members. Cognitive and physical function are probably affected less often and to a lesser extent.

Pages 238, 239

Part III

Communication in Family Medicine

15

Establishing Rapport
Pamela Jelly Boyers

1. The term "good bedside manner" is often used by patients when they are describing physicians to their friends. This term is exemplified by all the following characteristics and behaviors EXCEPT:

    A. A confident approach to the patient
    B. An acceptable personal appearance
    C. The wearing of scrubs
    D. Standing erect and moving briskly

Answer: C

Critique: Although competence is an important component of establishing a good and trusting physician-patient relationship, studies demonstrate that the physician's personal appearance is critical. A natural and concerned manner and a genuine smile go a long way toward reassuring the patient and establishing a friendly, yet professional, atmosphere. The physician's appearance is a significant outward manifestation of competence. White coats and conventional attire convey a reassuring and professional presence.

Page 249

2. Assisting the patient with his or her coat is considered to be a small but important courtesy in the physician-patient relationship. Other helpful behaviors that convey a genuine interest in the patient include all of the following EXCEPT:

    A. Correct pronunciation of the patient's name
    B. Reviewing the chart for information about the previous visit
    C. Using the patient's name twice in the first few minutes
    D. Calling the patient by his or her first name

Answer: D

Critique: Until a trusting physician-patient relationship is established, it is considered appropriate to refer to the patient by his or her last name and appropriate title. Overfamiliarity in the early encounters can lead to false expectations on the part of the patient and, to some, can seem disrespectful. However, much is accomplished by calling the patient the correct name with the correct pronunciation. If the physician reviews the chart for information from the previous visit, this is also very reassuring and conveys a sense of preparation and understanding of the problem. Information about the family can be kept in the margins of the chart and can prove to be very helpful as well as allowing for a genuine interest to be shown in the family and the work life of the patient.

Page 249

3. Mutual respect is a critical component of a trusting relationship. To establish this bond with a patient, a physician must do the following EXCEPT:

    A. Mirror the patient's feelings
    B. Objectively analyze the situation for diagnostic value
    C. Respect himself or herself first
    D. Speak highly of other physicians

Answer: A

Critique: A physician who shows a genuine respect for the patient's values and opinions will in turn be respected. If this approach is combined with concern and kindness and a sincere effort is made to understand the patient's difficulties, the patient is likely to respond positively to the physician's efforts. Although the ability to express empathy is vital, mirroring the patient's feelings would limit the objective impressions that are so necessary for an accurate diagnosis.

Page 250

4. A positive self-image is an important ingredient of being able to respect others. This is manifested by all of the following EXCEPT:

    A. Admitting limits of personal competence
    B. Feeling comfortable asking for help from a colleague in front of the patient
    C. Manifesting an image of omnipotence
    D. Freedom to establish personal relationships with patients

Answer: C

Critique: A physician who appears aloof and unfriendly often feels insecure within himself or herself. This stance gives the impression that the physician is "God-like" and results in the physician seeming remote and uncaring. This behavior sometimes arises from a fear of intimacy, and this anxiety prevents the physician from establishing a comfortable personal relationship with the patient (and others). A physician's effectiveness arises from the ability to analyze the psychological defenses that might interfere with the establishment of a successful physician-patient relationship.

Page 250

Questions 5–8 (True or False). The effectiveness of the physician-patient relationship is closely correlated with:

5. The degree of insight into one's limitations

6. The ability on the part of the physician to recognize his or her own emotions

7. The frequency with which the physician complains about the triviality of the patient's problems

8. The number of patients seen in the practice

Answers: 5-T, 6-T, 7-T, 8-T

Critique: The frequency with which a physician complains about the triviality of his or her patients' problems has been found to be related to the volume of patients seen and the degree to which the physician feels overburdened. This factor is, in turn, related to the degree to which the physician feels overburdened. The effectiveness of the physician is greatly determined by the physician's ability to understand and take care of his or her own emotional health. This involves the development of insight into his or her own emotions and an understanding of the accompanying reactions to patients.

Page 250

9. Patient satisfaction depends greatly on information received and on the degree to which the patient understands his or her illness. Factors that interfere with patient satisfaction include all of the following EXCEPT:

    A. Billing mistakes
    B. Appointment delays
    C. The telephone system
    D. Affective support
    E. All of the above

Answer: E

Critique: Patient satisfaction is closely tied to the physician's ability to explain clearly the medical findings and the treatment plan. A combination of this ability with a supportive attitude towards the patient's emotional concerns leads to the optimal situation. External factors, due to good practice management, such as accurate billing, timely appointments, and a responsive telephone system, ensure that most patients will feel satisfied with their medical care.

Page 250

10. All of the following techniques form the basis for the development of rapport with patients EXCEPT:

    A. Educating the patient about the disease process
    B. Conveying interest in the patient's well-being
    C. Motivating the patient to take part in his or her treatment
    D. Calling the patient on a regular basis

Answer: D

Critique: Calling the patient on a regular basis is unnecessary and might cause the physician to seem insecure. It is important, however, that the physician ensures that his or her practice has a responsive telephone system for the patient and also that the physician responds to telephone calls in a timely manner. Establishing an open channel for communication with face-to-face conversation with the patient remains the primary mode for establishing rapport.

Page 251

Questions 11–14 (True or False). Failure to establish rapport with the patient can:

11. Lead to an increase in malpractice suits

12. Increase the patient's uneasiness and apprehension

13. Help to protect the physician against transference problems

14. Keep encounters with the patient short

Answers: 11-T, 12-T, 13-F, 14-F

Critique: Studies of the physician-patient encounter have demonstrated that some of the longest interviews are due to failures in communication between the physician and the patient. Failures in communication can affect the outcome of treatment, and many complaints against physicians, including those that lead to legal action, stem from misunderstandings that arise in the relationship. Conscious attention to the development of a rapport with patients can lead to a positive outcome for the patient and the physician. A trust develops that can greatly ease the anxiety that accompanies any illness.

Page 252

Questions 15–18 (True or False). Establishing good communication with patients can be accomplished by:

15. Easy access to the physician

16. Prompt returning of telephone calls

17. Discouraging communication by telephone

18. Involving the office staff as an extension of your communication

Answers: 15-T, 16-T, 17-F, 18-F

Critique: Patients consider the easy gaining of access to the physician through early appointments or by telephone as a primary variable in patient satisfaction. In the early days of establishing a relationship with a physician, it is not uncommon for the patient to go through a testing time, especially regarding the issue of access. Although it is important to involve the office staff in a team approach to the patient, care needs to be taken that they do not totally substitute for the physician.

Page 251

19. To establish and maintain rapport involves:

    A. The recognition of a patient's true feelings
    B. The development of a sensitivity to subtle clues
    C. The differentiation of conscious and unconscious verbal and nonverbal clues
    D. The testing phase with the patient
    E. All of the above

Answer: E

Critique: Physicians who develop an alertness to the affective component of the patient's interactions can diagnose in biologic, psychological, and social terms. Conveying a genuine interest in the patient's concerns, for example, and paying attention to the verbal and nonverbal expression of feelings can lead to the early detection of depression. Noticing other subtle cues with facial expressions and breathing patterns can sometimes lead to a better understanding of the patient's symptoms.

Page 251

Questions 20–23 (True or False). Problems that seem trivial that patients bring to the physician's office should be regarded as:

20. A sign of psychosomatization on the part of the patient

21. A clue that the patient might be chemically addicted

22. A concern that the patient is unable to recognize directly

23. More suitable for an appointment with the office nurse

Answers: 20-F, 21-F, 22-T, 23-F

Critique: Although psychosomatization is frequently characterized by seemingly unremarkable complaints and findings, this should not be the initial diagnosis. Seemingly insignificant symptoms can be the expression of many issues, such as a lack of trust in the physician, a lack of insight on the part of the patient, or worries about his or her health in general. It is not uncommon for grieving people to experience fleeting symptoms that feel very real. Many individuals, including physicians, are not able to immediately connect somatization with feelings. They are unlikely to do so until they have been adequately reassured that there is no organic cause for the problem.

Page 252

Questions 24–28 (True or False). Which of the following verbal techniques is/are useful in the physician-patient encounter?

24. The use of medical terminology

25. Using medical jargon to describe the patient's illness

26. The use of slang to relate at the patient's level

27. Explaining the Latin derivation of the words used

28. Keeping explanations at a basic level

Answers: 24-F, 25-F, 26-F, 27-F, 28-T

Critique: Verbal communication accounts for about one third of the total communication in an encounter. Medical terminology should be avoided unless this terminology is very familiar to the patient. The use of medical jargon and slang can be offensive and seem patronizing. Special attention should be paid to the educational level of the patient and to his or her cultural background. Explanations should be kept at a basic level and should proceed only as rapidly as the patient's understanding permits.

Questions 29–32 (True or False). The effect of touch is considered to be therapeutic. Which of the following is/are true regarding touching a patient?

29. Touch can be good medicine.

30. Touch can break down some of the communication barriers.

31. Caution should be exercised not to use touch excessively.

32. Touch can be viewed as aggressive behavior.

Answers: 29-T, 30-T, 31-T, 32-T

Critique: There is a symbolic value to the act of touching. Patients often feel better after routine examinations. The laying on of hands has no scientific basis as a therapeutic tool; however, studies of primates have shown that touching gestures are considered nonaggressive and calming in nature. When used appropriately by the physician, touch can be facilitative and welcome.

33. (True or False) Mirroring is a technique used to establish confidence in a hysterical patient.

Answer: False

Critique: Mirroring is a sign that good communication is taking place. As a communication technique, it involves copying and reflecting the other's movements. To improve communication, some individuals consciously use the technique of mirroring the other person's body posturing. This technique has not been studied with patients with psychiatric or other affective disorders. It is not used to establish confidence in a hysterical patient. It is possible, however, that it might help as a technique to calm the mildly to moderately anxious patient.

34. It is said that the eyes are the most expressive part of the face. They are the most useful organ for identifying one of the following moods:

    A. Anger
    B. Fear
    C. Sincerity
    D. Depression

Answer: B

Critique: The eyes are probably the principal organs of expression and have been found to be better than the brow, forehead, or lower face for the accurate portrayal of fear. They are less accurate for anger and disgust. The eyes can also be used for clues to identify depression. Depression, especially in adolescent patients, is often masked by smiling; however, the astute physician will note that the eyes, brow, and forehead do not convey the same expression. Sincerity is expressed with the eyes. Good and frequent eye contact is a technique used to convey sincerity and the fact that the physician is truly listening.

Page 258

Questions 35–38 (True or False). It is important to be able to recognize the flirtatious patient and the flirtatious physician. Body language can be the greatest clue. Flirting behavior is manifested by:

35. The same body language behaviors in men and women

36. Preening gestures

37. Crossing the legs frequently

38. The use of "steepling"

Answers: 35-F, 36-T, 37-F, 38-F

Critique: Preening gestures can be signs of seductive behavior but are not necessarily so. Some preening is intended to be flirtatious, and some is unconscious behavior. Flirtatious behaviors in males and females differ, with the male usually utilizing gaze holding and head tilting. The female will cross her legs or stroke her arms or thighs. It is extremely important for the physician to recognize these behaviors in themselves or others before unknowingly encouraging the patient to respond in a sexual manner. Steepling is when a speaker joins his or her hands, with fingers extended and fingertips touching. It indicates confidence and assurance in the comments being made.

Pages 261 and 259 (steepling)

39. All of the following are reasonable interpretations of a perceived verbal-nonverbal mismatch, EXCEPT:

    A. The patient is not telling the truth.
    B. The patient may be in conflict.

    C. The patient is uncomfortable with a question.
    D. The patient is worried that he or she has a venereal disease.

Answer: D

Critique: The patient who is worried that he or she may have a venereal disease is more likely to exhibit other behaviors such as "door-knob" behavior or exhibit significant nonverbal discomfort. Several nonverbal behaviors, especially a verbal-nonverbal mismatch, are associated with lying. These behaviors include a light flick of the nose, a clearing of the throat, and avoidance of eye contact. Other clues that the patient might not be telling the truth are asymmetric facial expressions and a prolonged smile or expression of amazement. If the patient is in some inner conflict with what is being discussed, this incongruence is also sometimes experienced by the physician as a verbal-nonverbal mismatch.

40. The degree of comfort with intimate space is largely dependent on each of the following EXCEPT:

    A. The patient's cultural background
    B. The arrangement of the furniture in the physician's office
    C. The identity of the person who comes into the intimate space
    D. The number of symptoms that a patient experiences

Answer: D

Critique: There is a great deal of variation regarding the degree of comfort with intimate space. Cultural differences account for many of these differences, with the average American maintaining a protective "body bubble" of space about 2 feet in diameter. Intimate friends or spouses can invade this space without causing discomfort. The physician's desk can be a barrier to communication. In a family physician's office, the furniture should be arranged so that it does not impede effective communication.

Page 262

Questions 41–44 (True or False). A good physician recognizes hidden or masked communication. This capability aids in the diagnosis, because if not used:

41. Real concerns may go undetected.

42. The patient will be dissatisfied.

43. The patient fears that symptoms may be too trivial to mention.

44. It can help to avoid the "hand-on-the-doorknob syndrome."

Answers: 41-T, 42-T, 43-T, 44-T

Critique: If a physician listens only to the symptoms presented, the real concerns of the patient may go undetected. The result will be a dissatisfied patient. A patient who expresses dissatisfaction with his or her medical care may be dissatisfied because his or her real motivation in seeking care has not been illuminated. The patient's parting phrase might be the clue to the primary reason for his or her visit. The primary reason has not been withheld purposefully but has been hidden for a variety of possible reasons. The reason for the delay is often because the patient is seeking the courage to articulate his or her concerns. A patient with fears of cancer, for example, may fear that he or she is being irrational and be afraid of expressing his or her concerns.

Page 263

Questions 45–48 (True or False). A patient knows that his or her physician is listening well when the physician engages in the following behaviors:

45. Allowing a lot of time

46. Writing on the medical record at the same time

47. Giving feedback

48. Leaning forward

Answers: 45-F, 46-T, 47-T, 48-T

Critique: Good listening involves leaning forward and demonstrating a willingness to hear the speaker. To establish a climate that encourages the patient's willingness to share sensitive information is attained by being nonjudgmental, relaxed, and interested. It is helpful to remain quiet and allow the patient to do most of the talking. Lack of feedback during the encounter will make the patient feel as if the physician does not care about the problem. It is untrue to say that the longer the time taken to do a medical interview, the better will be the satisfaction level of the patient. It is also possible to write on the medical record during the interview in ways that do not interfere with listening.

49. The elderly patient may feel that his or her life is empty or meaningless. The family physician can help to alleviate these feelings by doing all of the following EXCEPT:

    A. Making a house call
    B. Having a sound knowledge of geriatric medicine
    C. Preserving a sense of dignity
    D. Making the patient's decisions for him or her

Answer: D

Critique: It is important to allow the older patient as much autonomy as possible. The geriatric patient will very much appreciate efforts made by the physician that enable him or her to maintain as much independence as possible. This includes independence in living and in making his or her own decisions. As well as being much appreciated, a house call also provides the physician with information about whether the patient is able to take care of himself or herself or is in need of assisted living. Fostering feelings of usefulness in the older patient greatly help to preserve the patient's sense of dignity.

16

Patient Compliance

Dana Nottingham

1. Approximately what percentage of patients will be noncompliant?

    A. 15%
    B. 30%
    C. 50%
    D. 75%

Answer: C

Critique: Physicians have a strong tendency to overestimate their patients' rate of compliance. Fifty percent is a representative statistic for the rate of compliance of patients in long-term therapy. Only about two thirds of those who continue under care take enough of their prescribed medication to achieve adequate blood pressure control, for example. Compliance with diets and lifestyle changes is even lower.

Page 269

2. Which of the following is correct regarding a patient's compliance with recommended treatments?

    A. Poor compliance is strictly the patient's fault.
    B. The patient's age, education level, and economic status affect his or her compliance.
    C. The more symptoms that a patient reports, the greater will be his or her compliance.
    D. No model has been developed that adequately explains or predicts a patient's behavior concerning compliance.

Answer: D

Critique: There is a natural tendency for the physician to believe that poor compliance is the patient's fault. However, there are many other factors leading up to the final act of pill taking that may have important effects on compliance behavior. With respect to the patient, such attributes as age, sex, marital status, education, intelligence, and economic status bear no consistent relationship with compliance. Two exceptions are the very young and very old, whose compliance characteristics tend to conform to those of their caregivers. Economic status can

affect access to medical care; however, once a patient is in care, it does not consistently affect compliance. Surprisingly, no relationship has been demonstrated between the severity of symptoms and compliance, but the more symptoms a patient reports, the lower his or her compliance is likely to be. In summary, no model has been developed as yet that adequately explains a person's behavior concerning compliance or gives a clear rationale for modifying it.

Page 269

3. (True or False) The following factors tend to increase compliance:

    1. The presence of a psychiatric disorder
    2. Increasing disability produced by a disease
    3. Having a chronic disease requiring long-term treatment
    4. Significant behavioral change required
    5. Prescribing the smallest possible number of drugs or treatments
    6. Prescribing medicines with few side effects
    7. Prescribing treatments with lower costs

Answers: 1-F, 2-T, 3-F, 4-F, 5-T, 6-F, 7-T

Critique: Psychiatric patients with schizophrenia, paranoid features, and personality disorders are less compliant than are other psychiatric patients—a fact that probably reduces the compliance of psychiatric patients as a whole below that of patients with nonpsychiatric disorders. Although the severity of symptoms is not related to compliance, increased disability produced by a disease appears to be associated with increased compliance. Chronic diseases that require long-term treatment, such as hypertension, have been shown clearly to result in increasingly poor compliance. This is more likely to be a function of the duration of the treatment regimen than the duration of the disease itself. On the whole, the greater the behavioral demands of a treatment, the poorer is the rate of compliance by the patient. In addition, it is quite clear that the greater the number of drugs or treatments prescribed for a patient, the greater is the probability of poor compliance. Although less important, patients are more likely to comply with a regimen requiring fewer, rather than more, daily doses. There is very little evidence, on the other hand, that side effects of treatment are a major cause of poor compliance. In fact, studies have shown that only 5 to 10% of patients have implicated side effects as being the reason for their noncompliance. Finally, the cost of treatment is an important barrier to compliance for many people.

Pages 270, 271

4. What things can the physician do to improve compliance?

1. Pick out the patients who will likely be poor compliers and concentrate efforts on them.
2. Emphasize the importance of continuity of care.
3. Really get to know their patients well so they will recognize when the patients are not complying.
4. Make sure patients are well satisfied with their care. CHOOSE ONE:

A. 1, 2, 3
B. 1, 3
C. 2, 4
D. 4
E. All of the above

Answer: C

Critique: Studies have shown that physicians using good clinical judgment are no better at detecting poor compliance in their patients than if they were flipping a coin. Furthermore, physicians do just as badly at estimating compliance in patients whom they have known for more than 5 years as they do with those whom they have known for shorter periods. Patients are more likely to comply with treatment if their expectations are met by the visit and if they are well satisfied with their care. The concept of a personal physician or the feeling of knowing a physician well has also been associated with increased compliance.

Page 271

5. (True or False) The following are ways to detect poor compliance:

1. Monitor for follow-up appointments.
2. Monitor the response to treatment.
3. Ask the patient directly.
4. Count pills.
5. Check serum drug levels.

Answers: 1-T, 2-T, 3-T, 4-T, 5-T

Critique: Although there is no guarantee that patients who keep appointments will comply with treatment, there is no doubt that those who do not appear for follow-up will not be in a position to comply with treatment. The importance of monitoring attendance cannot be overemphasized. Dropping out of care is one of the most frequent and most severe forms of noncompliance. Provided that the treatment prescribed is known to be efficacious, the failure of a patient to respond to treatment can be used as a readily available indicator of compliance levels. This method, however, is not infallible. When asked directly, about half of noncompliant patients will admit to missing at least some medication. However, they generally overestimate the amount of medication that they do take, therefore it is important to take into account that admission of any noncompliance implies a compliance rate of less than 80% or as low as 40% on average. If the physician approaches the patient with a face-saving, nonthreatening, nonjudgmental question, this technique will yield a higher proportion of accurate responses. As a method of proving a quantitative estimate of compliance over a period of time, pill counts can be relatively reliable as long as they are carried out in the patient's home with strict attention to bookkeeping. Unless the count can be carried out in such a manner that the patient is unaware of what is going on, it becomes a one-time-only procedure and is, therefore, not very practical for most clinical situations. In general, pill counts give higher estimates of compliance than do quantitative drug assays and lower (but more accurate) estimates than are given in patient self-reports. For some drugs, especially those with long serum half-lives that result in relatively steady serum levels, the measurement of serum levels can be an extremely useful indication of compliance. The caution is that there is a great deal of individual variation in drug absorption, metabolism, and excretion. In addition, serum levels of drugs with short half-lives give no information about long-term compliance.

6. Which of the following is correct?

A. If patients were well educated about their condition and its treatment, they would be near-perfect compliers.
B. It is possible to scare a patient into compliance.
C. The most successful way to improve compliance is to provide information and reinforcement and to involve family members.
D. Physicians, in general, do an effective job at improving compliance in their patients.

Answer: C

Critique: A popular misconception is that the only obstacle that stops patients from being near-perfect compliers is their ignorance of either the condition for which they are being treated or the treatment being used. Although there is some evidence that written instructions help to improve a patient's compliance for short-term regimens, even "mastery learning" has no beneficial effect on long-term compliance. The belief that it is possible to scare a patient into complying with treatment has also been dispelled. Furthermore, a survey of primary care physicians has shown that the methods that they employed to improve compliance were predominantly those that have been found lacking, and the methods that have been shown to be effective were not generally applied. Success for long-term treatments generally requires adopting tactics from at least two of the following areas: cognitive (clear information), behavioral (reminders and reinforcement), and social (involving family, friends, and providers).

Pages 273, 274

7. The main way to prevent poor compliance is to remove barriers to compliance, including:

1. A lot of time spent in the waiting room
2. Giving patients a specific time to return
3. Frequent dosing of medications
4. Allowing patients to become actively involved in their care

A. 1, 2, 3
B. 1, 3
C. 2, 4
D. 4
E. All of the above

Answer: B

Critique: The main thrust in the prevention of poor compliance is to remove barriers to compliance. Preventing patients from dropping out of care is of primary importance. Longer waiting times are associated with higher "no-show" rates, thus the physician should try to keep the patient's waiting time to a minimum. A system for follow-up that ensures that patients leave the office with a specific time for a future appointment rather than with instructions to call for an appointment in, for example, 3 months, makes detection of those who do drop out much easier. Simplification of the treatment regimen will remove another barrier to compliance. Three ways to do this would be to eliminate unnecessary medications, to prescribe medicines that need to be taken as few times daily as possible, and to prescribe the least amount of medication necessary to achieve the therapeutic goal. It has been shown that patients who feel that they are actively involved in their own care have better compliance rates than do those who are not actively involved. Negotiating care with patients, as well as encouraging them to take greater responsibility for their care by asking more questions of their physicians, results in improved attendance and better compliance in general.

Page 274

8. Which of the following interventions has been successful in treating poor compliance?

A. Prompt action to reschedule a patient who misses an appointment
B. Unit dose reminder pill packaging
C. Home visits
D. Providing care at the workplace
E. Group discussions

Answer: A

Critique: If a patient fails to keep an appointment, the receptionist or office nurse must act promptly to reschedule that patient. Personal contact with persistent nonattenders by the physician himself or herself and the use of outreach services, such as public health nurses, are other ways of "treating" nonattendance. None of the following has improved compliance when tested alone: special learning packages and pamphlets, special unit dose reminder pill packaging, counseling about medication and compliance by a health educator or nurse, visits to patients' homes, providing care at the workplace, self-monitoring of blood pressure, tangible rewards, or group discussions. Although these tactics have not worked alone, many have been part of more complex interventions that have been successful. Another important point to remember is that poor compliance is a chronic condition; therefore, treatment of noncompliance must continue as long as the prescribed regimen.

Page 274

9. The decision to apply tactics designed to change a patient's compliance behavior should meet several ethical standards. Among them are:

A. The diagnosis must be correct.
B. The prescribed therapy, as well as the method employed to improve compliance, must be of established efficacy.
C. Neither the illness nor the proposed treatment should be trivial.
D. The patient must be an informed and willing partner in any attempt to alter his or her rate of compliance.
E. All of the above

Answer: E

Critique: All of these criteria should be met.

Page 275

17

Patient Education

Dana Nottingham

1. Patient education may result in substantial benefits. Which of the following does it *increase?*

    1. Adherence to treatment regimens
    2. Morbidity and mortality
    3. Patient satisfaction and autonomy
    4. Medical costs

    A. 1, 2, 3 are correct
    B. 1 and 3 are correct
    C. 2 and 4 are correct
    D. 4 is correct
    E. All of the above

Answer: B

Critique: Patient education has been suggested as a way to increase adherence, to improve satisfaction, to lower cost, to reduce morbidity and mortality, to enhance quality of life, and to empower patients or increase their autonomy. Although the impact of education varies by the type of educational intervention and by the target outcome or the target population studied, careful reviewers have concluded that substantial benefits have been demonstrated from a wide range of strategies.

Page 278

2. (True or False) Results of patient education or health promotion that have an impact on the physician may include:

    1. Practice marketing through enhanced patient satisfaction
    2. Fewer unnecessary office visits and phone calls
    3. Increased liability risk
    4. More malpractice actions

Answers: 1-T, 2-T, 3-F, 4-F

Critique: For physicians, the direct benefits of education and health promotion efforts include practice marketing through enhanced patient satisfaction. There is also evidence that education reduces unnecessary office visits and phone contacts, which have become increasingly important as managed and capitated medical care have be-

come more common. Legal issues must also be considered. The current legal standard of informed consent holds the physician accountable for injuries resulting from undisclosed risks. Enhanced patient satisfaction that results from education, together with more realistic expectations, can contribute greatly to the prevention of malpractice actions. The process of patient education, together with its documentation, thus also serves as a method for reducing liability risk.

Page 279

3. Which of the following is true regarding the impending changes in the health care system in the United States?

    A. The paradigm has shifted from preventive care to curative care.
    B. Changes have been prompted by problems of access to care and the high cost of care.
    C. Changes have been prompted by the realization that encouraging patients to make lifestyle changes is not an effective intervention.
    D. Changes will not require much patient education to carry out.

Answer: B

Critique: It is clear that the health care system in the United States is in the midst of profound change. The major change has been prompted by problems of access to care and the high cost of care. At the same time, there are significant changes occurring based on a paradigm shift from curative care to preventive care. This paradigm shift was encouraged by the U.S. Preventive Services Task Force in 1989 when it pointed out that existing data "suggest that among the most effective interventions available to clinicians for reducing the incidence and severity of the leading causes of disease and disability in the United States are those that address the personal health practices of patients" (1989, p. xxii). Prevention must become the agenda of both patients and health care providers. The education of patients will be critical to the implementation of this paradigm.

Pages 279, 280

4. (True or False) Patient education is not always appropriate.

Answer: False

Critique: Patient education is always appropriate. It is hard to imagine a medical interaction in which education of the patient or his or her family cannot make a contribution. However, there are circumstances in which one must be sensitive to the ability of patients and families to benefit from the education. For example, people who have just been told of a major diagnosis, such as cancer, may not be able to deal with or remember further information given at that time, even if they request it. In these instances, it will be important to schedule additional contacts to continue the process.

Page 280

5. (True or False) Patient education is a separate part of the patient encounter, distinct from history taking, examination, and therapy.

Answer: False

Critique: Although it is possible to view patient education this way, the reality is that education is a critical thread throughout the fabric of high-quality primary care. When observing an excellent family physician, it is typically evident that education is incorporated continuously during the interaction with the patient, not segregated as a separate step.

Page 280

6. Opportunities for health education may exist through which of the following?

    1. School programs
    2. Workplace programs
    3. Community organizations and events
    4. Mass media

    A. 1, 2, and 3 are correct
    B. 1 and 3 are correct
    C. 2 and 4 are correct
    D. 4 is correct
    E. All of the above

Answer: E

Critique: There are many additional opportunities to get involved in health education. Health education, which is a regular part of curricula in schools, may also be found in workplace programs in many communities and is featured routinely in the mass media. These activities do not have to take a lot of time and effort and can begin with something small and manageable, such as a question and answer session. Family physicians who have become involved in health education benefit from the knowledge that their health messages are reaching a wider audience with greater potential impact from the related networking

in their community and from enhanced reputations leading to practice growth.

Pages 280, 281

7. Which of the following strategies yields the greatest benefits when applied to patient education?

    1. What? How? Why?
    2. Feedback, reinforcement, and individualization
    3. "Tell 'em what you're going to tell 'em. Tell 'em. Tell 'em what you told 'em."
    4. Facilitation, relevance, and use of multiple educational channels

    A. 1, 2, and 3 are correct
    B. 1 and 3 are correct
    C. 2 and 4 are correct
    D. 4 is correct
    E. All of the above

Answer: C

Critique: Fortunately, much is known about how to educate most effectively. Research has demonstrated consistently that benefits are greatest when interventions follow these sound educational principles: feedback, reinforcement, individualization, facilitation, relevance, and use of multiple educational channels. Feedback simply means that the patient is informed about progress toward goals and objectives. Reinforcement refers to encouragement or rewards for progress. Individualization takes into account the needs, desires, and characteristics of the patient and demands that specific goals and objectives be negotiated for each patient. Facilitation refers to materials, cues, or skill training that assist the patient in making changes. Relevance to the learner means that the content is appropriate for an individual patient's circumstances. Multiple educational channels imply combined learning strategies as well as a team approach to education.

Page 281

8. Which of the following is the most critical factor in changing health behavior? The patient's:

    A. Knowledge
    B. Health beliefs
    C. Support
    D. Motivation

Answer: D

Critique: Studies of health promotion have found that motivation for change (but not beliefs or efficacy) is clearly associated with behavioral responses to health promotion interventions. Health beliefs and self-efficacy have predicted motivation for change in most lifestyle areas. Perceived support was not found to be important in predicting motivation but did have associations with self-efficacy for some lifestyle areas, as did beliefs. These findings strongly suggest that motivation, or a state of interest in making a change, is an extremely important intervening step in the adoption of new behavior.

Page 282

9. (True or False) Which of the following describes effective patient education?

    1. It involves a cycle of assessment, planning, instructing, and evaluation.

    2. It must take into account the patient's current medical conditions, risk for future health problems, motivation to address any identified needs or behaviors, and existing understanding.

    3. It should be a collaborative process between the physician and the patient.

    4. The evaluation step is one that could sometimes be skipped.

    5. It is more a matter of time than it is of efficiency.

Answers: 1-T, 2-T, 3-T, 4-F, 5-F

Critique: Education is a dynamic process, most akin to a cycle of assessment, planning, instructing, and evaluation. A number of factors must be assessed, including the patient's current medical condition, risks for future health problems, and motivation to address any identified needs or behaviors. Ideally, this assessment should be a collaborative process between the physician and the patient, so that both become invested in its outcome. For motivated patients, it makes sense to proceed with cues, instruction, and skill training as appropriate. It is always important to establish the patient's existing understanding and preferences for learning before launching into a plan for education. The next step is to plan the delivery or process of education, which will include a joint decision on the use of various modalities based on preference and resources, as well as who will be involved. Once the education has been provided, a key step that unfortunately is often overlooked is to evaluate the behavior, skill, or knowledge that was targeted. This evaluation logically leads to another cycle of assessment, planning, and providing further education as needed. The trick is not to think that all of this must be accomplished in one 15-minute visit. In fact, conducting effective patient education is not so much a matter of time as it is a matter of efficiency. Collecting data for rational patient education planning is possible in a relatively small amount of time if it is woven into the fabric of routine care. In many instances, much information is already known to the family physician and can be utilized without further time spent in data gathering.

Pages 283, 284

10. (True or False) Physicians should not waste their time encouraging change in an unmotivated patient.

Answer: False

Critique: When patients are unmotivated, the physician should decide whether or not to try to increase motivation through an assessment and modification of beliefs, self-efficacy, and supports or barriers. At a minimum, an "open door" policy should be adopted. The physician must convey the message that he or she is willing and ready to help the patient make changes when the patient becomes motivated to make them. Motivation to change should be assessed on a regular basis as the patient is cared for over time. The key to avoiding frustration is to focus first on motivated patients, who will respond to brief, time-efficient messages and interventions that are well within the reach of busy practitioners. The satisfaction gained from these efforts can re-energize the physician to make attempts to expand activities to unmotivated patients. For unmotivated patients, a long-term view is often helpful. The goal is to change motivation in small increments over time and to be ready to detect a change in motivation that will allow for a meaningful change in behavior. The best strategy is to be nonjudgmental, to feel rewarded for small changes that the patient makes, to further encourage the patient, and to accept that some people will not change despite one's best efforts.

Pages 284, 285

11. Physicians often rely on printed material to augment verbal instructions, thus patient literacy becomes important. What aspect of literacy is the most crucial as it relates to patient education?

    A. Reading ability
    B. Spelling
    C. Reading comprehension
    D. Writing ability

Answer: C

Critique: National surveys have estimated a prevalence of functional illiteracy of 13 to 55%. Studies also have consistently found large discrepancies between the reading comprehension of the average patient and the ability levels needed to read patient education materials. Even when asked about it, illiterate patients generally do not admit to their deficiency voluntarily. Physicians have often used educational grade level attainment as a surrogate for reading comprehension, but this may overestimate reading comprehension by an average of three or four grade levels.

Page 286

12. The involvement of which of the following increases the impact of patient education?

    A. Physician
    B. Receptionist
    C. Nurse
    D. Office patient education committee
    E. All of the above

Answer: E

Critique: Formal studies and anecdotal reports have consistently indicated that involvement of all of the office staff in patient education makes the total impact all the more powerful and saves the physician's time. Depending on the physician's interest and the nature of the problem, the education can be given by the physician himself or herself or can be delegated to others. In larger practices, interested staff can form a "patient education committee" that sets priority areas for the practice, evaluates or develops printed materials and other resources, and uses a quality improvement process to foster higher quality patient education. Available community resources should also not be overlooked.

Page 286

13. Common pitfalls in patient education include which of the following?

    1. Establishing too much of an atmosphere of acceptance
    2. Failure to understand the patient's anxieties and fears
    3. Being too specific in the instructions
    4. Using medical jargon

    A. 1, 2, and 3 are correct
    B. 1 and 3 are correct
    C. 2 and 4 are correct
    D. 4 is correct
    E. All of the above

Answer: C

Critique: An atmosphere of acceptance, but not necessarily of approval, is the first prerequisite for effective communication. Physicians must demonstrate that they understand the patient's perspective, even if they do not agree with it. These crucial steps lead to teamwork with the patient toward achievement of common goals. Without the establishment of such an accepting atmosphere, patients will be reluctant to share feelings and other information about themselves. Understanding the patient's anxieties and fears is also important. Research has shown that mild to moderate fear can be motivating, whereas extreme fear tends to lead to denial and is therefore counterproductive. Medical jargon should also be avoided. Specificity and clarity are equally important principles. Specific instructions will help greatly to ensure that motivated patients will have the information they need to change their behavior effectively. A final tip for effective verbal instruction is to check continually the patient's understanding of what he or she has been told.

Page 287

14. (True or False) Printed patient education materials:

    1. Should always be preceded by verbal instruction
    2. Are desired by patients and often lead to improved outcomes
    3. Should contain accurate information
    4. Should be of appropriate content and format, at a reading level appropriate for the patients served by the practice, and presented clearly

Answers: 1-T, 2-T, 3-T, 4-T

Critique: Unfortunately, printed patient education materials are often used alone or without sufficient preceding verbal instruction, as a surrogate for provider-patient interaction. A great deal of research has shown that these materials are not effective when used in this manner. However, studies have also shown that printed materials are desired by patients and lead to improved outcomes

when given to supplement other instruction. It is important to recognize that physicians are responsible for the accuracy of any printed material that they distribute. Several issues that are important to consider before using existing materials are: (1) the content is appropriate; (2) the material is clearly presented, with a reading level appropriate for patients served by the practice; (3) additional copies of the material continue to be available for replenishing supplies, or the material should continue to be available for replenishing supplies or may perhaps go out of print; and (4) the format of the material is suitable for storage and display in whatever system is used in the practice.

Page 288

15. Several other modalities can be helpful adjuncts in patient education, such as:

    A. Models
    B. Anatomic charts
    C. Audiotape or videotape
    D. Computer-assisted instruction
    E. All of the above

Answer: E

Critique: It is generally helpful to supplement printed materials with models, anatomic charts, and other visual aids that can be used during the process of instruction. Alternative modalities include audiotape, videotape, and computer-assisted instruction. Use of videotape instruction has been shown to be quite good at increasing short-term knowledge and in role modeling, although it offers no advantages in the areas of long-term retention of information or adherence and has the disadvantage of relatively great expense. Computer-assisted instruction is an emerging technology that offers great promise.

Page 289

16. (True or False) The physician's waiting room should be just an attractive area with comfortable chairs and a magazine rack or a television.

Answer: False

Critique: One of the ways to be most effective in patient education is to view the practice setting in its totality as an educational experience for patients. From this perspective, health providers can examine critically each physical area and each staff person for his or her potential to contribute to patient education. For example, the waiting area need not be just an attractive area with comfortable chairs and a magazine rack or a television. Physicians can make available a rack of nonprescriptive education brochures, decorate the walls with posters that reinforce simple educational messages, and even play educational videotapes or use computer-assisted instruction. Examination rooms can also have posters and racks of printed material, particularly materials that patients might be embarrassed to pick up while others are watching.

Page 289

18

Interviewing Techniques

Betty Young

1. The patient's narrative can be enhanced by which one of the following strategies?

   A. Ask only direct questions.
   B. Suggest answers to your questions.
   C. Ask the patient to explain reasons for his or her answers.
   D. Use empathic responses to the patient's statements.
   E. Use nonverbal behavior to give negative feedback to the patient.

Answer: D

Critique: The patient's narrative is enhanced when the patient is given responsibility for sharing his or her medical history. The physician can promote this process by using facilitative responses, reflections, and empathic responses, rather than by asking direct questions.

Page 293

2. Which of the following statements is true regarding the angry patient?

   A. Anger is a natural result of frustration.
   B. Physicians usually have similar responses to the angry patient.
   C. Patients are usually unable to control their anger.
   D. Anger is rarely used to control the behavior of others.

Answer: A

Critique: Anger is the natural result of frustration in normal, healthy persons. Physicians vary in their ability to recognize anger and tolerate it in a patient. Physicians may need to learn how to be comfortable with an angry patient and how to help the patient overcome his or her frustration in a socially acceptable manner.

Page 297

3. Which of the following strategies is the most effective in helping patients feel more empowered in the interview process?

   A. Ask patients to complete a comprehensive health history questionnaire.
   B. Provide patients with educational materials.
   C. Ask patients their opinions.
   D. Ask patients if they have any questions.

Answer: C

Critique: One of the most effective strategies in helping patients feel more empowered in the interview process is for the physician to ask the patient his or her opinion and to respond to what the patient says. It is a method of acknowledging that the patient's opinion has value and relevance in the interview. It also promotes the active role of the patient in the interview process.

Page 292

4. Of the following physician behaviors, which one represents a barrier to patient involvement?

   A. Listens attentively
   B. Uses technical medical terms to explain the problem to the patient
   C. Explains the treatment and management plan
   D. Employs empathic responses
   E. Includes confrontation to clarify responses

Answer: B

Critique: Physician behaviors can become a barrier to patient empowerment or patient involvement in the interview. If the physician focuses the interview narrative on the disease rather than on the patient, the encounter may deteriorate into a series of questions that do not encourage the patient's involvement. Use of technical terms in the discussion of disease contributes to the patient's feelings of disempowerment.

Page 293

Questions 5–10 (True or False).

5. Direct questions that require a yes or no answer from the patient are very effective in obtaining a history of the patient's present illness.

6. Direct questions that require a yes or no answer from the patient provide for more efficient use of the physician's time than do other interviewing techniques.

7. More patient involvement in the interview process results in greater patient satisfaction.

8. "Critical listening" is a process by which physicians listen attentively and respond appropriately to patients who are being interviewed.

9. Patients form their first impressions of physicians within 20 seconds based on visual inputs, such as the physician's posture, dress, attitude, physical distance, sex, age, and body build.

10. Every communication has two components: the cognitive, or dictionary definition of the words used, and the affective or emotional tone of the communication. Physicians must necessarily focus most of their attention on the cognitive component.

Answers: 5-F, 6-F, 7-T, 8-T, 9-T, 10-F

Critique: Direct questions that require yes or no answers may not elicit the information that the patient wanted to give. The direct question approach does not give patients an opportunity to volunteer the information that they consider to be important. Direct questions are not considered to be an effective use of the physician's time. An interview consisting mainly of direct questions elicits little information per unit time, because most of the interview time is spent by the physician framing or asking questions that provide only specific bits of information. If the physi-

cian does not ask the one specific question that taps the necessary information, the interview may not result in pertinent data gathering. A number of research studies demonstrate that more patient involvement in the interview process results in greater patient satisfaction. It is important to encourage greater patient participation in the interview in order to enhance patient satisfaction and to obtain relevant data. Research studies also demonstrate that greater involvement of patients in their own medical care promotes better outcomes. Critical listening is an active process by which physicians demonstrate that they are indeed listening to the patient. This is accomplished by using facilitative responses that encourage the patient to further enlarge on the topic, by reflections that restate a portion of what the patient has said in order to encourage the patient further, and by empathic responses that help the patient to believe that the physician cares about his or her problems. Patients form their first impressions of the physician in the first 20 seconds based on visual input. Their first impression of the physician's dress, attitude, physical distance, sex, age, and body build, as well as the physician's voice pitch, volume, and expression, are noted quickly and judged by the patient based on the patient's own prejudices or past experiences. Every communication has two components: the cognitive component and the affective component or emotional tone of the communication. Physicians need to hear both components and to be able to respond to either component. If physicians respond only to the cognitive component or to words that the patients use, they may miss the intended meaning.

Pages 291–293, 295

Part IV

Practice of
Family Medicine

19

Clinical Problem Solving

David R. Rudy

1. One of the greatest challenges of primary care, particularly family practice, is the state of disorganization of the symptoms often presented to the practitioner. In order to make a "diagnosis" (classification of symptoms and signs into a recognizable pattern, representing a disease or syndrome), the practitioner must bring organization from such chaos. Which of the following is not a contributing factor in the initial disorganization, peculiar to primary care practice?

    A. Patients may present with more than one problem, not necessarily in the patient's order of priority nor of medical importance.
    B. The most sensitive problems may be expressed in indirect or cryptic language.
    C. The problem presented by the patient is not necessarily the same as the disease.
    D. The bell curve of normal variation can result in numerous false-positive laboratory findings.
    E. Much of the information presented is irrelevant to the problem (i.e., distracting "noise").

Answer: D

Pages 304, 305

Questions 2–6. The next five questions list various characteristics of disturbed health as defined by McWhinney. Answer A if the characteristic belongs to *illness* and B if the characteristic belongs to *disease.*

2. The patient complains of pressing chest pain, radiating down the left arm.

3. The patient notes burning epigastric pain that increases after the ingestion of coffee.

4. Exercise involving the rapid ascent of stairs causes demand on the myocardium to exceed the ability of the coronary circulation to accommodate to this demand, and the result is angina pectoris.

5. A woman is suffering from excruciating deep spinal pain and she has been ignoring a breast mass for 6 months, because she does not want to know what its significance might be.

6. Degeneration of malignant plasma cells results in punched-out bony lesions, severe osteoporosis, and bone pain.

Answers: 2-A, 3-A, 4-B, 5-A, 6-B

Critique: In question 2, the suffering constitutes the *illness* that accompanies angina pectoris (atherosclerotic vascular disease). In question 3, the suffering accompanies what is most likely to be peptic ulcer disease, which is yet to be diagnosed as such but definitely constitutes an *illness.* In question 4, the disease angina is induced by exercise. Suffering is not mentioned. The pathophysiology is described, but symptoms are not the focus of the discussion. Disease is not an illness without suffering of symptoms. In question 5, the *illness* is associated with what is most likely to be due to the disease—breast cancer with bone metastases. In question 6, a disease process is described without mention of symptoms. The disease is most likely to be multiple myeloma. Although pain is mentioned, it is presented as cognitive information and not in the context of a patient's complaint.

Pages 304, 305

Questions 7–10 (True or False). Diagnostic hypotheses are established by cues. They are ranked in descending order of problems to be ruled in or out. Answer the following questions T for true or F for false.

7. The physician should always investigate the most likely problem first, in the interest of economy.

8. The predictive value of a cue (e.g., a symptom or a sign) is dependent solely on the percentage of cases of the disease that would produce the cue.

9. For a given test that gives results along a continuum (e.g., blood sugar from 10 to 300 mg/dl), a variation of the established normal limit has opposite effects on sensitivity and specificity.

77

10.   The definition of specificity is the rate (percentage or fraction) of patients who do not have the disease in whom the test or cue is negative or absent.

Answers: 7-F, 8-F, 9-T, 10-T

Critique: The disease to be ruled out first may be the most likely, all other things being equal and costs of the tests being comparable. However, the first disease to be ruled out may just as often be the most serious in the near future, but not the most likely, such as appendicitis. The (positive) predictive value of a test or cue is dependent not only on sensitivity (and specificity) but also on prevalence, as will be illustrated in problems to be presented. Changing the arbitrary limit of normal, such as downward (e.g., for blood sugar) in order to diagnose a greater percentage (of diabetics), will also have the effect of decreasing specificity, thus more false-positive results will occur.

Pages 303, 304

11.   One of McWhinney's examples illustrates the different ranking diagnosis (depression) of the symptom *fatigue* by a family physician compared with the ranking diagnosis (anemia) made by a hematologist. This is reasonable and is an example of which one of the following phenomena?

A. Differing *sensitivity* of the cue, fatigue, in a family practice as opposed to a hematologist's referral practice
B. Differing *specificity* of the cue, fatigue, in a family practice as opposed to a hematologist's referral practice
C. Differing *prevalence* of the cue, fatigue, in a family practice as opposed to a hematologist's referral practice
D. Differing accuracy of a complete blood count in a family practice as opposed to a hematologist's laboratory
E. A family physician is less likely to be alert to the possibility of anemia than is a hematologist.

Answer: C

Critique: This illustrates well the differing applicability of prevalence to the usefulness of a test result or cue. In a family practice, the prevalence of depression may be as high as 2 to 5%, whereas *symptomatic* anemia may have a prevalence of one tenth to one twentieth as much; the opposite may be true in a hematologist's practice. The sensitivity of the cue, fatigue, is constant for each disease regardless of which physician diagnoses the symptom. However, the predictive value of fatigue as a single symptom will be markedly different in the two situations.

Pages 307, 308

Questions 12–15.   These questions apply to a disease whose prevalence is 10/1000. The *sensitivity* of a blood test for this disease is 95%; the *specificity* is 90%.

12.   In a population of 100,000, those with the disease will number:

A. 1
B. 10
C. 100
D. 1000
E. 10,000

13.   If all the population of 100,000 were tested by Ajax Labs, the number of people who would have a positive result for the disease would be:

A. 5
B. 950
C. 10,850
D. 90
E. 95

14.   In the population of 100,000, those who would have a negative test result would number:

A. 99,900
B. 90,000
C. 95
D. 89,915
E. 89,150

15.   The positive predictive value for the test is:

A. 5%
B. 10%
C. 8.8%
D. 95%
E. 90%

Answers: 12-D, 13-C, 14-E, 15-C

Result	Disease	No Disease	Totals
Positive	a 950	b 9900	c 10,850
Negative	d 50	e 89,100	f 89,150
Total	g 1000	h 99,000	i 100,000

Pages 309–312

Critique: The way to understand the foregoing concepts is to form a 3 × 3-inch table, as above. The columns (vertical) represent the presence of *disease, no disease,* and *totals* of the rows. The rows represent *positive* test results, *negative* test result, and *totals* of the columns. The table is best constructed by first placing the population number in cell *i* (100,000), which is the total for all columns and rows. Cell *g* contains the prevalence of the disease in the population of 100,000 (10/1000 = 1000/100,000). A test with a sensitivity of 95% will be positive in 950 of the 1000 persons with disease. This number is entered into cell *a*. The number of persons without disease is calculated by subtracting the number with disease from the population number and entering the result in cell *h*. The number of people with negative test results in those with no disease (true negative, cell *e*) is found by multiplying *h* by the specificity (90% = 0.9). From this point, all of the remaining cells may be filled in by calculating and balancing the numbers. The total of row totals and that of column totals is equal to 100,000 and so forth. It is then readily apparent that all positive test results are equal to 10,850. Answer C in question 13 is a figure that far overshadows the number of true positives. The predictive value of this positive test result is calculated by the number of true positive results, 950/the number of all positive results, 10,850 = 0.08755 = 8.8% (answer C in question 15). This figure illustrates graphically that the predictive value of a test may be quite mediocre even with an excellent sensitivity and a good specificity if the population at risk has a low prevalence. The false-positive test results in this example outnumber the true positive test results by more than 10:1. The total number of negative test results is $d + e = 89,150$ (answer E in question 14).

20

Infectious Diseases

Thomas Maddox

1. Antibiotic prophylaxis to prevent perioperative infections should:

    A. Be used for all surgical procedures
    B. Be continued for a minimum of 3 days
    C. Be administered at the time of or immediately prior to surgery
    D. Be started at least 5 half-lives prior to surgery so that a therapeutic level can be achieved
    E. Include the use of an oral antibiotic for any gastrointestinal surgery

Answer: C

Critique: Antibiotic prophylaxis for some procedures is indicated only when the patient has elevated risk factors that predispose him or her to develop postsurgical infections. Appropriate prophylactic use of antibiotics includes administration of the antibiotic immediately prior to the time of surgery and continued for no more than 24 hours after surgery. The antibiotic chosen should provide coverage for the most likely organisms to be encountered. Antibiotics given after inoculation of a wound are ineffective in preventing infection.

Page 324

2. Aminoglycoside antibiotics:

    A. Are well absorbed orally
    B. Have bacteriostatic activity
    C. Require dosage adjustments in patients with renal impairment
    D. Are not effective against aerobic gram-negative bacilli
    E. Work by inhibiting cell wall synthesis

Answer: C

Critique: Aminoglycosides are not absorbed orally and must be given parenterally. They have activity against most gram-negative bacilli and some staphylococci. Aminoglycosides are not metabolized and are excreted by the kidneys, requiring dosage adjustment in patients with renal dysfunction. Monitoring of blood levels during treatment is recommended. Aminoglycosides are bactericidal because they bind to ribosomes irreversibly.

Page 329

3. Match the following statements with the appropriate cephalosporins. (Each choice may be used more than once.)

    A. First-generation cephalosporins (e.g., cephadroxil, cephalexin)
    B. Second-generation cephalosporins (e.g., cefuroxime, cefaclor)
    C. Third-generation cephalosporins (e.g., cefotaxime, ceftriaxone)

    1. Good penetration into the cerebrospinal fluid (CSF)
    2. Weakest *Staphylococcus* coverage
    3. The most limited spectrum of activity against gram-negative organisms
    4. Provides coverage for *Haemophilus influenzae* but has no antipseudomonal activity

Answers: 1-C, 2-C, 3-A, 4-B

Critique: Cephalosporins are divided into first-, second-, and third-generation classes by virtue of the timing of their development and spectrum of activity. First- and second-generation cephalosporins are active against most gram-positive organisms. The second-generation agents are also active against *H. influenzae.* Third-generation cephalosporins have the weakest staphylococci coverage but are active against *Pseudomonas* species. Third-generation cephalosporins penetrate the CSF more reliably than do first- or second-generation cephalosporins. The spectrum of activity of oral second-generation cephalosporins makes them particularly useful in the treatment of lower respiratory tract infections when simpler and cheaper forms of therapy cannot be used due to allergy or resistance.

Page 332

4. (True or False) Patients should be cautioned against taking over-the-counter antacids while taking quinolone antibiotics.

Answer: True

Critique: Absorption of quinolone antibiotics is inhibited by antacids containing divalent cations (calcium, iron, zinc). H_2 receptor antagonists, however, do not inhibit absorption.

Page 334

5. (True or False) The elbow is the most commonly affected joint in children with septic arthritis.

Answer: False

Critique: The knee is the most common joint involved in both adults and children with septic arthritis.

Page 336

6. Which of the following is a predisposing risk factor for developing infective endocarditis?

   A. Congestive heart failure
   B. Atrial septal defect
   C. Chronic atrial fibrillation
   D. Atherosclerotic valvular disease
   E. Aortic stenosis

Answer: D

Critique: Intravenous drug use, prosthetic heart valves, rheumatic heart disease, and atherosclerotic valvular disease are important predisposing factors for developing infective endocarditis. Valvular lesions with a high-pressure gradient raise a patient's risk for bacterial seeding of heart valves. Congestive heart failure, atrial septal defects, chronic atrial fibrillation, and stenotic valvular lesions usually have low-pressure gradients, placing patients at low risk for bacterial seeding.

Page 340

7. Elevation of the protein level in CSF during meningitis is due to:

   A. Alteration in the blood-brain barrier
   B. Increase in the number of bacteria present
   C. Increase in the number of white blood cells present
   D. Not truly elevated in relation to the CSF glucose level
   E. Proteins in the cytoplasm released from injured glial cells

Answer: A

Critique: Inflammation of the meninges during infection causes the blood-brain barrier to become more permeable to plasma proteins. Normal neonatal CSF may have a protein content of up to 120 mg/dl. In adults, the CSF may have protein levels of greater than 300 mg/dl during a meningeal infection due to bacterial or fungal pathogens. The CSF may contain from 50 to 150 mg/dl of protein during viral meningitis.

Page 345

8. Regarding body temperature:

   A. Is mediated by the direct effect of angiotensin II
   B. Is controlled by the sympathetic nervous system
   C. Has a normal diurnal variation
   D. Results of blood cultures should be obtained before initiating antibiotics in febrile patients with neutropenia.
   E. A febrile illness that lasts for more than 3 days without an identifiable cause and negative cultures is classified as a fever of unknown origin (FUO).

Answer: C

Critique: Body temperature is maintained at an average of 98.6 degrees by the autonomic nervous system. There is a diurnal peak in body temperature in the late afternoon and early evening. Interleukin-1, released by monocytes and macrophages, exerts a direct effect on the thermoregulatory center to cause fever. FUO is, by definition, a febrile illness that lasts for more than 3 weeks and has no identifiable cause. A neutropenic patient who is febrile should be started on broad-spectrum antibiotics empirically because of the patient's susceptibility to the development of overwhelming sepsis.

Pages 349, 357

9. (True or False) In the United States, diarrheal diseases are among the five leading causes of death in children.

Answer: True

Critique: Diarrheal diseases are among the five leading causes of death in small children each year. In underdeveloped countries, death due to diarrheal diseases is the leading cause of death in infants.

Page 351

10. Treatment of infectious diarrhea includes:

   A. Increasing the intake of dairy products for children
   B. Antiperistaltic drugs (diphenoxylate, loperamide) for diarrhea caused by *Shigella*
   C. Oral antibiotics for uncomplicated *Salmonella*
   D. Oral antibiotics when pseudomembranous colitis is identified
   E. Prophylactic administration of antibiotics to prevent traveler's diarrhea

Answer: D

Critique: The most important aspect of treatment for diarrheal illnesses is adequate hydration. Children with diarrhea due to viral gastroenteritis should avoid milk products due to temporary lactase deficiency. Antiperistaltic drugs are contraindicated in patients with invasive diarrhea caused by organisms such as *Shigella, Salmonella,* and *Yersinia. Salmonella* is a self-limited disease, and supportive care is usually all that is necessary, unless bacteremia occurs. Treatment with antibiotics in otherwise healthy individuals prolongs the carrier state of *Salmonella* and raises the risk of person-to-person transmission. Use of antibiotics changes the normal bacterial flora of the bowel and provides an opportunity for overgrowth of *Clostridium difficile. C. difficile* produces a toxin that causes diarrhea, fever, and abdominal pain. This condition, called pseudomembranous colitis, is treated by oral metronidazole or vancomycin. Intravenous antibiotics are of no value in clearing *C. difficile.* The use of bismuth subsalicylate (Pepto-Bismol) has been shown to help to prevent infection with toxigenic strains of *E. coli.* Taking antibiotics prophylactically, however, may predispose the person to infection with resistant organisms and is not recommended.

Pages 352–355

11.   The most common organisms that cause otitis media in children younger than 3 years of age are:

   A. *Streptococcus pneumoniae, Mycoplasma pneumoniae,* and *Klebsiella*
   B. *S. pneumoniae, Haemophilus influenzae,* and *Moraxella catarrhalis*
   C. *Staphylococcus aureus, H. influenzae,* and *Escherichia coli*
   D. *M. pneumoniae, Chlamydia pneumoniae,* and *Nocardia asteroides*
   E. *M. catarrhalis, Pseudomonas aeruginosa,* and influenza A

Answer: B

Critique: Otitis media is the most common cause of infection in children younger than 3 years of age. Eustachian tube dysfunction (failure to drain secretions from the middle ear), caused by mucosal swelling and congestion of pharyngeal tissue, produces a favorable environment for bacterial growth within the middle ear. The most common organisms cultured from suppurative middle ear infections are *S. pneumoniae, H. influenzae,* and *M. catarrhalis.* Amoxicillin is the antibiotic of choice in the treatment of otitis media.

Page 359

12.   A 5-year-old girl presents to the emergency room with a fever (102° F orally), difficulty breathing, and difficulty swallowing, causing her to drool. Additional information or studies should include:

   A. Questioning the parent or guardian about a familial history of similar problems in the child's relatives
   B. Lateral soft tissue radiographs of the neck
   C. Complete neurologic examination with attention to a stiff neck and the presence of a gag reflex
   D. Cultures of the oropharynx for viruses and bacteria
   E. Giving the appropriate dose of an antipyretic and observing the child for further evidence of localized infection

Answer: B

Critique: This child is presenting with symptoms suggestive of epiglottitis. Epiglottitis usually occurs in children between 2 and 7 years of age, preceded by a sore throat, high fever, hoarseness, and respiratory distress. The child may be unable to handle his or her own secretions because of difficulty swallowing, causing him or her to drool. Difficulty breathing may also be seen in severe cases. Care should be taken when examining children with possible epiglottitis, because stimulation of the oropharynx may precipitate acute airway obstruction. Lateral soft tissue radiographs of the neck will show an enlarged epiglottis. There is no familial tendency for this infectious disease. An antipyretic may be appropriate for the child's fever, but the child needs immediate and aggressive antibiotic therapy for this potentially fatal infection. Use of a third-generation cephalosporin or cefuroxime is indicated as soon as the clinical diagnosis is made.

Page 360

13.   Which of the following is correct concerning lower respiratory tract infections:

   A. Many cases may be prevented by annual influenza vaccinations for persons at risk
   B. Blood cultures are not necessary in patients with suspected pneumonia when sputum cultures have been obtained.
   C. Prophylactic administration of antibiotics should not be given to patients with a history of chronic bronchitis due to the possible development of resistant organisms.
   D. *Klebsiella* pneumonia is the most common cause of pneumonia in adults.
   E. *Mycoplasma pneumoniae* is the most common cause of lower respiratory tract infections in children younger than 8 years of age.

Answer: A

Critique: Respiratory tract infections in the adult are caused by *Streptococcus pneumoniae* most frequently. Respiratory syncytial virus is the most common pathogen that causes lower respiratory tract infections in children. Persons at high risk for development of respiratory tract infections should receive an annual influenza vaccine. Pneumococcal vaccine is also recommended at least once. The use of prophylactic antibiotics is indicated for patients with chronic bronchitis to prevent recurrences of lower respiratory tract infections.

Pages 359–364

14.   In patients with sexually transmitted diseases:

   A. Males or females exposed to sexual partners known to have gonorrhea should be cultured and treated if positive.
   B. Penicillin G is the treatment of choice for gonorrhea.
   C. Venereal Disease Research Laboratory (VDRL) titers may continue to be positive even after adequate therapy for syphilis.
   D. Toxic shock syndrome is seen only during menses.
   E. Herpes simplex type 1 only affects the oral mucosa.

Answer: C

Critique: Most sexually transmitted diseases have continued to increase annually, despite education efforts for prevention. Several strains of *Neisseria gonorrhoeae* have developed resistance to penicillin. For this reason, ceftriaxone, cefixime, or ciprofloxacin are preferred therapies for uncomplicated gonorrhea. Persons known to have been exposed to a sexual partner with gonorrhea should be treated and have cultures taken at the same visit. Follow-up cultures should be done approximately 1 week after treatment to ensure clearance of infection. Even after adequate therapy for syphilis, the VDRL nontreponemal antibody test may continue to be positive. Toxic shock syndrome, caused by *Staphylococcus aureus* and some strains of *Streptococcus pyogenes,* was first recognized in association with tampon use. Toxic shock syndrome now, however, is predominantly nonmenstrual and is seen as frequently in men as in women. Herpes simplex type 1 is capable of producing infection in both oral and genital mucosal surfaces and is responsible for up to 15% of all genital herpes infections.

Pages 368–370, 372, 373

15. (True or False) Acute rheumatic fever is a frequent complication of impetigo due to group A streptococci.

Answer: False

Critique: Impetigo is most commonly caused by *Streptococcus pyogenes* (group A) or *Staphylococcus aureus.* Acute poststreptococcal glomerulonephritis may occur after impetigo due to *S. pyogenes.* The strains of group A streptococci that cause impetigo do not typically cause acute rheumatic fever. Acute rheumatic fever may be seen as a sequela of pharyngeal infections due to group A streptococci.

Page 375

16. Which of the following statements regarding tuberculosis is correct?

    A. Tuberculosis is usually spread via fomites.
    B. Miliary tuberculosis results from direct invasion of the *Mycobacterium tuberculosis* organism to adjacent organs.
    C. A Ghon complex refers to calcified lymph nodes.
    D. Erythema of greater than 10 mm is always a positive reaction to an intradermal purified protein derivative (PPD).
    E. Joint involvement is the most common form of extrapulmonary tuberculosis.

Answer: C

Critique: Tuberculosis is caused by *M. tuberculosis.* It is spread by inhalation of aerosolized droplets. Fomites are not usually responsible for transmission. Miliary tuberculosis refers to dissemination of the tuberculosis organisms throughout the body by hematogenous spread. Ghon complexes are lymph nodes that have been infected by the tubercle bacillus and calcify upon resolution of primary infection. Intradermal skin testing with PPD is done to screen for possible tuberculosis infection. Interpretation of PPD reactions is dependent upon the patient's risk factors for development of tuberculosis. Reactions of greater than 15 mm are considered to be a positive reaction in individuals with no other health-related problems. A reaction of greater than 5 mm may be considered positive in patients with human immunodeficiency virus (HIV) infection, a recent history of exposure to tuberculosis, or an abnormal chest radiograph. Extrapulmonary tuberculosis is often seen in patients with HIV infection. The lymph node is the most common area involved in extrapulmonary tuberculosis.

Pages 376–378

17. A 32-year-old woman is diagnosed as having an acute urinary tract infection. You would be correct in telling her:

    A. The most common cause is bacteria that enter the bladder by hematogenous spread.
    B. A urinary tract infection is often an overgrowth of the usual normal flora of the bladder.
    C. Urinary tract infections are often related to sexual activity.
    D. *Klebsiella* and *Proteus mirabilis* are the most common bacteria that cause a majority of urinary tract infections.
    E. There is no need for treatment of asymptomatic bacteriuria in pregnant women.

Answer: C

Critique: Escherichia coli is the most common bacteria responsible for urinary tract infections. Most urinary tract infections are caused by bacteria entering the normally sterile bladder via ascent through the urethra. Trauma to the external urethra, such as that which occurs during sexual intercourse, can increase the possibility of bacteria entering the bladder. Asymptomatic bacteriuria in pregnancy should still be treated because of an increased risk of nephritis in the mother. Neonatal complications of bacteriuria in pregnancy include prematurity, perinatal death, stillbirth, and intrauterine growth retardation.

Pages 380, 381

18. Which of the following is characteristic of congenital rubella syndrome?

    A. Low birthweight
    B. Hydrocephaly
    C. Limb malformations
    D. Renal dysfunction
    E. Dental malformations

Answer: A

Critique: Both temporary and permanent problems are associated with congenital rubella syndrome. Temporary manifestations include low birthweight, thrombocytopenia, and hepatosplenomegaly. Permanent manifestations are deafness, cataracts, and patent ductus arteriosus. Developmental problems, including mental retardation, behavior disorders, and seizures, can also be seen.

Page 389

19. (True or False) A person who is susceptible may contract chickenpox after exposure to someone with herpes zoster (shingles).

Answer: True

Critique: Varicella-zoster virus causes chickenpox (varicella) as a primary illness. After reactivation, the varicella-zoster virus can migrate along a dermatome to cause shingles (herpes zoster). Lesions that occur with zoster shed the varicella-zoster virus. Persons who are susceptible may contract chickenpox after exposure to these lesions.

Page 390

20. Influenza vaccination is indicated for which of the following patients?

    A. A 46-year-old man with a history of smoking
    B. A 62-year-old healthy woman
    C. A 29-year-old man with HIV infection
    D. A 14-year-old girl with a seizure disorder
    E. A 5-year-old child attending day care

Answer: C

Critique: Annual vaccination of individuals at risk for the development of influenza is recommended. Individuals considered at highest risk include adults and children with chronic cardiovascular or pulmonary diseases. Residents of nursing homes, all individuals older than 65 years of age, patients with renal dysfunction, anemia, immunosuppression, and adults and children with diabetes mellitus are all considered to be at modest risk. Children on long-term aspirin therapy are also considered to be at modest risk. Physicians, nurses, medical care personnel, and family members who have extensive contact with high-risk patients should also be vaccinated to prevent transmission of influenza to patients.

Page 362

21. (Matching) Match the item with the appropriate disease. (Each item may be used only once.)

    A. *Pneumocystis carinii* pneumonia (PCP)
    B. Lyme disease
    C. Measles
    D. Psittacosis
    E. Traveler's diarrhea
    F. Infective endocarditis
    G. Coccidioidomycosis

    1. Deer tick
    2. Roth spots
    3. Birds
    4. HIV
    5. Travel to the Southwest
    6. Koplik's spots
    7. Toxigenic *Escherichia coli*

Answers: 1-B, 2-F, 3-D, 4-A, 5-G, 6-C, 7-E

Critique: Lyme disease is transmitted by the deer tick (genus *Ixodes*) and is caused by the spirochete *Borrelia burgdorferi*. Retinal infarctions, known as Roth spots, are oval hemorrhages with central pallor seen in patients with infective endocarditis. Psittacosis is a nonbacterial source of lower respiratory tract infection. Birds are a frequent source of psittacosis infections. Patients with HIV infection are at increased risk of PCP. This may be prevented with the prophylactic use of trimethoprim-sulfamethoxazole. Coccidioidomycosis, found in the Southwest United States, is a fungal agent responsible for pneumonia. Koplik's spots are bluish gray specks on an erythematous base on the buccal mucosa. Koplik's spots are associated with measles. Traveler's diarrhea, which is caused by strains of *E. coli* that produce an enterotoxin, is often associated with travel to tropical or semitropical countries.

Pages 337, 340, 354, 363, 387

21

Care of the Adult HIV-1-Infected Patient

Michael B. Weinstock

1. Concerning the epidemiology of human immunodeficiency virus (HIV) disease, which of the following is true?

   A. In 1992, HIV was the leading cause of death among men 25 to 44 years of age.
   B. In 1992, HIV was the leading cause of death among women 25 to 44 years of age.
   C. Due to increased education, the rates of HIV infection in women and adolescents are decreasing.
   D. The largest risk factor in the transmission of HIV to women is intravenous drug use.

Answer: A

Critique: In 1992, HIV was the leading cause of death among men 25 to 44 years of age and the fourth leading cause of death in women of the same age group. The year 1993 marked the first year that heterosexual transmission was a risk factor in more than 50% of women with acquired immunodeficiency syndrome (AIDS).

Page 393

2. Which of the following routes of transmission of HIV has been identified?

   A. Hepatitis B vaccine
   B. Contact with tears or sweat
   C. Contact with semen
   D. Insect vectors
   E. All of the above

Answer: C

Critique: None of the aforementioned factors have been implicated as routes of transmission except contact with semen. Other things that have *not* been implicated include contact with environmental surfaces, changing diapers, hugging, shaking hands, sneezing, RhoGAM, heat-treated factor VIII, and immunoglobulin preparations. Educating patients to this fact will help to dispel myths and fears about HIV disease.

Page 396

3. According to the 1993 revised classification system for HIV infection, which of the following patients is considered to have AIDS?

   A. An HIV-positive patient with persistent generalized lymphadenopathy
   B. An HIV-positive patient with idiopathic thrombocytopenic purpura
   C. An HIV-positive patient with oral hairy leukoplakia
   D. An HIV-positive patient with recurrent pneumonia
   E. An HIV-positive patient with vulvovaginal candidiasis

Answer: D

Critique: Recurrent pneumonia in patients with HIV disease is among the several new conditions listed in the Centers for Disease Control and Prevention (CDC) 1993 revised classification system for AIDS. Others include invasive cervical cancer, pulmonary *Mycobacterium* tuberculosis, and CD4+ lymphocyte counts of less than 200 cells/mm^3. The other choices listed occur more frequently in patients with HIV and, when seen, should prompt consideration of testing for HIV but would not by definition classify a patient as having AIDS.

Page 395

4. Concerning the occupational rate of nosocomial transmission following parenteral exposure from infected patients, which of the following is correct?

A. The risk of transmission of HIV is approximately 3.2% (60 infections in more than 2008 needle sticks).
B. The risk of transmission of HIV is approximately 0.32% (6 infections in more than 2008 needle sticks).
C. The risk of transmission is the same whether the needle is hollow or solid.
D. The risk of cutaneous hepatitis B virus infection is approximately 10%.

Answer: B

Critique: The risk of transmission of HIV is approximately 0.32% (6 infections in more than 2008 needle sticks). The risk of transmission of hepatitis B under similar circumstances is 25%. Factors that increase the possibility of transmission include intramuscular injections, injections of blood, large-bore hollow needles, patient viremia, and the immune status of the recipient health care worker. The risk from mucous membrane contact or inoculation of nonintact skin is approximately 5%. Universal precautions should be used when there is a possibility of exposure to blood or body fluids.

Pages 395, 396

5. All of the following should be included in post-test counseling EXCEPT:

A. The meaning of the test result
B. Appropriate measures to prevent or decrease the risk of transmission of HIV
C. Advising the patient not to engage in homosexual intercourse
D. Informing the patient about appropriate medical and health care support services
E. The benefits of partner notification and a mechanism for referral

Answer: C

Critique: Pretest and post-test counseling are important, regardless of the test result. The complexity of post-test counseling warrants against giving HIV test results over the telephone for considerations of confidentiality and complete information. The counseling should be done in an informative, impartial, and nonjudgmental manner. The other choices listed should all be included in post-test counseling.

Pages 396, 397

6. Which of the following is true concerning serologic testing?

A. The best ambulatory test is a polymerase chain reaction (PCR), because it directly detects the presence of a virus.
B. If the Western blot test result is positive, it is confirmed by an enzyme-linked immunosorbent assay (ELISA) test.
C. Approximately 95% of patients will develop an antibody response within 5.8 months of the initial infection.

D. The median time for the production of detectable antibodies in the host is 6 months.
E. All patients with a positive serologic test result for HIV should receive a serologic test for AIDS.

Answer: C

Critique: If result of the ELISA is positive, it is confirmed by the Western blot test. Neither test is 100% sensitive or specific because they are limited by a "reliance" on host antibody production and on the absence of host cross-reacting antibodies. The median time for host production of detectable antibodies is 2.1 months, and 95% of patients will develop an antibody response within 5.8 months of the initial infection. Although the PCR detects a viral presence, its use in the ambulatory setting is limited by time, expense, and expertise in interpreting the results. All of the tests available to date detect infection with HIV, not AIDS per se.

Page 397

7. Which of the following is/are true concerning HIV and women?

A. Women are more likely to develop invasive candidal infections than disseminated Kaposi's sarcoma.
B. Breast milk is capable of transmitting HIV.
C. HIV may be passed during artificial insemination.
D. The use of zidovudine (AZT) during pregnancy reduces the vertical transmission of HIV.
E. All of the above.

Answer: E

Critique: One of the most significant advances in the last several years has been the discovery that the use of zidovudine during pregnancy reduces the vertical transmission rate of HIV. The reduction in transmission may be up to two thirds (~25% with a placebo and ~8% with AZT). Women frequently develop recurrent bacterial pneumonias, pelvic inflammatory disease (PID), and cervical dysplasia.

Pages 398, 399

8. Which of the following is true concerning tuberculosis prophylaxis?

A. Patients should receive prophylaxis for *Mycobacterium* tuberculosis if the PPD skin test shows a 5-mm or greater induration.
B. Patients should receive prophylaxis for *M. tuberculosis* only if the PPD skin test result is 10 mm or greater induration.
C. PPD skin testing cannot be interpreted if the patient has had a bacille Calmette-Guérin (BCG) vaccine.
D. PPD skin testing is worthless because many patients are anergic.
E. Patients with positive PPD skin test results should be treated with isoniazid for 6 months.

Answer: A

Critique: Patients with HIV and a PPD skin test result of 5 mm or greater induration should receive 1 year of isoniazid (or rifampin) prophylaxis regardless of age and regardless of prior vaccine with BCG. A negative PPD test result is not sufficient to rule out tuberculosis, because many patients are anergic; however, a positive test result is helpful. Side effects of isoniazid include hepatitis, peripheral neuropathy, nausea, diarrhea, and hyperglycemia.

Pages 400, 401, 403, 405–407

9. Which of the following vaccines should *not* be given to patients with HIV?

    A. Pneumovax
    B. Influenza
    C. Oral poliovirus (OPV)
    D. Hepatitis B
    E. Tetanus toxoid

Answer: C

Critique: The inactivated poliovirus vaccine (IPV) should be given to HIV-infected patients who were not vaccinated as children instead of the OPV. The IPV should also be given to household contacts. The yellow fever vaccine is not recommended for patients with HIV. The other vaccines listed are safe to give.

Page 401

10. Which is true concerning zidovudine (AZT)?

    A. Although it was the first nucleoside analogue approved for treatment of HIV, it is not currently used because the new antiretrovirals (ddI, ddC, d4T) work better.
    B. The drug is viricidal.
    C. The drug should be started when HIV infection is diagnosed.
    D. Side effects include anemia, granulocytopenia, nausea, headache, and myalgias.
    E. The drug must be stopped if the patient becomes macrocytic.

Answer: D

Critique: None of the HIV treatment regimens currently available is viricidal, and zidovudine continues to be a mainstay of therapy. Indications for starting antiretroviral therapy are a CD4+ count with fewer than 200 cells/mm^3 or *symptomatic* HIV infection with CD4+ count of higher than 500 cells/mm^3. Zidovudine is usually the initial therapy. Zidovidine induces macrocytosis, and this may be used to measure compliance. All of the side effects listed earlier may be caused by zidovudine.

Pages 402, 405

11. John R. is a 32-year-old man who is HIV positive. Although he has been asymptomatic, his CD4+ count has been slowly drifting downward. His last two counts were 182 cells/mm^3 and 174 cells/mm^3. In addition to initiating therapy with zidovudine (AZT), you also advise him that he should receive prophylaxis for *Pneumocystis carinii* pneumonia (PCP). Which of the following is true?

    A. The first line drug of choice for PCP prophylaxis is aerosolized pentamidine.
    B. Although trimethoprim-sulfamethoxazole has improved morbidity, it has not affected survival rates.
    C. Patients with allergic manifestations from trimethoprim-sulfamethoxazole should stop the medication immediately and should never be restarted on it.
    D. Patients should not be started on PCP prophylaxis until the CD4+ count drops to 100 cells/mm^3.
    E. For patients unable to tolerate trimethoprim-sulfamethoxazole secondary to allergic reactions, desensitization protocols are available.

Answer: E

Critique: Trimethoprim-sulfamethoxazole is the drug of choice for PCP prophylaxis and should be started when the CD4+ count drops to 200 cells/mm^3. This drug is inexpensive and has very low breakthrough rates when patients are compliant. The dose is one double-strength tablet per day or one double-strength tablet three times per week. Other medications for PCP prophylaxis include dapsone, aerosolized pentamidine isethionate, and the combination of sulfadoxine and primethamine (Fansidar).

Pages 402–405

Questions 12–17. Match the following opportunistic infections with first-line treatment:

    A. Ganciclovir
    B. Trimethoprim-sulfamethoxazole
    C. Benzathine penicillin
    D. Pyrimethamine plus leucovorin (folinic acid) plus sulfadiazine
    E. Ketoconazole
    F. Clotrimazole

12. *Pneumocystis carinii* pneumonia

13. *Toxoplasma gondii* encephalitis

14. *Treponema* syphilis, primary

15. *Candida* stomatitis

16. *Candida* esophagitis

17. Cytomegalovirus retinitis

Answers: 12-B, 13-D, 14-C, 15-F, 16-E, 17-A

Critique: Trimethoprim-sulfamethoxazole is the first-line medication for treatment *and* prophylaxis of PCP.

In patients being treated for PCP, if the P_{O_2} is less than 70 mm Hg, add prednisone (40 mg orally twice a day for 5 days; then 40 mg/day for 5 days; then 20 mg/day for 11 days). Treatment of toxoplasmic encephalitis is often initiated on an empirical basis to avoid a stereotactic brain biopsy to differentiate from lymphoma or progressive multifocal leukoencephalopathy (PML).

18. Concerning cytomegalovirus (CMV) retinitis, which of the following is correct?

    A. CMV retinitis occurs in 25% of patients, usually when CD4+ lymphocyte counts are less than 50 cells/mm³.
    B. Current treatment requires induction and lifelong maintenance therapy.
    C. Toxicities of ganciclovir include neutropenia, thrombocytopenia, confusion, central nervous system (CNS) symptoms, adjustment for patients with renal failure.
    D. Toxicities of foscarnet include renal failure, anemia, liver enzyme elevation, seizures, and decreased calcium levels.
    E. All of the above.

Answer: E

Critique: Ganciclovir and foscarnet are used to treat CMV retinitis, although neither is viricidal and each has many side effects. Current treatment requires induction and lifelong maintenance therapy. The oral formulation of ganciclovir has recently been approved.

Pages 406, 407

Questions 19–21. Match the medications with their major toxicities:

    A. Peripheral neuropathy, aphthous ulcers, pancreatitis, pruritus, and headaches
    B. Pancreatitis, peripheral neuropathy, and diarrhea
    C. Anemia, granulocytopenia, nausea, headache, and myalgias

19. Zidovudine (AZT)

20. Didanosine (ddI)

21. Zalcitabine (ddC)

Answers: 19-C, 20-B, 21-A

Critique: It is important to be aware of the unique side effects and interactions of medications commonly prescribed to patients with HIV and AIDS. Patients taking ddI who develop abdominal pain should immediately stop the medication, and pancreatitis should be excluded as an etiology. Both ddI and ddC can cause peripheral neuropathy in addition to distal symmetrical polyneuropathy (DSP), a common complication in patients with AIDS. The interaction of zidovudine and ganciclovir may cause synergistic bone marrow suppression.

Pages 406–408

22

Pulmonary Medicine

Edward T. Bope and Peter Nalin

Questions 1–4 (True or False). The routine use of chest radiographs is particularly important for:

1. Screening for early evidence of lung cancer in asymptomatic people who smoke cigarettes

2. Screening for asymptomatic tuberculosis infection

3. Improving the overall management of patients with chronic obstructive pulmonary disease (COPD) with clinical evidence of worsening

4. Evaluating possible causes of persistent cough

Answers: 1-F, 2-F, 3-T, 4-T

Critique: Chest radiographs are not a screening tool for lung cancer in smokers. Chest radiographs are a helpful diagnostic study in smokers with symptoms suggestive of lung cancer. Chest radiographs are not screening tools for tuberculosis. They are helpful in the clarification of patients with positive purified protein derivative (PPD) results, whether or not they are otherwise symptomatic. They can also help in evaluating COPD patients or patients with persistent cough.

Page 411

Questions 5–8 (True or False). True statements about respiratory function tests include:

5. Spirometry in the office practice is useful in the assessment of bronchospasm.

6. Pulse oximetry is a useful noninvasive method for determining the partial pressure of oxygen in the blood.

7. Arterial blood gases provide information about the degree of metabolic compensation for respiratory dysfunction.

8. Expected values for forced vital capacity (FVC) and forced expiratory volume in 1 second (FEV_1) are determined by the weight and sex of the individual.

Answers: 5-T, 6-F, 7-T, 8-T

Critique: Spirometry can quantify the degree of bronchospasm quickly and cost effectively in the office setting. Pulse oximetry noninvasively determines the percent oxygen saturation. Determination of the partial pressure of oxygen is obtained from arterial blood gases. Arterial blood gases are the best way of assessing states of acidosis and alkalosis. Weight and gender are used to determine expected values for forced vital capacity and FEV_1.

Page 412

9. A 52-year-old man presents to the office with the recent onset of a nonproductive cough. He has never smoked tobacco products and has had only intermittent exposure to passive smoke at work. He denies fever, chills, weight loss, and hemoptysis. In seeking an explanation for his cough, which one of the following findings would be a likely cause?

    A. Chronic use of H_2-blockers for peptic ulcer disease

    B. Recent addition of an angiotension-converting enzyme (ACE) inhibitor to his hypertensive medications

    C. Use of acetaminophen with codeine for a recent fractured ankle

    D. Occasional use of prochlorperazine (Compazine) suppositories for nausea associated with a migraine headache

Answer: B

Critique: H_2-blockers can reduce cough and bronchospasm resulting from nocturnal reflux. ACE inhibitors may cause a cough in approximately 10% of patients. Codeine is a narcotic cough suppressant. Prochlorperazine does not cause a cough.

Pages 412, 413

10. In which of the following clinical problems is an exudative pleural effusion likely to occur?

    A. Congestive heart failure

B. Atelectasis
C. Lymphatic obstruction due to a malignancy
D. Nephrotic syndrome (hypoalbuminemia)

Answer: C

Critique: The increased hydrostatic venous pressure of congestive heart failure induces a transudative effusion. The diminished intravascular oncotic pressure of nephrotic syndrome also induces a transudative effusion, as does atelectasis, which intensifies the negative intrapleural pressure. Malignancies that obstruct lymphatic drainage cause exudative effusions.

Page 413

11. In ambulatory patients, pleural fluid first accumulates in the:

A. Anterior thorax
B. Posterior thorax
C. Medial thorax
D. Lateral thorax

Answer: B

Critique: Pleural fluid first accumulates posteriorly in ambulatory patients.

Page 413

12. A 40-year-old migrant farm worker from the southwestern region of the United States presents with increasing shortness of breath, cough, and occasional sharp stabbing chest pain. He has not taken his temperature, but he feels warm some of the time. He smokes one pack of unfiltered cigarettes per day and drinks heavily on weekends. He has dullness over the right lower chest, and a chest radiograph shows a moderate-sized pleural effusion. A diagnostic thoracentesis reveals significant eosinophils in the fluid. Your differential diagnosis should include all of the following EXCEPT:

A. Tuberculosis
B. Coccidioidomycosis
C. Viral pleuritis
D. Recurrent pulmonary embolus
E. Recurrent pancreatitis

Answer: E

Critique: Not only can eosinophils in pleural fluid signify tuberculosis and coccidioidomycosis, but eosinophils can also indicate viral pleuritis and a pulmonary embolism in the differential diagnosis. They are not found in pancreatitis.

Page 414

13. Acute onset of pleuritic chest pain with cough, fever, and hypoxia would lead you to suspect pulmonary embolus. Pneumonia caused by which of the following organisms is a common imitation:

A. *Streptococcus* pneumonia
B. *Haemophilus influenzae*
C. *Klebsiella* pneumonia

D. *Moraxella catarrhalis*
E. All of the above

Answer: A

Critique: Pneumococcal pneumonia can easily mimic the quick onset and pleuritic quality of a pulmonary embolus. Since fever is a symptom shared by both, it will not differentiate. The other organisms would not cause a similar symptom complex.

Pages 416, 417

Questions 14–17 (True or False). Answer true or false for each of the following options with regard to bronchiolitis:

14. It is most frequently seen in children 1 to 3 years of age.

15. Cases occur predominantly between Janaury and May.

16. Respiratory syncytial virus is the only agent identified in bronchiolitis.

17. Rhinorrhea, respiratory distress, and wheezing are common signs.

Answers: 14-F, 15-T, 16-F, 17-T

Critique: Bronchiolitis is a disease seen most commonly in children from 2 to 12 months of age. Respiratory syncytial virus is the most common etiologic agent and is the cause in 80% of cases in epidemic months (January to May) and a little over 50% during the nonepidemic months. Several other organisms can cause bronchiolitis. The most striking of the findings are rhinorrhea, respiratory distress, and wheezing. Bronchiolitis can easily be confused with pneumonia and gastric aspirations.

Page 421

18. Which of the following would be the correct treatment plan for an asymptomatic pregnant patient who has recently converted from a negative tuberculosis (TB) skin test to a positive skin test:

A. Isoniazid alone
B. Rifampin alone
C. No treatment until after delivery
D. Isoniazid and rifampin
E. Isoniazid, rifampin, and pyrazinamide

Answer: A

Critique: The correct regimen for a recent asymptomatic TB converter who is pregnant is isoniazid. Isoniazid and rifampin can be used without fear of teratogenicity. Ethambutol should be added if drug resistance is suspected in active disease.

Pages 424, 425

Questions 19–22 (True or False). Which of the following factors make a solitary nodule more likely to be a cancer rather than a benign lesion:

19. Age over 35

20. Presence of calcification

21. Size greater than 4 cm

22. History of smoking

Answers: 19-T, 20-F, 21-T, 22-T

Critique: A solitary pulmonary nodule is more likely to be a carcinoma if it has the following associated factors: the patient is older than 35 years of age, absence of calcifications, size greater than 4 cm, and a history of smoking. Another worrisome sign is an increasing size.

Page 435

23. (True or False) As a cure for bronchogenic carcinoma, surgery is the best modality.

Answer: True

Critique: Of patients with bronchogenic carcinoma, 90% will die of their disease. The small percentage who survive owe their cure to surgical resection of the tumor. Obviously many factors go into deciding if the patient is a surgical candidate, such as the size and location of the tumor as well as the severity of the concomitant disease.

Page 438

24. (True or False) The proper management of a pneumothorax is a chest tube as soon as possible.

Answer: False

Critique: While a chest tube will resolve a pneumothorax, it is not always necessary. Some cases of small spontaneous pneumothorax can be managed with observation and serial x-rays.

Page 435

25. Select the drug that has been reported to cause interstitial pneumonitis.

    A. Nonsteroidal anti-inflammatories
    B. Nitrofurantoin
    C. Coumadin
    D. Inhaled corticosteroids
    E. Calcium channel blockers

Answer: B

Critique: The drug most typically encountered causing interstitial pneumonitis in a family practice would be nitrofurantoin. The other drugs listed have not been shown to cause this disease.

Page 431

Questions 26–29 (True or False). Which of the following are true concerning COPD?

26. Both chronic bronchitis and emphysema are forms of COPD.

27. Long-term oxygen use has not been shown to improve the quality of life.

28. Bacteria play a large role in exacerbations.

29. Pneumococcal vaccination and annual influenza vaccination are important management.

Answers: 26-T, 27-F, 28-F, 29-T

Critique: Both emphysema and chronic bronchitis qualify as COPD. Long-term oxygen use has been shown to improve both the quality and duration of life. The role of bacteria in the deterioration or exacerbation of the patient with COPD is unclear, with studies arguing both sides. Good management would include vaccinating with pneumoccal vaccine and annual influenza vaccine.

Pages 427, 428

23

Otolaryngology

Gregory H. Blake

1. The parent of a 15-month-old male noted the onset of temperature to 101.5° F, a barking cough, and inspiratory stridor. On examination, his respiratory rate was 35 breaths/min with inspiratory stridor and the chest was clear. The most likely diagnosis is:

    A. Croup
    B. Supraglottitis
    C. Peritonsillar abscess
    D. Foreign body aspiration
    E. Juvenile laryngeal papillomatosis

Answer: A

Critique: All the conditions noted occur in children. Croup usually presents in children younger than 2 years of age and occurs in epidemics in late fall or early winter. Children present with fever, barking cough, inspiratory stridor, and hoarseness over a 24-hour period. With the exception of inspiratory stridor and tachypnea, the results of the physical examination are negative. Supraglottitis usually occurs in children younger than 6 years of age and presents with an abrupt onset of fever greater than 102° F, severe sore throat, and dysphagia. The physical examination reveals difficulty swallowing secretions, tachypnea, and the use of accessory muscles of respiration. Peritonsillar abscess presents with acute pharyngitis progressing to difficulty in swallowing. The patient will have fever, mild dehydration, increased oral secretions, and trismus. The physical examination reveals a swollen tonsil that is displaced toward the midline and downward. Foreign body aspiration most commonly presents in small children, who may have coughing and intermittent or constant stridor, wheezing, or cyanosis. The physical examination reveals any combination of tachypnea, cyanosis, stridor, and wheezing. Unless their condition is complicated by pneumonia, patients are afebrile. Juvenile laryngeal papillomatosis almost always presents in children by 4 years of age with major voice changes and hoarseness.

Page 441

2. The most frequent cause of supraglottitis in children is:

    A. β-Hemolytic *Streptococcus*
    B. *Streptococcus pneumoniae*
    C. *Haemophilus influenzae*
    D. Parainfluenza virus
    E. *Staphylococcus aureus*

Answer: C

Critique: *H. influenzae* is almost always the cause of supraglottitis in children. In adults, β-hemolytic *Streptococcus, Pneumococcus,* and *S. aureus* may cause supraglottitis. Parainfluenza virus usually causes croup.

Page 441

3. Which of the following therapeutic regimens is best for the management of supraglottitis?

    A. Cool-mist ultrasonic humidifier, racemic epinephrine
    B. Oral ampicillin, low-flow oxygen with humidified air
    C. Low-flow oxygen and intubation
    D. Parenteral metronidazole, humidified air with low-flow oxygen
    E. Sulbactam-ampicillin, low-flow oxygen with humidified air

Answer: E

Critique: Supraglottitis is a life-threatening condition that may result in respiratory embarrassment from a swollen epiglottis blocking air flow. For this reason, all patients should be admitted to the hospital for parenteral antibiotics and observation. Because of the relative occurrence of ampicillin-resistant *Haemophilus influenzae,* antibiotic choices include sulbactam-ampicillin (Unasyn), cefuroxime (Zinacef), ceftriaxone (Rocephin), or chloramphenicol. Humidified air with low-flow oxygen should be administered. Close observation of the patient is essential because airway compromise may progress suddenly to obstruction and require emergency intubation.

Page 441

4. A 25-year old white woman comes to the clinic and reports having had symptoms of nasal obstruction and clear nasal discharge intermittently for the past 6 years. An examination reveals mild swelling of the nasal mucosa. Her only other problem is mild anxiety. Which of the following is the most likely diagnosis?

    A. Viral rhinitis
    B. Vasomotor rhinitis
    C. Allergic rhinitis
    D. Choanal atresia

Answer: B

Critique: Vasomotor rhinitis is due to dilatation of nasal vessels and consequent nasal discharge. It occurs more commonly in adolescents and young adults, in women, and those suffering from chronic anxiety. Vasomotor rhinitis presents with nasal obstruction and clear nasal discharge. Viral rhinitis occurs once or twice a year in adults. It is typically caused by rhinoviruses and peaks in September, January, and April. Allergic rhinitis usually begins before a person is 20 years of age and may occur seasonally in response to pollen antigens or perennially in response to house dust, animal dander, or food. In addition to nasal discharge, allergic rhinitis presents with sneezing and increased lacrimation. Choanal atresia is congenital blockage of one or both posterior choanae and would have manifested nasal obstruction at birth.

Pages 461, 462

5. A 16-year-old African-American male comes to clinic complaining of right ear ache and fever to 102° F. He describes fullness and tenderness to touch behind the ear. He has a history of chronic suppurative otitis media. The physical examination reveals postauricular erythema, tenderness, and slight swelling. Which of the following is the most likely diagnosis?

    A. Chronic suppurative otitis media
    B. Lateral sinus thrombophlebitis
    C. Acute mastoiditis with periosteitis
    D. Cholesteatoma
    E. Acute mastoid osteitis

Answer: C

Critique: The first stage of acute mastoiditis is consistent with acute otitis media. The second stage of acute mastoiditis involves spread of the infection to the periosteum covering the mastoid process. It presents with fever, otalgia, postauricular erythema, tenderness, and slight swelling. Acute mastoid osteitis involves a progression, with the pinna being displaced outward and downward, and swelling of the posterior superior ear canal wall. Lateral sinus thrombophlebitis results from inflammation in the adjacent mastoid. Mural thrombi may become infected and occlude the lumen. Patients will present with high, spiking fevers and chills and signs of increased intracranial pressure. A cholesteatoma is keratinizing stratified squamous epithelium within the middle ear or pneumatized portion of the temporal bone. Signs and symptoms are usually absent for years. A continuous foul-smelling discharge and progressive hearing loss are the usual presenting signs.

Pages 454–456

6. Acoustic neuromas:

    A. Typically present with progressive intermittent dizziness
    B. Result in conductive hearing loss
    C. Account for approximately 30% of brain tumors
    D. Produce unilateral, progressive hearing loss
    E. Respond well to chemotherapy

Answer: D

Critique: Acoustic neuromas account for approximately 8% of all brain tumors. They typically present with gradual, progressive, unilateral sensorineural hearing loss with poor speech discrimination. Approximately 10% of patients will present with episodic vertigo. Acoustic neuromas are usually removed surgically.

Page 457

7. A 32-year-old pilot notes severe pain and decreased hearing in his left ear several hours after landing a plane from a rapid descent. Otoscopy reveals a vascular injection and a small hemorrhage of the tympanic membrane, but there is no evidence of blood in the middle ear. What is the most appropriate plan of treatment?

    A. Confirm the hearing loss with an audiogram.
    B. Prescribe a course of topical and systemic decongestants.
    C. Prescribe a long-acting antihistamine of choice.
    D. Refer the patient to an otolaryngologist for a myringotomy.

Answer: B

Critique: This patient is experiencing barotrauma to his left ear. Factors favoring the development of barotrauma are swelling of the nasopharyngeal end of the eustachian tube secondary to an upper respiratory infection or allergy, ignorance of the need to equalize pressure, rapid rate of descent, and sleeping during descent. Symptoms that may vary in intensity include severe pain, decreased hearing, a sense of fullness, low-pitched tinnitus, and, occasionally, vertigo. When a sensation of fullness is first noted, the Valsalva maneuver may help. Topical and systemic decongestants may be helpful. Antihistamines are not likely to help, and only a limited number are approved for use by pilots. If a hemotympanum is present, a myringotomy can be performed if the pilot must immediately return to flight.

Pages 458, 459

8. Upper facial pain, discharge, visual dysfunction, headaches, fever, and chronic cough are manifestations of:

    A. Ethmoid sinusitis
    B. Frontal sinusitis
    C. Viral rhinitis
    D. Vasomotor rhinitis
    E. Allergic rhinitis

Answer: A

Critique: Since the ethmoid sinus is separated from the eye and the brain by only a thin bony wall, patients with ethmoid sinusitis will manifest symptoms and complications from both areas. A patient with frontal sinusitis will present with headaches that are worse in the mornings, mucopurulent discharge, and fever. The patient with viral rhinitis may present with a low-grade fever, nasal discharge, headache, and nonproductive cough but will lack visual signs. Vasomotor rhinitis is caused by dilatation of nasal vessels with consequent discharge. Allergic rhinitis may be complicated by sinusitis but presents as an itching of the nose and eyes, sneezing, nasal obstruction, watery nasal discharge, and increased lacrimation.

Pages 462–464

9. A 52-year-old African-American man complains of persistent nasal stuffiness. He has a history of seasonal allergies and vasomotor rhinitis. The physical examination reveals enlarged, meaty, obstructive turbinates. Spraying the nose with ephedrine fails to produce a decongestant effect. What is the most likely diagnosis?

    A. Allergic rhinitis
    B. Chronic vasomotor rhinitis
    C. Viral rhinitis
    D. Maxillary sinusitis
    E. Chronic hypertrophic rhinitis

Answer: E

Critique: Chronic hypertrophic rhinitis is the end stage of repeated viral rhinitis, allergic rhinitis, vasomotor rhinitis, and rhinitis medicamentosa. It manifests as enlarged, meaty, obstructive turbinates. The diagnosis is confirmed by a lack of decongestant effect after spraying the nose with a topical sympathomimetic solution (ephedrine). Surgical management is usually the only effective treatment for this condition.

Page 467

10. A 14-year-old white female has a 24-hour history of sore throat, fever, headache, and odynophagia. She denies nasal congestion or cough. The physical examination reveals patchy, purulent tonsillar exudate with petechiae in the soft palate and tender anterior cervical adenopathy. The most likely cause of her symptoms is:

    A. Gonococcal pharyngitis
    B. Chlamydial pneumonia
    C. Viral upper respiratory tract infection
    D. Group A, β-streptococcal tonsillitis
    E. Mycoplasmal pharyngitis

Answer: D

Critique: A patient with streptococcal pharyngitis presents with a sore throat, fever, and odynophagia. The patient may complain of myalgias, arthralgias, abdominal pain, headache, or vomiting. On physical examination, pharyngeal erythema, soft palate petechiae, tender anterior cervical adenopathy, and a patchy, purulent tonsillar exudate may occur. If cough and rhinorrhea were present, a viral etiology would be much more likely. Lower respiratory tract signs and symptoms including cough, dyspnea, or rales would support pneumonia.

Page 467

11. A 48-year-old white woman reports the sensation that food "sticks" in her lower esophagus. She denies pain or weight loss. She does not smoke or drink alcohol. Which of the following is most consistent with her complaints?

    A. Diffuse esophageal spasms
    B. Achalasia
    C. Zenker's diverticulum
    D. Squamous cell carcinoma
    E. Esophagitis

Answer: B

Critique: Achalasia results from a decreased number of ganglion cells in Auerbach's mesenteric plexus, resulting in diminished or absent peristalsis. Patients most frequently report the sensation of food "sticking" in the lower esophagus. Regurgitation is common, but pain is infrequent. Diffuse esophageal spasms result from failure of the muscular contractions to follow the usual peristaltic pattern in the distal half of the esophagus. Patients complain of dysphagia accompanied by substernal pain mimicking angina. Zenker's diverticulum is a pharyngo-esophageal pouch that is typically seen in elderly men. It causes regurgitation of food, foul odor, dysphagia, and aspiration. Squamous cell carcinoma manifests with dysphagia of solid foods, then liquids, and weight loss, hoarseness, cough, and pneumonia. Esophagitis may be associated with dysphagia, but usually pyrosis is a prominent complaint.

Pages 469, 470

12. Chronic bronchitis, excessive alcohol ingestion, cigarette smoking, and extended speaking are contributing factors for:

    A. Acute laryngitis
    B. Laryngomalacia
    C. Chronic laryngitis
    D. Vocal cord paralysis
    E. Laryngeal webs

Answer: C

Critique: Chronic laryngitis results from using the voice for extended speaking or singing. Chronic bronchitis, excessive alcohol ingestion, and cigarette smoking are contributing factors. Acute laryngitis is usual of viral etiology and produces a mild, self-limited illness. Laryngomalacia causes an inspiratory stridor in infancy that usually resolves by 12 to 18 months of age. It results from a soft, floppy laryngeal skeleton and immature neuromuscular function. Vocal cord paralysis is usually a congenital abnormality or a result of lesions affecting the recurrent laryngeal nerve. Laryngeal webs can be glottic, subglottic, or supraglottic. They produce changes ranging from mild hoarseness to aphonia to stridor and gross obstruction.

Pages 470, 471

13. A 62-year-old white man reports a 2-month history of hoarseness and weight loss. The physical examination is negative for adenopathy. Which of the following is the most likely cause of his problem?

A. Glottic carcinoma
B. Supraglottic carcinoma
C. Laryngeal papillomatosis
D. Subglottic stenosis
E. Subglottic hemangioma

Answer: A

Critique: Laryngeal cancer can arise from the true vocal cords (glottic), the false vocal cords and epiglottis (supraglottic), or the piriform sinuses and vallecula (marginal). The clinical presentation and prognosis vary depending on the tumor's origin. Glottic carcinoma presents with hoarseness early and has a cure rate more than 90% for T1 lesions. Supraglottic and marginal laryngeal cancers present with a sensation of a lump in the throat, dysphagia, or an asymptomatic neck node mass. This type of cancer has an 85% cure rate for T1 lesions. Laryngeal papillomatosis, caused by the human papillomavirus, presents as multiple lesions in young adults or a single wart in older adults. These lesions cause a major voice change and hoarseness. Subglottic stenosis results from prolonged infant intubation, external trauma, burns, and granulomatous disease. Stridor is a common presenting sign. Subglottic hemangiomas result in stridor.

Page 472

14. Which one of the following statements is true concerning Sjögren's syndrome?

A. The parotid gland is not involved.
B. Typical findings include xerostomia, keratoconjunctivitis, and a connective tissue disorder.
C. This syndrome does not respond to systemic corticosteroids.
D. The syndrome frequently leads to salivary gland cancer.

Answer: B

Critique: Sjögren's syndrome consists of the triad of xerostomia, keratoconjunctivitis, and a connective tissue disorder. The parotid glands are diffusely enlarged with a firm, irregular contour. The diagnosis is confirmed by increased gamma globulins, rheumatoid factor, or antinuclear antibodies. The recommended early treatment is corticosteroids and symptomatic treatment of symptoms with artificial tears and saliva. Malignant degeneration of the salivary gland cells is not part of the syndrome.

Page 478

Questions 15–19. Match each of the following malignancies with the appropriate lettered option. Each lettered response may be used once, more than once, or not at all.

A. Tobacco and alcohol use
B. Exposure to nickel or wood dust
C. Both A and B
D. Neither A nor B

15. Malignant tumors of the nose

16. Salivary gland malignancies

17. Melanoma

18. Cancer of the tongue

19. Squamous cell carcinoma of the ear

Answers: 15-B, 16-D, 17-D, 18-A, 19-D

Critique: Exposure to nickel, wood dust, or Thorotrast are major etiologic factors for malignant neoplasms of the nose. Cancer of the tongue is related to tobacco and alcohol usage. Exposure to solar radiation predisposes a patient to melanomas and squamous cell carcinoma of the ear.

Pages 465, 469, 1073

Questions 20–22. Match the following statements about congenital cysts of the neck with the most appropriate response from the list of lettered options. Each lettered response may be used once, more than once, or not at all.

A. Branchial cleft cyst
B. Thyroglossal duct cyst
C. Both A and B
D. Neither A nor B

20. Usually located immediately inferior to the hyoid bone

21. Usually located along the anterior border of the sternocleidomastoid

22. Usually becomes apparent after the first decade of life

Answers: 20-B, 21-A, 22-A

Critique: The branchial apparatus is a series of segmental arches separated by external grooves and internal pouches that develop during the fourth week of intrauterine life. Disorders in neonatal development can lead to the appearance of cysts, draining sinuses, or lymphatic vascular tumors. Branchial cleft cysts appear as smooth, round, nontender masses along the anterior border of the sternocleidomastoid muscle. They become apparent after the first decade of life when slow fluid accumulation or infection leads to their discovery. Thyroglossal duct cysts are usually located immediately inferior to the hyoid bone but can be located anywhere from the submental region to the suprasternal notch. These cysts typically become apparent as a painless, midline neck mass during the first decade of life.

Page 476

Questions 23–26. Oral problems may be a manifestation of systemic disease. Match each of the following clincial findings with the most likely associated systemic illness. Each lettered response may be used once, more than once, or not at all.

A. Diabetes mellitus
B. Ascorbic acid deficiency
C. Addison's disease

D. Acromegaly
E. Kwashiorkor

23. Swollen gingival tissue that bleeds easily

24. Dryness of the tongue and gingival hypertrophy

25. White or very dark-appearing mucosa

26. Acute necrotizing gingivitis with atrophy of papillae of the tongue

Answers: 23-B, 24-A, 25-C, 26-E

Critique: Diabetes mellitus frequently causes tongue dryness in addition to gingival bleeding, hypertrophy, and purple discoloration. Addison's disease often results in white or very dark-appearing oral mucosal pigmentation. Acromegaly causes mandibular hyperplasia and marked enlargement of the tongue. Ascorbic acid deficiency results in swollen gingival tissue that bleeds easily. Kwashiorkor, severe protein depletion, results in an acute necrotizing gingivitis, candidiasis, atrophy of the papillae of the tongue, and cracking of the skin at the angle of the mouth.

Page 468

Questions 27–30. Match each of the following numbered statements related to face and deep neck infections with the most likely involved deep neck or facial space. Each lettered response may be used once, more than once, or not at all.

A. Pharyngomaxillary space
B. Retropharyngeal space
C. Submandibular space
D. Parotid space
E. Masticator space

27. Refusal of food followed by fever and respiratory obstruction

28. Trismus and swelling over the angle of the mandible

29. Fever, sore throat, and pain on swallowing

30. Skin redness and fluctuance or swelling of the mouth and tongue

Answers: 27-B, 28-E, 29-A, 30-C

Critique: Infections in the deep neck are defined by bony structures and fascial envelopes. Most infections are caused by streptococcal species, but *Staphylococcus aureus* and anaerobes can be significant pathogens. Pharyngomaxillary space infections encompass the space bounded by the hyoid bone, the temporal bone, the lateral pharyngeal wall, and the mandible. Patients initially present with fever, sore throat, and pain on swallowing. Retropharyngeal space infections occur in tissues deep to the posterior pharyngeal well, including the nose, sinuses, and adenoids. Typical presentations for infections of the retropharyngeal space are refusal of food followed by fever and respiratory obstruction. Submandibular space infections are bound by the floor of the mouth and the

deep cervical fascia between the mandible and the hyoid bone. Presentations typically include redness of the skin and fluctuance or mouth and tongue swelling. Parotid space infections encompass the parotid gland. Masticator space infections occur just anterior to the pharyngomaxillary space. They present with trismus and swelling over the angle of the mandible.

Pages 475, 476

Questions 31–35 (True or False). An 8-year-old white male comes for evaluation after failing an audiometric screening test at school. His mother reports that he plays radios louder than others at home and that frequently he states that he does not hear well when people talk to him. Which of the following are risk factors for sensorineural hearing loss?

31. Gestational history of toxoplasmosis

32. Premature birth

33. Third-generation cephalosporin treament for septicemia

34. Mumps

35. Maternal thyrotoxicosis

Answers: 31-T, 32-T, 33-F, 34-T, 35-T

Critique: Sensorineural hearing loss in children may go undetected for years. Once detected, a work-up must be conducted to determine the cause. Maternal infections that can affect the fetus and cause hearing loss include rubella, cytomegalovirus, toxoplasmosis, influenza, syphilis, and herpes simplex types 1 and 2. Perinatal events producing hypoxia and hearing loss include placenta previa, abruptio placentae, prolonged difficult labor, nuchal or prolapsed cord, and prematurity. Aminoglycoside antibiotics destroy the hair cells and stria vascularis of the inner ear, producing an irreversible hearing loss. Postnatal viral infections caused by adenovirus, chickenpox, Epstein-Barr virus, herpes zoster oticus, influenza, measles, mumps, encephalitis, and viral hepatitis can cause hearing loss. Mumps is the leading cause of acquired unilateral sensorineural hearing loss in children. Maternal thyrotoxicosis, diabetes mellitus, and pseudohypoparathyroidism predispose the fetus to hearing damage.

Page 447

Questions 36–40 (True or False). A 48-year-old African-American woman presents to the clinic with tinnitus and hearing loss. Which of the following characteristics favor a diagnosis of Meniere's disease?

36. Occurs more commonly in men

37. Typically occurs around 65 years of age

38. Vertigo tends to lessen over time as hearing loss worsens.

39. Smoking cessation should reduce the frequency of attacks.

40. Frequently follows an episode of acute suppurative otitis media

Answers: 36-F, 37-F, 38-T, 39-T, 40-F

Critique: Meniere's disease describes the coexistence of recurrent vertigo, tinnitus, and hearing loss. It occurs most frequently in women around 50 years of age. Typically, the vertigo will lessen over time, while the hearing loss worsens due to the gradual destruction of the vestibular and cochlear receptor sites. Long-term management to reduce the frequency of attacks includes smoking cessation, decreased caffeine consumption, and a low-salt diet. Labyrinthitis, resulting from extension of infection within the temporal bone, and not Meniere's disease, is a complication of acute suppurative otitis media.

Pages 449, 450

Questions 41–45 (True or False). Which of the following statements are true concerning otitis media with effusion?

41. It usually develops secondary to obstruction of the eustachian tube, barotrauma, or radiotherapy.

42. It involves positive pressure within the middle ear.

43. It is the most common cause of hearing loss in children.

44. Eighty percent of patients with otitis media will be effusion free within 4 weeks.

45. Insertion of pressure-equalizing tubes is indicated for effusions lasting 3 months or more.

Answers: 41-T, 42-F, 43-T, 44-F, 45-T

Critique: Otitis media with effusion develops secondary to eustachian tube obstruction, barotrauma, or radiotherapy. The fluid may be either serous or mucoid. Its pathogenesis involves negative pressure within the middle ear, resulting in mucosal absorption of middle ear gas. Otitis media with effusion is the most common cause of hearing loss in children. Eighty percent of patients with otitis media with effusion will be effusion free within 2 months. If the effusion persists longer than 3 months, the insertion of pressure-equalizing tubes is indicated. Up to 20% of patients may require repeated placement of pressure-equalizing tubes.

Page 454

Questions 46–50 (True or False). Which of the following statements are true concerning presbycusis?

46. It is characterized by a bilateral, symmetrical, neurosensory hearing loss in frequencies above 2000 Hz.

47. Initially, only conversational speech is impaired.

48. There is difficulty in discriminating consonant sounds.

49. Two thirds of the population older than 65 years of age are significantly affected.

50. Hearing aids are not typically effective.

Answers: 46-T, 46-F, 48-T, 49-F, 50-F

Critique: Presbycusis results from aging of the auditory system. It results in a bilateral, symmetrical, neurosensory hearing loss in frequencies above 2000 Hz. Initially, conversation is not impaired because the speech frequencies of 500 to 2000 Hz are not involved. Patients complain of difficulty in understanding speech because of a decreased ability to discriminate consonants. Approximately one third of the population over 65 years of age has a significant impairment. Most individuals can be helped with a properly fitted hearing aid.

Page 460

Questions 51–55 (True or False). Which of the following are true statements about acute sinusitis?

51. Frequent swimming is a predisposing factor.

52. Streptococci are a common causative organism.

53. Maxillary sinusitis may cause tooth pain.

54. Ciprofloxacin is the treatment of choice.

55. Antral washings are usually necessary in the management of most cases.

Answers: 51-T, 52-T, 53-T, 54-F, 55-F

Critique: Acute sinusitis has multiple predisposing factors, including allergic rhinitis, deviated nasal septum, foreign body, and swimming. Systemic predisposing factors are diabetes, malnutrition, and blood dyscrasias. The most common causative organisms in adults are *Streptococcus pneumoniae* and *Haemophilus influenzae*. In children, *Moraxella catarrhalis* is another important causative organism. Maxillary sinusitis frequently results in maxillary toothaches. Amoxicillin or trimethoprim with sulfamethoxazole is effective against the majority of organisms. Amoxicillin with clavulanate (Augmentin), cefuroxime axetil (Ceftin), and second-generation macrolides are good alternative therapies. Antral washings are not necessary to treat acute sinusitis.

Pages 462, 463

Questions 56–60 (True or False). A 7-year-old white female reports swelling of her right parotid gland. Which of the following statements are true concerning salivary gland disease in children?

56. Viral parotitis is usually caused by the mumps virus.

57. Viral parotitis is most frequently complicated by pneumonia.

58. Purulent saliva drains from the parotid gland duct in viral parotitis.

59. Viral parotitis has a 7-day incubation period.

60. Encephalitis, orchitis, and deafness are important complications of viral parotitis.

Answers: 56-T, 57-F, 58-F, 59-F, 60-T

Critique: The most common cause of parotid gland swelling in children is mumps or viral parotitis. Mumps is a febrile illness resulting in painful parotid gland enlargement and a red punctum at the opening of the duct inside the cheek with clear saliva. The mumps virus usually causes viral parotitis, but echovirus and coxsackie virus A have been cultured. Mumps has an incubation period of 18 to 21 days post exposure. Encephalitis, orchitis, and deafness are important complications of viral parotitis; however, pneumonia is not a complication.

Page 477

24

Allergy

William Jorgenson

1. Of the four basic classifications of allergic reactions, the one resulting from an immunoglobulin (Ig)E-bound antibody complex is a:

    A. Type I reaction *IgE bound to mast or Basal cell.*
    B. Type II reaction
    C. Type III reaction
    D. Type IV reaction

Answer: A

Critique: All the aforementioned are listed in the Coombs and Gell classifications of allergic reactions, but only type I reactions involve the IgE complex bound to either mast cells or basophils. Type II and type III reactions involve circulatory IgG, IgM, and complement activation. Type IV reaction does not involve an antibody reaction but rather is based on sensitized T cells.

Page 481

2. The most common type of allergic rhinitis seen in the population of patients treated by family physicians is:

    A. Perennial allergic rhinitis
    B. Seasonal allergic rhinitis
    C. Rhinitis medicamentosa
    D. Vasomotor rhinitis

Answer: B

Critique: Allergic rhinitis is a common problem seen in primary care. When it occurs episodically and is frequently associated with seasonal changes and pollination, it is called seasonal allergic rhinitis. When symptoms are present on a more continuous basis, it is called perennial allergic rhinitis. Rhinitis medicamentosa and vasomotor rhinitis are neither inflammatory nor allergic diseases. Rhinitis medicamentosa is a chronic reactive vasodilatation caused by excessive use of topical decongestants. Perennial allergic rhinitis is seen in half as many patients younger than 20 years of age as in seasonal allergic rhinitis. Vasomotor rhinitis is a vasodilatation and secretory problem manifested by a physical or irritating trigger (i.e., cold air, odors, or smoke). Nonallergic rhinitis with eosinophilia (NARES) is another cause of perennial rhinitis but has no evidence of an allergic trigger or allergy by skin testing; however, eosinophils are present in nasal secretions.

Pages 462, 483–485

3. Which of the following measures, employed in a preventative mode for the management of chronic asthma, should be considered as foundation therapy for children and adults?

    A. Regular use of a peak flow meter
    B. Daily use of β_2-agonist
    C. Cromolyn sodium
    D. Glucocorticoid inhalation
    E. Ipratropium bromide inhalation

Answer: A

Critique: Monitoring peak flows is an important part of the management of chronic asthma in children and adults. Peak flow meters are inexpensive and afford the patient and physician the ability to assess pulmonary function on a regular basis. They can alert the individual to changes in pulmonary function that often occur prior to an acute exacerbation and before the need arises for urgent intervention. Daily use of β_2-agonists as primary therapy for chronic asthma is contraindicated. Overemphasis on these agents has been implicated recently in the increased mortality and morbidity associated with asthma. Cromolyn sodium is considered to be the drug of choice for children younger than 10 years of age. Glucocorticoid inhalations may be used in patients with chronic asthma older than 10 years of age, especially as an alternative to chronic oral steroids. Ipratropium bromide is most useful in patients with bronchospasm associated with chronic bronchitis and emphysema. Its beneficial effects in typical asthmatics is not clearly defined.

Pages 492–494

4. Symptoms of exercise-induced asthma include mild chest tightness, irritation, and cough. Individuals may wheeze overtly and become severely short of breath and disabled when severe hypoxia is present. The most useful method for evaluation of exercise-induced asthma in a primary care office is a(n):

A. Chest x-ray
B. Methacholine provocation test
C. Exercise challenge test
D. Treadmill exercise tolerance test
E. Arterial blood gas before and after exercise

Answer: C

Critique: In a primary care office setting, an exercise challenge test with pre and post exercise pulmonary function tests is a very reliable method to evaluate a patient suspected of having exercise-induced asthma. A decrease in the peak expiratory flow rate of 10% or a 12% decrease in forced expiratory volume in 1 second (FEV_1) is necessary to make the diagnosis. The chest x-ray may be of some use in newly diagnosed asthmatic patients but does not define exercise-induced asthma. The methacholine provocation test, which is an excellent test to exclude asthma in questionable cases, is time consuming and carries some risk. It is best left to specialty practices. The treadmill stress test is used mainly to evaluate patients with suspected coronary artery disease. Arterial blood gas measures are useful in monitoring severe asthmatic patients to assess the need for intubation and aggressive therapy.

Pages 482, 494

5. An evaluation of drug allergy can be best evaluated by:

A. Radioallergosorbent test (RAST)
B. Readministering a suspected drug
C. Leukocyte cytotoxicity
D. Lymphocyte stimulation test
E. Mast cell histamine release

Answer: B

Critique: In vivo testing is the most reliable method of evaluating clinical reactions due to drug allergy. The best method is to readminister the drug to see if the clinical reaction can be reproduced. Due to inherent risks, confirmation is usually not necessary unless treatment is essential or there is no alternative drug. In vitro tests, including RAST, lymphocyte stimulation tests, mast cell histamine release, and leukocyte cytotoxicity, are generally unreliable.

Page 501

6. Patients with the classic urticarial lesions that do not fade over a relatively short period of time (a few hours) are suspect for:

A. Acute urticaria
B. Chronic urticaria
C. Vasculitis
D. Food allergies
E. Allergic contact dermatitis

Answer: C

Critique: Normally urticaria resolves spontaneously over a short period of time. Whether acute or chronic,

the wheals appear rather abruptly and slowly fade over a few hours. Persistent lesions should raise the suspicion of an underlying vasculitis. Allergic contact dermatitis is a pruritic eruption that starts as erythema and progresses to a vesiculobullous lesion. It is mediated by a type IV reaction. Food allergies normally remain for 2 to 3 days.

Pages 497–499

7. Asthma is a reversible obstructive disorder of the tracheobronchial tree that is characterized by paroxysmal episodes of respiratory distress interspersed with periods of well-being. Asthma is also an inflammatory process involving all of the following EXCEPT:

A. Mucosal edema
B. Marked eosinophilia
C. Mucous production
D. Increased vascular permeability
E. Bronchial muscular contraction

Answer: B

Critique: Numerous biochemical mediators of inflammation have been identified as being important in the pathophysiology of asthma. They combine to produce the inflammatory changes that are characteristic of asthma, including mucosal edema, increased mucous production, and bronchial smooth muscle spasm. Eosinophilia, although common in asthmatics, is not a cardinal feature and its presence is not essential for the disease to manifest.

Page 487

8. A 16-year-old female presents with a history of intermittent acute asthma. Most of her attacks respond to a β-agonist administered via a meter-dosed inhaler. Additional information necessary to evaluate the severity of her asthma includes all of the following EXCEPT:

A. Frequency of attacks
B. Duration of an attack
C. Intensity of associated symptoms
D. Symptom-free interval
E. Family history of asthma or atopy

Answer: E

Critique: The clinical characteristics of acute asthma attacks are important parts of the history to obtain to confirm the diagnosis and assess the severity of the problem. All of the following—frequency, duration, intensity, symptom-free interval, and response to previous medication—are related to severity. A family history of asthma or atopy is common in individuals with asthma and may help with the diagnosis but does not provide any information about the severity of illness.

Page 488

9. Common food allergens include all of the following EXCEPT:

A. Milk
B. Eggs
C. Legumes

D. Shellfish
E. Disaccharides

Answer: E

Critique: Although any food is potentially allergenic, the most common ones include milk, eggs, nuts and legumes, shellfish and other fish, wheat, chocolate, and pork. The diagnosis of a food allergy depends primarily on the history. Avoidance is the mainstay of food "allergy" treatment. The "true" elimination diet is effective in both identifying the culprit food as well as in proving the return of symptoms when the food is reintroduced into the diet. Simple sugars and disaccharides are small molecules and are unlikely to be allergens; however, lactose can be a source of intolerance to milk and milk products.

Pages 502, 503

10. Symptomatic control of allergic rhinitis includes all of the following; however, use should be limited to no more than 3 days' duration for:

A. Antihistamines
B. Oral α-adrenergic drugs
C. Topical vasoconstrictors
D. Topical glucocorticoids
E. Normal saline nose spray

Answer: C

Critique: Use of topical vasoconstrictors is best limited to no more than 3 days consecutively to prevent rebound engorgement and rhinitis medicamentosa. Antihistamines are effective when used regularly during exacerbations and are best used prior to exposure. The effectiveness of antihistamines may be enhanced with concomitant use of oral α-adrenergic decongestants. Nasal glucocorticoids are effective for antihistamine failures but may take up to 3 weeks to exert an effect.

Page 485

11. Asthma in pregnancy improves in one third of patients; slightly more than one third remain the same; and less than one third worsen. Uncontrolled asthma leading to hypoxemia is a greater risk to the fetus than are any of the usual drugs used in the treatment of asthma. Of the following drugs used to treat asthma, which has NOT been established as safe in pregnancy?

A. β-Agonists
B. Theophylline
C. Cromolyn sodium
D. Antihistamines
E. Decongestants

Answer: E

Critique: Treatment of severe asthma in pregnancy is important to prevent hypoxemia. Therapy with theophylline has not been associated with teratogenicity. Cromolyn can be used safely to prevent asthma attacks. Certain antihistamines (i.e., diphenhydramine, tripelennamine, chlorpheniramine) can be used judiciously but should be used sparingly in the first trimester. Inhaled β-agonists can be used; however, in large doses or orally, β-agonists may theoretically affect uterine contractions. No decongestants have been established as safe during pregnancy, but pseudoephedrine is considered the safest oral decongestant of this group.

Page 495

Questions 12–15 (Matching). Match the following Coombs-Gell type of reaction with the corresponding clinical manifestation. Each option may be used once, more than once, or not at all.

A. Type I
B. Type II
C. Type III
D. Type IV

12. Serum sickness reaction

13. Anaphylaxis

14. Contact dermatitis

15. Transfusion reactions

16. Autoimmune hemolytic anemia

Answers: 12-C, 13-A, 14-D, 15-B, 16-B

Critique: The common clinical problems seen in primary care can be identified with the various types or classes of allergic reactions. This separation allows better understanding of the mechanisms of action as well as the antigen-antibody reaction involved. Serum sickness reactions are type III reactions involving circulating antigen-antibody complexes along with complement-induced tissue injury. Anaphylaxis, a type I reaction, is mediated through IgE antibodies. Contact dermatitis results from a cell-mediated type IV reaction. Transfusion reactions and autoimmune hemolytic anemias are type II reactions involving immune complexes bound to tissue and complement activation.

Page 482

Questions 16–19 (True or False). Features of allergic drug reactions include:

16. Prior exposure to the agent without an adverse effect

17. Frequent occurrence in a large portion of the population

18. Occurrence of a reaction several days after a subsequent exposure to the agent

19. Production of similar reactions by small quantities of the suspected drug

20. A wide range of clinical manifestations that are easily confused with side effects of the drug in question

Answers: 16-T, 17-F, 18-T, 19-T, 20-F

Critique: True drug interactions, although not seen routinely in primary care, are important just the same. Patient education and instruction on avoidance can be lifesaving. Patients need to realize that subsequent exposure to even small amounts of previous allergy-producing drugs can have disastrous consequences. Patients also need to know that allergic reactions may take some time to occur after a subsequent exposure. Usually the first exposure to the agent is not associated with any adverse effects. Drug reactions are usually restricted to a limited number of syndromes that are commonly accepted as allergic in nature and are distinct from other side effects of the drug.

Pages 501–503

Questions 20–24 (True or False). The clinical history is the most important component in the evaluation of a patient with a suspected allergic problem. The history should address common sources of allergens including:

20. Home heating

21. Pets

22. Household furnishings

23. Laundry detergents

24. Bedding

Answers: 20-T, 21-T, 22-T, 23-T, 24-T

Critique: A careful history of exposure to allergens common in both home and work environments is essential when evaluating the potentially allergic patient. In the home, heating ducts, pets, household furnishings, detergents, and bedding are all important areas to cover in detail. In the work environment, concern for air pollution, chemical irritation, physical demands, and job stresses are important.

Page 482

Questions 18–22. Match each of the following treatment strategies with the most appropriate lettered option. Each option may be used once, more than once, or not at all.

   A. Anaphylactic shock
   B. Cardiogenic shock
   C. Both A and B
   D. Neither A and B

18. Intubation if respiratory effort is compromised

19. Immediate administration of epinephrine

20. Administration of intravenous fluids to restore intravascular volume

21. Immediate administration of intravenous corticosteroids

22. Administration of intravenous dopamine to maintain blood pressure

Answers: 18-C, 19-A, 20-C, 21-D, 22-B

Critique: Anaphylactic shock is a life-threatening reaction that requires the immediate administration of epinephrine. Both anaphylactic shock and cardiogenic shock require stabilization and restoration of intravascular volume, airway management, and oxygenation. Intravenous diphenhydramine may be helpful to control angioedema in anaphylactic shock. Vasopressor agents used in the treatment of cardiogenic shock, such as dopamine, isoproterenol, or norepinephrine, are rarely required for anaphylactic shock. If intravenous fluids (sometimes several liters are required) do not restore blood pressure in anaphylactic shock, isoproterenol has advantages over other commonly used vasopressors because it is also a bronchodilator. Glucocorticoids may be beneficial to suppress a late-phase reaction in anaphylaxis; however, glucocorticoids are never indicated in the first few minutes of resuscitation.

Pages 500, 501

25

Parasitology and Travel Medicine

Victor S. Sierpina

1. Which of the following statements about parasitic diseases is correct?

 A. Asymptomatic infection does not need treatment.
 B. Parasitic infections are found primarily in developing countries.
 C. Parasitic infections are confined to lower socioeconomic classes.
 D. Water treatment and sanitation have decreased gastrointestinal parasitic infections.

Answer: D

Critique: Individuals unknowingly may harbor parasites; however, symptomatic and asymptomatic parasitic diseases should be treated because of the threat to public health. The public commonly, but incorrectly, assumes that parasitic diseases are confined to developing countries and lower socioeconomic classes. As much as 20% of the American population harbor some parasite. Public health management of water and sanitation has greatly reduced the number of gastrointestinal parasitic infections.

Page 506

2. Which of the following protozoans that inhabit the gastrointestinal tract produces clinical disease in immunocompetent hosts?

 A. *Cyclospora cayetanensis*
 B. *Isospora belli*
 C. *Enterocystozoon* species (*Microsporidium*)
 D. *Cryptosporidium parvum*

Answer: A

Critique: A number of protozoans can be found in stool; however, only four, *Entamoeba histolytica, Balantidium coli, Giardia lamblia,* and *Cryptosporidium parvum,* are significant pathogens in immunocompetent hosts. *C. cayetanensis, I. belli,* and *Enterocystozoon* species (*Microsporidium*) are pathogenic in immunosuppressed individuals.

Pages 506, 507

Questions 3–4. A 25-year-old female patient presents to your office with a 2-week history of abdominal bloating, flatulence, and diarrhea. She has no history of irritable bowel or other chronic medical conditions; however, she noted the onset of the symptoms about 1½ weeks after returning from a backpacking trip to Colorado where she drank water from a mountain stream.

3. Which of the following is the most likely diagnosis for her condition?

 A. Shigellosis
 B. Giardiasis
 C. Mercury toxicity
 D. Cryptosporidiosis

Answer: B

Critique: This is a classic example of water-borne diarrheal illness. The suspected water source of the probable infection as well as the incubation period suggest giardiasis. The other infections have less incubation time and present with more severe symptoms. Mercury toxicity is also more acute but seems less likely because of the postulated source of stream water.

Pages 507–509

4. Which of the following is an appropriate treatment for this condition?

 A. Loperamide 2 mg tid until symptoms resolve
 B. Amoxicillin 500 mg tid for 10 days
 C. Metronidazole 250 mg tid for 2 weeks
 D. Mebendazole 100 mg—single dose

Answer: C

Critique: Metronidazole is the treatment of choice for giardiasis in adults. Furazolidone is a good alternative in children. Paromomycin, a nonabsorbed aminoglycoside can be substituted in the case of pregnant women. Loperamide is used to control diarrhea and has no antimicrobial activity. Resistance has limited the usefulness of amoxicillin in treating bacterial pathogens. Mebendazole is effective in treating enterobiasis (pinworms).

Pages 508, 515

5. Which one of the following results from an infected intermediate host that is a source of food for humans?

    A. Giardiasis
    B. Amebiasis
    C. Cryptosporidiosis
    D. Taeniasis

pork tapeworm Taenia solium

Answer: D

Critique: Taeniasis is transmitted through infected meat, generally pork, which has ingested the ova. The organism then develops in the pig and is introduced into the human gut when the infected, undercooked pork is ingested. The other organisms are water-borne infections, and although an intermediate host may be involved (e.g., Giardia), it is not required.

Pages 507, 508, 511–512

6. Which of the following is the causative organism in cysticercosis?

    A. *Ascaris lumbricoides*
    B. *Entamoeba histolytica*
    C. *Taenia solium*
    D. *Enterobius vermicularis*

Answer: C

Critique: Cysticercosis, the larval stage of *T. solium* (pork tapeworm), results from the migration of oncospheres to various body tissues. The organism is endemic in many areas of the world. Central and South American reservoirs are important sources of disease in the United States in immigrants and close contacts. Clinical manifestations depend on the tissue involved. Neurocysticercosis is the most important clinical condition caused by *T. solium*. It is a common cause of adult onset seizures in endemic areas.

Page 511

7. A mother brings her 4-year-old child in for examination because she notes that the child is scratching around her anus and complaining of itching. On physical examination, you notice some superficial excoriations in the perirectal region but no other significant findings. The child appears alert and healthy. Which one the following is commonly used to confirm the diagnosis?

    A. Scotch tape test
    B. Two-week clinical trial of mebendazole
    C. Stool for ova and parasites
    D. Anoscopy

Answer: A

Critique: Based on the history, the most likely diagnosis is pinworms. This can be easily and inexpensively diagnosed with the application of Scotch tape on the perianal area at night with application to a microscope slide the next morning. The ova of *Enterobius vermicularis* are easily visible on the slide. Both pyrantel pamoate and mebendazole are effective for killing adult worms.

Page 516

8. A 42-year-old man, who recently returned from a 3-month religious sabbatical to India, comes to your office with a jar containing a worm that he passed in his stool. This specimen is about 1 foot long. He has had episodes of abdominal pain and cramps since returning from his trip. Of the following all are true EXCEPT:

    A. The specimen is most likely to be *Ascaris lumbricoides.*
    B. Treatment usually requires combination therapy with mebendazole.
    C. Bowel perforation is the most common gastrointestinal complication.
    D. This parasite is frequently an opportunistic infection in patients with acquired immunodeficiency syndrome (AIDS).

Answer: A

Critique: The description of the size of worm, the probable area of infection, and the symptoms certainly suggest ascariasis. Ascariasis is estimated by the World Health Organization (WHO) to be the most common parasitic disease in the world. Mebendazole, pyrantel pamoate, and levamisole are commonly used as single agents for therapy and yield cure rates of at least 80%. Intestinal obstruction is a serious complication in heavy infestations. Perforation, leading to peritonitis or abscess, can occur but is an uncommon event. Although ascariasis may occur in persons with AIDS, it is not particularly associated with this disease nor is it considered to be an opportunistic infection.

Pages 516–518

9. Which one of the following organisms can be associated with coughing, wheezing, and hypersensitivity pneumonitis?

    A. *Enterobius vermicularis*
    B. *Ascaris lumbricoides*
    C. *Pediculus humanus humanus*
    D. *Giardia lamblia*
    E. *Balantidium coli*

Answer: B

Critique: Of the gastrointestinal pathogens listed, *A. lumbricoides* is the only one known to leave the gut and infect other tissue. *A. lumbricoides* is well known to migrate to the lungs, where it induces a hypersensitivity reaction and asthmatic attacks. Pulmonary infiltrates can be seen on x-ray, and the patient may have a cough, bloody sputum, dyspnea, fever, and other systemic signs. *P. humanus humanus,* the common body lice, is an ectoparasite and does not infect the pulmonary system.

Pages 516–518

Questions 10–12. A 40-year-old grade school teacher presents to your office with a complaint of intense itching. The areas of the skin that are affected include the hands, under the breasts, and along the waistline. An examination reveals small papulovesicular lesions in the interdigital webs of the fingers and marked excoriations of several areas with erythema.

10. The differential diagnosis could include all of the following EXCEPT:

    A. Dyshidrotic eczema
    B. Contact dermatitis
    C. Scabies
    D. Pityriasis rosea

Answer: D

Critique: Although the clinical description suggests scabies, both dyshidrotic eczema and contact dermatitis can present as intensely pruritic and papulovesicular dermatoses. Pityriasis rosea is a macular rash with oval, salmon-colored, truncal lesions that can be scaly and pruritic but not vesicular.

11. Which one of the following would help to confirm the most likely diagnosis in this patient?

    A. A KOH scraping of the skin
    B. A skin biopsy
    C. Unroofing a lesion and checking a sample under the microscope for parasites
    D. A Wood light examination

Answer: C

Critique: A scabies infestation is characterized by burrows that contain the offending organism and its feces. This creates the intensely pruritic lesions in the dermis. Placing mineral oil on the site and then scraping it with a scalpel onto a microscope slide is often diagnostic. The KOH and Wood light examination are helpful in fungal infections of the skin, which this does not resemble. A skin biospy is more helpful in longer-standing, undiagnosed dermatoses.

12. Pleased with your rapid diagnosis and effective treatment of the patient's condition (noted in the previous question), this same teacher returns a few weeks later with a complaint of "dandruff." On examining her hair and scalp, you note a number of whitish, tan-colored flecks adhering to her hair strands. The scalp itself is neither peeling or scaling. Which of the following would you recommend as part of the management of this problem?

    A. Comb out her hair with a fine-toothed comb.
    B. Use an over-the-counter preparation for dandruff.
    C. Use 1% hydrocortisone lotion on the scalp.
    D. Consultation with a dermatologist.

Answer: A

Critique: Because the scalp is not scaling, dandruff or the more accurate diagnosis of seborrheic dermatitis is not present here. The fact that the lesions are located on the hair shafts is indicative of head lice. The nits should be combed out with a fine-toothed comb, and a single application of shampoo containing permethrin or lindane is generally curative. The treatment of this common condition is well within the realm of a family physician and does not require a referral.

Pages 518, 519

13. Proper prophylaxis regimens for malaria in chloroquine-resistant areas of the world include:

    A. Pyrimethamine-sulfadoxine (Fansidar) 3 tablets weekly for 8 weeks
    B. Mefloquine (Lariam) 250 mg/wk starting 1 week prior and continuing 4 weeks after travel
    C. Sulfamethoxazole-trimethoprim (Septra) 1 tablet daily for the course of the travel
    D. Ciprofloxacin (Cipro) 500 mg bid starting 1 week before travel and continuing for 4 weeks after travel.

Answer: B

Critique: With the emergence of chloroquine-resistant malarial organisms in many areas of the world, it is essential to check a recent source such as the Centers for Disease Control and Prevention (CDC) Yellow Book for recommendations for malarial prophylaxis in many countries. With the exception of the Middle East, western Central America, Haiti, and the Dominican Republic, chloroquine resistance is common and mefloquine is becoming the drug of choice for prophylaxis.

Pages 524, 525

14. A 45-year-old woman presents to your office with a history of abdominal cramping and bloody diarrhea for the last 3 days. On further questioning, she tells you that she had been on a 2-week vacation touring Mexico and Central America. She occasionally ate some of the local foods, especially fresh fruits and salads, but was careful about her drinking water. She has felt well for the past month after returning from her trip until the current symptoms started 3 days ago. She has no other history of travel or exposures to infectious agents. Of the following organisms, which one is most likely to cause her symptoms?

    A. Norwalk virus
    B. Enterotoxigenic *Escherichia coli*
    C. *Salmonella* species
    D. *Giardia lamblia*
    E. *Entamoeba histolytica*

Answer: E

Critique: All of these agents have been associated with traveler's diarrhea; however, the long incubation time and the bloody stool make the *Amoeba* the most likely culprit. The virus and bacterial species listed would have a much earlier presentation. *Giardia* also incubates more quickly and is rarely the cause of bloody diarrhea. In a case in which the history does not narrow the number of organisms, empirical treatment may make the patient more comfortable while awaiting laboratory results. An antidiarrheal such a loperamide, imodium, or bismuth subsalicylate would be useful in the absence of blood. A reasonable additional therapy would be an antibiotic to cover the bacterial pathogens, most commonly *E. coli.* Currently, ciprofloxacin is considered to be the antibiotic of choice for this organism, and it will also cover *Shigella.* Sulfamethoxazole-trimethoprim or doxycycline are traditional and cheaper alternative therapies. If the stool specimen showed a parasite, the treatment could be revised to include specific therapy for the identified organism.

Page 525

Questions 15–18 (True or False). A 33-year-old woman arrives in your office with a 1-year history of abdominal pain and diarrhea, which has recently been increasing in intensity. Her past history includes admission to the hospital 1 year ago for dehydration due to *Cryptosporidium.* Her social history is notable in that her husband died 5 years ago of a "lymphoma."

The physical examination reveals patchy white lesions on the oral mucosa and epigastric and midabdominal tenderness to palpation. The examination is otherwise unremarkable. Which of the following tests is pertinent to the evaluation of this patient's abdominal pain and diarrhea?

15. Stool examination for ova and parasites

16. Stool culture and sensitivity

17. Complete blood count (CBC) and blood chemistry profile

18. Human immunodeficiency virus (HIV) antibody

Answers: 15-T, 16-T, 17-T, 18-T

Critique: The 1-year persistence of diarrhea with a history of *Cryptosporidium* suggests an immunocompromised patient. The social history of death from lymphoma of her spouse points to a possible risk factor. (Did her husband die of primary lymphoma or was it associated with AIDS?) Another opportunistic infection (*Candida*) really builds the case further for an immunocompromised host. In fact, this actual case study did show a persistent *Cryptosporidium* infection in a patient who was HIV-positive and died of complications of AIDS within the year.

Page 509

Questions 19–22 (True or False). A 3-year-old Hispanic child is brought to your office by his mother. Through a translator, you learn that the child moved from Mexico to the United States at 1 year of age. According to the mother, he has always been healthy; however, he has not done well in the past year. He has seemed irritable and has had episodes of nausea, vomiting, and diarrhea. He seems tired frequently and is not growing as well as his brothers did when they were the same age. On examination you note a smaller-than-average child, with pale nailbeds and conjunctiva. His abdomen seems diffusely tender, although without localization. An evaluation of this child should include:

19. Complete blood count

20. Tuberculosis (TB) skin test

21. Stool for ova and parasites

22. Computed tomography (CT) scan of the abdomen

Answers: 19-T, 20-T, 21-T, 22-F

Critique: This child certainly has the potential for a number of conditions. A good history and physical examination can be supplemented by appropriate testing including the CBC, TB skin test, and stool for ova and parasites. The systemic symptoms suggest a rather generalized process, and the history of moving from a Third World country widens the differential from what one might usually expect. A CT scan of the abdomen at this time would not be helpful or cost-effective.

Page 517

Questions 23–26 (True or False). In the preceding case history, organisms that could be identified in the stool and that could explain this child's illness include:

23. *Ascaris lumbricoides*

24. *Entamoeba histolytica*

25. *Isospora belli*

26. *Taenia solium*

Answers: 23-T, 24-T, 25-F, 26-T

Critique: *A. lumbricoides, E. histolytica,* and *T. solium* are endemic in Third World areas and can cause constitutional symptoms. *I. belli* is a benign commensal and would not be considered abnormal in the stool.

Pages 506, 507, 511, 517

Questions 27–31 (True or False). Reasons why a patient might come in for an evaluation prior to foreign travel include which of the following?

27. To update routine and special immunizations

28. For advice about risk factors endemic in the area of travel

29. For prophylactic medications (e.g., for diarrhea or malaria)

30. To review current medical problems and medications prior to travel

31. To obtain a referral for medical care overseas in case of an emergency

Answers: 27-T, 28-T, 29-T, 30-T, 31-T

Critique: Although there are a multitude of possibilities for which a physician might be consulted prior to travel, all of the aforementioned are typical issues. Examples of other reasons for a pre-travel visit could include a prescription for sleeping medication, such as triazolam (Halcion), zolipidem tartrate (Ambien), melatonin, to help deal with jet lag, various certificates of health and immunization, discussion of protection from the sun, and education about behavioral measures to avoid traveler's diarrhea.

Pages 521–525

Questions 32–35 (True or False). A 50-year-old executive comes to your office for a pre-travel examination. He is planning a business trip to Mexico that is critical to his company. He will be visiting potential factory sites in remote areas. Appropriate steps at this time include:

32. Prescribe ciprofloxacin 500 mg qd for the course of his trip.

33. Start malaria prophylaxis 1 week prior to his departure.

34. Provide a list of safe foods and beverages for prevention of traveler's diarrhea.

35. Administer hepatitis B vaccine.

Answers: 32-T, 33-T, 34-T, 35-F

Critique: Generally, a pre-travel visit can include a risk assessment and counseling for risk reduction as well as appropriate preventive and therapeutic measures. In this case, the patient is on a "critical" mission and cannot afford to be sick during his stay. Thus, prophylactic antibiotics can be started along with the other measures. Hepatitis A prophylaxis in the form of immunoglobulin or hepatitis A vaccine could also be given. Hepatitis B is not likely to be a high-risk issue, even if he could get the series of three injections in time.

Pages 521, 524–526

Questions 36–39 (True or False). True statements about his trip include:

36. Tap water and ice made from tap water are safe for consumption.

37. Mexico is a high-risk country for traveler's diarrhea.

38. Loperamide can be used safely if there is blood in the stool.

39. Immune serum globulin may be administered to prevent hepatitis A.

Answers: 36-F, 37-T, 38-F, 39-T

Critique: Mexico is certainly a high-risk area for traveler's diarrhea. The need for clear-cut counseling regarding items such as ice and tap water is especially important for this patient's safety. Although loperamide can be helpful to treat diarrhea, a bloody stool indicates a more serious inflammation (e.g., amebiasis or shigellosis) and needs definitive treatment. Loperamide may worsen these conditions. Immune serum globulin is effective in preventing hepatitis A. If time allows, hepatitis A vaccine can be administered.

Page 525

Questions 40–44 (True or False). Safe foods or beverages for prevention of traveler's diarrhea include:

40. Beer or wine

41. Freshly peeled fruits

42. Well-cooked meats and fish, hot on serving

43. Green salads

44. Bread or crackers

Answers: 40-T, 41-F, 42-T, 43-F, 44-T

Critique: It is very important for travelers to understand the concept of what is and is not a safe food. Selected examples are often the best way to convey that information. In this list, bottled beverages and cooked and dry foods are good examples of safe foods. Moist materials such as peeled fruits (unpeeled are safe) and fresh vegetables have a significant risk of carrying and conveying infected organisms such as *Escherichia coli*, amoebas, giardia, and other bacteria, viruses, or parasites.

Page 525

26

Obstetrics

Bill G. Gegas

1. Post-pill amenorrhea that lasts longer than 6 months occurs in:

    A. Less than 1% of women
    B. Approximately 10% of women
    C. Approximately 40% of women
    D. Approximately 60% of women

Answer: A

Critique: Many women are concerned about the effects of oral contraceptives on their menstrual cycle and fertility. Prolonged (greater than 6 months) amenorrhea occurs in fewer than 1% of women who have used contraceptives.

Page 529

2. The preconception control of hyperglycemia results in:

    A. Lower rates of spontaneous abortion
    B. Reduction in macrosomia
    C. Reduction in stillbirths
    D. All of the above

Answer: D

Critique: In addition to the aforementioned benefits, one study has found that preconception control of hyperglycemia is also related to a reduction in congenital malformations.

Page 529

3. When a pregnant woman contracts rubella in the first trimester, prospective studies have demonstrated that the risk of fetal anomalies is:

    A. 25%
    B. 50%
    C. 75%
    D. 100%

Answer: A

Critique: Rubella infections during pregnancy can result in stillbirths, spontaneous abortion, or congenital rubella syndrome. The risk of fetal anomalies is 25% if the mother is infected in the first trimester, compared with less than 1% if the mother is infected in the second trimester.

Page 530

4. The risk of spina bifida and other neural tube defects can be reduced by consuming:

    A. Niacin
    B. Thiamine
    C. Ascorbic acid (vitamin C)
    D. Folic acid

Answer: D

Critique: The Centers for Disease Control and Prevention (CDC) recommended in 1993 that all women of childbearing age who are capable of becoming pregnant consume 0.4 mg/day of folic acid. In addition, women with a history of neural tube defects in previous pregnancies should begin taking 4 mg/day of folic acid at least 1 month prior to conception and during the first 3 months of pregnancy.

Page 531

5. Extreme obesity increases the risk of:

    A. Gestational diabetes
    B. Hypertension
    C. Macrosomia
    D. All of the above

Answer: D

Critique: In addition to diabetes, hypertension, and macrosomia, the obese woman is also at increased risk for dysfunctional labor and shoulder dystocia.

Page 534

6. The risk of oligohydramnios increases when the total amniotic fluid index (the cumulative measurement of fluid pockets from all four quadrants by ultrasound) is less than:

    A. 5 cm
    B. 6 cm

C. 7 cm

D. 8 cm

Answer: A

Critique: An amniotic fluid index (AFI) of less than 5 cm is indicative of oligohydramnios, which may signal a maternal or fetal complication. Further investigation or testing is recommended.

Page 536

7. Uterine evacuation by sharp curettage may result in dense uterine synechiae, causing amenorrhea. This is known as:

A. Kallmann's syndrome

B. Meigs' syndrome

C. Asherman's syndrome

D. McCune-Albright syndrome

Answer: C

Critique: Asherman's syndrome can be a complication of sharp curettage and is less commonly seen now due to vacuum curettage techniques. Kallmann's syndrome is primary amenorrhea secondary to inadequate release of gonadotropin-releasing hormone. Meigs' syndrome is the triad of ovarian tumors, ascites, and hydrothorax. McCune-Albright syndrome is the association of fibrous dysplasia of the skeletal system with cutaneous pigmentation and precocious pubertal development. It is an endocrinologic disorder that is more common in girls.

8. Herpes gestationis is a disease of late pregnancy and the puerperium that results in severe pruritus and widespread ulcerations of the skin. The etiology is:

A. Unknown

B. Herpes simplex I

C. Herpes simplex II

D. Epstein-Barr virus

Answer: A

Critique: Herpes gestationis is a poorly named disease of unknown etiology but is not caused by the herpes virus. Accurate diagnosis may require a skin biopsy, and the condition may be severe enough to warrant terminating the pregnancy.

Page 539

9. All pregnant women should undergo screening for gestational diabetes by giving them a 50-g glucose load when they are between 26 and 28 weeks' gestation. These patients should undergo a 3-hour glucose tolerance test if the 1-hour blood glucose is greater than:

A. 120 mg/dl

B. 125 mg/dl

C. 130 mg/dl

D. 135 mg/dl

Answer: D

Critique: All women should undergo a 3-hour glucose tolerance test if the 1-hour blood glucose is greater than 135 mg/dl. If the 3-hour test is abnormal, immediate counseling regarding diet is indicated and high-risk care should be initiated.

Page 544

10. "Rhinitis of pregnancy" is a particularly troublesome condition for many pregnant women. The etiology of this nasal and sinus congestion is:

A. Viral

B. Bacterial

C. Hormonal

D. Allergic

Answer: C

Critique: Estrogen induces hyperemia of all mucous membranes and may cause partial blockage of the nasal passages and sinuses, even without infection or underlying allergies.

Page 545

11. Neonates of women who have active hepatitis B or are chronic carriers should, at birth, receive:

A. First dose of hepatitis vaccine only

B. Hepatitis B hyperimmune globulin only

C. Both hepatitis vaccine and hyperimmune globulin

D. Both hepatitis vaccine and interferon therapy

Answer: C

Critique: There is evidence that the combination of hepatitis vaccine and hyperimmune globulin given to the neonate shortens the disease and prevents carrier status of hepatitis B. Interferon has no role in this condition.

Page 545

12. The Bishop method for scoring the cervix consists of five parameters, which are given a value from 0 to 3. This method allows the clinician to distinguish a very unfavorable cervix for induction from a more favorable one. A score that is considered to be highly favorable for induction is:

A. 6

B. 7

C. 8

D. 9

Answer: D

Critique: Factors included in the Bishop scoring system of the cervix are dilatation, effacement, station, consistency, and position of the cervical os. A score of 9 or greater is highly favorable for induction.

Page 548

13. A nonstress test is a noninvasive technique for monitoring the fetus. If the fetus does not respond, it is considered to be nonreactive, which may suggest fetal sleep or fetal compromise. A nonreactive test:

A. Should be followed by immediate cesarean section

B. Should be followed by amniocentesis
C. Should be followed by transfer of the patient to a center that treats high-risk cases
D. Should be repeated in 8 hours

Answer: D

Critique: A nonreactive nonstress test should be repeated in 8 hours and, if still nonreactive, the patient should undergo a biophysical profile. Although the other options may eventually be needed, they would not be the initial course of action.

Page 550

14. Intrauterine growth retardation is defined as a weight:

A. Below the 10th percentile of expected weight by ultrasound
B. Below the 20th percentile of expected weight by ultrasound
C. Below the 30th percentile of expected weight by ultrasound
D. Below the 40th percentile of expected weight by ultrasound

Answer: A

Critique: Estimated fetal weight by ultrasound requires measurements of the biparietal diameter, head and abdominal circumference, and femur length. A weight below the 10th percentile of expected weights for the population suggests intrauterine growth retardation.

Page 552

15. Cocaine usage is associated with an increase in the frequency of:

A. Placenta previa
B. Multiple gestation
C. Abruptio placentae
D. Ectopic pregnancy

Answer: C

Critique: Placental abruption is seen with increased frequency in women who use cocaine. Women with an abruption should be considered for drug screening. The other choices are not associated with cocaine usage.

Page 551

16. The most common cause of postpartum hemorrhage in the first 4 to 6 hours is:

A. Cervical laceration
B. Uterine relaxation
C. Uterine rupture
D. Retained placenta

Answer: B

Critique: The most common cause of postpartum hemorrhage in the first 4 to 6 hours is uterine relaxation. Uterine rupture is rare, and although lacerations and retained placental fragments do occur, they should be considered after massage and oxytocic agents have been tried.

Page 563

17. The most common cause of uterine inversion is:

A. Precipitous delivery
B. Multiple gestation
C. Excessive traction on the umbilical cord
D. Fundal pressure applied during delivery

Answer: C

Critique: Spontaneous inversion of the uterus almost never occurs, and in virtually all cases this condition is due to excessive traction on the umbilical cord. The condition is corrected by immediately replacing the uterus. The other choices are not predisposing causes of inversion.

Page 565

27

Care of the Newborn

Camille Leugers

1. Which of the following screening blood tests to identify congenital diseases or illness would be meaningless if collected immediately after delivery?

    A. Assay for phenylalanine
    B. Thyroid-stimulating hormone (TSH)
    C. Blood glucose
    D. Serologic test for syphilis

Answer: A

Critique: The use of routine neonatal thyroid screening tests (T_4 or TSH) in developed countries has significantly decreased the morbidity associated with undiagnosed congenital hypothyroidism. Routine syphilis serology should be performed in all infants, although positive results may not reflect disease in the infant. Blood phenylalanine levels are used to screen for phenylketonuria, but it is important that screening occur after the infant has had a milk feeding to avoid a false-negative result.

Pages 584–586

2. With few exceptions, all mothers should be encouraged to breast-feed. Counseling about breast-feeding prior to the mother being discharged from the hospital may improve success. Which of the following suggestions would you make to a new mother to help her breast-feed successfully?

    A. Maternal anxiety or nervousness should not affect lactation.
    B. Premature babies may not be able to suck actively enough to stimulate lactation and should be formula-fed instead.
    C. Supplemental feedings should be encouraged in the first few days of life in order to prevent dehydration.
    D. Feeding on demand is better than scheduled feedings.

Answer: D

Critique: In most cases, confident mothers have no problems nursing healthy babies. Demand feeding is recommended to match the milk supply with the infant's need and to minimize the infant's frustration. Babies with health problems, such as prematurity, may not suck actively enough to stimulate lactation through the release of prolactin; however, the use of a breast pump may stimulate lactation and allow the challenged neonate to receive the benefits of colostrum from expressed milk via tube feedings if needed. Supplemental feedings with formula may decrease the chance of successful breast-feeding and should be discouraged. Expressed and stored breast milk is an excellent alternative when direct breast-feeding is not possible.

Pages 591, 592

3. Ms. P. is a 28-year-old G_3P_3 who delivered a healthy, full-term baby girl 2 weeks ago. She is a single parent and has two older children who are 4 and 5 years of age and who live at home with her. Her fiancé also resides in the home and is a first-time parent. This is a fussy baby, unlike her first two children who the mother describes as easy-going. She has not established a good routine of breast-feeding yet. Ms. P. is somewhat frustrated and admits to bouts of tearfulness, especially when the baby cries. She has heard of various remedies for colic and wonders what to do about it. The infant weighed 4100 g at birth and now weighs 4300 g. Which of the following options would be the most appropriate approach at this time?

    A. Advise that she stops breast-feeding because of the infant's poor weight gain.
    B. Advise the parents to start the infant on an over-the-counter remedy for colic.
    C. Explore each parent's understanding of colic and how each parent deals with the infant's crying spells.
    D. Advise the mother that her crying spells may be negatively affecting her baby.
    E. Prescribe an antidepressant for unresolved post-partum depression.

Answer: C

Critique: The infant's weight gain at this point is not worrisome and should not be a reason to discontinue breast-feeding. Colic is poorly understood pathophysiologically, and no pharmacologic remedy offers consistent relief. It is important to explore the parents' concerns about colic and investigate the possibility of an abusive response to crying. While post-partum depression is common, it does not imply poor maternal-infant bonding or incapacity. Symptoms of post-partum depression should be explored further, and the new mother should be encouraged to report worsening or persistent symptoms. Treatment at this time is not warranted.

Pages 591, 592

4. Mr. L. is the father of a 3-week-old male infant, whom you saw last week at a routine 2-week visit. The infant had regained his birthweight and was settling into a comfortable routine. Today the father calls and reports that on awakening from a nap the infant's rectal temperature is 100° F. You should advise the father to:

    A. Unbundle the child for 20 minutes, recheck the temperature, and report this to the nurse.
    B. Bring the child in for a visit this morning.
    C. Report to the hospital for direct admission and a sepsis work-up.
    D. Give an appropriate dose of acetaminophen and recheck the temperature in 2 hours.

Answer: B

Critique: Fever in the neonatal period is extremely important and should not be managed over the telephone. Unbundling the child in your office, in addition to taking a thorough history and doing a thorough examination, is prudent. A temperature that resolves with unwrapping the infant, in the case of an infant who is feeding well, behaving normally, and has a normal physical examination, can be managed with observation. If the temperature has not resolved with unbundling, a thorough laboratory investigation is required, and management should be based on a repeat examination and results of laboratory tests. Infants are often admitted to the hospital for empirical antibiotic therapy pending culture results.

Pages 592, 593

5. Which one of the following statements is correct regarding resuscitation of the infant with meconium-stained amniotic fluid?

    A. Suctioning should be done as rapidly as possible because the neonate is more sensitive to hypoxia than is the adult.
    B. Suctioning efforts should be abandoned once the infant has begun breathing.
    C. "Terminal" passage of meconium presents the greatest risk for meconium aspiration syndrome in the neonate.
    D. Sudden deterioration in a meconium-stained baby should prompt investigation of a pulmonary air leak.

Answer: D

Critique: The ball-valve action of meconium in the airways can lead to the development of an air leak and

pneumothorax. Deterioration of an infant with meconium staining should suggest the possibility of these complications. Suctioning should be done thoroughly, preferably prior to stimulating the respiratory gasp, because the neonate is less sensitive to hypoxia than is the adult. The trade-off between prolonged hypoxia and decreased risk of meconium aspiration syndrome favors suctioning. Suctioning should continue even if the infant has begun to breathe. About 10% of deliveries are complicated by meconium in amniotic fluid, but the passage of meconium terminally in the birth process presents the least risk for an adverse outcome.

Page 595

6. Which one of the following statements regarding the ventilation of a neonate during resuscitation is correct?

    A. Initial oxygen concentrations should be as low as possible while monitoring oxygenation in the neonate.
    B. The ventilatory rate should be approximately 50 breaths/min.
    C. Bag-and-mask ventilation should be used in infants in whom diaphragmatic hernia is suspected.
    D. Intubation should be the initial goal in resuscitation of the apneic neonate.

Answer: B

Critique: Initial use of 100% oxygen at a ventilatory rate of 50 breaths/min via bag-and-mask is recommended. Oxygen concentration can be diminished, as resuscitative efforts continue, guided by monitoring the neonate, to lessen the risk of retrolental fibroplasia and bronchopulmonary dysplasia. Intubation should be used in an infant with a scaphoid abdomen, suggesting a diaphragmatic hernia to prevent air from entering the gut and making pulmonary ventilation even more difficult. Otherwise, bag-and-mask ventilation is the choice in initial resuscitative efforts.

Pages 595, 596

7. Which of the following is one of the most common causes of bleeding in an otherwise well newborn?

    A. Disseminated intravascular coagulation
    B. Consumptive thrombocytopenia
    C. Vitamin K deficiency
    D. Liver failure

Answer: C

Critique: Disseminated intravascular coagulation, consumptive thrombocytopenia, and liver failure are the most frequent causes of bleeding in the ill newborn. The most common causes of bleeding in the healthy newborn are immune thrombocytopenia, vitamin K deficiency, hemophilia, and anatomic vascular anomalies.

Page 604

8. Which of the following is characteristic of physiologic jaundice?

    A. It occurs in fewer than 20% of all full-term babies.
    B. It typically presents on the first post-partum day.

C. Peak bilirubin levels occur within 1 week.
D. Unconjugated bilirubin levels over 20 mg/dl are commonly observed in full-term infants with physiologic jaundice.

Answer: C

Critique: Physiologic jaundice is common and occurs in half of full-term infants and more than half of premature infants. It peaks and recedes within the first week of life. Unconjugated bilirubin levels exceeding 15 mg/dl constitute exaggerated physiologic jaundice. Jaundice presenting in the first 24 hours of life is not physiologic and should prompt further investigation.

Pages 604, 605

9. You have just delivered a 3300-g female infant with a 5-minute Apgar score of 8 because of central cyanosis that has persisted for 25 minutes. The infant is crying, moving vigorously, and otherwise looks well. This may be a physiologic finding, but you are concerned about a number of more serious causes of central cyanosis in this infant, including all of the following EXCEPT:

A. Sepsis
B. Heart failure
C. Choanal atresia
D. Polycythemia

Answer: C

Critique: Causes of persistent central cyanosis are numerous and are the result of the presence of 3 g/dl or more of unsaturated hemoglobin in arterial blood. Central cyanosis persisting for longer than 20 minutes in a noncrying infant is not physiologic; potential causes include polycythemia, right-to-left shunting, methemoglobinemia, and heart failure. Choanal atresia is characterized by central cyanosis that paradoxically clears with crying.

Pages 571, 572

10. Neonatal resuscitation differs from adult resuscitation in several ways. A solid understanding of these differences is important in order to successfully care for the critically ill neonate. All of the following statements regarding neonatal resuscitation are true EXCEPT:

A. Rapid volume expansion is critical in restoring neonatal cardiac output.
B. Vascular access is more easily obtained in the newborn than in the adult.
C. Supplemental oxygen must be administered more carefully to prevent hyperoxemia.
D. Arterial blood gas determinations may be more difficult to obtain, and acceptable sampling sites differ.

Answer: A

Critique: Because stroke volume is relatively fixed in the neonate, volume expansion to increase preload will not have a significant effect on cardiac output. In addition, rapid volume expansion can cause dilatation of the ductus arteriosus or periventricular hemorrhage in the prema-

ture infant. Vascular access is readily available in the newborn through the umbilical artery or vein. Care must be taken to avoid hyperoxemia, especially in premature infants. Even brief periods may lead to retrolental fibroplasia and blindness. Arterial gases are sometimes difficult to obtain in the newborn. Brachial and femoral arteries should be avoided.

Pages 594, 595

Questions 11 and 12. You are called to the newborn nursery to examine a jittery, irritable infant who is now 18 hours old. She was born by elective repeat cesarean section to a 32-year-old G_2P_2 woman whose prenatal course was remarkable only for poor weight gain and cigarette smoking. The infant's blood glucose is normal, but a drug screen shows the presence of cocaine.

11. Other symptoms of cocaine withdrawal in the neonate include all of the following EXCEPT:

A. Sedation
B. Seizures
C. Diarrhea
D. Diaphoresis
E. Vomiting

12. Which one of the following substances does **NOT** cause the drug withdrawal syndrome described above?

A. Alcohol
B. Phenytoin
C. Phenobarbital
D. Benzodiazepines
E. Narcotics

Answers: 11-A, 12-B

Critique: Seizures, diarrhea, diaphoresis, vomiting, hyperventilation, and hypertonicity can all be seen in drug withdrawal syndromes. Sedation is seen in infants with drug exposure syndromes (e.g., babies of drug-treated epileptic mothers). Alcohol, phenobarbital, benzodiazepines, and narcotics can cause the aforementioned withdrawal syndrome. Methadone can cause the same symptoms, although the onset may not occur for days or weeks from birth. Exposure to phenytoin can cause sedation in the neonate.

Page 602

Questions 13–16 (Matching). Appropriate pharmacologic resuscitation of the newborn requires knowledge of proper medications, dosages, and routes of administration. Match each of the following statements with the most appropriate response from the options listed below. Each lettered option may be used once, more than once, or not at all.

A. Naloxone
B. Epinephrine
C. Both A and B
D. Neither A nor B

13. Can be delivered via endotracheal tube

14. Can be given subcutaneously or intramuscularly

15. Should be given for persistent bradycardia (heart rate <80)

16. Should be considered in resuscitation of the depressed neonate

Answers: 13-C, 14-A, 15-B, 16-A

Critique: Both naloxone and epinephrine can be administered via an endotracheal tube, and naloxone can be administered subcutaneously or intramuscularly provided that perfusion is adequate. Bradycardia that persists despite adequate ventilation and cardiac compressions can be treated with epinephrine, 0.01 to 0.03 mg/kg, and repeated every 5 minutes. Depressed infants should be treated with naloxone if narcotics have been given to the mother within 4 hours of delivery, or if the mother may have self-administered narcotics prior to hospitalization.

Pages 597, 598

Questions 17–21 (Matching). Match each of the numbered statements below with the most appropriate option from the following list. Each lettered option may be used once, more than once, or not at all.

    A. Respiratory distress syndrome (hyaline membrane disease)
    B. Meconium aspiration syndrome
    C. Both A and B
    D. Neither A nor B

17. Extracorporeal membrane oxygenation (ECMO) has proved useful in some cases.

18. Chest radiographs show perihilar streaking.

19. Pneumothorax is a common complication.

20. Characterized by grunting, intercostal retractions, and nasal flaring

21. Use of synthetic human surfactant has been highly effective.

Answers: 17-C, 18-D, 19-B, 20-C, 21-A

Critique: Respiratory distress syndrome (hyaline membrane disease) and meconium aspiration syndrome are characterized by signs of respiratory distress, including grunting, nasal flaring, and retractions. In both conditions ECMO has been used as a salvage procedure, sometimes with a good outcome. Chest radiographs show perihilar streaking in transient tachypnea of the newborn and a "ground-glass" appearance in respiratory distress syndrome. Pneumothoraces are common in meconium aspiration syndrome because of air-trapping caused by the ball-valve action of meconium collections in the airways. Human surfactant has been used successfully in respiratory distress syndrome but not in meconium aspiration.

Pages 599, 600

Questions 22–26 (Matching). Match each of the following statements with the best response from the lettered options listed below. Each option may be used once, more than once, or not at all.

    A. Early onset sepsis
    B. Late onset sepsis
    C. Both A and B
    D. Neither A nor B

22. Group B β-hemolytic *Streptococcus* is a common pathogen.

23. *Haemophilus influenzae* is a common pathogen.

24. Ampicillin and an aminoglycoside may be used in the treatment of this problem.

25. *Listeria monocytogenes* is a common pathogen.

26. Third-generation cephalosporins may be used in the treatment of this problem.

Answers: 22-C, 23-B, 24-C, 25-B, 26-C

Critique: The organisms that cause sepsis and present in the first 5 days of life (early-onset sepsis) are maternal gut flora, including group B β-hemolytic streptococci and *L. monocytogenes.* A wider variety of pathogens are responsible for late-onset sepsis. These pathogens include the pathogens seen in early-onset sepsis as well as *S. pneumoniae* and *H. influenzae.* Traditionally, both early and late sepsis have been treated with ampicillin and an aminoglycoside. Third-generation cephalosporins have increasingly come to replace these older agents because of a broader spectrum of coverage and the increasing resistance of some organisms.

Pages 601, 602

Questions 27–30 (Matching). Examination of the skin in the newborn often yields clues to underlying illness or disease. Match the following skin lesions with the associated conditions listed below. Each lettered option may be used once, more than once, or not at all.

    A. Congenital rubella
    B. Sturge-Weber syndrome
    C. Group B streptococcal infection
    D. Neurofibromatosis
    E. Salmon patches

27. Transient capillary hemangioma of the forehead, glabella, or eyelids

28. Light to dark brown macules distributed over the trunk and axillae

29. Diffusely distributed purplish subcutaneous nodules

30. A spreading petechial rash involving the face, trunk, and limbs

Answers: 27-E, 28-D, 29-A, 30-C

Critique: The intradermal hematopoiesis of congenital rubella causes purplish subcutaneous nodules, which are described as having a "bluberry muffin" appearance. Sturge-Weber syndrome is characterized by a permanent port wine stain, usually in the trigeminal distribution, and capillary hemangioma of the meninges, which can result in seizure disorder and retardation. Salmon patches, "stork bites," and flame nevi are terms that apply to transient capillary hemangiomas of the forehead, glabella, or eyelids. Sometimes the term flame nevus is applied to a port wine stain. Isolated, small (<1.5 cm) pigmented lesions can be a routine finding, but multiple, larger café au lait spots and often small axillary lesions should raise the possibility of neurofibromatosis, prompting further investigation. A diffuse petechial rash that is spreading suggests the possibility of sepsis, whereas a fixed petechial eruption on the presenting part is not an uncommon finding in the normal newborn.

Pages 573–577

Questions 31–34 (True or False). An evaluation of the newborn should include assignment of Apgar scores. Which of the following statements about Apgar scores are true?

31. A 1-minute Apgar score greater than 9 is uncommon.

32. 1- and 5-minute Apgar scores less than 7 are predictive of illness in the neonate.

33. A score of 3 or less at 1 minute is a good predictor of the need for prolonged resuscitation.

34. A decrease in Apgar scores from 1 to 5 minutes predicts illness in the neonate.

Answers: 21-T, 32-F, 33-T, 34-T

Critique: A 1-minute Apgar score of 9 is common due to physiologic acrocyanosis. An infant with an Apgar score of 7 at 1 minute will usually need no special stimulation, whereas a score of 7 at 5 minutes, or a score that has fallen from 1 to 5 minutes, predicts illness in the neonate. Prolonged resuscitative efforts can be predicted from a 1-minute Apgar score of 3 or less.

Pages 570–572

Questions 35–39 (True or False). You are in the hospital to see your patient, who is a first-time mother. Last night you delivered her full-term, 3700-g male infant after a difficult labor characterized by a prolonged second stage. The baby is doing well in all other respects, but on examination you note a cephalohematoma. The mother is understandably concerned about her son, and you seek to reassure her. True statements about cephalohematomas include:

35. They are caused by rupture of small, subperiosteal vessels.

36. Occasionally they can be associated with an underlying skull fracture.

37. Skull radiographs are recommended to rule out an underlying skull fracture.

38. The swelling is easily distinguished from caput succedaneum on physical examination, because cephalohematomas do not cross suture lines.

39. Surgical drainage is the treatment of choice for a cephalohematoma to prevent prolonged neonatal jaundice.

Answers: 35-T, 36-T, 37-F, 38-T, 39-F

Critique: Cephalohematomas are caused by the rupture of small, subperiosteal vessels, and they do not cross suture lines, unlike the swelling of caput succedaneum. They are usually not present at birth but present as a slowly enlarging, nondiscolored mass under the scalp. About 1 in 20 cephalohematomas overlie a skull fracture, but radiographs are not routinely recommended. The resorption of the old blood in the cephalohematoma can be associated with prolonged neonatal jaundice, but surgical drainage is not recommended because of the risk of infection. Resorption usually occurs over 2 to 12 weeks.

Page 578

Questions 40–43 (True or False). Rhinorrhea in the neonatal period:

40. Is a relatively common condition

41. May suggest a congenital syphilis infection

42. Can be associated with a skull fracture

43. May be associated with a congenital rubella infection

Answers: 40-F, 41-T, 42-T, 43-F

Critique: Rhinorrhea is uncommon in the neonatal period. Congenital syphilis can produce rhinorrhea, which is commonly referred to as "snuffles." A basilar skull fracture can produce cerebrospinal fluid rhinorrhea. Congenital rubella infection does not typically present with nasal discharge.

Page 580

Questions 44–48 (True or False). Patient education about newborn safety is an important aspect of care of the newborn. Which of the following are important safety risks in the neonatal period?

44. Airway obstruction

45. Motor vehicle accidents

46. Thermal injury

47. Child abuse

48. Animal bites

Answers: 44-T, 45-T, 46-T, 47-T, 48-T

Critique: To some extent all of the listed problems are preventable causes of injury and death in the neonatal period. Parents should be counseled about car safety and appropriate use of car seats and safety restraints, safe use of pacifiers, adjusting the temperature of the hot water heater to prevent accidental scalding, and keeping pets away from the infant. Child abuse is another important cause of injury and death in the newborn.

Page 590

Questions 49–53 (True or False). You are seeing a 28-year-old juvenile diabetic who is planning to start a family and wonders what risks her infant might face. She has historically had good control of blood sugar and has not yet suffered any complications of diabetes. Which of the following statements are true regarding risks to the infant of a diabetic mother?

49. Increased risk of birth defects

50. Increased risk of respiratory distress syndrome

51. Increased risk of anemia

52. Increased risk of idiopathic seizure disorder

53. Increased incidence of shoulder dystocia

Answers: 49-T, 50-T, 51-F, 52-F, 53-T

Critique: Infants of diabetic mothers face a number of additional risks, including increased risk of birth defects, birth trauma, respiratory distress syndrome, and hypoglycemia. Shoulder dystocia is a concern due to fetal macrosomia and may result in birth trauma such as a broken clavicle. Hypoglycemia may present as seizures; however, idiopathic seizure disorders are not associated with infants of diabetic mothers. There is no evidence that anemia is a greater risk for infants of diabetic mothers.

Page 603

Questions 54–58 (True or False). Overproduction of heme is one of the possible causes of neonatal jaundice. Causes of overproduction of heme include:

54. Biliary obstruction

55. Metabolic disorders

56. Polycythemia

57. ABO incompatibility

58. Intestinal obstruction

Answers: 54-F, 55-F, 56-T, 57-T, 58-F

Critique: The overproduction of heme can be caused by reabsorption of extravasated blood, such as in a cephalohematoma; by hemolysis, either acute or chronic; or by polycythemia. Undersecretion of bilirubin, which is found in some metabolic disorders or biliary obstruction, and underexcretion of bilirubin, which is secondary to intestinal obstruction, are other causes of neonatal jaundice.

Pages 604, 605

28

Growth and Development

Clyde A. Addison

1. A mother brings her 2-year-old daughter to the clinic. She is concerned that her baby has stopped growing. The child is in the 50th percentile for height and weight and has remained on her growth curve for height and weight. You notice that she is 34 inches tall today and that her height has not changed from 3 months ago. The most appropriate action at this time is to:

 A. Obtain bone films of the hand and wrist to verify her true age.
 B. Order thyroid studies to further evaluate the cause of her stunted growth.
 C. Reassure the mother that linear growth in toddlers can occur in increments and re-examine the child in 3 months.
 D. Obtain a family history regarding short stature or skeletal abnormalities.
 E. Despite an adequate weight, increase the child's caloric intake.

Answer: C

Critique: Each child has a different rate of maturation. Thus, if a child falls off the growth curve, one might obtain films of the hand and wrist to rule out short stature or constitutional growth delay. In this case, the child has remained on the growth curve; thus, she will probably show an increase in length within the next 3 months. Linear growth in infants has been shown to occur in incremental bursts, rather than continuously. Although thyroid studies may be ordered in the event of bone age immaturity, these studies are not indicated at this time. Although hereditary factors and diet are important in growth and development, neither taking a detailed family history nor increasing the caloric intake would be appropriate in this case.

Page 611

2. The first sign of puberty in boys is:

 A. Growth of pubic hair
 B. Testicular and scrotal growth
 C. Phallic enlargement
 D. Growth of axillary hair
 E. Deepening of the voice

Answer: B

Critique: Scrotal and testicular growth are followed by the appearanc of pubic hair within 6 months, then phallic enlargement within 12 to 18 months. Axillary hair does not appear until 2 years following scrotal and testicular growth.

Page 617

3. The first sign of puberty in females is the appearance of:

 A. Breast buds
 B. Menstruation
 C. Pubic hair
 D. Axillary hair

Answer: A

Critique: The breast bud is the first sign of puberty in girls. Breast buds are followed by growth of pubic and axillary hair. Menstruation occurs at a later stage of pubertal development.

Page 617

4. Which one of the following statements about pubertal development is correct?

 A. Boys reach peak height velocity later than girls do.
 B. Pubic hair appears earlier in males than in females.
 C. In both sexes, the length of the trunk is the first parameter to reach adult size.
 D. Pubertal males achieve greater shoulder and hip breadth than do pubertal females.
 E. Female menstrual cycles start with the first ovulation.

Answer: A

Critique: The timing of pubertal development for individuals is highly variable; however, the sequence is quite specific. It is also different for males and females. Boys reach peak height velocity later than do girls, thus accounting for their generally taller stature. Pubic hair tends to appear earlier in females than in males. Head, hands, and feet reach adult size first, followed by the legs, and finally the trunk, which accounts for much of the pubertal growth spurt. Pubertal males achieve wider shoulders, whereas pubertal females achieve wider hips. The first menstrual cycles of a pubertal female are often irregular, anovulatory cycles.

Pages 616–618

5. Which one of the following vitamin supplements is likely to benefit certain breast-fed infants?

    A. Vitamin A
    B. Vitamin B
    C. Vitamin C
    D. Vitamin D
    E. Vitamin E

Answer: D

Critique: Only small amounts of vitamin D are present in human milk; therefore, breast-fed babies who are darkly pigmented or who receive little exposure to sunlight may benefit from an additional 400 units/day of vitamin D.

Page 620

6. Intrinsic factors that influence childhood developmental outcomes include:

    A. Intrauterine events
    B. Infectious agents
    C. Temperament
    D. Traumatic exposures
    E. Chemical exposures

Answer: C

Critique: Although no one is certain that absolute reliance on certain factors will lead to either a positive or negative developmental outcome, most child development researchers have concluded that developmental outcomes are a product of intrinsic and extrinsic factors. Intrinsic child factors include genetic potential and temperament; whereas extrinsic environmental factors include intrauterine, infectious, traumatic, chemical, and sociocultural factors.

Page 622

7. A drawback to developmental surveillance is that:

    A. The caregiver does not seek input from other professionals.
    B. Attendance to parental concerns is minimal.
    C. There are no standardized guidelines.
    D. No provisions are made for longitudinal tracking.
    E. Interpretation of findings within the context of the child's well-being is rarely accomplished.

Answer: C

Critique: The concept of developmental surveillance was introduced to monitor child development. It conains four key components: (1) eliciting and attending to parental concerns, (2) longitudinal tracking of children's developmental progress, (3) seeking input from other professionals involved with the child, and (4) interpretation of all findings within the context of the child's well-being. Although this method is quick and inexpensive, there are no standardized guidelines. There is, therefore, a danger that many children with significant delays may be missed.

Page 624

8. Which of the following is **NOT** associated with temperament:

    A. Adaptability
    B. Industry
    C. Mood
    D. Rhythmicity
    E. Distractibility

Answer: B

Critique: As part of the child's psychosocial development, there are many theories, including personality development, that help us to understand this difficult concept. For instance, Iroquoian's psychosocial stages are widely referenced and contain eight stages that represent different life events. These events are seen as crises that require the integration of personal needs with sociocultural demands. Industry versus inferiority (8 to 12 years of age) finds the caregiver working with the school to ensure that the child is achieving his or her abilities and feeling a sense of competence rather than inferiority. Temperament is an additional factor in child behavior. There are three basic temperament profiles based on nine temperament characteristics. Adaptability, industry, rhythmicity, and distractibility are four of the nine temperament characteristics. The remaining characteristics are activity, approach or withdrawal, intensity, attention span or persistence, and sensory threshold.

Page 627

9. In relation to temperament characteristics and profiles, activity refers to:

    A. Immediate reaction of the child to stimuli
    B. Regularity of physiologic functions
    C. Negative responses of mild intensity to new stimuli
    D. Frequency and speed of involvement
    E. Amount of external stimulation required to evoke a response

Answer: D

Critique: Temperament is believed to be an inborn trait that influences how an infant interacts with and learns from his or her environment. Nine characteristics of temperament are described. Activity refers to the frequency and speed of involvement that an infant or child demonstrates with a task or stimulus. Rhythmicity refers to the regularity of physiologic functions. The immediate reaction of the child to stimuli and negative responses of mild intensity to new stimuli are parts of the approach or withdrawal phenomenon. The sensory threshold reflects the amount of external stimulation required to evoke a response.

Pages 626, 627

10. The measles epidemic of 1989 to 1991 was caused by:

    A. An influx of unvaccinated immigrants
    B. Children not being vaccinated at the recommended age
    C. The increased cost of vaccinations to single-parent families
    D. No organized effort to vaccinate all children
    E. The normal cyclic recurrence of disease

Answer: B

Critique: The measles epidemic of 1989 to 1991 was caused by children not being vaccinated at the recommended age despite reasonably well organized efforts. Individual cost is usually not an issue. With adequate "herd" immunity, the influx of a relatively small number of unvaccinated individuals would not account for an epidemic. Although infectious diseases may be cyclical, widespread immunity will still be effective in preventing epidemics.

Page 627

11. Absolute contraindications to vaccinations include:

    A. Localized erythema at the site of injection
    B. Current antimicrobial treatment
    C. Recent exposure to an infectious disease
    D. Anaphylactic reaction to the vaccine
    E. Minor febrile illness

Answer: D

Critique: Unless an individual is immunosuppressed, the only true contraindication listed earlier is an anaphylactic reaction to the vaccine or to one of its components.

Page 628

12. Patients with acquired immunodeficiency syndrome (AIDS) should **NOT** receive:

    A. Oral polio vaccine
    B. Diphtheria, pertussis, tetanus vaccine
    C. *Haemophilus influenzae* type B conjugate vaccine
    D. Hepatitis B virus vaccine
    E. Acellular pertussis vaccine

Answer: A

Critique: Immunosuppressed individuals should not be given live virus vaccines such as OPV, because the endogenous immune system is already compromised.

Page 628

13. A single mother recently moved to your practice area from another state. She delivered a healthy 8 lb 2 oz baby girl 2 months ago. Her baby received her first hepatitis B vaccine within 24 hours of delivery. In a routine history for your files, you note that the baby was seen in the local emergency department due to difficulty breathing and an urticarial rash. From your review of the emergency department records, you note that the infant was inappropriately given undercooked scrambled eggs 1 week ago. Her mother tearfully states that she was told to tell you about this, because this could affect her baby's immunizations. She presents today for an initial visit and to discuss the immunization question. At the appropriate time, which of the following vaccines should be administered with extreme caution and only under a special protocol?

    A. Measles, mumps, and rubella (MMR) vaccine
    B. Oral polio vaccine
    C. Diphtheria, acellular pertussis, and tetanus vaccine
    D. *Haemophilus influenzae* type B conjugate vaccine

Answer: A

Critique: An anaphylactic reaction to egg ingestion is an absolute contraindication to the MMR vaccine. Egg proteins (antigens) are present in this vaccine. Protocols are available to administer MMR to individuals with an allergy to egg antigens, but this requires extreme caution. Of note, egg proteins are also present in the yellow fever vaccine, which poses a significant problem for people traveling abroad, who require this vaccination. Skin testing in adults is sometimes warranted.

Page 628

14. What is the safest anatomic site to administer vaccines to an infant in the first year of life?

    A. Superior lateral gluteal area
    B. Center of the deltoid
    C. Superior lateral thigh area
    D. Inferior gluteal area near the midline

Answer: C

Critique: For adults, the superior lateral gluteal area, well away from the sciatic nerve, or the deltoid are safe sites to administer intramuscular injections. In infants, however, the safest place to administer vaccinations is the superior lateral thigh area, which is well away from the sciatic nerve and its branches.

Page 629

15. A new parent calls your office 2 days after her 2-month-old baby received his vaccines. She is concerned because the infant is fussy and has a temperature of 102.5° F. She denies any seizure activity and states that the baby is eating well. The most likely cause of the febrile reaction is:

    A. *Haemophilus influenzae* type B conjugate vaccine
    B. Hepatitis B vaccine
    C. Oral polio vaccine

D. Diphtheria, pertussis, and tetanus (DTP) vaccine
E. MMR vaccine

Answer: D

Critique: The DTP is the one most likely to cause a mild febrile morbidity. It is also associated with mild "fussiness." Neither of these is an absolute contraindication to the next series of vaccinations with DTP. However, persistent inconsolable crying lasting for more than 3 hours or a fever higher than 40.5° C (105° F) is a true contraindication to the vaccination series with DTP. Acetaminophen, at the time of vaccination and every 4 hours thereafter for 24 hours, may reduce the likelihood of a febrile reaction. MMR is not a concern here, because it is not indicated until 15 months of age.

Pages 628, 629

Questions 16–20 (True or False). Compared with children of familial short stature, children with constitutional short stature:

16. Are more likely to be male

17. Tend to be short at birth

18. Follow the normal growth curve from birth but at the fifth percentile or lower

19. Have a bone age equal to their height age

20. Reach puberty at an appropriate time

Answers: 16-T, 17-F, 18-F, 19-T, 20-F

Critique: Short stature is a concern for parents and children alike. If an organic cause has been excluded, the clinician must differentiate constitutional short stature from familial short stature. Children with constitutional short stature tend to be male; are normal in length at birth; have a bone age equal to height age; demonstrate a downward shift in growth rate during the first 2 years of life then stabilize at 4 to 5 cm/yr; and reach puberty at a somewhat later time than do most children.

Page 616

Questions 21–24 (True or False). Human milk is of higher quality than cow's milk due to:

21. Secretory immunoglobulin (Ig) A antibodies

22. Lactose as the main source of carbohydrate

23. Higher concentrations of essential and sulfur-containing amino acids

24. Higher sodium concentration

Answers: 21-T, 22-F, 23-T, 24-F

Critique: The best source of nutrition for an infant during the first year of life is human breast milk. Human milk is superior to cow's milk because it contains immunologically active substances, including IgA antibodies,

higher-quality protein containing higher concentrations of essential and sulfur-containing amino acids, and a lower solute load. Lactose is the primary sugar in both breast milk and cow's milk.

Pages 619, 620

Questions 25–29 (True or False). Parents bring their 15-month-old son in for a well-child examination. His immunizations are current, and he has had no significant illness. His height and weight are at the 50th percentile. The parents are concerned because he has not started to walk on his own. He will walk around objects while holding on and will walk if the parents hold both his hands. To determine if the child's development is progressing normally, you perform a developmental assessment. Which of the following activities should this child be doing at this age?

25. Stacks two cubes

26. Names multiple body parts

27. Feeds self with utensils

28. Follows one-step commands

29. Draws a line with a crayon after a demonstration

Answers: 25-T, 26-F, 27-T, 28-T, 29-T

Critique: Developmental testing is an important part of practice and should always be addressed when a parent raises a concern. Although many children take their first few steps by 15 months, this child does not seem significantly delayed. By 15 months you could expect this child to stack two cubes, point to a few body parts, feed himself with utensils, follow simple commands, and draw a line after a demonstration. Speech develops later.

Page 623

Questions 30–34 (True or False). Which of the following vaccines are contraindicated in an individual who has had a serious allergic reaction to neomycin?

30. MMR vaccine

31. Oral polio vaccine

32. Diphtheria, acellular pertussis, and tetanus vaccine

33. *Haemophilus influenzae* type B conjugate vaccine

34. Intramuscular polio vaccine (IPV)

Answers: 30-T, 31-F, 32-F, 33-F, 34-T

Critique: An anaphylactic reaction to neomycin or streptomycin is a true contraindication for IPV. MMR is contraindicated after an anaphylactic reaction to neomycin. The other vaccines are not developed in systems that retain small amounts of antibiotics.

Page 628

Questions 35–38 (True or False). Which of the following statements about immunization practices and recommendations are correct?

35. A 15-month-old child who is currently being treated with amoxicillin for otitis media with effusion should not receive the schedule immunizations.

36. *Haemophilus influenzae* type B conjugate vaccine is contraindicated in a 2-month-old child with well-controlled seizures.

37. Preterm infants can safely receive regularly scheduled immunizations.

38. IPV can safely be substituted for OPV when a member of the recipients' household is immunosuppressed.

Answers: 35-F, 36-F, 37-T, 38-T

Critique: Penicillin-derived antibiotics have no adverse effect on the infant when used in conjunction with the vaccines. *H. influenzae* type B vaccine currently shows no true contraindication to its use. However, a caveat should be noted. If this vaccine is in the combined form with DPT (Tetramune), contraindications to DPT would naturally exclude this formulation also. IPV does not have a contraindication for immunosuppressed household members as does OPV; however the type of immunity conveyed to the recipient differs and he or she should receive OPV whenever it becomes feasible.

Page 628

29

Childhood and Adolescence

Janice Kelly Smith

1. Questions about the dietary habits of children should include an evaluation of risk factors for anemia. Which one of the following statements regarding iron deficiency anemia in childhood is correct?

    A. Iron deficiency anemia is most likely to be detected by 6 months of age.
    B. Serum ferritin is a more sensitive and specific test for iron deficiency anemia than for hemoglobin or hematocrit.
    C. Iron deficiency anemia has no effect on behavior and development.
    D. A microcytic anemia not responsive to iron therapy is most likely due to sickle cell disease.

Answer: B

Critique: Iron deficiency anemia is rarely detected before 8 to 10 months of age, because it takes several months to deplete the maternal iron stores. Although ferritin is a much more specific and sensitive test, it is more expensive and thus is not used as routinely. The hematocrit is not lowered until the iron stores are already depleted. It is important to screen for and detect iron deficiency anemia because it does have some effect on learning and behavior. Thalassemia is the second most common cause of microcytic anemia and is most commonly found in children of Mediterranean, Asian, or black heritage. Sickle cell anemia is usually normocytic.

Page 639

2. Which one of the following statements is correct regarding screening for lead in children 2 years of age and younger?

    A. A level less than 15 μg/dl is considered to be no risk.
    B. A fingerstick sample is as reliable as a venous sample.
    C. Screening is recommended for all children at approximately 24 months of age.

    D. Screening should be repeated until age 14 for all children living in housing built before 1960.

Answer: C

Critique: Lead poisoning has become a major public health concern, not only because of its increasing detection but also because of studies that have shown significant cognitive deficits, behavior disorders, and slowed growth in children with levels above 10 μg/dl. Screening is therefore recommended for all children at ages 9 to 12 months, and again at 24 months, and subsequently for those with identified risk factors or previous elevated levels. The fingerstick method is less reliable because of potential contamination from environmental lead. Screening is not recommended for children older than 6 years of age, because the incidence is markedly decreased and also the effect on learning and development are most pronounced at younger ages.

Page 640

3. Which of the following statements regarding lipid screening in childhood is correct?

    A. All children older than 2 years of age should be offered screening.
    B. All children older than 2 years of age with a strong family history of hypercholesterolemia or premature heart disease should be offered screening.
    C. Children with a cholesterol level above the 50th percentile of cholesterol readings for children should be targeted for intervention.
    D. Parents should be instructed to put their children on 2% or less milk fat as soon as they are weaned from breast or formula, regardless of their risk.

Answer: B

Critique: Only children with a strong family history of premature heart disease or hyperlipidemia need be screened, although even this remains controversial. The current recommendations are that those with a cholesterol level above the 95% level of acceptability should be targeted for special management. This would be a level above 200 mg/dl. All children need some fat in their diet, and it is not recommended to put children on low-fat milk until after the second birthday.

Page 640

4. A mother of a 2-year-old child is expecting her second child in 2 months. She has questions regarding the recommendations for safety seats for both her 2-year-old, who now weighs 26 lb, and the new sibling. Which one of the following statements is correct?

   A. The 2-year-old child can safely use a toddler's seat.
   B. The infant must be carried in a special infant seat but can face either backwards or forwards.
   C. Child safety seats are required for all children who weigh less than 50 lb.
   D. Once a child is big enough to use a seat belt, the child should always use the shoulder harness as well.

Answer: A

Critique: Child safety seats are required by law in all states. Infants who weigh less than 17 lb must ride in an approved seat and must always face the rear of the vehicle. A toddler's seat can be used after a child weighs 17 to 20 lb. These seats face forward and must be used until the child weighs 40 to 44 lb. At that time, the child can sit in an approved booster seat or with a regular lap belt. The shoulder harness should not be used in children under 4½ feet tall.

Page 641

5. A 2-year-old child is brought into your office by her mother for a routine check-up. Included in this visit are height and weight measurements, a review of the child's dietary habits, and a review of her immunization status. She received diphtheria, pertussis, and tetanus (DPT) vaccine and *Haemophilus influenzae* type B (HIB) at 2, 4, and 6 months, and a measles, mumps, and rubella (MMR) vaccine at 15 months. Which of the following immunizations should be offered at this visit?

   A. Oral polio virus (OPV) vaccine
   B. DPT vaccine only
   C. Second MMR vaccine
   D. DPT and HIB booster

Answer: D

Critique: By 24 months of age, a child should have received four doses of DPT and HIB. Only three doses of OPV are required until age 4. The second dose of MMR can be given at either the 4- to 5-year-old visit or at the prepubertal visit. This is intended to booster potentially waning immunity from the first vaccination, which would not be expected by age 2.

Page 642

6. Anticipatory guidance is an important part of all well-child care and should be incorporated into every visit.

Each of the following statements regarding primary prevention in childhood is true EXCEPT:

   A. The child's developmental stage is closely related to his or her risk of certain injuries.
   B. The most common type of accidents that result in fatalities are motor vehicle accidents, half of which result in pedestrian deaths.
   C. Drownings are rare in the bathroom at home.
   D. A hot water heater setting of 125° F is recommended to avoid severe burns from tap water.

Answer: C

Critique: It is important to assess the child's developmental stage in order to anticipate the hazards that pose the biggest threat to the child's health and to teach the parents how to avoid or beware of these hazards. Motor vehicle accidents account for the largest number of fatal accidents, with drownings following in second place. A large number of the drownings occur in pools and bathtubs, thus careful supervision of bath time is mandatory. Water heated over 125° F can result in severe burns.

Pages 641, 642

Questions 7–10. A 4-year-old black male is brought to your office with a 2-day history of tiring easily, cough that is worse at night-time, and also the complaint of a vague stomach ache. He has no history of asthma but has had two episodes of acute bronchitis, the first at 18 months of age. On physical examination, he is in no acute distress, and his vital signs are: heart rate of 104 beats/min; respiratory rate of 30 per minute; temperature of 100° F. The head, eyes, ears, nose, throat (HEENT) examination is unremarkable except for a mildly erythematous pharynx. A few small cervical nodes are palpable. Auscultation of the chest reveals bilateral expiratory wheezes, with a prolonged expiratory phase. No nasal flaring or retractions are noted.

7. All of the following should be considered in the differential diagnosis EXCEPT:

   A. Acute bronchitis
   B. Asthma
   C. Foreign body aspiration
   D. Acute laryngotracheitis (croup).

Answer: C

Critique: Acute bronchitis, asthma, and croup could all present in this manner. With acute bronchitis, you might expect more productive cough, although in a 4-year-old child this is often difficult to ascertain. Wheezing can infrequently accompany a case of acute bronchitis, secondary to acute inflammation of the airways. Croup is most common in children from ages 1 to 5, with a peak incidence at age 2. It is usually characterized by a barking cough but can also present as above. An upper respiratory infection alone does not cause shortness of breath and audible wheezing, although it could certainly be a trigger for asthma. A foreign body aspiration is more likely to present with an acute onset of dyspnea and with unilateral wheezes, although atypical presentations can occur.

Pages 644–646

8. The first line of treatment could include all of the following EXCEPT:

    A. Nebulizer treatment with albuterol
    B. Antibiotics
    C. Cromolyn sodium spinhaler treatment
    D. Subcutaneous epinephrine

Answer: C

Critique: All of the aforementioned choices are used in the acute treatment of asthma, except cromolyn sodium. Cromolyn sodium is used as a prophylactic drug because of its anti-inflammatory properties but offers no benefit in this setting. Nebulized albuterol can be given every 20 minutes for a total of three doses. Subcutaneous epinephrine is used much less but can be used if a nebulizer machine is not available. Epinephrine, 1:1000, can be used in a dosage of 0.01 mg/kg, up to a total single dose of 0.3 mg. Underlying upper and lower respiratory tract infections can frequently trigger an asthma attack, therefore antibiotics are sometimes indicated if the clinical situation warrants their use. Likewise, acute bronchitis can cause reversible airway obstruction, and β-agonists can be an adjunct to treatment of the bronchitis.

Pages 644–646

9. The child responds to your initial treatment. Which of the following would be most appropriate for short-term management of this child?

    A. Oral albuterol
    B. Oral steroids
    C. Metered-dose inhaler (MDI) of a β-agonist
    D. Oral theophylline

Answer: A

Critique: Oral albuterol is usually well tolerated in a child this age, whereas a 4-year-old child's gross motor skills are usually not adequate to use an MDI. Oral steroids are not indicated in this patient who had a good initial response to β-agonists. Oral theophylline can be used but is less well-tolerated. Oral theophylline must be more carefully monitored with blood levels and will require a loading dose.

Pages 645, 646

10. The child has subsequently had four or five similar episodes per year and is missing school frequently. All of the following are acceptable management options and should be discussed with the patient and family EXCEPT:

    A. Discussion of possible triggers and their avoidance
    B. Use of oral steroids for maintenance therapy
    C. Use of a cromolyn sodium spinhaler three to four times a day

    D. Use of inhaled steroids daily
    E. Use of daily theophylline

Answer: B

Critique: Long-term maintenance treatment of chronic asthma requires a history of potential triggers, which might include cigarette smoke in this particular patient as well as pets, dust mites, foods, stressors, and climatic changes. Cromolyn sodium and steroids are both useful in the prevention of asthma exacerbations because of the underlying inflammation present in the airways of asthmatics. Inhaled steroids are safe to use in children and can be employed for maintenance. Oral steroids, because of their side effect profile and affect on growth, should be avoided in the prevention of attacks; however, they can be quite useful in acute disease for short-term therapy. Theophylline is also used for long-term maintenance therapy but is used less often since the advent of these other drugs.

Pages 645, 646

11. Adolescents seek health care less often than do younger children. Some of the reasons why they are less likely to seek care include all of the following EXCEPT:

    A. Issue of confidentiality
    B. Economics
    C. Transportation
    D. Less concern about their health than other age groups

Answer: D

Critique: Adolescents, in fact, see themselves as needing more comprehensive health care and express more concern over health-related issues than would be expected. Confidentiality is a very real concern and must be addressed up front, especially if the physician also provides care for other family members. Adolescents may not have the financial resources to obtain care, especially if they do not want their parents to know the reasons why they are seeking care. Transportation is also a problem for the younger adolescent who does not want his or her family to know about a visit to the doctor. Being sensitive to these issues can help the physician in providing services for this age group.

Pages 647, 648

12. Indicators of increased risk for early sexual activity in adolescence include all of the following EXCEPT:

    A. Tanner stages 4 to 5
    B. Presence of a steady boyfriend or girlfriend
    C. History of sexual abuse
    D. Low self-esteem

Answer: D

Critique: Studies have demonstrated that adolescents who have a steady boyfriend or girlfriend and who are more developed physically (i.e., Tanner stages 4 to 5) are more likely to initiate sexual activity at an earlier age than are their same-age but less physically developed counterparts. More than 60% of girls who become pregnant as teenagers report a history of sexual abuse, usually by a close family member. A study of the relationship between self-esteem, sexual activity, and pregnancy dispelled the popular misconception that pregnant teenagers have lower levels of self-esteem. In fact, there was no difference between the two groups.

Pages 654, 655

Further Reading

Robinson RB, Frank DI: The relation between self-esteem, sexual activity, and pregnancy. Adolescence 29: 113, 1994.

13. When comparing the proportion of cases of AIDS in adolescents with the proportion in adults, all of the following statements are true EXCEPT:

   A. There is a higher proportion of females to males in the adolescent population.
   B. Heterosexually acquired cases make up a greater proportion of cases in adolescents.
   C. Minorities comprise a higher proportion of the cases in adolescents compared with adults.
   D. Intravenous (IV) drug use is not a risk factor for AIDS in the teenage group.

Answer: D

Critique: All of the first three statements regarding AIDS incidence levels are true, which means that we should be even more diligent about cautioning our teenage patients about the risks of sexual activity. Many still perceive it primarily as a disease of homosexual males. IV drug abuse is a risk factor in all age groups, although it is not found as commonly in teenagers.

Page 656

Questions 14–16. Match each of the following statements, with the associated microorganism from the following list. Each choice may be used once, more than once, or not at all.

   A. *Streptococcus pneumoniae*
   B. Viruses
   C. Parainfluenza viruses
   D. *Moraxella catarrhalis*

14. The most common bacterial pathogen in childhood otitis media

15. Causes more than 80% of all cases of acute pharyngitis

16. The pathogen responsible for most cases of croup in childhood

Answers: 14-A, 15-B, 16-C

Critique: *Streptococcus* pneumonia is the leading cause of bacterial otitis media, followed closely by *Haemophilus influenzae* and *M. catarrhalis*. The most common pathogen, however, is probably a virus. Acute pharyngitis, as well as other upper and lower respiratory tract infections, is also most commonly caused by viruses. Parainfluenza virus is thought to be the major etiologic agent of croup.

Pages 642, 643

Questions 17–19. Match each of the following statements with the correct antibiotic from the following list. Each choice may be used once, more than once, or not at all.

   A. Amoxicillin
   B. Erythromycin
   C. Ceftriaxone
   D. Ciprofloxacin

17. Can be used for a one-dose treatment of acute otitis media in children

18. Most common first-line treatment for acute otitis media in children

19. Can be used for prophylaxis in children with recurrent otitis media

Answers: 17-C, 18-A, 19-A

Critique: Although a single dose of intramuscular (IM) ceftriaxone has been found to be effective in the treatment of acute otitis media, oral amoxicillin is still one of the most commonly used drugs for first-line treatment as well as for prophylaxis of recurrent infections. Erythromycin alone has not been as effective, although in combination with trimethoprim-sulfamethoxazole, it is quite effective. In general the fluoroquinolones are contraindicated in children.

Page 643

Questions 20–22. A 14-year-old white female presents to your office for her immunization update. During the visit you ask her about school, her extracurricular activities, her relationships with peers and parents, then about any risk-taking behaviors. She reluctantly admits to occasionally having a few drinks on weekends, and after more gentle probing, she admits to once having had sexual relations while under the influence of alcohol. You explain to her that although she only had sex the one time, she is at some increased risk for developing a sexually transmitted disease (STD). Match each of the following statements with the correct answer from the following list. Each choice may be used once, more than once, or not at all.

   A. Chlamydia
   B. Gonorrhea
   C. Both A and B
   D. Neither A nor B

20. The most common STD in this age

21. Has a predilection for the columnar epithelium on the immature cervix of an adolescent female

22. Is usually asymptomatic in males

Answers: 20-A, 21-C, 22-A

Critique: Chlamydia has been found to be the most common STD in adolescents, prompting clinicians to recommend routine screening of all sexually active female teen-agers. It frequently occurs in conjunction with gonorrhea; therefore, these are usually both part of a routine examination. Both gonorrhea and chlamydia have a predilection for the immature cervix. Oral contraceptives may offer some protection against these STDs by virtue of the fact that they lead to a maturation of the cervical epithelium. Chlamydia infections in males are frequently asymptomatic, thus making it difficult to recognize and treat the infection. All contacts of a female diagnosed with chlamydia should be treated for the disease.

Pages 655, 656

Questions 23–25. After discussing the risks of STDs with this patient, you turn to a discussion of other risks of sexual activity, including pregnancy. Match each of the following statements with the correct contraceptive method from the following list. Each choice may be used once, more than once, or not at all.

A. Oral contraceptives
B. Levonorgestrel-releasing implants (Norplant)
C. Intrauterine device
D. Condoms

23. Provide the best protection against STDs

24. Most common side effect is irregular menstrual bleeding.

25. Have an increased incidence of ectopic pregnancy, pelvic inflammatory disease (PID), and infertility in later years associated with their use.

Answers: 23-D, 24-B, 25-C

Critique: Although condoms provide the best protection against STD transmission in sexually active teenagers, they are frequently used improperly and sporadically and provide less protection against unwanted pregnancy. Norplant is a long-acting levonorgestrel-releasing implant that provides protection for 5 years and theoretically is ideal for this age group because it does not require remembering to take a pill or use of condoms. However, this implant has fallen out of favor because of frequent reports of irregular menstrual bleeding. The intrauterine device is contraindicated for teenagers because of the increased incidence of PID, infertility, and ectopic pregnancy.

Pages 654, 655

30

Behavioral Problems in Children and Adolescents

Arch G. Mainous III

Questions 1–4. Match the following types of attachment with the appropriate scenario:

    A. Disoriented-disorganized
    B. Anxious-resistant
    C. Secure
    D. Avoidant pattern

1. An infant discovers that she is separated from her mother. The infant expresses little distress at this situation and is somewhat wary of contact with her mother when she reappears.

2. An infant discovers that she is separated from her mother. The infant becomes particularly agitated and begins to cry. When the mother reappears the infant is soothed and the crying quickly stops.

3. An infant discovers that she is separated from her mother. The infant becomes particularly agitated and begins to cry. When the mother reappears, the infant stares blankly at the parent and looks away with a glazed appearance.

4. An infant discovers that she is separated from her mother. The infant becomes particularly agitated and begins to cry. When the mother reappears, the infant remains agitated and is not easily comforted.

Answers: 1-D, 2-C, 3-A, 4-B

Critique: The main developmental task of infancy is the establishment of trust versus mistrust. Emotional attachment of the infant to the caregiver is very important to later healthy emotional development. Most infants develop secure attachments with their caregivers. In secure attachments, although the infant will have separation anxiety, the infant will be quickly soothed and comforted by the caregiver. In avoidant pattern attachments, when children are separated from caregivers they tend to express little distress and may even avoid contact with the caregiver when he or she reappears. Infants with anxious-resistant attachments are agitated when separated from a caregiver but are not quickly relieved when they return. This pattern of attachment may be related to later oppositional defiant disorders. The disoriented-disorganized pattern of attachment is characterized by infant behaviors like staring blankly when a parent approaches. This form of attachment seems to be linked to the development of dissociative disorders.

Pages 660, 661

5. (True or False) Evaluate each of the following statements according to its appropriateness in management of attachment problem behavior:

1. Note nonjudgmentally the behavior of concern, and educate the parent about the behavior that most infants would display in that particular situation.

2. Tell parents that the baby is the most important thing in their lives and that any needs that they have for social interaction are unimportant now that they have a baby.

3. Look for evidence of abuse toward the baby but do not investigate parental abuse history if the baby demonstrates no signs of abuse.

4. List the cues that babies give for help, and acknowledge that some cues may be irritating to adults.

Answers: 1-T, 2-F, 3-F, 4-T

Critique: Assessment, early detection, and intervention for management of attachment behavior problems are important tasks in prenatal and well-baby visits. It is important that the physician identify the strengths of the parents and the stressors in their environment that may influence infant and child behavior. Parents must be educated on normal infant behavior. Physicians should also investigate the parents' history of abuse or violence, because this may predispose them to aggressive or abusive parenting styles. The physician must also educate the parents on their own affiliation and social support needs and the importance of not becoming socially isolated.

Pages 661, 662

6. Which of the following characteristics has been shown to be related to an infant's likelihood of having colic?

    A. Dysthymia
    B. Feeding method
    C. Gender
    D. Parents' socioeconomic status

Answer: A

Critique: Colic is a syndrome of excessive crying that causes considerable concern among parents. The causes of colic are not well understood. Investigations into several of the possible etiologies (e.g., cow's milk protein allergy, gastrointestinal dysmotility) have yielded conflicting data. The feeding method, gender of the infant, and parent's socioeconomic status do not seem to be related to colic. Some evidence exists to suggest that colicky babies are dysthymic. A comprehensive history should be undertaken for infants with colic and may suggest a likely cause.

Further Reading

Rautava P, Helenius H, Lehtonen L: Psychosocial predisposing factors for infantile colic. BMJ 307:600–604, 1993.
Rakel RE (ed.), 5th ed.: Textbook of Family Practice. Philadelphia, WB Saunders, 1995, pp 662, 663.
Treem WR: Infant colic: A pediatric gastroenterologist's perspective. Pediatr Clin North Am 41:1121–1138, 1994.

7. (True or False) Evaluate the following characteristics of infant sleep:

1. Newborn babies sleep about 16 hr/day.

2. By 3 months of age only about 30% of infants have concentrated their sleep during the night.

3. A newborn baby's sleep patterns go from an alert state to rapid eye movement (REM) sleep without non-REM sleep.

4. Infants awaken intermittently during the night.

Answers: 1-T, 2-F, 3-T, 4-T

Critique: Parents commonly experience frustration about infant sleep patterns. Education of parents regarding normal sleep patterns is an important task of the family physician. Newborn babies sleep about 16 hr/day and go from alert states to REM activity, missing out on the stages of non-REM sleep. Infants tend to awaken intermittently during the night, and by 3 months of age 70% of infants have concentrated their sleep during the night.

Page 663

8. Which one of the following attributes is *not* characteristic of encopresis?

    A. Thirty to 50% of children with encopresis have abnormal or prolonged external anal sphincter contraction while straining to defecate.
    B. Encopresis is always the result of chronic constipation.
    C. Treatment regimens for encopresis should include establishing a structured toilet routine.
    D. Encopresis usually occurs in children older than 4 years of age.

Answer: B

Critique: Encopresis is repeated, involuntary defecation into one's clothing. This definition assumes that individuals have some voluntary control over defecation. Thus, encopresis is usually observed in children older than 4 years of age. Although encopresis is often the result of chronic constipation, recent evidence suggests that encopresis can exist without constipation. Further evidence suggests that a substantial number of children with encopresis have abnormal or prolonged external anal sphincter contraction during defecation. An important part of treatment of encopresis is the establishment of a structured toileting program.

Page 664

9. The symptom complex of inattention, impulsivity, and overactivity inappropriate for one's developmental age is characteristic of which one of the following disorders?

    A. Generalized anxiety disorder
    B. Adjustment disorder
    C. Attention deficit/hyperactivity disorder (ADHD)
    D. Oppositional defiant disorder

Answer: C

Critique: The symptom complex of inattention, impulsivity, and hyperactivity are characteristic of the diagnosis of ADHD. ADHD is frequently comorbid with anxiety, oppositional defiant behavior, depression, and substance abuse in adolescents and young adults. Adjustment disorders are reactions to identifiable stressors that may result in depression, anxiety, or conduct disturbances. These reactions in adjustment disorders should diminish within 6 months.

Page 665

10. (True or False) Evaluate the following characteristics of ADHD:

1. ADHD is equally prevalent in boys and girls.

2. A high incidence of alcoholism is present in the parents of children with ADHD.

3. ADHD exhibits approximately 10 to 15% prevalence in school-aged children.

4. Afflicted children eventually outgrow ADHD.

Answers: 1-F, 2-T, 3-F, 4-F

Critique: ADHD is a very common condition encountered in primary care. The prevalence in the school-aged population is estimated at 3 to 5%, with boys being significantly more likely than girls to have the condition. Long-term follow-up studies indicate that symptoms of ADHD persist into adulthood. A high incidence of alcoholism and mental disorders (e.g., hysteria affective disorders, depression) exists among parents of children with ADHD.

Further Reading

Mannuzza S, Klein RG, Bessler A, et al: Adult outcome of hyperactive boys: Educational achievement, occupational rank, and psychiatric status. Arch Gen Psychiatry 50:565–576, 1993.

Rakel RE: Textbook of Family Practice. Philadelphia, WB Saunders, 1995, p 665.

Zametkin AJ: Attention-deficit disorder: Born to be hyperactive? JAMA 273:1871–1874, 1995.

11. Which of the following rating scales is *not* used to evaluate children for ADHD?

  A. Minnesota Multiphasic Personality Inventory (MMPI)
  B. Child Behavior Checklist
  C. Yale Children's Inventory
  D. Conners' Teacher Rating Scale

Answer: A

Critique: Although rating scales are part of the standard evaluation of children suspected of ADHD, the MMPI is not used to evaluate children for ADHD.

Page 666

12. (True or False) Evaluate the following statements regarding treatment of children with ADHD:

1. At least 70% of children who are given methylphenidate have a successful response.

2. An electrocardiogram is recommended prior to starting methylphenidate.

3. Once ADHD has been diagnosed, psychopharmacologic therapy is the only necessary treatment.

4. Clonidine is effective in children with comorbid Tourette's syndrome.

Answers: 1-T, 2-F, 3-F, 4-T

Critique: Psychopharmacologic therapy should be considered as only one part of the treatment plan, and only after ADHD has been diagnosed. Stimulants like methylphenidate are commonly used and have shown successful responses in approximately 70% of children. For children in whom stimulant medication is not indicated, tricyclic antidepressants are used. An electrocardiogram is not recommended prior to stimulant medication but is recommended prior to beginning tricyclic antidepressant medication. Clonidine is effective in children with ADHD who also have Tourette's syndrome.

Pages 667, 668

Questions 13-16. Match the following conditions with the appropriate characteristic:

  A. Oppositional defiant disorder
  B. Conduct disorder

13. Overt verbal confrontational behavior

14. Prevalence increases with age

15. Confrontational behavior that tends to result in personal harm or property damage

16. Covert antisocial behavior

Answers: 13-A, 14-B, 15-B, 16-B

Critique: Although oppositional defiant disorder and conduct disorder have some similarities, they have several important differences. Conduct disorder tends to start later than does oppositional defiant disorder, and conduct disorder increases in prevalence with age. Oppositional defiant disorder is characterized by overt verbal confrontations (e.g., arguments with adults, refusal to comply), whereas conduct disorder behavior tends to result in physical harm or property damage and tends to be of a covert, concealing nature.

Page 669

17. Which one of the following statements is true of childhood depression?

  A. Appetite changes and weight loss are common symptoms in young children.
  B. Complaints of headaches and stomachaches are common symptoms in young children.
  C. Antidepressants are highly effective in treatment of childhood depression.
  D. The course of childhood depression is dictated solely by genetic characteristics.

Answer: B

Critique: Although major depression is relatively rare in children, depressive symptoms are not uncommon in older children. Expression of depression tends to differ between children and adults, with appetite changes and weight loss being rare in children and complaints of headaches and stomachaches being common symptoms. A genetic component seems to play a role in childhood depression but does not solely determine the course of the illness. The child's living environment influences the course of childhood depression.

Pages 670, 671

18. Which one of the following statements is true in adolescent depression?

  A. Appetite changes and weight loss are common symptoms in adolescents.
  B. Antidepressants demonstrate 90% effectiveness in adolescents.
  C. A depressed teenager is less likely than an adult to commit suicide.
  D. Psychotropic medications should be initiated after the depression has persisted for at least 1 month.

Answer: A

Critique: Unlike depression in children, adolescents tend to have symptoms similar to those of adults, including appetite loss and sleep disturbance. Further, depressed adolescents are at least as likely as depressed adults to commit suicide. However, as in children, antidepressant medication has not been shown to be effective and, when used, should not be initiated until after the depression has persisted for at least 6 months.

Pages 672, 673

19. Refusal to maintain a minimally normal body weight (≥15% below expected body size), an intense fear of gaining weight, and a misconception of body size are characteristics of which one of the following disorders in adolescents?

    A. Obsessive-compulsive disorder
    B. Bulimia nervosa
    C. Dysthymia
    D. Anorexia nervosa

Answer: D

Critique: Anorexia nervosa and bulimia nervosa are eating disorders in adolescents. Anorexia nervosa is characterized by a refusal to maintain a minimally normal body weight (85% of normal for height and age; another standard designates a body mass index of ≤17.5 kg/m²), while bulimia nervosa is characterized by binge eating followed by inappropriate purging behaviors (e.g., self-induced vomiting, misuse of laxatives). The bulimic typically maintains body weight at or above minimum normal standards. A disturbance in perception of body weight and size is an essential feature of both eating disorders. If the individual exhibited obsessions and compulsions toward things other than food, body shape, or weight, he or she could have an additional diagnosis of obsessive-compulsive disorder. As with other mood disorders, a common symptom of dysthymia is reduced appetite and weight loss.

Further Reading

Rakel RE: Textbook of Family Practice. Philadelphia, WB Saunders, 1995, p 673.
Selzer R, Bowes G, Patton G: When is an adolescent too thin (Letter)? Am J Psychiatry 152:813–814, 1995.

20. (True or False) Evaluate the following regarding anorexia nervosa:

1. Anorexia nervosa is equally prevalent among boys and girls.

2. The age at onset is 15 to 20 years of age.

3. Tachycardia is a common physical finding.

4. Low blood urea nitrogen (BUN) is a common laboratory finding.

Answers: 1-F, 2-F, 3-F, 4-T

Critique: Anorexia nervosa is much more common in girls than in boys, with the highest risk group being middle and upper-middle class white females. The age of onset is 12 to 16 years, while the age of onset for bulimia nervosa is later at 15 to 20 years of age. Common physical and laboratory findings of individuals with anorexia nervosa are bradycardia, hypocholesterolemia, and low BUN levels.

Page 673

31

Office Surgery

Gary W. Kearl

1. (True or False) The following pre-existing medical problems may decrease the safety of office surgery:
1. Hypertension
2. Skin infections
3. Diabetes
4. Anxiety
5. Human immunodeficiency virus (HIV)

Answers: 1-F, 2-T, 3-T, 4-F, 5-T

Critique: Addressing specific areas of a patient's history (e.g., history of seizures, angina pectoris, cardiac arrhythmias) will enhance the patient's safety during office surgery. Identification and control of pre-existing conditions that suppress the patient's immune response (e.g., diabetes, HIV, and immunosuppressive drugs) may help to prevent postoperative infectious complications. However, many pre-existing diseases such as hypertension and chronic anxiety do not increase preoperative risk.

Pages 675, 676

2. The preoperative evaluation before an extensive office surgical procedure should include:

A. Screening for hepatitis B
B. A complete blood count
C. A resting electrocardiogram (ECG)
D. A posteroanterior and lateral chest x-ray
E. A serum chemistry panel

Answer: B

Critique: The preoperative evaluation of a patient who will be undergoing office surgery usually does not require laboratory testing. However, if the procedure is **extensive** or involves a vascular area, then a complete blood count with a differential, prothrombin time, partial thromboplastin time, and bleeding time should suffice for patients without a family history of coagulopathies. There is no need to obtain serum chemistries, hepatitis B screening, a chest x-ray, or a resting ECG for patients who are scheduled for office surgery.

Pages 675, 676

3. (True or False) Compared with local (injectable) anesthetics, topical anesthetics offer:

1. Decreased patient discomfort during administration
2. Similar depth of anesthesia
3. Decreased duration of anesthetic effect
4. Improved anesthesia of mucous membranes
5. Protection from hypersensitivity reactions

Answers: 1-T, 2-F, 3-T, 4-T, 5-F

Critique: Eutectic mixture of local anesthetic (EMLA) cream is currently the best topical anesthetic for use in small areas. *Tetracaine, adrenaline, cocaine* (TAC) is another useful topical anesthetic. Compared with injectable anesthetics, topical anesthetics do not produce any discomfort and generate a superior level of anesthesia over mucosal surfaces. However, depending on the type of agent, injectable anesthetics produce deeper, longer lasting anesthetic effects. Hypersensitivity reactions are uncommon but can occur in response to the use of either topical or local anesthetics.

Pages 675, 676

Further Reading

Derksen DJ, Pfenninger JL: Local anesthesia. *In* Pfenninger JL, Fowler GC (Eds): Procedures for Primary Care Physicians. St. Louis, MO, Mosby-Year Book, 1994, pp 135–140.
Dery W: Topical anesthesia. *In* Pfenninger JL, Fowler GC (Eds): Procedures for Primary Care Physicians. St. Louis, MO, Mosby-Year Book, 1994, pp 141–144.

Questions 4–8. Match each numbered statement with the correct lettered term listed below.

A. Local infiltration
B. Digital block
C. Both
D. Neither

4. Sodium bicarbonate can reduce the pain of administration of this form of anesthesia.

5. Epinephrine should NEVER be used with this form of anesthesia.

6. The skin surface should be numbed first by injecting anesthetic into the intradermal space.

7. This form of anesthesia can prevent distortion of anatomic landmarks.

8. This form of anesthesia may be injected intravenously.

Answers: 4-C, 5-B, 6-C, 7-B, 8-D

Critique: Local (injectable) anesthetics are extremely useful in a wide variety of clinical situations. The local infiltration technique is simpler to perform and usually requires less anesthetic. The digital block produces less distortion of the local anatomy and a larger area of anesthesia (particularly in the digits). Injection of local anesthetics causes pain from the needle and from the irritating effect of the low pH of the anesthetic solution on tissue. Addition of sodium bicarbonate (in a ratio of 1:10) can reduce the pain of the injection by buffering the acidity of the anesthetic without altering the speed of onset or the duration of the anesthesia. Epinephrine is frequently pre-mixed with local anesthetic to reduce bleeding and prolong the anesthetic effect. However, a mixture of local anesthetic and epinephrine should NEVER be used in a digital block because of the possibility of tissue necrosis. During both procedures, surface anesthesia of the injection site should be obtained by injecting a small quantity of the anesthetic solution into the intradermal space. The physician should always draw back on the plunger of the syringe prior to injecting any anesthetic to avoid intravenous administration and systemic toxicity.

Page 680

Further Reading

Derksen DJ, Pfenninger JL: Local anesthesia. *In* Pfenninger JL, Fowler GC (Eds): Procedures for Primary Care Physicians. St. Louis, MO, Mosby-Year Book, 1994, pp 135–140.
Moy JG, Pfenninger JL: Peripheral nerve blocks and field blocks. *In* Pfenninger JL, Fowler GC (Eds): Procedures for Primary Care Physicians. St. Louis, MO, Mosby-Year Book, 1994, pp 145–155.

Questions 9–12. Match each numbered statement with the correct lettered term listed below.

    A. Benzodiazepine sedatives
    B. Narcotic analgesics
    C. Both
    D. Neither

9. Can provide retrograde amnesia

10. Can produce respiratory suppression

11. Can be reversed by administering nalmefene

12. Can be reversed by administering flumazenil

Answers: 9-A, 10-C, 11-B, 12-A

Critique: Benzodiazepines improve pain control during office surgery by causing sedation. The benzodiazepine

midazolam can also produce retrograde amnesia that may be beneficial to some patients. Narcotic analgesics improve pain control by blocking pain receptors in the central nervous system. Both classes of medications can produce clinically significant respiratory depression that is worsened when these two classes of drugs are used at the same time. Although *flumazenil* can be used to reverse benzodiazepine sedation, it has not been shown to be effective in treating benzodiazepine-induced hypoventilation. *Naloxone* and *nalmefene* are narcotic antagonists that can be used to reverse the toxic effects of narcotics. (An older product, *nalorphine,* was withdrawn from the United States' market in 1978 because it was not a pure opiate antagonist.) Since these agents also reverse the analgesic effects of opiates, they should *not* be used to reverse drowsiness unless opiate-induced respiratory depression is also present.

Page 680

Further Reading

Clinical Pharmacology, version 1.5. Gold Standard Multimedia, Inc., 1995.

Questions 13–17. Match each numbered statement with the correct lettered term listed below.

    A. Simple wound closure
    B. Layered wound closure
    C. Both
    D. Neither

13. Best method for closure of skin wounds in areas where the skin tension is high

14. Best method for closure of the majority of skin wounds

15. Excess suture tension from this method of wound closure (at the wound edge) can retard wound healing and promote infection.

16. Surface sutures from this technique can produce scarring if left in place too long.

17. Best method for closure of skin wounds on the trunk or extremity

Answers: 13-B, 14-A, 15-C, 16-C, 17-D

Critique: Although simple (one-layered) wound closure is usually sufficient for repairing most skin wounds, layered closure is required when there is increased tension at the site of the wound. Care must be taken to avoid suturing the edges of the wound together so tightly that capillary blood flow at the wound edge is disrupted and healing is delayed. Skin sutures should also be removed and replaced with adhesive strips as soon as possible to avoid surface scarring. Finally, lacerations of the trunk or extremity should be repaired with continuous, subcuticular, absorbable sutures.

Page 681

18. (True or False) True statements about suturing lacerations include:

1. Skin areas with greater vascularity tolerate less tension at the wound edges.
2. Undermining of the skin should be avoided because this retards wound healing.
3. Sutures made from synthetic material generally provoke less inflammation.
4. External facial sutures should be removed in 3 to 4 days.
5. Sutures placed in fatty tissue layers hold poorly.

Answers: 1-T, 2-F, 3-T, 4-T, 5-T

Critique: Sutures are used to hold the edges of the wound together, prevent bleeding, and promote wound healing. Wound healing is accomplished by fibroblasts that migrate into the wound and deposit collagen fibers that help to reunite the edges of the wound. Although vascular tissues heal more quickly than do nonvascular tissues, excess wound tension can retard the flow of blood to the wound and retard healing. Permanent sutures are unnecessary for wound healing, and synthetic sutures (which provide less inflammation) produce less scarring. Nevertheless, external sutures can produce scarring in as few as 4 days. Accordingly, facial wounds should be repaired with subcuticular stitches if the wound tension is such that external sutures would have to be left in place for more than 4 days.

Page 681

19. Incision and drainage of a cutaneous collection of purulent material is a common office procedure. This procedure involves each of the following EXCEPT:

A. Application of warm compresses to the skin overlying the collection of pus
B. Cleansing of the skin overlying the collection of pus with a topical anesthetic
C. Infiltration of the skin overlying the collection of pus with a local anesthetic
D. Incision of the skin overlying the collection of pus using a scalpel
E. Irrigation of the cavity with a 50 : 50 mixture of sterile water and hydrogen peroxide

Answer: C

Critique: A cutaneous abscess often requires incision and drainage (I&D) to prevent bacteremia or septicemia. The site for the I&D should be prepared by application of warm compresses (which encourage the development of fluctuance) and a topical antiseptic (which helps to prevent secondary infection following an I&D procedure). The skin overlying the abscess should be anesthetized using EMLA cream because local infiltration of anesthetic solutions is largely ineffective owing to the abnormal pH of infected tissues. The incision is usually made with a no. 11 scalpel, and the cavity is irrigated with a 50 : 50 solution of sterile water and hydrogen peroxide followed by a half-strength solution of povidone-iodine.

Pages 682, 683

Questions 20–24. Match each numbered statement with the correct lettered term listed below.

A. Excisional biopsy
B. Shave biopsy
C. Both
D. Neither

20. Used to make or confirm a diagnosis

21. Removes a full-thickness specimen

22. Anesthetic is *not* necessary.

23. Contraindicated for melanomas

24. Does not require suturing

Answers: 20-C, 21-A, 22-D, 23-B, 24-B

Critique: Skin biopsies are used to make or confirm a diagnosis for definitive treatment. Both techniques require use of a topical or local anesthetic. The *shave biopsy* technique, however, does not require suturing and is used to remove small skin lesions that do not require a complete thickness specimen for either diagnosis or treatment. The *excisional biopsy* technique, on the other hand, is reserved for larger skin lesions that require a full dermal thickness specimen such as a melanoma.

Pages 683, 684

Further Reading

Snell G: Skin biopsy. *In* Pfenninger JL, Fowler GC (Eds): Procedures for Primary Care Physicians. St. Louis, MO, Mosby-Year Book, 1994, pp 20–26.

25. To minimize scar formation when performing excisional skin biopsies, it is important to:

A. Keep the length of the incision as short as possible.
B. Undermine the edges of the incision prior to suturing.
C. Make the incision perpendicular to relaxed skin tension lines.
D. Pull the edges together with forceps or hemostats while suturing.
E. Make an elliptical incision with a length to width ratio of 2 : 1.

Answer: B

Critique: In order to minimize scarring from an excisional biopsy, the incision should be elliptical and parallel to the (relaxed) skin tension lines. The corner angles of the ellipse should form a 30-degree angle, and the length to width ratio of the incision should be 4 : 1. Although there may be a significant gap between the tissue margins following the removal of the biopsy specimen, use of hemostats or forceps should be avoided because they tend to damage the edges of the wound. If there is pronounced tension when the margins are brought together, undermining the wound edges can release this tension and prevent scarring.

Pages 680, 681, 684

Further Reading

Snell G: Skin biopsy. *In* Pfenninger JL, Fowler GC (Eds): Procedures for Primary Care Physicians. St. Louis, MO, Mosby-Year Book, 1994, p 24.

26. (True or False) Compared with the skin of younger individuals, the skin of older persons:
1. Tolerates greater wound tension
2. Has greater vascularity
3. Wound strength develops more slowly
4. Closure with adhesive strips is superior to closure with sutures

Answers: 1-F, 2-F, 3-T, 4-T

Critique: The skin of geriatric patients requires special care during surgery because their skin is thinner, has fewer capillary loops, and heals more slowly. Accordingly, compared with younger persons, the skin of elderly patients tolerates lower wound tension and heals better with adhesive strips than sutures.

Pages 681, 682

Questions 27–32. Match each numbered statement with the correct lettered term listed below.

    A. Simple lacerations
    B. Complex lacerations
    C. Both
    D. Neither

27. Short, shallow, straight

28. Use of a braided suture to repair

29. Irregular, long, deep

30. Emotionally stressful for the victim

31. Carries a higher risk of infection

32. Easy to anesthetize

Answers: 27-A, 28-D, 29-B, 30-C, 31-B, 32-A

Critique: Traumatic incisions of the skin are classified as either *simple* or *complex,* depending on their configuration. Lacerations are usually emotionally stressful, particularly when the victim is a child. *Simple* lacerations are relatively short, straight, and shallow; however, *complex* lacerations are longer, more irregular, and involve structures below the subcutaneous tissues. As a result, simple lacerations are easier to clean and anesthetize, whereas *complex lacerations* are more easily infected and scar more readily. A monofilament suture should be used to close *simple* and *complex* lacerations because a braided suture increases the risk of wound infection.

Page 684

33. Bleeding from lacerations should *not* be controlled by:

    A. Clamping the tissue underlying the bleeding
    B. Application of direct pressure to the wound
    C. Use of pressure dressings after wound closure
    D. Use of ligatures
    E. Suturing the wound

Answer: A

Critique: One of the goals of laceration care is to stop bleeding. The physician should *never* attempt to *blindly* clamp a bleeding site in the wound, because this may cause nerve, vascular, or tissue damage. Direct pressure to the wound before closure will usually stop most non-pulsatile bleeding. Although ligatures may also be used to control bleeding, suturing the wound will usually suffice to stop persistent bleeding. Following closure, pressure dressings can help to prevent further bleeding.

Page 684

Further Reading

Snell G: Laceration repair. *In* Pfenninger JL, Fowler GC (Eds): Procedures for Primary Care Physicians. St. Louis, MO, Mosby-Year Book, 1994, pp 12–19.

34. Treatment of a subungual hematoma includes each of the following EXCEPT:

    A. Application of warm packs to the affected nail
    B. Making a hole in the affected nail with an electrical cautery
    C. Melting a hole in the affected nail with a heated paper clip
    D. Cutting a hole in the affected nail with a scalpel blade
    E. Complete removal of the affected nail

Answer: A

Critique: Treatment of a subungual hematoma consists of decompression of the nailbed by evacuation of the hematoma. This can usually be accomplished by creating a hole in the affected nail with the heated tip of an electrical cautery instrument, the heated end of an unwrapped paper clip wire, or the tip of a no. 15 scalpel blade. In instances of a subungual hematoma arising from a nailbed laceration, it may be necessary to remove the nail of the affected digit entirely to prevent a post-traumatic nail deformity. Application of warmth would probably worsen the pain by increasing blood flow into the hematoma.

Page 685

Further Reading

Peggs JF: Subungual hematoma evacuation. *In* Pfenninger JL, Fowler GC (Eds): Procedures for Primary Care Physicians. St. Louis, MO, Mosby-Year Book, 1994, pp 47–49.

35. (True or False) True statements about the following problems of the nails and digits include:
1. Most cases of onychomycosis are resistant to oral antifungal agents.
2. Conservative treatment of an ingrown toenail (e.g., soaks, elevation of the affected side of the

nail, and use of antibiotics) is effective if applied at an early stage of the problem.

3. Partial excision of an ingrown toenail often provides inadequate treatment.
4. Surgery of the nails and digits can usually be accomplished without the use of a local anesthetic.

Answers: 1-F, 2-T, 3-T, 4-F

Critique: Onychomycosis of the nails does respond to an antifungal agent but may require up to 18 months for complete resolution of the infection. Although conservative treatment can improve ingrown toenails, surgical treatment is often required to effect complete resolution of this problem. Partial excision of an ingrown toenail is more difficult to manage postoperatively and often fails to resolve the problem. The digits are too well innervated to be operated on without a digital block.

Pages 685, 686

Questions 36–42. Match each numbered statement with the correct lettered term listed below.

A. External hemorrhoids
B. Internal hemorrhoids
C. Both
D. Neither

36. Consist of vascular tissues located within the anal canal

37. Caused by dysplastic changes in the overlying tissue

38. The most common symptom is pain.

39. Can be treated surgically without pain

40. Treatment usually includes hydrocortisone cream.

41. The most common symptom is painless bleeding.

42. The most common finding is thrombus formation.

Answers: 36-C, 37-D, 38-A, 39-B, 40-C, 41-B, 42-A

Critique: Hemorrhoids are vascular tissues that line the anal canal and help cushion the passage of the stool during defecation. Hemorrhoids that originate from above the dentate line are classified as "internal" and those that originate from below the dentate line are "external." Unlike polyps, hemorrhoids are not caused by dysplastic changes within the overlying anal mucosa but are the result of venous distention due to increased pressure generated within the anal canal from straining caused by constipation. The most common symptom arising from an internal hemorrhoid is painless rectal bleeding, whereas the most common symptom from an external hemorrhoid is pain. The most common finding in external hemorrhoids is venous thrombosis. Although the primary treatment for internal and external hemorrhoids is hydrocortisone cream, the most important treatment is to soften stools by increasing dietary fiber. Surgical treatment of internal hemorrhoids

is painless because the anal mucosa above the dentate line contains minimal innervation.

Pages 686, 687

43. (True or False) True statements about the surgical care for the following gynecologic problems include:

1. An I&D of a Bartholin's gland cyst followed by insertion of a Word catheter usually results in satisfactory resolution of this problem.
2. Cervical biopsies are usually obtained from cervical tissue that stains dark brown following the application of Lugol's solution.
3. Total excision of a Bartholin's gland cyst is usually necessary to adequately treat this problem.
4. Cervical biopsies may be performed without the aid of a colposcope.
5. Endometrial biopsies normally require some form of regional anesthesia.

Answers: 1-T, 2-F, 3-F, 4-T, 5-F

Critique: A Bartholin's gland cyst arises from a blockage of the drainage duct. A simple I&D of the cyst will produce immediate relief, but insertion of a Word catheter is necessary in order to prevent a recurrence. In most cases, complete excision of the cyst is unnecessary. Cervical biopsies are used to evaluate abnormal cervical lesions and Papanicolaou smears. Lugol's solution can be applied to the cervix to help identify sites for cervical biopsies. Lugol's solution is taken up by normal cervical tissue and allows the physician to selectively biopsy abnormal areas without the use of a colposcope. The endometrial biopsy is used to evaluate the cause of abnormal uterine bleeding. The patient does not usually need anesthesia for an endometrial biopsy unless cervical dilation is required in order to pass the biopsy instrument through the endocervical canal into the uterine cavity.

Pages 687, 688

Questions 44–48. Match each numbered statement with the correct lettered term listed below.

A. Benign breast lesions
B. Malignant breast lesions
C. Both
D. Neither

44. Tenderness helps to distinguish this lesion.

45. Fifty percent of these are identified by the patient.

46. These feel round, smooth, firm, and mobile.

47. These feel flat, rough, hard, and immobile.

48. These should be evaluated with needle aspiration.

Answers: 44-D, 45-C, 46-A, 47-B, 48-C

Critique: Fifty percent of abnormal breast lumps are detected by patients. The presence or absence of tenderness does not reliably indicate malignant potential. *Benign* lesions are typically round, smooth, firm, and mobile to the touch. *Malignant* lesions are flat, rough, hard, and immobile. Despite these characteristics, the physical examination has limited ability to distinguish between benign and malignant lumps. As a result, the method of choice for evaluating breast lumps is needle aspiration.

Pages 688, 689

49. A breast mass with overlying erythema and induration of the skin and ill-defined margins is a manifestation of a:

    A. Breast abscess
    B. Malignant breast tumor
    C. Fibroadenoma of the breast
    D. Breast cyst

Answer: B

Critique: Breast cancer is an inflammatory disease that may present with signs suggestive of an abscess. However, unlike a breast abscess, the resultant mass will feel hard and gritty and will not be accompanied with a fever. Classic "orange peel" changes and ulceration of the skin are late signs that signify advanced disease. Breast fibroadenomas and cysts may occur within the same breast. Fibroadenomas tend to be rubbery and firm with well-circumscribed edges. Breast cysts vary in size during the menstrual cycle; they are often tender and may spontaneously disappear.

Pages 688, 689

Questions 50–55. Match each numbered statement with the correct lettered term listed below.

    A. Needle aspiration
    B. Open biopsy
    C. Both
    D. Neither

50. Best procedure for evaluation of a cystic mass

51. Best procedure for evaluation of a solid mass

52. Should be performed in an outpatient surgery center

53. Can be performed in the physician's office

54. Produces a histologic specimen

55. Produces a cytologic specimen

Answers: 50-A, 51-B, 52-B, 53-A, 54-B, 55-A

Critique: A needle aspiration procedure is the easiest method for evaluating a breast lump. Although it is safe to perform in the office and does not require expensive equipment, this procedure only yields cytologic speci-

mens. Moreover, needle aspiration has an approximate 15% false-negative rate for identifying malignancies. An open biopsy provides a true histologic specimen but may require more extensive anesthesia, more expensive equipment, and assistance. As a result, open biopsies are usually performed by general surgeons in an outpatient surgery center.

Page 689

Further Reading

Hogle HH: Breast biopsy. *In* Pfenninger JL, Fowler GC (Eds): Procedures for Primary Care Physicians. St. Louis, MO, Mosby-Year Book, 1994, pp 714–717.

56. (True or False) True statements about the use of *cryosurgery* include:
    1. Local anesthesia is necessary for adequate pain control.
    2. Cryosurgery heals well, producing minimal or no scarring.
    3. Cryosurgery can be used to remove any benign skin lesion.
    4. Cryosurgery cannot be used to remove malignant skin lesions.
    5. Postoperative infection following cryosurgery is very rare.

Answers: 1-F, 2-T, 3-F, 4-F, 5-T

Critique: Cryosurgery is used to destroy skin lesions through focused application of intense cold, which results in partial-thickness thermal injury. Cryosurgery is easy to use, does not require any local anesthesia (although nonsteroidal antiinflammatory drugs help relieve postoperative pain), produces minimal or no scarring, and has a very low potential for postoperative infection. Cryosurgery cannot be used to treat subcutaneous lesions or large (greater than 1 cm) cutaneous lesions. Moreover, it should not be used around the scalp or eyebrows, because it will destroy the hair follicles and result in a permanent bald spot. It should not be used to treat melanomas but can be used to destroy basal cell carcinomas and actinic keratoses.

Page 690

Further Reading

Hocutt JE: Cryosurgery. *In* Pfenninger JL, Fowler GC (Eds): Procedures for Primary Care Physicians. St. Louis, MO, Mosby-Year Book, 1994, pp 102–120.

57. (True or False) Compared with conventional surgical techniques, *laser* surgery:
    1. May aggravate healing by stimulating keloid formation
    2. Is safer for the physician and the support staff

3. Has limited applicability to family practice
4. Is not superior except for specific surgical problems

Answers: 1-T, 2-F, 3-T, 4-T

Critique: Although laser surgery has gained widespread acceptance within many surgical subspecialties, it has not proved to be superior to most of the conventional office surgery techniques that are used by family physicians. In fact, laser surgery equipment is costly, takes up more space, and generates unpleasant fumes that can cause health problems for the physician and support staff. As a result, lasers have only limited applicability for most family physicians.

Pages 690–694

Further Reading

Rasmusen JE, Pfenninger JL: Laser therapy. *In* Pfenninger JL, Fowler GC (Eds): Procedures for Primary Care Physicians. St. Louis, MO, Mosby-Year Book, 1994, pp 84–90.

32

Gynecology

Gary W. Kearl

1. Risk factors for cervical neoplasia include each of the following EXCEPT:

    A. Genital human papilloma virus (HPV) infection
    B. History of alcohol use
    C. History of an abnormal Papanicolaou smear
    D. More than two lifetime sexual partners
    E. Initiation of sexual activity before age 20

Answer: B

Critique: Use of alcohol has been associated with an increased risk of breast cancer but is not linked with an increased risk of cervical cancer. HPV has been implicated as the causative agent of cervical cancer; however, many HPV infections are subclinical. Accordingly, any patient with a history of an abnormal Papanicolaou smear, multiple sexual partners, or initiation of sexual activity before the age of 20 should be classified as being at high risk for eventual development of cervical cancer and should receive an annual cervical screening.

Pages 696, 700

Further Reading

Ferenczy A: Epidemiology and clinical pathology of condylomata acuminata. Am J Obstet Gynecol 172:1333, 1995.

2. A 32-year-old single woman presents to the emergency room for evaluation and treatment of a head laceration. She is accompanied by her boyfriend, and she reports that she "accidentally slipped" and fell and struck her head against a wooden chair, causing the laceration. On examination, you note that her upper arms have several fresh bruises and that she has a swollen, bruised eyelid. You should do each of the following EXCEPT:

    A. Document the full extent of the patient's injuries in the medical chart.
    B. Interview the patient alone and ask about her relationship with her boyfriend.
    C. Provide the patient with information regarding local "safe" shelters.
    D. Express concern to the boyfriend about the nature of the patient's injuries.

    E. Document a possible diagnosis of domestic violence in the medical chart.

Answer: D

Critique: Domestic violence and *spouse abuse* are terms applied to violence that occurs between partners in an ongoing relationship, whether or not the partners are married. Victims of domestic violence are frequently manipulated psychologically by their abusers. Accordingly, if the victim is accompanied by the perpetrator of the abuse, she may be unwilling to openly disclose the true cause of her injuries. As a result, physicians should be sensitive to the possibility of domestic violence whenever the pattern of physical injuries does not fit the initial history. If a victim of domestic violence is accompanied by the perpetrator of the abuse, the physician should attempt to interview the victim alone and provide her with emotional support and access to a shelter where she can be protected from further abuse. The perpetrator should never be informed of a diagnosis of domestic violence or spouse abuse without the victim's consent.

Page 695

Further Reading

Goldberg WG, Tomlanovich MC: Domestic violence victims in the emergency department—new findings. JAMA 251:3264, 1984.

Questions 3–6. Anticipatory guidance is based on the patient's current position in the life cycle. Match the numbered stages of the life cycle listed below with the correct lettered options listed below:

    A. Developing self-image
    B. Choice of career
    C. Work satisfaction
    D. End-of-life issues

3. Elderly

4. Adolescents

5. Older adults

6. Young adults

Answers: 3-D, 4-A, 5-C, 6-B

Critique: Although there is some overlap among the issues facing individuals in each stage of the life cycle, each age group has unique issues to cope with. End-of-life issues are most acute for the elderly, whereas development of self-image is particularly important for adolescents. Older adults are often confronted with concerns about job satisfaction, whereas young adults are often more concerned with choosing and establishing a career.

Page 695

7. Papanicolaou screening has proved to be very effective in reducing deaths from cervical cancer. It is an excellent screening test for each of the following reasons EXCEPT:

A. It is easy to perform.
B. It is relatively inexpensive.
C. It is well accepted by patients.
D. It has a low false-positive rate.
E. It has a high false-negative rate.

Answer: E

Critique: The cervical Papanicolaou smear is used to screen for cervical cancer, the most common cause of cancer in women. The Papanicolaou test permits identification of premalignant and malignant lesions of the cervix at a stage at which treatment is both effective and acceptable to patients. Moreover, the Papanicolaou test is acceptable to women, easy to perform, and relatively inexpensive. Although the Papanicolaou test has a low false-positive rate, it can underestimate the severity of cervical lesions. For this reason, cervical abnormalities identified by the Papanicolaou test must be further evaluated by other means.

Pages 696, 700

Questions 8–12. (True or False). Cervical cancer screening:

8. Should begin when a woman decides to become sexually active

9. Can be discontinued after a woman has had three negative test results

10. Is conducted at intervals of 1 to 3 years depending on the patient's risk

11. Should include the collection of cervical endothelial cells

12. May be stopped if the patient is in a monogamous sexual relationship

Answers: 8-T, 9-F, 10-T, 11-T, 12-F

Critique: Cervical cancer is a disease that occurs in sexually active women. Consequently, cervical screening should begin when a women becomes sexually active. Cervical screening is usually conducted annually but may

be performed less frequently if the patient has had three negative test results and is considered to be at low risk for developing cervical cancer. The presence of endothelial cells on the Papanicolaou smear is a marker for an adequate sample of cervical cells. Even if a woman has only one sexual partner, she still needs to be screened regularly for cervical cancer, particularly if her partner has other sexual partners.

Page 697

Questions 13–17. The older Papanicolaou system of reporting cervical cytology differs from the newer Bethesda system in several ways. Match each numbered statement listed below with the correct lettered term:

A. Papanicolaou system
B. Bethesda system
C. Both A and B
D. Neither A nor B

13. Includes specific criteria for atypical cells

14. Includes five categories for Papanicolaou examination results

15. Provides a description of the adequacy of the sample

16. Localizes cervical lesions

17. Assesses the severity of premalignant lesions

Answers: 13-B, 14-C, 15-B, 16-D, 17-B

Critique: The Bethesda system of reporting cervical cytology was developed to replace the older Papanicolaou reporting system. Both systems include five categories of Papanicolaou results. However, unlike the Papanicolaou system, the Bethesda system includes explicit criteria for cellular atypia and dysplasia and provides a description of the adequacy of the smear. Neither system is able to localize cervical lesions. As a result, cervical abnormalities must be evaluated further using colposcopy or cervicography.

Pages 697, 698

Questions 18–21. The Bethesda system of reporting cervical or vaginal cytologic diagnoses includes two categories of premalignant lesions. Match the numbered cytologic features listed below to the correct lettered classification.

A. Low-grade *squamous intraepithelial lesions* (SIL)
B. High-grade *squamous intraepithelial lesions* (SIL)

18. Cervical intraepithelial neoplasia stage I (CIN I) (mild dysplasia)

19. CIN II (moderate dysplasia)

20. CIN III (severe dysplasia)

21. Atypical cervical cells associated with HPV

Answers: 18-A, 19-B, 20-B, 21-A

Critique: The Bethesda system of cytology reporting reflects current understanding of the pathophysiology of cervical transformation. The system includes only two categories (low or high grade) of premalignant squamous intraepithelial lesions. Low-grade SIL includes cytologic abnormalities associated with cervical HPV infections and CIN I (mild dysplasia). High-grade SIL includes cervical cells with CIN 2 and 3 (moderate or severe dysplasia).

Pages 697, 698

Questions 22–26. (True or False) The family physician must ensure that patients receive adequate cervical screening. Therefore, the family physician:

22. Must ensure collection and preservation of an adequate Papanicolaou smear

23. Supervises the reading of the Papanicolaou smear be the cytotechnician

24. Collects relevant patient information (e.g., last menstrual period, past use of hormone)

25. Decides whether to follow or evaluate the patient further

26. Assesses the quality of the Papanicolaou smear

Answers: 22-T, 23-F, 24-T, 25-T, 26-F

Critique: Cervical screening is fraught with many problems. The family physician is responsible for collecting, preserving, and forwarding the Papanicolaou smear to a reputable cytology laboratory on a regular basis. The family physician should also collect and forward all relevant clinical information and make a final determination of whether to continue following a patient or evaluate the patient through further examinations or consultations. The cytopathologist is responsible for personally reading or supervising the reading of the Papanicolaou smear by a qualified cytotechnician. The cytopathologist is also responsible for maintaining a laboratory quality assurance program and for assessing the appearance and adequacy of the smear.

Page 698

27. A colposcopic evaluation of cervical abnormalities includes each of the following EXCEPT:

    A. Application of Monsel's solution to highlight abnormal cells
    B. Application of vinegar solution to highlight abnormal cells
    C. Examination of the vulva, vagina, and cervix for abnormal cells
    D. Visualization of the entire squamocolumnar junction for abnormal cells
    E. Application of Lugol's solution to highlight abnormal cells

Answer: A

Critique: The colposcope is an optical device that permits a magnified view of the surface of the female genital tract. A complete colposcopic evaluation includes an examination of the vulva, vagina, and cervix for dysplastic or malignant tissues. A satisfactory colposcopic examination includes visualization of the entire squamocolumnar junction. Acetic acid (vinegar) and Lugol's solutions are used to highlight abnormal cervical tissues for possible biopsy. Monsel's solution is used to stem bleeding from cervical biopsy sites.

Page 699

28. Atypical cervical cells are caused by each of the following EXCEPT:

    A. Infection
    B. Repair
    C. Metaplasia
    D. Dysplasia
    E. Air drying

Answer: C

Critique: Atypical cells on a Papanicolaou smear are a marker for genital infections by HPV, *Trichomonas*, *Chlamydia*, etc.; cellular repair following injury to the cervix; cervical dysplasia; and improper Papanicolaou smear collection technique (air drying). Metaplasia is a physiologic process and does not produce atypia.

Page 699

29. A 24-year-old sexually active female patient presents with a vaginal discharge and genital itching. A physical examination including visual inspection of the vulva, vagina, and cervix is remarkable only for a thin watery vaginal discharge. A microscopic examination of a potassium hydroxide (KOH) slide and saline "wet prep" of the discharge is remarkable only for numerous white blood cells (WBCs). Her Papanicolaou smear demonstrates koilocytotic atypia. The most likely cause of her symptoms is:

    A. Bacterial vaginosis
    B. Subclinical HPV infection
    C. *Candida*
    D. Poor hygiene
    E. *Trichomonas*

Answer: B

Critique: Each of the choices listed above could cause the patient's symptoms. However, a saline wet preparation should demonstrate "clue cells" in the case of bacterial vaginosis, or motile *Trichomonas* organisms in the presence of *Trichomonas* infection. *Candida* infection should demonstrate budding yeast on a KOH slide. Poor hygiene might produce genital itching and discharge but would not be expected to produce koilocytosis on a Papanicolaou smear. HPV is the most prevalent viral sexually transmitted disease (STD) encountered currently. The peak age for acquiring genital HPV infections is 20 to 25 years. Moreover, as many as 95% of genital HPV infections may be subclinical (e.g., not associated with condylomata). Although the Papanicolaou smear may demonstrate candidal species and trichomonads, koilocytosis is the best morphologic marker for HPV infection.

Pages 696, 700, 703–707

Further Reading

Ferenczy A: Epidemiology and clinical pathology of condylomata acuminata. Am J Obstet Gynecol 172:1336, 1995.

30. Menstruation occurs in response to:

    A. Action of follicle-stimulating hormone (FSH)
    B. Production of progesterone by theca cells
    C. Action of luteinizing hormone (LH)
    D. Production of estrogen by granulosa cells
    E. Falling ovarian steroid levels

Answer: E

Critique: The menstrual cycle involves a complex interaction between the hypothalamus, pituitary, ovary, and endometrium. FSH, produced by the anterior pituitary, causes production of estrogen by the theca cells of the ovary. Estrogen stimulates maturation of one or more ovarian follicles and proliferation of the endometrial lining. Rising estrogen levels stimulate a "mid-cycle" surge of LH that triggers ovulation and production of progesterone by the granulosa cells of the ovary. Lack of conception results in an abrupt fall of ovarian steroid levels that triggers menstruation.

Page 701

Questions 31–36. Match the numbered causes of abnormal vaginal bleeding listed below with the correct lettered causes.

    A. Menorrhagia
    B. Metrorrhagia
    C. Menometrorrhagia

31. Uterine fibroids

32. Anovulatory cycles

33. Threatened abortion

34. Oral contraceptives

35. Intrauterine device (IUD)

36. HPV

Answers: 31-A, 32-C, 33-C, 34-B, 35-A, 36-B

Critique: Menorrhagia refers to regular but heavy menstrual bleeding. Use of an IUD and uterine fibroids are common causes of this type of bleeding. Metrorrhagia refers to menstrual-type vaginal bleeding that occurs more frequently than normal. Oral contraceptives may produce intermenstrual (breakthrough) bleeding. Genital infections such as HPV may also produce metrorrhagia. Menometrorrhagia refers to irregular but heavy or prolonged vaginal bleeding. This pattern of bleeding is observed when anovulatory cycles result in endometrial

hyperplasia from unopposed estrogen secretion. A threatened abortion might also produce this type of bleeding.

Pages 701, 702

37. Each of the following may cause amenorrhea EXCEPT:

    A. Sheehan's syndrome
    B. Turner's syndrome
    C. Asherman's syndrome
    D. Anorexia nervosa
    E. Ovarian cancer

Answer: E

Critique: Amenorrhea is defined as an absence of menses for at least 6 months. Sheehan's syndrome (infarction of the anterior pituitary following a postpartum hemorrhage) is a rare cause of amenorrhea due to panhypopituitarism. Turner's syndrome results in amenorrhea from gonadal dysgenesis. Asherman's syndrome results in amenorrhea due to endometrial scarring following a dilatation and curettage. Anorexia nervosa can produce amenorrhea from excessive loss of body fat. Ovarian cancer does not normally produce amenorrhea.

Page 702

Questions 38–41. Match each of the numbered conditions listed below with the correct lettered treatments.

    A. Metronidazole 500 mg bid for 7 days
    B. Topical estrogen
    C. Topical clotrimazole
    D. Metronidazole 2 g in a single dose

38. Bacterial vaginosis

39. Candidal vulvovaginitis

40. Trichomoniasis

41. Atrophic vaginitis

Answers: 38-A, 39-C, 40-D, 41-B

Critique: Bacterial vaginosis is the most commonly diagnosed cause of vaginitis. Oral metronidazole is the drug of choice, but intravaginal metronidazole gel or clindamycin cream can also be used. Candidal infections usually respond to clotrimazole, miconazole, or nystatin. Candidal infections that persist after imidazole treatment may be caused by non-albicans species and may require treatment with terconazole. *Trichomonas* also responds to oral metronidazole, but it can usually be treated with a single (2 g) oral dose. Atrophic vaginitis results from estrogen deficiency and is seen most commonly in menopausal women. It can be treated with topical estrogen or estrogen replacement therapy.

Pages 703–707

Questions 42–45. Match each of the numbered conditions listed below with the correct lettered major clinical manifestations.

A. Malodorous, watery, greenish discharge
B. Itchy, thick, white discharge with erythematous mucosa
C. Malodorous, thick, gray-white discharge
D. Clear watery discharge with friable mucosa

42. Bacterial vaginosis

43. Candidal vulvovaginitis

44. *Trichomonas* vaginitis

45. Atrophic vaginitis

Answers: 42-C, 43-B, 44-A, 45-D

Critique: Bacterial vaginosis is caused by anaerobic and gram-negative bacteria. Patients usually complain of a malodorous (fishy), sticky gray-white discharge. Candidal vulvovaginitis is primarily caused by *Candida albicans* and produces an itchy, thick white discharge that is adherent to erythematous mucosa. *Trichomonas* is a flagellated protozoan that produces a malodorous, greenish watery vaginal discharge. Atrophic vaginitis is caused by low estrogen levels and produces a clear, watery discharge and friable atrophic mucosa.

Pages 703–707

Questions 46–49. Match each of the numbered descriptions listed below with the correct lettered condition.

A. Acute pelvic pain
B. Chronic pelvic pain
C. Both A and B
D. Neither A nor B

46. Frequently associated with depression

47. Frequently associated with fever

48. Can include a pelvic mass

49. May present with a vaginal discharge

Answers: 46-B, 47-A, 48-C, 49-A

Critique: Acute pelvic pain is often caused by an ascending genital tract infection. Although symptoms of acute pelvic pain are nonspecific, treatment usually includes the administration of antibiotics. Chronic pelvic pain often involves other pelvic structures besides the reproductive tract and is often associated with depression. Both forms of pain can be caused by a pelvic mass.

Pages 707–709

50. Characteristics associated with ectopic pregnancy include all of the following EXCEPT:

A. Use of an IUD increases the risk.
B. Positive but declining serum hCG titer
C. Intrauterine pregnancy

D. High risk of maternal death
E. Pelvic pain can occur.

Answer: C

Critique: Ectopic pregnancy is an increasingly common source of acute pelvic pain. IUD use, progestin-only oral contraceptives, and a history of pelvic inflammatory disease (PID) or tubal surgery are risk factors for developing ectopic pregnancy. Patients can present with amenorrhea, vaginal bleeding, and pelvic pain. An undiagnosed ruptured ectopic pregnancy carries a mortality rate of 30%. The presence of an intrauterine pregnancy makes a concurrent ectopic pregnancy unlikely.

Page 708

51. A 19-year-old female patient presents with lower pelvic pain. She has always had regular periods and denies any history of dysmenorrhea. She is sexually active but uses condoms and denies any history of STDs or amenorrhea. On physical examination, she has a nontender, freely moveable, and unilateral adnexal mass. Her findings are most likely due to:

A. A tubo-ovarian abscess
B. A uterine fibroid
C. An ectopic pregnancy
D. A functional ovarian cyst
E. Endometriosis

Answer: D

Critique: Although there are a number of causes for a pelvic mass, the patient's age, history, and physical findings are most suggestive of a functional ovarian cyst. A tubo-ovarian abscess is unlikely in a patient without a history of STD or PID. Uterine fibroids can mimic ovarian cysts but are usually asymptomatic in young women. Ectopic pregnancy is usually associated with amenorrhea. Endometriosis can create an adnexal mass but is usually associated with recurrent dysmenorrhea.

Page 708

52. Additional work-up of the patient in question 51 should include each of the following EXCEPT:

A. Pregnancy test
B. Pelvic ultrasound
C. Cervical cultures for gonorrhea and chlamydia
D. Empirical trial of oral contraceptives
E. Papanicolaou smear

Answer: E

Critique: Although this patient appears to have a functional ovarian cyst, a negative result on a pregnancy test would help to rule out an ectopic pregnancy. Moreover, a pelvic ultrasound could help to confirm whether or not the mass is cystic and could help to rule out the possibility of a tubo-ovarian abscess from a subacute form of PID. Cervical cultures for gonorrhea and chlamydia would also help to rule out the possibility of a tubo-ovarian abscess from PID. If the ultrasound revealed that the mass appears to be "functional," then an empirical course of oral contraceptives should cause the cyst to regress. A Papanicolaou smear would not be helpful in this situation.

Page 709

53. Menopause is associated with each of the following EXCEPT:

    A. Recurrent hot flashes and moodiness
    B. Vaginal dryness and dyspareunia
    C. Increased serum cholesterol levels
    D. Low FSH and LH levels
    E. Increased risk of fractures

Answer: D

Critique: During menopause the ovaries become less responsive to gonadotropin stimulation, resulting in high levels of FSH and LH and lower levels of estrogen. Declining estrogen produces multiple symptoms and physical changes: hot flashes, moodiness, vaginal dryness, and dyspareunia. Menopausal patients also develop an increased risk of cardiovascular disease due to rising levels of low-density lipoprotein (LDL) cholesterol and a decline in high-density lipoprotein (HDL) cholesterol; and an increased risk of hip and vertebral fractures because of osteoporosis.

Page 710

54. (True or False) Estrogen replacement therapy (ERT) has been shown to be effective for:

    1. Relieving the symptoms of menopause
    2. Decreasing the risk of breast cancer
    3. Decreasing the risk of cardiovascular disease
    4. Improving glycemic control
    5. Decreasing the risk of osteoporosis

Answers: 1-T, 2-F, 3-T, 4-F, 5-T

Critique: ERT is effective at relieving the symptoms of menopause and decreasing the risk of osteoporosis and cardiovascular disease. The propensity of ERT to increase or decrease breast cancer risk remains controversial. Studies have appeared that indicate increased, decreased, and no effect on breast cancer risk. If there is a risk, these studies appear to indicate that the hazard is small for average-risk women, constituting a relative risk of under 1.5. This risk must be weighed against the comparatively large cardiovascular and musculoskeletal benefits of ERT. Clinicians must also consider that ERT might cause estrogen-sensitive breast cancers to grow more rapidly. Finally, ERT exerts no significant effect on glucose metabolism.

Page 711

Further Reading

Colditz GA, Hankinson SE, Hunter DJ, et al: The use of estrogens and progestins and the risk of breast cancer in postmenopausal women. N Engl J Med 332:1589–1593, 1995.
Colditz GA, Stampfer MJ, Willett WC, et al: Prospective study of estrogen replacement therapy and risk of breast cancer in postmenopausal women. JAMA 264:2648–2653, 1990.
Henderson BE, Paganini-Hill A, Ross RK: Decreased mortality in users of estrogen replacement therapy. Arch Intern Med 151:75–78, 1991.
Kergkvist L, Adami HO, Persson I, et al: The risk of breast cancer after estrogen and estrogen-progestin replacement. N Engl J Med 321:293–297, 1989.
Steinberg KK, Thacker SB, Smith SJ, et al: A meta-analysis of the effect of estrogen replacement therapy on the risk of breast cancer. JAMA 265:1985–1990, 1991.

55. (True or False) The following regimens of ERT would be appropriate in a menopausal woman with an intact uterus:

    1. Transdermal estrogen 0.05 mg twice weekly
    2. Estrogen 0.625 mg/day during days 1 to 25; progesterone 10 mg/day during days 14 to 25 each month
    3. Estrogen 0.625 mg/day, progesterone 2.5 mg/day
    4. Conjugated estrogen 0.3 mg/day
    5. Estrogen 0.625 mg/day, progesterone 2.5 mg/day during days 1 to 14

Answers: 1-F, 2-T, 3-T, 4-F, 5-T

Critique: There are numerous ERT regimens. Women with an intact uterus should receive a combination of estrogen and progesterone in either a continuous or sequential fashion. Estrogen alone (even in low dose) is not appropriate because of the increased risk of uterine cancer.

Page 711

56. Each of the following is a risk factor for pelvic relaxation, EXCEPT:

    A. Multiparity
    B. Obesity
    C. Giving birth to a macrosomic infant
    D. Chronic coughing or straining
    E. Cesarean section

Answer: E

Critique: Pelvic relaxation results from damage to pelvic ligaments and muscles. Multiparity, giving birth to macrosomic infants, obesity, and chronic coughing or straining all result in increased stress on pelvic structures. Cesarean delivery protects against pelvic relaxation. Menopause can aggravate mild pelvic relaxation.

Page 712

Questions 57–61. Match each of the numbered descriptions listed below with the correct lettered condition.

    A. Anatomic stress incontinence
    B. Urge incontinence
    C. Both A and B
    D. Neither A nor B

57. Results in unwanted release of urine

58. Caused by detrusor muscle instability

59. Occurs while coughing or straining

60. Caused by neurologic injury

61. Associated with pelvic relaxation

Answers: 57-C, 58-B, 59-A, 60-D, 61-A

Critique: Anatomic stress incontinence is caused by pelvic relaxation and results when bladder pressure exceeds urethral sphincter pressure. Anatomic stress incontinence is aggravated by increased intra-abdominal pressure.

Urge incontinence is caused by uninhibited detrusor muscle contractions. Although both forms of incontinence result in unwanted release of urine, no neurologic dysfunction is involved.

Page 712

33

Contraception

Cynda Johnson

Questions 1–5. Match each of the following options with the most appropriate statement regarding oral contraceptives:

    A. Combined oral contraceptives (OCs)
    B. Progestin-only OCs
    C. Both A and B
    D. Neither A nor B

1. An excellent contraceptive option for a breast-feeding woman.

2. A hormone-containing pill intended to be taken every day of the cycle.

3. The failure rate in a typical user of the method is about 3%.

4. OCs should be discontinued periodically to decrease risk associated with usage of the method.

5. OCs are contraindicated in the 40-year-old woman who smokes.

Answers: 1-B, 2-B, 3-C, 4-D, 5-A

Critique: As stated in the text, the mini pill is used commonly in lactating women, and the milk supply is not reduced. Mini pills are taken every day of the month with no seven-day hiatus. There is no evidence of a need to discontinue OCs periodically. The risks associated with combined OC use do not appear to be related to the length of the time that a woman is on the pill. The risk of arterial events associated with combined OC use appears to be confined to older women with risk factors, especially cigarette smokers. The mortality risk is primarily among women older than 35 years of age; combined OCs are contraindicated for this group of women.

Pages 716, 721

Questions 6–10. (True or False) The following methods of birth control have a failure rate of less than 1% in the typical user.

6. Combined oral contraceptives

7. TCu 380A intrauterine device (IUD)

8. Dcpo-Provera (medroxyprogesterone)

9. Norplant

10. Cervical cap

Answers: 6-F, 7-T, 8-T, 9-T, 10-F

Page 716

11. Newer progestins with apparently fewer androgenic effects include all of the following EXCEPT:

    A. Norgestimate
    B. Norethindrone
    C. Desogestrel
    D. Gestodene

Answer: B

Critique: Several new progestins with less androgenic effects include desogestrel, norgestimate, and gestodene. Norethindrone is an older progestin found in many currently used oral contraceptives.

Page 716

12. When initially selecting a combined oral contraceptive for a low-risk patient, which ONE of the following doses of ethinyl estradiol is optimal for the estrogen component?

    A. 30 μg
    B. 80 μg
    C. 20 μg
    D. 50 μg

Answer: A

Critique: A pill with less than 50 μg should be used initially; however, there is an increased pregnancy rate with the 20-μg pills.

Page 720

Questions 13–18. Match the following options with the most appropriate statements:

A. Depo-Provera
B. Diaphragm
C. Combined oral contraceptives
D. Norplant

13. There is an increased incidence of urinary tract infection in some users.

14. Users who become pregnant have a reduced risk of ectopic pregnancy.

15. The expected return of fertility takes longer than with other methods.

16. The most common reason for discontinuing this method is persistence of irregular vaginal bleeding or spotting.

17. Unexpected spotting should prompt an evaluation for *Chlamydia* infection.

18. Decreased incidence of sexually transmitted diseases (STDs) in users of this method.

Answers: 13-B, 14-C, 15-A, 16-D, 17-C, 18-B

Critique: Use of the diaphragm is associated with an increased incidence of urinary tract infection in some women. One of the noncontraceptive benefits of combined oral contraceptives is a decreased number of ectopic pregnancies. The return of fertility after the use of Depo-Provera is delayed for at least 3 months after the last injection, and the median time to conception is 10 months. There is no evidence that Depo-Provera causes permanent infertility. The risk for *Chlamydia trachomatis* infection of the cervix is higher among women who use oral contraceptives than among nonusers. Irregular bleeding patterns including spotting, frequent bleeding, and scanty bleeding are common with Norplant. Bleeding problems are by far the main reason for which patients request the removal of Norplant. At least one study suggests that female-dependent barrier contraceptives might confer better STD protection for women than do male condoms.

Pages 718, 719, 721, 722, 724, 725

19. Use of oral contraceptives is clearly associated with *decreased* risk of which ONE of the following cancers?

A. Breast
B. Liver
C. Cervical
D. Ovarian

Answer: D

Critique: Use of oral contraceptives appears to reduce the risk of endometrial cancer by 50% and that of ovarian cancer by 40%. There is probably no increased risk of breast cancer; however, some studies suggest a slightly increased risk of breast cancer among younger women. It is unclear whether there is any change in the incidence of cancer of the cervix in women on oral contraceptives. Liver cancer, although still extremely rare, is increased in incidence among women taking oral contraceptives.

Page 717

Questions 20–25. Match the following options with the appropriate female hormones:

A. Progestins
B. Estrogens
C. Both A and B
D. Neither A nor B

20. Associated with increase in high-density lipoprotein cholesterol (HDL)

21. Associated with increase in low-density lipoprotein cholesterol (LDL)

22. Associated with a decreased risk of endometrial cancer

23. A headache is a common side effect.

24. Use in contraceptive dosages is teratogenic.

25. May aggravate acne

Answers: 20-B, 21-A, 22-A, 23-B, 24-D, 25-A

Critique: Although combined oral contraceptives also show a decrease in the incidence of endometrial cancer, the progestin component accounts for this result. Depot therapy with medroxyprogesterone (Depo-Provera) reduces the risk of endometrial cancer by about 80%. Headache is a symptom that is often associated with the estrogen component of combined oral contraceptives and may be decreased with a low-dose estrogen pill. Authorities differ as to whether women with migraine headaches are candidates for estrogen-containing oral contraceptives at all. However, there is consensus that progressive or severe headaches should prompt discontinuation of oral contraceptives. Because of experience with high-dose progestins and diethylstilbestrol taken early in pregnancy, there has been concern that oral contraceptives might cause congenital anomalies. However, careful study has failed to reveal convincing evidence that exposure to contraceptive doses of estrogens or progestins early in pregnancy is teratogenic. The more androgenic progestins (norgestrel and levonorgestrel) in combined oral contraceptives may aggravate acne. However, acne improves on the combined oral contraceptives, probably from the estrogen component.

Pages 717, 718, 722

26. Drugs reported to increase combined oral contraceptive failure rates include all of the following drug categories EXCEPT:

A. Benzodiazepines
B. Antibiotics
C. Anticonvulsants
D. Mineral oils

Answer: A

Critique: All of the agents noted, except for the benzodiazepines, have been associated with an increased risk of oral contraceptive failure.

Page 719, Table 33–3

Questions 27–29. (True or False) The following represent conditions for which combined oral contraceptive pill (OCP) use confers some degree of protection or improved outcomes.

27. Iron deficiency anemia

28. Pelvic inflammatory disease

29. Migraine headaches

Answers: 27-T, 28-T, 29-F

Critique: Decreased risk of pelvic inflammatory disease is a noncontraceptive benefit of OCPs. Iron deficiency anemia is also less common among OCP users than among nonusers. Some experts believe that migraine headaches are actually a contraindication to use of oral contraceptives because of the possibility that use of OCPs might actually increase the frequency or severity of a vascular headache.

Pages 718, 719

Questions 30–34. (True or False) The following are absolute contraindications to use of combined oral contraceptives.

30. Diabetes

31. Hypertension

32. Coronary artery disease

33. Acute hepatitis

34. Liver neoplasm

Answers: 30-F, 31-F, 32-T, 33-T, 34-T

Critique: Diabetes is listed as a condition that may make oral contraceptive use less desirable, but in fact in many cases it is the best form of birth control for diabetic women, in whom preventing pregnancy may be very important. Similar arguments can be given for patients who have hypertension. Coronary artery disease is a contraindication to the use of oral contraceptives. It is usually desirable to stop combined contraceptives until the liver enzymes return to normal in a case of acute hepatitis. Liver neoplasm, either benign or malignant, is a contraindication to use of oral contraceptives.

Page 720

35. Which ONE of the following is true about the levonorgestrel implant (Norplant)?

    A. The optimal timing for insertion is in the first 14 days of the menstrual cycle.
    B. It is a good contraceptive method for women on anticonvulsants.

    C. The physician should schedule more time for insertion than removal.
    D. After 5 years the capsules should be removed even if the patient is having no side effects from the method.

Answer: D

Critique: The optimal timing for insertion of the implant is within the first 5 to 7 days of the menstrual cycle. It is believed that women taking anticonvulsant medications probably should consider other methods of contraception, because anticonvulsants may render these implants less effective. Much more time is required for removal than for insertion. After 5 years the capsules should be removed, because the contraceptive effect decreases rapidly after that time period.

Page 721

36. Which ONE of the following would be the preferred method of contraception in an obese woman with anovulation and dysfunctional uterine bleeding?

    A. Depo-Provera
    B. Norplant
    C. Progestin only pill
    D. Copper-containing IUD

Answer: A

Critique: Depo-Provera is a very good choice for a patient who has anovulation and dysfunctional uterine bleeding. This is a very common scenario in the obese woman. Norplant is not a good choice for this patient, because individuals who already have dysfunctional uterine bleeding will likely continue to be unhappy, considering that the greatest side effect of the Norplant is irregular, unexpected bleeding. The same could be said for progestin only birth control pills. Finally, a copper-containing IUD, if anything, will cause increased irregular bleeding and will certainly not normalize the bleeding pattern.

Pages 121–123

Questions 37–42.
    A. TCU-380A IUD
    B. Progestasert IUD
    C. Both A and B
    D. Neither A nor B

37. Highly effective, reversible form of contraception

38. Interference with implantation is major mechanism of action

39. Multiyear use

40. Impregnated with barium making it radiopaque

41. IUD preferred in the nulliparous woman

42. Increased menstrual blood loss

Answers: 37-C, 38-D, 39-A, 40-C, 41-B, 42-A

Critique: Both IUD types provide highly reversible contraception, and it is now believed that IUDs do not work primarily by interference with implantation but by preventing fertilization of the ovum. The Progestasert IUD must be changed annually; the copper TCU-380A can be left in for 10 years. If the IUD string cannot be found, both IUDs are radiopaque and can be located by x-ray. Only the Progestasert is approved for use in nulliparous women. Finally, the IUDs that contain progestins usually decrease menstrual blood loss, whereas there is an increase in blood loss associated with the copper-containing IUD.

Page 722

43. Which ONE of the following is a contraindication to use of the IUD?

  A. High risk for sexually transmitted diseases
  B. Breast-feeding
  C. 6 weeks post partum
  D. Nulliparity

Answer: A

Critique: An IUD is a very good choice for a breast-feeding woman. Although an IUD can be placed earlier than 6 weeks post partum, thereafter, insertion is extremely safe. As noted earlier, the Progestasert can be used in nulliparous women; however, the IUD is contraindicated in women who are at high risk for STDs.

Page 723

44. All of the following statements regarding vaginal barrier contraception are true EXCEPT:

  A. Typical-use efficacy and optimal-use efficacy are nearly identical.
  B. These methods provide some protection against STDs.
  C. Systemic effects are minimal.
  D. The woman's partner may help in the placement of these devices.

Answer: A

Critique: The typical-use efficacy and perfect-use efficacy are quite disparate in the vaginal barrier methods, because they are dependent on coitus.

Pages 716, 723, 724

45. Of the following statements regarding male condoms, all are true EXCEPT:

  A. A patient or his partner may be sensitive to the latex material of which the condom is made.
  B. "Natural" membrane condoms are preferred over latex condoms for preventing the spread of STDs.
  C. The condom is considered to be a coitus-dependent form of contraception.
  D. If lubrication is needed, KY jelly or contraceptive foam may be used with the condom.

Answer: B

Critique: Latex condoms are known to provide better protection than do membrane condoms against STDs.

Page 724

Questions 46–49. Match the following options with the appropriate numbered statements:

  A. Bilateral tubal ligation
  B. Vasectomy
  C. Both A and B
  D. Neither A nor B

46. Must be considered a permanent method of sterilization

47. Effectiveness of 100%

48. Generally an office procedure

49. Effective immediately after the procedure has been carried out

Answers: 46-C, 47-D, 48-B, 49-A

Critique: The patient should never select one of these methods with the intention that it will be reversible. Proper evaluation and counseling are essential. Both of these methods are highly effective: the failure rate of female sterilization is 0.4%, and the failure rate for male sterilization is 0.15%. One of the advantages of the vasectomy over the tubal ligation is that it is an office procedure and can be done under local anesthesia. Azoospermia is not immediate after vasectomy. About 12 to 20 ejaculations are required to clear the genital tract of viable sperm. Unprotected intercourse should not occur until a specimen of semen reveals no viable sperm.

Pages 716, 726

50. Which ONE of the following may NOT be used for postcoital fertility control?

  A. Combination oral contraceptive pills
  B. Mifepristone
  C. Depo-Provera
  D. IUD

Answer: C

Critique: Each of these other methods, if used correctly, can be used in postcoital fertility control. Oral contraceptives are the most common choice and are the easiest to use.

Page 727

51. Which ONE of the following would be the optimal contraceptive choice for an adolescent with a history of *Chlamydia* infection and one therapeutic abortion?

  A. Condom and oral contraceptive
  B. Diaphragm and condom
  C. Female condom
  D. Depo-Provera

Answer: A

Critique: The combination of a condom and oral contraceptive would be particularly useful in this patient both to prevent spread of STDs and as a very reliable combination for contraception. This patient would probably not be a reliable diaphragm user and would need better contraception. The diaphragm and condom would provide superior contraception when used together, but the couple would need to use them consistently; her history of an elective abortion suggests that such an expectation might prove overly optimistic. The female condom is also dependent on coitus. It would provide good protection from STDs but only if used every time. It does not have a high rate of effectiveness in preventing pregnancy. Depo-Provera provides excellent contraception but provides no protection from STDs.

34

Interpretation of the Electrocardiogram

Michael D. Hagen

Questions 1–3. The heart can be considered an electrical "dipole," with an isoelectric plane passing through the heart. The electrocardiogram (ECG) measures the heart's electrical activity via electrodes attached to the limbs and the chest. Match the appropriate limb lead with the potential that lead will measure in the normal heart.

    A. Right arm electrode (or lead)
    B. Left arm electrode (or lead)
    C. Both A and B
    D. Neither A nor B

1. A negative potential

2. A positive potential

3. A neutral, or zero, potential

Answers: 1-A, 2-B, 3-D

Critique: The heart represents an electrical dipole with an isoelectric region or plane passing through the heart's center. Electrodes placed above the plane will measure negative potentials; those placed below the plane measure positive potentials. In the normal heart, the right arm electrode will demonstrate negative potentials. Similarly, the left arm lead will measure positive potentials. The limb leads are either above or below the isoelectric plane and therefore will not demonstrate neutral potential in the normal heart.

Further Reading

Vallbona C: Interpretation of the electrocardiogram. *In* Rakel RE (ed.): Textbook of Family Practice, 5th ed. Philadelphia, WB Saunders, 1995, p 729.

4. The P wave of the ECG represents which one of the following electrical phenomena?

    A. Repolarization of the ventricles
    B. Repolarization of the atria
    C. Depolarization of the ventricles
    D. Depolarization of the atria

Answer: D

Critique: The wave forms displayed on the ECG represent voltages developed by depolarization and repolarization of the myocardium. The P wave reflects depolarization of the atria. The QRS wave depicts depolarization of the ventricles. The T wave indicates repolarization of the ventricles. Atrial repolarization is usually masked by the QRS wave.

Further Reading

Vallbona C: Interpretation of the electrocardiogram. *In* Rakel RE: Textbook of Family Practice, 5th ed. Philadelphia, WB Saunders, 1995, p 730.

5. (True or False) Which of the following represents scalar analysis of an ECG?

    A. Assessment of the PR interval
    B. Assessment of the QRS wave duration
    C. Assessment of wave shape and amplitude in multiple leads
    D. Assessment of the QT interval

Answers: A-T, B-T, C-F, D-T

Critique: Electrocardiographic wave shapes and amplitudes are used in assessing ECG patterns or pattern analysis. The PR interval indicates the time required for a sinus impulse to depolarize the atria, travel through the atrioventricular (AV) node, and through the bundle branches. The QT interval describes the time required for both ventricular depolarization and repolarization. The QRS duration depicts the time required for ventricular depolarization once the depolarizing impulse has arrived over the bundle branches. These intervals and durations all represent components of scalar analysis.

Further Reading

Vallbona C: Interpretation of the electrocardiogram. *In* Rakel RE: Textbook of Family Practice, 5th ed. Philadelphia, WB Saunders, 1995, p 730.

Questions 6–8. Match the following electrophysiologic phenomena with their corresponding electrocardiographic representations:

    A. Atrial depolarization
    B. Ventricular depolarization
    C. Atrial repolarization
    D. Ventricular repolarization

6. The QRS wave

7. The T wave

8. The P wave

Answers: 6-B, 7-D, 8-A

Critique: The P wave represents atrial depolarization. The QRS wave depicts ventricular depolarization and usually masks repolarization of the atria. The T wave represents ventricular depolarization.

Further Reading

Vallbona C: Interpretation of the electrocardiogram. *In* Rakel RE (ed.): Textbook of Family Practice, 5th ed. Philadelphia, WB Saunders, 1995, p 730.

9. Which of the following frontal plane QRS axes indicate left axis deviation?

    A. +45 degrees
    B. +80 degrees
    C. −45 degrees
    D. +180 degrees

Answer: C

Critique: The potentials measured in the limb leads provide a means for estimating the mean QRS axis in the frontal plane. The normal axis lies between 0 and +90 degrees. An axis between 0 and −90 degrees indicates left axis deviation. Axes between +90 and +180 degrees denote right axis deviation. Extreme right axis deviation exists when the mean QRS axis lies between +180 and −90 degrees.

Further Reading

Vallbona C: Interpretation of the electrocardiogram. *In* Rakel RE: Textbook of Family Practice, 5th ed. Philadelphia, WB Saunders, 1995, p 732.

10. (True or False) Assume that you have read an ECG and determined that the mean QRS axis is +75 degrees in the frontal plane. Which of the following would represent an abnormal T axis in this context?

    A. +60 degrees
    B. −20 degrees
    C. +135 degrees
    D. +30 degrees

Answers: A-T, B-F, C-F, D-T

Critique: The T wave axis in the frontal plane should lie within +60 degrees counterclockwise and +40 degrees clockwise of the QRS axis. Axes of +60 and +30 degrees satisfy this criterion. For a QRS axis of +75 degrees, a T axis of −20 degrees represents excessive counterclockwise rotation. Similarly, +135 degrees indicates excessive clockwise deviation from the QRS axis.

Further Reading

Vallbona C: Interpretation of the electrocardiogram. *In* Rakel RE: Textbook of Family Practice, 5th ed. Philadelphia, WB Saunders, 1995, p 732.

11. In Figure 34–1, the mean QRS axis in the frontal plane is:

    A. −30 degrees
    B. +90 degrees
    C. +120 degrees
    D. +60 degrees

Answer: D

Critique: The simplest method for determining the frontal plane mean QRS axis is to scan the ECG limb leads for an isoelectric (i.e., QRS waveform displacement above the baseline equal to displacement below the baseline) tracing. In this ECG, lead aVL demonstrates an isoelectric QRS complex. This indicates that the mean QRS axis is perpendicular to this lead, either +60 or −120 degrees. The positive QRS complexes in leads I, II, and III indicate that the axis points downward and to the left. This yields an axis of +60 degrees.

Further Reading

Vallbona C: Interpretation of the electrocardiogram. *In* Rakel RE: Textbook of Family Practice, 5th ed. Philadelphia, WB Saunders, 1995, pp 731, 732.

12. Examine Figure 34–2. The frontal plane mean QRS axis for this tracing is:

    A. +120 degrees
    B. −40 degrees
    C. −90 degrees
    D. 0 degrees

Answer: B

Critique: The frontal plane mean QRS axis for this tracing is approximately −40 degrees. The QRS complex in lead II is nearly isoelectric, which means that the QRS axis is nearly perpendicular to this lead. This means that the axis is close to either −30 or +150 degrees. The QRS in leads aVF and III are negative, which indicates that the axis points upward and to the left; therefore, the axis must be close to −30 degrees. Note, however, that the QRS in lead II is not completely isoelectric; the net deflection is slightly negative, which indicates that the axis is slightly to the left of −30 degrees or about −40 degrees.

Further Reading

Vallbona C: Interpretation of the electrocardiogram. *In* Rakel RE: Textbook of Family Practice, 5th ed. Philadelphia, WB Saunders, 1995, pp 731, 732.

13. For the tracing in question 12, the frontal plane mean T axis is:

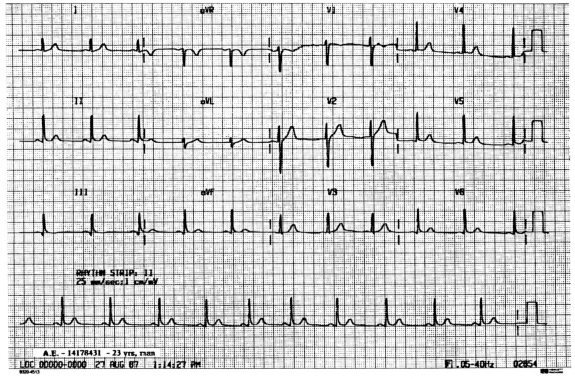

Figure 34–1 (Reproduced with permission from Rakel RE [Ed]: Textbook of Family Practice, 5th ed. Philadelphia, WB Saunders, 1995, p 734.)

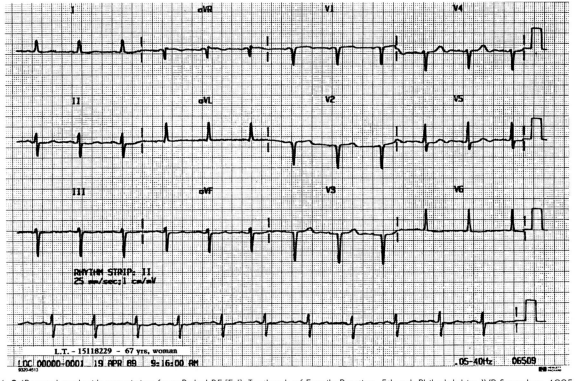

Figure 34–2 (Reproduced with permission from Rakel RE [Ed]: Textbook of Family Practice, 5th ed. Philadelphia, WB Saunders, 1995, p 735.)

A. +90 degrees
B. −40 degrees
C. +120 degrees
D. +60 degrees

Answer: D

Critique: The T wave is isoelectric in lead aVL; therefore, the mean T axis must be either +60 or −120 degrees. Because the T wave deflection is positive in lead II and slightly positive in lead aVF, the T axis lies to the left and downward. The axis is therefore +60 degrees.

Further Reading

Vallbona C: Interpretation of the electrocardiogram. *In* Rakel RE: Textbook of Family Practice, 5th ed. Philadelphia, WB Saunders, 1995, pp 731, 732.

14. Which of the following characteristics do you find in Figure 34–3?

A. Left ventricular strain
B. Right atrial hypertrophy
C. Left axis deviation
D. Left ventricular hypertrophy

Answer: A

Critique: The tracing exhibits left ventricular strain. The largest limb lead QRS deflection appears in lead I, where the QRS is positive. The T wave is negative in this lead, fulfilling one criterion for strain. Additionally, the mean QRS axis is approximately +15 degrees, while the T wave

axis is to the right of +90 degrees, or about +120 degrees. The tracing demonstrates a normal mean QRS axis and shows no evidence of right atrial hypertrophy or left ventricular hypertrophy.

Further Reading

Vallbona C: Interpretation of the electrocardiogram. *In* Rakel RE: Textbook of Family Practice, 5th ed. Philadelphia, WB Saunders, 1995, pp 733, 738, 744.

15. In the normal heart, the transition from a negative to positive QRS deflection occurs where in the precordial (V_1 to V_6) leads?

A. V_1–V_2
B. V_2–V_3
C. V_4–V_5
D. V_5–V_6

Answer: B

Critique: In the normal heart, the precordial leads will demonstrate negative QRS complexes in leads V_1 and V_2. Transition from negative to positive should occur between leads V_2 and V_3 (i.e., V_4, V_5, and V_6 should demonstrate positive QRS complexes).

Further Reading

Vallbona C: Interpretation of the electrocardiogram. *In* Rakel RE: Textbook of Family Practice, 5th ed. Philadelphia, WB Saunders, 1995, p 737.

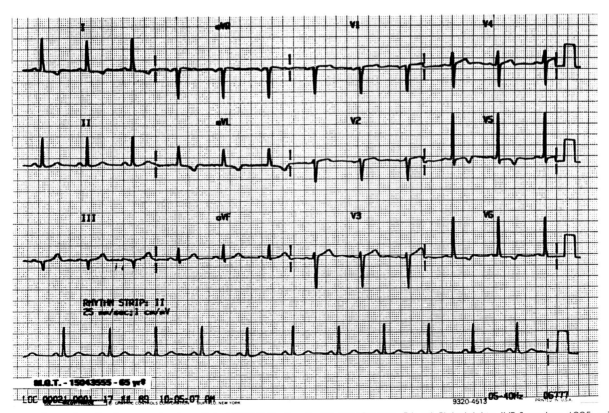

Figure 34–3 (Reproduced with permission from Rakel RE [Ed]: Textbook of Family Practice, 5th ed. Philadelphia, WB Saunders, 1995, p 736.)

16. Of the following, which is **not** a criterion for considering left ventricular hypertrophy on an ECG?

    A. Left axis deviation
    B. QRS magnitude >1.5 mv (15 mm) in the lead of mean axis
    C. S_1 plus R_5 <3.5 mv (35 mm)
    D. QRS duration between 0.08 second and 0.12 second

Answer: C

Critique: Several criteria exist for diagnosis of left ventricular hypertrophy on the ECG. If the S wave magnitude in lead V_1 plus the R wave magnitude in V_5 is greater than 3.5 mv (35 mm), the reader should consider left ventricular hypertrophy. Left axis deviation, QRS magnitude greater than 1.5 mv (15 mm), and normal QRS duration are criteria for diagnosing left ventricular hypertrophy. The Estes criteria provide a semiquantitative method for determining the presence of left ventricular hypertrophy. Presence of the criteria yields points: 4 points indicate probable left ventricular hypertrophy; 5 points signify definite left ventricular hypertrophy. The criteria and associated points are:

- Amplitude of the R wave or S wave in limb leads ≥2 mv (20 mm); or S wave in I, V_1, or V_2 ≥3 mv (30 mm); or R wave in V_5 or V_6 >3 mv (30 mm): 3 points
- ST segment changes with digitalis: 1 point
- ST segment changes without digitalis: 2 points
- Left atrial enlargement: 3 points
- Left axis deviation of ≥ −30 degrees: 2 points
- QRS duration greater than 0.09 second: 1 point
- Intrinsicoid deflection in V_5 or V_6 >0.05 second: 1 point

Further Reading

Vallbona C: Interpretation of the electrocardiogram. *In* Rakel RE (ed.): Textbook of Family Practice, 5th ed. Philadelphia, WB Saunders, 1995, p 738.
Watanabe AM, Ryan T: Electrocardiography, stress testing, and ambulatory monitoring. *In* Kelley WN (Ed): Essentials of Internal Medicine. Philadelphia, JB Lippincott, 1994, p 62.

17. (True or False) Figure 34–4 meets the following criteria for left ventricular hypertrophy (assume that the patient is not taking digitalis).

    A. QRS duration greater than 0.09 second
    B. Left axis deviation of ≥ −30 degrees
    C. ST segment changes without digitalis
    D. Left atrial enlargement
    E. Amplitude of R or S wave in limb leads ≥2 mv (20 mm)

Answers: A-T, B-T, C-T, D-F, E-T

Critique: The QRS duration is about 0.10 to 0.11 second, and the frontal plane mean QRS axis is −30 degrees on the basis of the isoelectric QRS in lead II with negative QRS deflection in aVF. The tracing exhibits marked ST segment changes in the lateral chest leads (V_5 and V_6). Additionally, the R wave amplitude is 2.1 mv (21 mm) in lead aVL, and the S wave amplitude is 2.3 mv (23 mm)

in lead III. The tracing does not demonstrate left atrial enlargement. Using the Estes point system, the tracing yields 8 points. This score indicates definite left ventricular hypertrophy. Additionally, S_1 plus R_5 equals 5.5 mv (55 mm), which also suggests left ventricular hypertrophy.

Further Reading

Vallbona C: Interpretation of the electrocardiogram. *In* Rakel RE: Textbook of Family Practice, 5th ed. Philadelphia, WB Saunders, 1995, p 738.
Watanabe AM, Ryan T: Electrocardiography, stress testing, and ambulatory monitoring. *In* Kelley WN (Ed): Essentials of Internal Medicine. Philadelphia, JB Lippincott, 1994, p 62.

18. (True or False) Figure 34–5 displays the following characteristics seen in right ventricular hypertrophy:

    A. Normal QRS duration
    B. Right axis deviation
    C. Right ventricular strain pattern
    D. R_1 >0.7 mv (7 mm)

Answers: A-T, B-T, C-T, D-T

Critique: The tracing displays a QRS duration of about 0.08 second. The frontal plane mean QRS axis is +120 degrees (the QRS is isoelectric in aVR, which indicates an axis of +120 when considered with the positive QRS deflection in aVF), which indicates right axis deviation. A strain pattern exists in the anterior chest leads. The R wave magnitude in lead V_1 is substantially greater than 0.7 mv.

Further Reading

Vallbona C: Interpretation of the electrocardiogram. *In* Rakel RE: Textbook of Family Practice, 5th ed. Philadelphia, WB Saunders, 1995, pp 739, 740.

19. Of the following options, which one is **not** a criterion for diagnosing left bundle branch block on an ECG?

    A. QRS duration prolongation (>0.12 second)
    B. Slurring of the QRS complex in several leads
    C. Right axis deviation
    D. Posterior axis in the horizontal plane (i.e., in the V leads)

Answer: C

Critique: QRS prolongation, QRS slurring, and posterior axis in the horizontal plane all occur with left bundle branch block. The ECG will demonstrate left rather than right axis deviation.

Further Reading

Vallbona C: Interpretation of the electrocardiogram. *In* Rakel RE: Textbook of Family Practice, 5th ed. Philadelphia, WB Saunders, 1995, pp 740, 741.

20. (True or False) Figure 34–6 demonstrates the following characteristics of left bundle branch block:

    A. Left axis deviation
    B. Left ventricular strain pattern

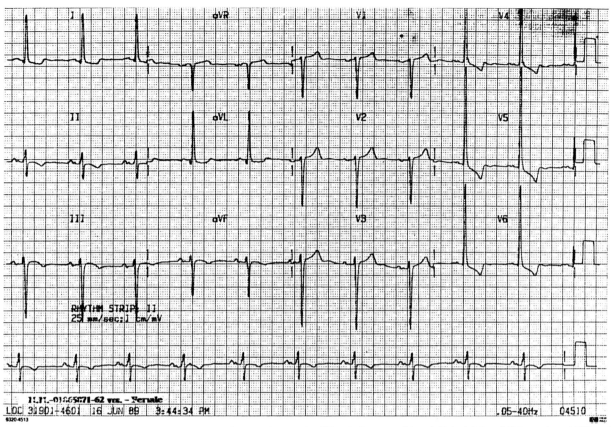

Figure 34–4 (Reproduced with permission from Rakel RE [Ed]: Textbook of Family Practice, 5th ed. Philadelphia, WB Saunders, 1995, p 739.)

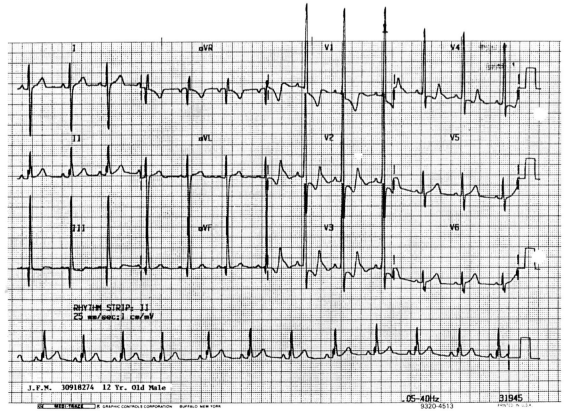

Figure 34–5 (Reproduced with permission from Rakel RE [Ed]: Textbook of Family Practice, 5th ed. Philadelphia, WB Saunders, 1995, p 740.)

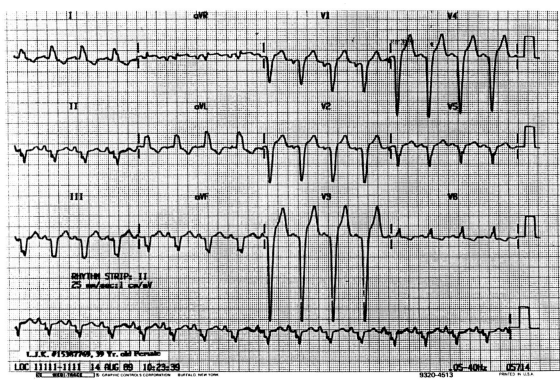

Figure 34–6 (Reproduced with permission from Rakel RE [Ed]: Textbook of Family Practice, 5th ed. Philadelphia, WB Saunders, 1995, p 742.)

   C. Normal QRS magnitude in a lead parallel to the QRS axis
   D. Slurring of QRS complexes

Answers: A-T, B-T, C-T, D-T

Critique: The tracing demonstrates a mean frontal plane QRS axis of −60 degrees. The ECG also displays strain and QRS slurring in several leads. The QRS magnitude is normal in aVL, the lead closest to the mean QRS axis.

Further Reading

Vallbona C: Interpretation of the electrocardiogram. *In* Rakel RE: Textbook of Family Practice, 5th ed. Philadelphia, WB Saunders, 1995, pp 740, 741.

21. All of the following represent criteria for left anterior hemiblock (also called left anterior fascicular block) **except:**

   A. Right axis deviation
   B. Q wave in lead aVL
   C. Normal magnitude QRS complexes
   D. QRS duration <0.12 second

Answer: A

Critique: The left bundle branch divides into two fascicles: superior and inferior. Because of the heart's position in the chest, these fascicles assume anterior and posterior configurations, respectively, with respect to the ECG. In left anterior hemiblock, initial ventricular depolarization forces extend downward and to the right, sometimes writing a Q wave in lead I. As the area served by the anterior fascicle depolarizes subsequently, ventricular forces

swing back to the left and superiorly. This sequence writes an initial R wave with a deep S wave in lead III. Unless ventricular hypertrophy coexists with the hemiblock, QRS complexes should demonstrate normal magnitude. QRS duration will be less than 0.12 second.

Further Reading

Vallbona C: Interpretation of the electrocardiogram. *In* Rakel RE: Textbook of Family Practice, 5th ed. Philadelphia, WB Saunders, 1995, pp 742, 743.

22. (True or False) Statements regarding characteristics demonstrated in Figure 34–7 include:

   A. Left axis deviation
   B. Ventricular strain pattern
   C. QRS duration of 0.14 second
   D. RSR in lead V_1

Answers: A-F, B-T, C-F, D-T

Critique: This tracing demonstrates right axis deviation, with a mean frontal plane QRS axis of +120 degrees. The QRS duration is about 0.10 second, and lead V_1 displays an RSR' pattern. These findings are consistent with right bundle branch block. Note that if the QRS duration is between 0.10 second and 0.12 second, this constellation constitutes an *incomplete* right bundle branch block. A QRS duration of 0.12 second or longer would indicate a complete right bundle branch block.

Further Reading

Bundle branch blocks. *In* Lipman BC, Cascio T: ECG Assessment and Interpretation. Philadelphia, FA Davis, 1994, pp 160–162.

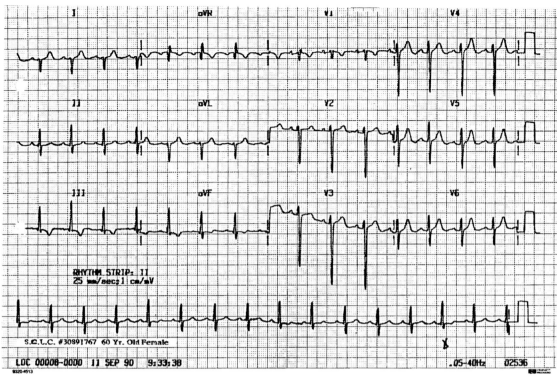

Figure 34–7 (Reproduced with permission from Rakel RE [Ed]: Textbook of Family Practice, 5th ed. Philadelphia, WB Saunders, 1995, p 741.)

Vallbona C: Interpretation of the electrocardiogram. *In* Rakel RE: Textbook of Family Practice, 5th ed. Philadelphia, WB Saunders, 1995, pp 741, 742.

23. Figure 34–8 exhibits which one of the following conditions?

    A. First-degree AV block
    B. Left bundle branch block
    C. Right axis deviation
    D. Bifascicular block
    E. Left posterior hemiblock

Answer: D

Critique: This ECG demonstrates left axis deviation (mean QRS axis −45 degrees), right bundle branch block, and limb lead findings consistent with a left anterior hemiblock. This tracing therefore exhibits bifascicular block. The PR interval is normal, thus ruling out first-degree AV block. The QRS duration is normal, which rules out a left bundle branch block. The tracing does not exhibit findings of a left posterior hemiblock.

Further Reading

Vallbona C: Interpretation of the electrocardiogram. *In* Rakel RE: Textbook of Family Practice, 5th ed. Philadelphia, WB Saunders, 1995, pp 740–744.

24. All of the following represent criteria for ECG evidence of right atrial enlargement EXCEPT:

    A. P wave duration of <0.08 second
    B. Positive P wave in lead aVL
    C. Vertical P wave axis
    D. P wave magnitude >0.25 mv (2.5 mm)

Answer: B

Critique: Criteria for right atrial enlargement include a P wave duration of 0.08 second or less, vertical axis or right axis deviation, P wave magnitude of greater than 0.25 mv (2.5 mm), and a negative P wave in lead aVL. The P wave axis would have to lie to the left of +60 degrees to yield a positive P wave in lead aVL and thus would not meet criteria for right atrial enlargement.

Further Reading

Vallbona C: Interpretation of the electrocardiogram. *In* Rakel RE: Textbook of Family Practice, 5th ed. Philadelphia, WB Saunders, 1995, pp 744–746.

25. All of the following represent ECG criteria for left atrial enlargement EXCEPT:

    A. A biphasic P wave in lead V_1
    B. Two small P wave axes separated by 30 to 60 degrees
    C. Duration of P wave <0.08 second
    D. Presence of a "double-humped" P wave in lead II

Answer: C

Critique: The P wave represents depolarization potentials from both atria. In left atrial enlargement, the larger left atrium depolarizes later than the normal right atrium. Thus the ECG displays an initial P wave axis of about +60 degrees (reflecting right atrial depolarization) and a second P wave component with an axis to the left (reflecting left atrial depolarization) of the initial forces. This phenomenon results in a double-humped P wave in lead II and biphasic P wave in the lead V_1. The duration of

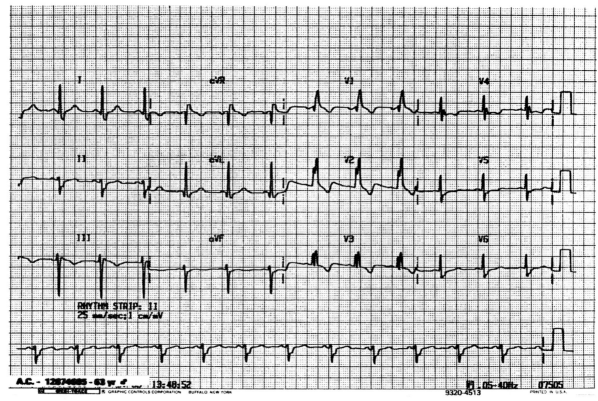

Figure 34-8 (Reproduced with permission from Rakel RE [Ed]: Textbook of Family Practice, 5th ed. Philadelphia, WB Saunders, 1995, p 745.)

the P wave is usually longer than 0.08 second in the context of left atrial enlargement.

Further Reading

Vallbona C: Interpretation of the electrocardiogram. *In* Rakel RE: Textbook of Family Practice, 5th ed. Philadelphia, WB Saunders, 1995, pp 746, 747.

26. (True or False) Axis changes associated with myocardial infarction include:

A. The ST segment axis points **away** from the area of injury.
B. The T wave axis points **toward** the area of ischemia.
C. The axis of the initial forces of the QRS complex points **toward** the area of injury.

Answers: A-F, B-F, C-F

Critique: With a completed myocardial infarction, the dead tissue produces no potentials, and the initial QRS forces will point away from the infarcted tissue. This writes a Q wave in the ECG leads associated with the damaged area. Similarly, the T wave axis points away from an area of ischemia, leading to T wave inversion. The ST segment axis points toward an area of injury, displayed as ST segment elevation.

Further Reading

Vallbona C: Interpretation of the electrocardiogram. *In* Rakel RE: Textbook of Family Practice, 5th ed. Philadelphia, WB Saunders, 1995, pp 748, 749.

Questions 27–29. Match the following ECG characteristics with the time at which they might most likely be observed in an evolving myocardial infarction.

A. T wave inversion
B. Deep and wide Q waves
C. Both A and B
D. Neither A nor B

27. Acute myocardial infarction (within 1 week of onset)

28. Subacute myocardial infarction (between 1 and 8 weeks of onset)

29. Old myocardial infarction (more than 8 weeks after onset)

Answers: 27-C, 28-C, 29-B

Critique: During the acute phase of a myocardial infarction, prominent ST segment elevation or depression should appear. T wave inversion can also appear during the acute phase. Additionally, Q waves might also be seen. In the subacute phase, the ECG can demonstrate both T wave inversion and Q waves. Eight weeks after the initial infarction, deep and wide Q waves should persist. Note that a normal ECG can display insignificant Q waves, usually in leads I and aVL and the lateral chest leads. Insignificant Q waves have less than 0.04-second duration and less than 25% of the magnitude of the associated R wave.

Further Reading

Myocardial infarction. *In* Lipman BC, Cascio T: ECG Assessment and Interpretation. Philadelphia, FA Davis, 1994, pp 195–200.
Vallbona C: Interpretation of the electrocardiogram. *In* Rakel RE (ed.): Textbook of Family Practice, 5th ed. Philadelphia, WB Saunders, 1995, pp 749, 750.

30. Anterior or anteroseptal myocardial infarction is caused by occlusion of which one of the following coronary arteries?

    A. Dominant right coronary artery
    B. Circumflex coronary artery
    C. Left anterior descending coronary artery
    D. Terminal portion of the left anterior descending coronary artery

Answer: C

Critique: The left anterior descending coronary artery supplies the anterior or anteroseptal myocardium. Occlusion of the circumflex coronary artery leads to infarction in the heart's lateral wall. Occlusion of a dominant right coronary artery results in inferior wall infarction; occlusion of a dominant left coronary artery can have the same result. Terminal left anterior descending coronary arterial occlusion leads to apical infarction.

Further Reading

Myocardial infarction. *In* Lipman BC, Cascio T: ECG Assessment and Interpretation. Philadelphia, FA Davis, 1994, pp 200–206.
Vallbona C: Interpretation of the electrocardiogram. *In* Rakel RE (ed.): Textbook of Family Practice, 5th ed. Philadelphia, WB Saunders, 1995, p 750.

31. Elevated ST segments, negative T waves, or QS complexes in leads V_1 and V_2 indicate infarction of which portion of the myocardium?

    A. Inferior diaphragmatic
    B. Posterior
    C. Apical
    D. Anterior or anteroseptal

Answer: D

Critique: Elevated ST segments, negative T waves, or QS complexes in V_1 and V_2 leads indicate infarction of the anterior or anteroseptal region of the myocardium. A true posterior infarction would display ST segment depression anteriorly, with positive T waves and R waves in the anterior leads. Apical infarction is associated with ST segment and T wave changes in lead I and will demonstrate a Q wave in lead I with old infarctions.

Further Reading

Vallbona C: Interpretation of the electrocardiogram. *In* Rakel RE: Textbook of Family Practice, 5th ed. Philadelphia, WB Saunders, 1995, p 750.

32. Elevated ST segments, negative T waves, and Q waves in leads II, III, and aVF are found in an infarction of which portion of the myocardium?

    A. Posterior
    B. Anterior or anteroseptal
    C. Inferior (or diaphragmatic)
    D. Anterolateral

Answer: C

Critique: Elevated ST segments, negative T waves, and Q waves in leads II, III, and aVF indicate inferior or diaphragmatic myocardial infarction. A true posterior myocardial infarction would display ST segment depression anteriorly, with positive T waves and R waves in the anterior chest leads. Anterior or anteroseptal infarctions would display elevated ST segments, negative T waves, or QRS complexes in the anterior leads. An anterolateral infarction would demonstrate ECG changes in leads I and aVL and the lateral chest leads (V_5 and V_6).

Further Reading

Myocardial infarction. *In* Lipman BC, Cascio T: ECG Assessment and Interpretation. Philadelphia, FA Davis, 1994, pp 202, 203.
Vallbona C: Interpretation of the electrocardiogram. *In* Rakel RE (ed.): Textbook of Family Practice, 5th ed. Philadelphia, WB Saunders, 1995, p 750.

33. Figure 34–9 demonstrates infarction in which portion of the myocardium?

    A. Inferior (or diaphragmatic)
    B. Posterior
    C. Anterolateral
    D. Anterior or anteroseptal

Answer: D

Critique: This tracing demonstrates elevated ST segments in the anterior or anteroseptal chest leads, indicating acute anterior or anteroseptal myocardial infarction. The tracing also demonstrates poor R wave progression.

Further Reading

Myocardial infarction. *In* Lipman BC, Cascio T: ECG Assessment and Interpretation. Philadelphia, FA Davis, 1994, pp 201, 202.
Vallbona C: Interpretation of the electrocardiogram. *In* Rakel RE (ed.): Textbook of Family Practice, 5th ed. Philadelphia, WB Saunders, 1995, pp 750–751.

34. Figure 34–10 demonstrates which one of the following?

    A. Acute anteroseptal myocardial infarction
    B. Old posterior myocardial infarction
    C. Acute anterolateral myocardial infarction
    D. Old inferior wall myocardial infarction

Answer: D

Critique: This tracing shows deep Q waves in leads II, III, and aVF; these findings indicate an old inferior wall myocardial infarction. An acute anteroseptal infarction would demonstrate ST segment changes in the anterior chest leads. An old posterior infarction would show prominent R waves in the anterior chest leads. An acute anterolateral infarction would cause ST segment elevation in leads I and aVL and the lateral chest leads.

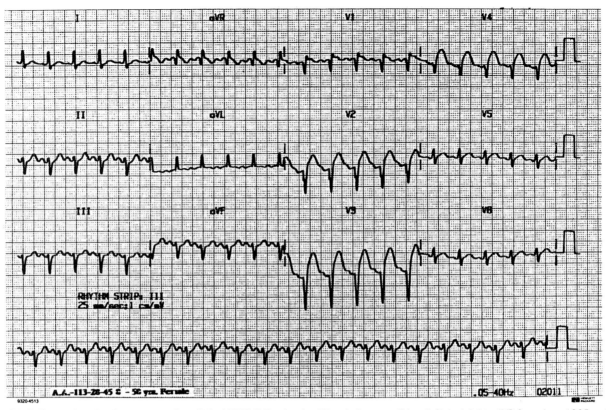

Figure 34–9 (Reproduced with permission from Rakel RE [Ed]: Textbook of Family Practice, 5th ed. Philadelphia, WB Saunders, 1995, p 751.)

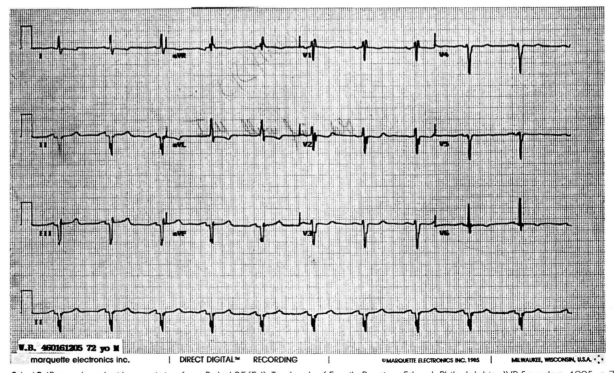

Figure 34–10 (Reproduced with permission from Rakel RE [Ed]: Textbook of Family Practice, 5th ed. Philadelphia, WB Saunders, 1995, p 753.)

Further Reading

Myocardial infarction. *In* Lipman BC, Cascio T: ECG Assessment and Interpretation. Philadelphia, FA Davis, 1994, pp 200–208.
Vallbona C: Interpretation of the electrocardiogram. *In* Rakel RE (ed.): Textbook of Family Practice, 5th ed. Philadelphia, WB Saunders, 1995, pp 750–753.

35. A 35-year-old man presents with a history of low-grade fever and myalgias for several days. During the past 24 hours, he has developed substernal chest pain that seems worse with deep inspiration. He also notes some relief when he sits up and leans forward. You perform an ECG in your office (Fig. 34–11). The most likely diagnosis for this scenario and ECG is:

A. Acute inferior myocardial infarction
B. Acute anteroseptal ischemia
C. Acute pericarditis
D. Acute posterior myocardial infarction

Answer: C

Critique: The clinical history and ECG findings are most consistent with acute pericarditis. The tracing demonstrates mild ST segment elevation in leads I, II, and aVL and in the anterior chest leads. No significant Q waves exist, and the ST segment axis approximates that of the QRS complex. Acute inferior myocardial infarction would demonstrate more pronounced ST segment changes inferiorly; additionally, Q waves and T wave inversion should appear if the process had been ongoing for several days. Anteroseptal ischemia would demonstrate ST segment depression rather than ST segment elevation. An acute posterior infarction should also demonstrate negative ST segments in the anterior chest leads.

Further Reading

Vallbona C: Interpretation of the electrocardiogram. *In* Rakel RE: Textbook of Family Practice, 5th ed. Philadelphia, WB Saunders, 1995, p 754.

36. You are performing a preparticipation sports examination on a 25-year-old man. He has no cardiac symptoms or complaints of chest pain. At his request, you perform an ECG, shown in Figure 34–12. The most likely diagnosis in this setting is:

A. Pericarditis
B. Inferior myocardial infarction
C. Early repolarization
D. Anterolateral ischemia

Answer: C

Critique: The tracing demonstrates ST segment elevation in leads II, III, and aVF and in several anterior V leads. The patient has no symptoms to suggest myocardial infarction, ischemia, or pericarditis. Of the options presented, early repolarization represents the most likely explanation for the ECG findings.

Further Reading

Vallbona C: Interpretation of the electrocardiogram. *In* Rakel RE (ed.): Textbook of Family Practice, 5th ed. Philadelphia, WB Saunders, 1995, p 754.

37. A 50-year-old man with a history of a documented myocardial infarction 3 years ago has just transferred his care to your practice. You perform an ECG as part of your examination. At present, the patient has no cardiac symptoms and has had none since the acute event. In view of his history, the patient's tracing (Fig. 34–13) demonstrates which of the following?

A. Inferior myocardial infarction
B. Acute pericarditis
C. Posterior myocardial infarction
D. Ventricular aneurysm

Answer: D

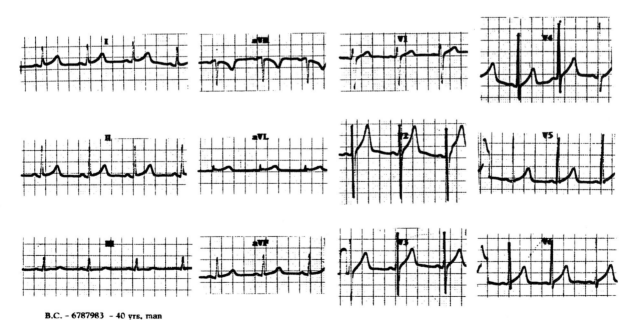

B.C. - 6787983 - 40 yrs. man

Figure 34–11 (Reproduced with permission from Rakel RE [Ed]: Textbook of Family Practice, 5th ed. Philadelphia, WB Saunders, 1995, p 754.)

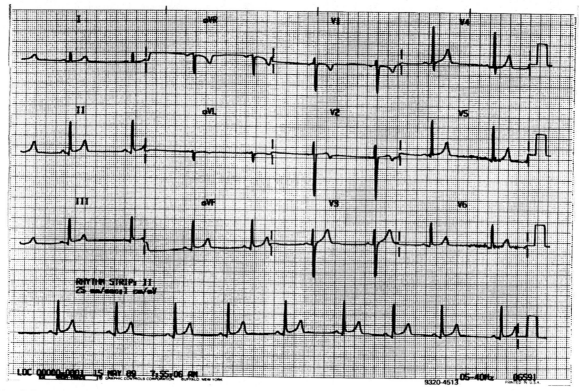

Figure 34–12 (Reproduced with permission from Rakel RE [Ed]: Textbook of Family Practice, 5th ed. Philadelphia, WB Saunders, 1995, p 755.)

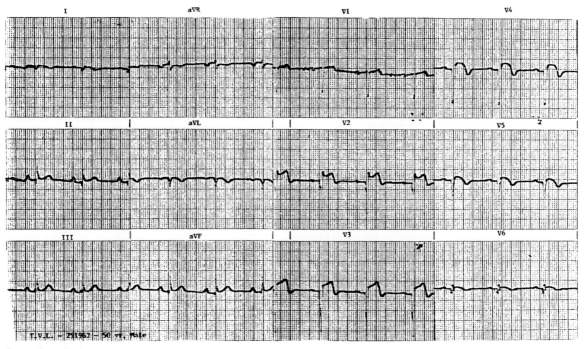

Figure 34–13 (Courtesy of Dr. H. Starke, Baylor College of Medicine, Houston, Tx.)

Critique: The tracing displays marked ST segment elevation in the precordial leads, along with QRS waves in V_3, V_4, and V_5. These findings are consistent with an old anterior or anteroseptal infarction with ventricular aneurysm formation. The patient's lack of symptoms and other ECG findings militate against the other options.

Further Reading

Vallbona C: Interpretation of the electrocardiogram. *In* Rakel RE: Textbook of Family Practice, 5th ed. Philadelphia, WB Saunders, 1995, p 755.

38. Of the following, which are true statements regarding criteria for diagnosing ischemia on an ECG?

    A. Upsloping ST segment
    B. ST segment depression lasting less than 0.08 second
    C. ST segment axis opposite of the QRS axis in the frontal plane
    D. ST segment axis same as the QRS axis in the horizontal plane

Answer: C

Critique: ST segment depression associated with ischemia displays downsloping or a horizontal appearance rather than upsloping. The depression should persist more than 0.08 second beyond the J point. The ST segment axis points away from the mean QRS axis in the frontal plane; this will yield depressed ST segments in leads with positive QRS complexes. The ST segment axis in the horizontal plane will also point away from the QRS axis, yielding ST segment depression in the lateral chest leads.

Further Reading

Vallbona C: Interpretation of the electrocardiogram. *In* Rakel RE (ed.): Textbook of Family Practice, 5th ed. Philadelphia, WB Saunders, 1995, pp 755–757.

39. Criteria for ECG diagnosis of dextrocardia include all of the following EXCEPT:

    A. Negative T waves in lead aVL
    B. Left axis deviation
    C. Negative T waves in the chest leads
    D. Negative QRS waves in the chest leads

Answer: B

Critique: Dextrocardia, one component of situs inversus, yields ECG findings that represent "mirror image" characteristics compared with the normal heart. The tracing will demonstrate right axis deviation, negative T waves in aVL, and negative T waves and QRS complexes in the chest leads.

Further Reading

Vallbona C: Interpretation of the electrocardiogram. *In* Rakel RE (ed.): Textbook of Family Practice, 5th ed. Philadelphia, WB Saunders, 1995, pp 757, 758.

40. (True or False) Statements regarding ECG findings obtained with reversed arm leads include:

    A. Lead I displays a mirror image of the normal pattern.
    B. Lead aVR will display a normal pattern.
    C. The horizontal plane and frontal plane QRS axes agree.
    D. T waves will appear normal in the chest leads.

Answers: A-T, B-F, C-F, D-T

Critique: When the right and left arm leads are reversed, the axes demonstrated by the limb leads and chest leads will disagree. Thus, the T waves in the chest leads will display their normal configuration but appear opposite to normal in the limb leads. Lead aVR will look like a normal aVL, and aVL will demonstrate the pattern expected for a normal aVR. The horizontal plane QRS axis (determined in the normally applied chest leads) will disagree with the frontal plane QRS axis (determined from the limb leads).

Further Reading

Vallbona C: Interpretation of the electrocardiogram. *In* Rakel RE: Textbook of Family Practice, 5th ed. Philadelphia, WB Saunders, 1995, pp 758, 759.

41. Causes of prolonged PR intervals include all of the following EXCEPT:

    A. Digitalis
    B. AV block due to coronary artery disease
    C. Diphtheria
    D. Wolff-Parkinson-White syndrome

Answer: D

Critique: Digitalis, AV block secondary to coronary disease, and diphtheria can all produce prolonged PR intervals. Wolff-Parkinson-White syndrome produces short PR intervals.

Further Reading

Vallbona C: Interpretation of the electrocardiogram. *In* Rakel RE: Textbook of Family Practice, 5th ed. Philadelphia, WB Saunders, 1995, pp 759–761.

42. (True or False) The following can produce prolonged QT intervals on the ECG.

    A. Hypocalcemia
    B. Hypokalemia
    C. Quinidine
    D. Digitalis

Answers: A-T, B-T, C-T, D-T

Critique: All of the listed drugs can produce prolonged QT intervals. Alternatively, hypercalcemia and hyperkalemia can shorten the QT interval.

Further Reading

Vallbona C: Interpretation of the electrocardiogram. *In* Rakel RE (ed.): Textbook of Family Practice, 5th ed. Philadelphia, WB Saunders, 1995, p 760.

43. An ECG demonstrates a measured QT interval of 0.34 second, and the RR interval is 0.72 second (18 mm). Which of the following is the corrected QT (QT_c)?

    A. 0.54 second
    B. 0.48 second
    C. 0.40 second
    D. 0.36 second
    E. 0.34 second

Answer: C

Critique: Several methods exist for correcting the QT interval for heart rate. Tables exist that provide corrected QT intervals for given heart rates. One commonly used formula relates the QT_c to the square root of the RR interval: $QT_c = QT/\sqrt{(RR)}$. In this example, the RR interval is 0.72, and the square root of the RR interval is 0.85. The QT_c is then equal to 0.34/0.85, or 0.40. The QT_c should be equal to or less than 0.44 second.

Further Reading

Generation of ECG waveforms. *In* Lipman BC, Cascio T: ECG Assessment and Interpretation. Philadelphia, FA Davis, 1994, pp 49, 50.
Goldberger AL: Electrocardiography. *In* Isselbacher KJ, Braunwald E, Wilson JD, et al (Eds): Harrison's Principles of Internal Medicine, 13th ed. New York, McGraw-Hill, 1994, pp 954–972.
Vallbona C: Interpretation of the electrocardiogram. *In* Rakel RE: Textbook of Family Practice, 5th ed. Philadelphia, WB Saunders, 1995, p 760.

44. Electrocardiographic criteria for diagnosing Wolff-Parkinson-White syndrome include all of the following EXCEPT:

    A. Short PR interval
    B. Presence of a delta wave
    C. Short QT interval
    D. Prolonged QRS duration

Answer: C

Critique: Wolff-Parkinson-White syndrome produces a prolonged QT interval rather than a short QT interval. All the other listed characteristics represent criteria for diagnosing Wolff-Parkinson-White syndrome.

Further Reading

Vallbona C: Interpretation of the electrocardiogram. *In* Rakel RE: Textbook of Family Practice, 5th ed. Philadelphia, WB Saunders, 1995, pp 760–763.

Questions 45–47. Match the following characteristics with the associated ECG diagnosis:

    A. Wolff-Parkinson-White syndrome
    B. Lown-Ganong-Levine syndrome
    C. Both A and B
    D. Neither A nor B

45. Shortened PR interval

46. Delta wave present

47. Normal QT interval

Answers: 45-C, 46-A, 47-B

Critique: Lown-Ganong-Levine and Wolff-Parkinson-White syndromes occur as a result of abnormal passage

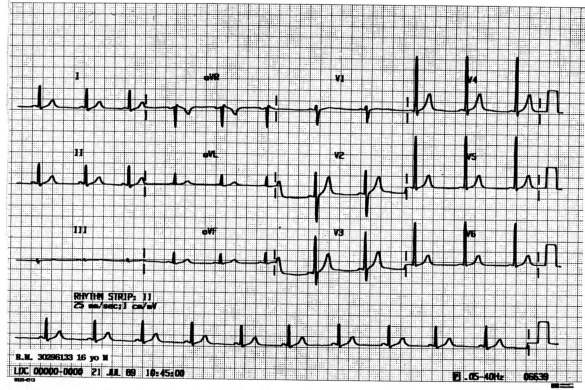

Figure 34–14 (Reproduced with permission from Rakel RE [Ed]: Textbook of Family Practice, 5th ed. Philadelphia, WB Saunders, 1995, p 762.)

of atrial impulses around the AV node via accessory bundles. In Wolff-Parkinson-White syndrome, impulses travel around the AV node via the bundle of Kent. In Lown-Ganong-Levine syndrome, impulses traverse the bundle of James. In both instances, the ECG demonstrates shortened PR intervals. The QT interval is prolonged in Wolff-Parkinson-White syndrome but is normal in Lown-Ganong-Levine syndrome. Wolff-Parkinson-White syndrome presents delta waves, whereas Lown-Ganong-Levine does not. Both syndromes predispose to tachyarrhythmias. Lown-Ganong-Levine syndrome is also called the short PR interval syndrome.

Further Reading

Vallbona C: Interpretation of the electrocardiogram. *In* Rakel RE: Textbook of Family Practice, 5th ed. Philadelphia, WB Saunders, 1995, pp 760–763.

48. (True or False) True statements regarding Figure 34–14 include which of the following?

A. Delta waves are present.
B. The QT_c interval is prolonged.
C. A shortened PR interval is present.
D. The QRS interval is prolonged.

Answer: C

Critique: This tracing represents an example of Lown-Ganong-Levine syndrome. No delta waves appear here. The measured QT appears to be approximately 0.40 second; the RR interval is about 0.92 second (23 mm). These values yield a QT_c of approximately 0.42 second, which is normal. The PR interval is slightly less than 0.12 second, which is short. The QRS duration is 0.08 second, which is normal.

Further Reading

Vallbona C: Interpretation of the electrocardiogram. *In* Rakel RE: Textbook of Family Practice, 5th ed. Philadelphia, WB Saunders, 1995, pp 760–763.

35

Cardiovascular Disease and Arrhythmias

Michael D. Hagen

Cardiovascular Disease

1. Match the following clinical characteristics with the appropriate syndrome:

    A. Down syndrome
    B. Turner's syndrome
    C. Both A and B
    D. Neither A nor B

1. Endocardial cushion and ventricular septal defects

2. Coarctation of the aorta and bicuspid aortic valves

3. Aortic dissection

Answers: 1-A, 2-B, 3-D

Critique: Down syndrome is associated with endocardial cushion defects and ventricular septal defects. Turner's syndrome is associated with coarctation of the aorta and bicuspid aortic valves. Marfan's syndrome is associated with aortic dissection.

Further Reading

Braunwald E: Approach to the patient with heart disease. *In* Isselbacher KJ, Braunwald E, Wison JD, et al: Harrison's Principles of Internal Medicine. New York, McGraw Hill, 1994.
Friedman WF, Child JS: Congenital heart disease in the adult. *In* Isselbacher KJ, Braunwald E, Wison JD, et al: Harrison's Principles of Internal Medicine. New York, McGraw-Hill, 1994.
Yakubov SJ, Bope ET: Cardiovascular disease and arrhythmia: Cardiovascular disease. *In* Rakel RE: Textbook of Family Practice. Philadelphia, WB Saunders, 1995, p 764.

2. Match the following physical findings with the appropriate clinical condition:

    A. Hypercholesterolemia

    B. Hyperthyroidism
    C. Both A and B
    D. Neither A nor B

1. Lipid-filled plaques around the eyes

2. Blue sclerae

3. Exophthalmos

Answers: 1-A, 2-D, 3-B

Critique: Xanthelasma represent lipid-filled plaques around the eyes and are seen in hypercholesterolemia. Blue sclerae can be seen in connective tissue disorders, such as osteogenesis imperfecta, Marfan's syndrome, and Ehlers-Danlos syndrome.

Further Reading

Yakubov SJ, Bope ET: Cardiovascular disease and arrhythmia: Cardiovascular disease. *In* Rakel RE: Textbook of Family Practice. Philadelphia, WB Saunders, 1995, p 764.

3. When measuring a patient's blood pressure, the systolic pressure is indicated by which of the following Korotkoff sounds?

    A. First appearance of a tapping sound as the cuff is deflated
    B. Change of tapping sounds to soft rumbling sounds
    C. Change of sounds from soft rumbling to loud murmur
    D. Disappearance of sounds

Answer: A

Critique: The Korotkoff sounds appear over the brachial artery as a blood pressure cuff, which is inflated around the upper arm, is deflated. The initial tapping sound heard as the cuff deflates correlates with systolic blood pressure. The disappearance of sounds occurs at the diastolic blood pressure.

Further Reading

Yakubov SJ, Bope ET: Cardiovascular disease and arrhythmia: Cardiovascular disease. *In* Rakel RE: Textbook of Family Practice. Philadelphia, WB Saunders, 1995, p 764.

4. (True or False) Conditions associated with pulsus paradoxus include which of the following?

    A. Pericardial tamponade
    B. Asthma
    C. Chronic obstructive pulmonary disease
    D. Pleural effusion

Answers: A-T, B-T, C-T, D-T

Critique: Pulsus paradoxus consists of a greater than 10 mm drop in systolic blood pressure with inspiration. All of the conditions listed can demonstrate pulsus paradoxus.

Further Reading

Yakubov SJ, Bope ET: Cardiovascular disease and arrhythmia: Cardiovascular disease. *In* Rakel RE: Textbook of Family Practice. Philadelphia, WB Saunders, 1995, p 765.

5. A height of the jugular venous pulse meniscus of 5 cm above the sternal angle corresponds with a central venous pressure of:

    A. 6 cm H_2O
    B. 8 cm H_2O
    C. 10 cm H_2O
    D. 12 cm H_2O

Answer: C

Critique: The height of the jugular venous meniscus above the sternal angle provides an estimate of the central venous pressure. The sternal angle lies approximately 5 cm above the right atrium; therefore, the jugular venous pulse height plus 5 cm approximates the central venous pressure. In this example, the 5-cm jugular venous pulse meniscus would correspond to a central venous pressure of about 10 cm H_2O.

Further Reading

Yakubov SJ, Bope ET: Cardiovascular disease and arrhythmia: Cardiovascular disease. *In* Rakel RE: Textbook of Family Practice. Philadelphia, WB Saunders, 1995, p 765.

6. Match the jugular venous wave with the appropriate physiologic phenomenon:

    A. "a" wave
    B. "v" wave
    C. Both A and B
    D. Neither A nor B

1. Fall in right atrial pressure as the tricuspid valve opens

2. Contraction of the atria

3. Flow of blood into right atrium with the tricuspid valve closed

Answers: 1-D, 2-A, 3-B

Critique: Close observation of the jugular venous pulse will disclose several waveforms. Contraction of the atria causes the "a" wave; the "v" wave occurs as blood rushes into the right atrium against a closed tricuspid valve in systole. Opening of the tricuspid valve causes a rapid decline in atrial pressure as blood rushes from the right atrium; this causes the "y descent" wave.

Further Reading

Yakubov SJ, Bope ET: Cardiovascular disease and arrhythmia: Cardiovascular disease. *In* Rakel RE: Textbook of Family Practice. Philadelphia, WB Saunders, 1995, p 765.

7. Conditions associated with *increased* intensity of the first heart sound include all of the following EXCEPT:

    A. Hypertension
    B. Thyrotoxicosis
    C. Mitral stenosis
    D. Prolonged PR interval

Answer: D

Critique: Hypertension, thyrotoxicosis, and mitral stenosis can all produce accentuated first heart sounds. A prolonged PR interval is associated with decreased first sound intensity.

Further Reading

Yakubov SJ, Bope ET: Cardiovascular disease and arrhythmia: Cardiovascular disease. *In* Rakel RE: Textbook of Family Practice. Philadelphia, WB Saunders, 1995, p 765.

8. The normal second heart sound consists of two identifiable components. Match the clinical conditions with the appropriate second heart sound pattern:

    A. Paradoxical splitting of the second sound
    B. Wide splitting of the second sound with preserved respiratory variation
    C. Both A and B
    D. Neither A nor B

1. Right bundle branch block

2. Pulmonic stenosis

3. Left bundle branch block

4. Aortic stenosis

5. Atrial septal defect

Answers: 1-B, 2-B, 3-A, 4-A, 5-D

Critique: Right bundle branch block and pulmonic stenosis can both produce wide splitting of the second sound with preserved respiratory variation. Left bundle branch block and aortic stenosis, by delaying aortic valve closure, can produce paradoxical splitting. Atrial septal defect is associated with fixed splitting of the second heart sound.

Further Reading

Yakubov SJ, Bope ET: Cardiovascular disease and arrhythmia: Cardiovascular disease. *In* Rakel RE: Textbook of Family Practice. Philadelphia, WB Saunders, 1995, p 765.

9. (True or False) Conditions that might be associated with a third heart sound include which of the following:

    A. Dilated congestive heart failure
    B. Thyrotoxicosis
    C. Aortic insufficiency
    D. Atrial septal defect

Answers: A-T, B-T, C-T, D-T

Critique: The third heart sound occurs as a result of rapid filling and expansion of the ventricles in diastole. Conditions that increase ventricular blood flow or volume can cause a third heart sound. Dilated congestive heart failure, thyrotoxicosis, atrial septal defect, and aortic insufficiency can all be associated with a third heart sound.

Further Reading

Yakubov SJ, Bope ET: Cardiovascular disease and arrhythmia: Cardiovascular disease. *In* Rakel RE: Textbook of Family Practice. Philadelphia, WB Saunders, 1995, pp 765, 766.

10. You are conducting a sports physical examination on an adolescent. During your cardiac examination, you detect a murmur that you feel is quite loud, but you don't detect a palpable thrill. Such a murmur would constitute what grade of intensity?

    A. Grade 1
    B. Grade 2
    C. Grade 3
    D. Grade 4
    E. Grade 5

Answer: C

Critique: The examiner describes the murmur as quite loud, but without an associated palpable thrill. The absence of a thrill rules out options D and E. The examiner's description rules out option A, because a grade 1 murmur would be much less intense. A grade 2 murmur would exhibit moderate intensity compared with this examiner's description.

Further Reading

Yakubov SJ, Bope ET: Cardiovascular disease and arrhythmia: Cardiovascular disease. *In* Rakel RE: Textbook of Family Practice. Philadelphia, WB Saunders, 1995, p 766.

11. Match the clinical condition with the associated murmur characteristic:

    A. Midsystolic ejection quality murmurs
    B. Holosystolic regurgitant quality murmurs
    C. Both A and B
    D. Neither A nor B

1. Begins with the first heart sound (S_1)

2. Has a crescendo-decrescendo waveform

3. Associated with aortic stenosis

4. Associated with anemia and thyrotoxicosis

Answers: 1-B, 2-A, 3-A, 4-A

Critique: Midsystolic murmurs begin after the first heart sound (S_1) and end before the second heart sound (S_2). Holosystolic murmurs begin with S_1 and extend to, or end before, S_2 depending upon the pressure across the opening that causes the murmur. Systolic ejection quality murmurs have a crescendo-decrescendo waveform. Aortic stenosis produces a systolic ejection quality murmur. High-flow states such as anemia and thyrotoxicosis can also produce systolic ejection murmurs.

Further Reading

Yakubov SJ, Bope ET: Cardiovascular disease and arrhythmia: Cardiovascular disease. *In* Rakel RE: Textbook of Family Practice. Philadelphia, WB Saunders, 1995, pp 766, 767.

12. During a cardiac examination, you note a decrescendo quality murmur, which is heard best in early diastole over the cardiac apex and in the right second intercostal space along the sternum. Of the following, the most likely cause of this murmur is:

    A. Mitral stenosis
    B. Aortic stenosis
    C. Mitral regurgitation
    D. Aortic regurgitation
    E. Tricuspid regurgitation

Answer: D

Critique: Mitral and tricuspid regurgitation would be heard in systole rather than in diastole. Similarly, the murmur of aortic stenosis would occur in systole. Mitral stenosis would occur later in diastole than described here. Aortic regurgitation fits best with the murmur description.

Further Reading

Yakubov SJ, Bope ET: Cardiovascular disease and arrhythmia: Cardiovascular disease. *In* Rakel RE: Textbook of Family Practice. Philadelphia, WB Saunders, 1995, pp 766, 767.

13. (True or False) Causes of continuous cardiac murmurs include which of the following?

    A. Aortic stenosis
    B. Patent ductus arteriosus

C. Coarctation of the aorta
D. Tricuspid insufficiency

Answers: A-F, B-T, C-T, D-F

Critique: Isolated aortic stenosis (in the absence of insufficiency) produces systolic murmurs. Isolated tricuspid insufficiency also produces systolic murmurs. Patent ductus arteriosus, because of the arteriovenous gradient that persists during both systole and diastole, can produce continuous murmurs. Coarctation of the aorta can also produce such murmurs.

Further Reading

Yakubov SJ, Bope ET: Cardiovascular disease and arrhythmia: Cardiovascular disease. *In* Rakel RE: Textbook of Family Practice. Philadelphia, WB Saunders, 1995, pp 766, 767.

14. (True or False) For murmurs associated with the following conditions, which murmurs tend to **increase** with isometric exercise?

    A. Ventricular septal defect
    B. Aortic stenosis
    C. Hypertrophic cardiomyopathy
    D. Mitral insufficiency

Answers: A-T, B-F, C-F, D-T

Critique: Isometric exercise, by increasing systolic blood pressure and systemic resistance, increases blood flow from high to low pressure circuits in the heart. This would lead to increased intensity of the murmurs associated with mitral insufficiency and ventricular septal defect. Similarly, isometric exercise ameliorates the systolic aortic outflow constriction seen with hypertrophic cardiomyopathy and will thus attenuate the associated murmur. Likewise, isometric exercise will lessen the pressure gradient across a stenotic aortic valve and similarly diminish the associated murmur.

Further Reading

Yakubov SJ, Bope ET: Cardiovascular disease and arrhythmia: Cardiovascular disease. *In* Rakel RE: Textbook of Family Practice. Philadelphia, WB Saunders, 1995, p 767.

15. Assuming upright posture from a recumbent position will **increase** the intensity of the murmur associated with which ONE of the following conditions?

    A. Tricuspid insufficiency
    B. Mitral insufficiency
    C. Pulmonic stenosis
    D. Hypertrophic cardiomyopathy

Answer: D

Critique: Assuming an upright from lying position decreases venous return to the heart and thus diminishes blood flow momentarily through the heart. This will diminish the murmurs of tricuspid and mitral insufficiency and pulmonic stenosis. The associated flow permits constriction of the outflow tract in hypertrophic cardiomyopathy and will, therefore, increase the intensity of the murmur associated with this abnormality.

Further Reading

Yakubov SJ, Bope ET: Cardiovascular disease and arrhythmia: Cardiovascular disease. *In* Rakel RE: Textbook of Family Practice. Philadelphia, WB Saunders, 1995, pp 767, 768.

16. (True or False) True statements regarding the association of cigarette smoking with cardiovascular disease include which of the following?

    A. Smoking increases the risk of premature death and/or myocardial infarction.
    B. Smoking decreases plasma fibrinogen levels in smokers.
    C. The risk of a coronary event remains constant after discontinuing smoking.
    D. Cigarette smoking contributes to approximately 350,000 deaths annually in the United States.

Answers: A-T, B-F, C-F, D-T

Critique: Cigarette smoking represents a modifiable risk factor that has a tremendous health impact. Approximately 350,000 deaths annually are attributable to smoking. Smoking increases an individual's risk of myocardial death or premature death. Plasma fibrinogen levels are increased in smokers rather than decreased. One year after discontinuing smoking, an ex-smoker's risk of a coronary event declines by approximately 50%.

Further Reading

Yakubov SJ, Bope ET: Cardiovascular disease and arrhythmia: Cardiovascular disease. *In* Rakel RE: Textbook of Family Practice. Philadelphia, WB Saunders, 1995, pp 766, 767.

17. (True or False) True statements regarding the association of high-density lipoprotein (HDL), low-density lipoprotein (LDL), and total cholesterol with the risk of coronary disease include which of the following?

    A. Elevated HDL is associated with increased coronary risk.
    B. Elevated LDL is associated with increased coronary risk.
    C. Reductions of total cholesterol confer decreased coronary risk.
    D. A 1% reduction in total cholesterol is associated with a 2% reduction in the risk of a coronary event.

Answers: A-F, B-T, C-T, D-T

Critique: A number of studies have confirmed the relationship between altered cholesterol metabolism and coronary heart disease. Elevated HDL confers reduced coronary heart risk. LDL elevations increase coronary risk. Several secondary prevention trials have demonstrated that lowering total cholesterol reduces coronary risk. The Framingham Heart Study and the Coronary Primary Prevention Trial suggest that each 1% decrease in the total cholesterol lowers coronary heart disease risk by 2%.

Further Reading

Yakubov SJ, Bope ET: Cardiovascular disease and arrhythmia: Cardiovascular disease. *In* Rakel RE: Textbook of Family Practice. Philadelphia, WB Saunders, 1995, p 769.

18. According to the National Cholesterol Education Program (NCEP), appropriate initial management for a total cholesterol level of 240 mg/dl (6.20 mmol/l) and a LDL level of 130 mg/dl (3.35 mmol/l) in a patient without known heart disease or risk factors should include all of the following EXCEPT:

    A. Instruct in a step 1 dietary therapy.
    B. Counsel to increase physical activity.
    C. Re-evaluate the patient's lipid status annually.
    D. Initiate lovastatin (Mevacor) therapy.

Answer: D

Critique: According to the NCEP guidelines, a total cholesterol level of 240 mg/dl should be evaluated further with lipoprotein analysis. For a patient with an LDL level of 130 mg/dl without known heart disease or risk factors, the clinician should provide instruction in a step 1 diet, encourage the patient to increase physical activity, and re-evaluate the patient annually. Pharmacotherapy, such as cholestyramine or lovastatin, would be inappropriate for such a patient according to NCEP guidelines.

Further Reading

U.S. Public Health Service: Cholesterol screening in adults. Am Fam Physician 51:129–136, 1995.
Yakubov SJ, Bope ET: Cardiovascular disease and arrhythmia: Cardiovascular disease. *In* Rakel RE: Textbook of Family Practice. Philadelphia, WB Saunders, 1995, pp 769, 770.

19. Under definitions developed by the Joint National Committee on Detection, Evaluation, and Treatment of High Blood Pressure, Fifth Report (JNC V), stage 1 hypertension is defined as which ONE of the following?

    A. Systolic blood pressure < 130 mm Hg and diastolic blood pressure < 85 mm Hg
    B. Systolic blood pressure 130–139 mm Hg and diastolic blood pressure 85–89 mm Hg
    C. Systolic blood pressure 140–159 mm Hg and diastolic blood pressure 90–99 mm Hg
    D. Systolic blood pressure 160–179 mm Hg and diastolic blood pressure 100–109 mm Hg
    E. Systolic blood pressure 180–209 mm Hg and diastolic blood pressure 110–119 mm Hg

Answer: C

Critique: The JNC V report introduced a staging system for describing the severity of hypertension. Stage 1 hypertension consists of a systolic blood pressure of 140 to 159 mm Hg and a diastolic blood pressure of 90 to 99 mm Hg. If the systolic and diastolic pressures fall into different stages, the higher stage should be used to describe the severity of the elevation.

Further Reading

Fifth report of the Joint National Committee on Detection, Evaluation, and Treatment of High Blood Pressure. Arch Intern Med 153:154–183, 1993.
Yakubov SJ, Bope ET: Cardiovascular disease and arrhythmia: Cardiovascular disease. *In* Rakel RE: Textbook of Family Practice. Philadelphia, WB Saunders, 1995, pp 770, 771.

20. For a systolic blood pressure of 130 to 139 mm Hg and a diastolic blood pressure of 85 to 89 mm Hg, the JNC V report recommends which one of the following:

    A. Evaluate or refer to a source of care within 1 week.
    B. Recheck the blood pressure in 2 years.
    C. Confirm the blood pressure within 2 months.
    D. Recheck the blood pressure in 1 year.

Answer: D

Critique: The Fifth Report of the Joint Committee on Detection, Evaluation, and Treatment of High Blood Pressure recommended that a systolic blood pressure of 130 to 139 mm Hg and a diastolic blood pressure of 85 to 89 mm Hg be rechecked in 1 year.

Further Reading

Fifth report of the Joint National Committee on Detection, Evaluation, and Treatment of High Blood Pressure. Arch Intern Med 153:154–183, 1993.
Yakubov SJ, Bope ET: Cardiovascular disease and arrhythmia: Cardiovascular disease. *In* Rakel RE: Textbook of Family Practice. Philadelphia, WB Saunders, 1995, pp 770, 771.

21. The fifth report of the Joint National Committee on the Detection, Evaluation, and Treatment of High Blood Pressure recommends that all of the following be included in initial diagnostic testing for new hypertensives EXCEPT:

    A. Urinalysis
    B. Blood glucose
    C. Serum creatinine
    D. Urinary metanephrines
    E. Total cholesterol and HDL cholesterol

Answer: D

Critique: In addition to a history and physical examination, the JNC V report recommends that evaluation of the new hypertensive patient should include urinalysis, glucose level, serum creatinine, and total and HDL cholesterol, uric acid, serum triglycerides, serum potassium and calcium levels, a complete blood count, and an electrocardiogram. The JNC V does not include urinary metanephrines in this initial evaluation.

Further Reading

Fifth report of the Joint National Committee on Detection, Evaluation, and Treatment of High Blood Pressure. Arch Intern Med 153:154–183, 1993.
Yakubov SJ, Bope ET: Cardiovascular disease and arrhythmia: Cardiovascular disease. *In* Rakel RE: Textbook of Family Practice. Philadelphia, WB Saunders, 1995, pp 770, 771.

22. A 45-year-old man has developed stage 2 hypertension, and lifestyle modification has not lowered his blood pressure. His initial evaluation revealed no evidence of cardiovascular disease. He plays tennis several times weekly and jogs on weekends. Because his blood pressure remains elevated, you have decided to initiate pharmacotherapy. Of the following therapeutic options, all represent reasonable choices for initial therapy EXCEPT:

A. Angiotensin-converting enzyme inhibitors (e.g., enalapril)
B. Calcium channel blockers (e.g., nifedipine)
C. Centrally acting α-agonists (e.g., clonidine)
D. β-Adrenergic blockers (e.g., propranolol)

Answer: D

Critique: This patient represents an otherwise healthy, physically active man. Of the options listed, the β-adrenergic agents represent the least preferable choice because of the potential impact that these drugs might have on his recreational athletic activities.

Further Reading

Yakubov SJ, Bope ET: Cardiovascular disease and arrhythmia: Cardiovascular disease. *In* Rakel RE: Textbook of Family Practice. Philadelphia, WB Saunders, 1995, pp 770–775.

23. True statements regarding exercise ^{201}Tl testing for coronary artery disease include all of the following EXCEPT:

A. Thallium "hot spots" appear in poorly perfused areas of myocardium.
B. Fixed perfusion defects represent a prior myocardial infarction (MI).
C. Resting electrocardiographic abnormalities represent a valid indication for an exercise thallium evaluation.
D. Redistribution of blood flow on comparison of resting and exercise scans indicates significant coronary artery stenosis.

Answer: A

Critique: Thallium enters myocardial cells in proportion to perfusion; poorly perfused myocardium appears as "cold spots" on a thallium scan. Fixed defects indicate a prior MI. A resting electrocardiographic abnormality represents one of the indications for conducting thallium scanning rather than electrocardiographic stress testing. Blood flow redistribution, as seen on a comparison of resting and exercise thallium scans, indicates significant coronary artery stenosis. During exercise, blood shunts away from diseased coronary artery segments toward lower resistance normal vessels. Thus, a scan taken when the patient is at rest will appear different from that taken during exercise.

Further Reading

Yakubov SJ, Bope ET: Cardiovascular disease and arrhythmia: Cardiovascular disease. *In* Rakel RE: Textbook of Family Practice. Philadelphia, WB Saunders, 1995, pp 776, 777.

24. In situations in which patients cannot undergo treadmill stress testing, certain drugs can be used to perform "pharmacologic" stress testing. Match the following pharmacologic agents with their *primary* mode of action in stress testing.

A. Adenosine
B. Dipyridamole

C. Both A and B
D. Neither A nor B

1. Act(s) by inducing coronary artery vasodilatation.

2. Act(s) by increasing heart rate and myocardial oxygen consumption.

Answers: 1-C, 2-D

Critique: Both adenosine and dipyridamole act by inducing vasodilatation. Because nonatherosclerotic vessels dilate more readily than do diseased arteries, these agents cause blood to shunt away from areas supplied by stenotic coronary arteries. The areas of the myocardium that are supplied by these diseased vessels will, therefore, demonstrate less perfusion than surrounding normally perfused tissue. As the effects of these agents dissipate, the perfusion differential should diminish, thus demonstrating reversible defects on the thallium scan. Dobutamine increases myocardial oxygen consumption and heart rate; those areas supplied by diseased coronary arteries will demonstrate echocardiographic abnormalities in response to dobutamine stimulation.

Further Reading

Yakubov SJ, Bope ET: Cardiovascular disease and arrhythmia: Cardiovascular disease. *In* Rakel RE: Textbook of Family Practice. Philadelphia, WB Saunders, 1995, pp 776, 777.

25. Lifestyle modifications that should be attempted in patients with coronary artery disease include all of the following EXCEPT:

A. Low-cholesterol, low-fat diet
B. Discontinue cigarette smoking
C. Weight loss
D. Decrease exercise

Answer: D

Critique: Patients who have coronary artery disease should attempt to undergo lifestyle changes that can limit the progress of the atherosclerotic process. Patients should be instructed in low-fat, low-cholesterol meal plans. If the patient smokes, the clinician should encourage the patient to discontinue use of cigarettes. Weight loss should be recommended for overweight patients. Coronary patients should be encouraged to engage regularly in moderate exercise.

Further Reading

Yakubov SJ, Bope ET: Cardiovascular disease and arrhythmia: Cardiovascular disease. *In* Rakel RE: Textbook of Family Practice. Philadelphia, WB Saunders, 1995, p 778.

26. β_1-Adrenergic blocking drugs have been demonstrated to improve survival after an MI and have demonstrated effectiveness in lowering blood pressure. Lipid solubility affects central nervous system side effects associated with use of β-blockers. Of the following β-blocking agents, all exhibit low lipid solubility EXCEPT:

A. Acebutalol
B. Atenolol
C. Propranolol
D. Nadolol

Answer: C

Critique: Acebutalol, atenolol, and nadolol exhibit relatively low lipid solubility. Propranolol exhibits high lipid solubility.

Further Reading

Wallin JD, Shah SV: β-Adrenergic blocking agents in the treatment of hypertension: Choices based on pharmacological properties and patient characteristics. Arch Intern Med 147:654–659, 1987.
Yakubov SJ, Bope ET: Cardiovascular disease and arrhythmia: Cardiovascular disease. *In* Rakel RE: Textbook of Family Practice. Philadelphia, WB Saunders, 1995, p 778.

27. (True or False) True statements regarding the physiologic effects of calcium channel blockers include which of the following?

A. Decrease vascular tone
B. Positive inotropic effects
C. Increase sinoatrial (SA) node conduction time
D. Increase coronary blood flow

Answers: A-T, B-F, C-F, D-T

Critique: The calcium channel blockers decrease vascular tone and increase coronary blood flow. They decrease sinoatrial conduction time and generally have negative inotropic effects, although the different classes of calcium channel blockers vary in this regard. The dihydropyridine class (e.g., nifedipine, amlodipine, nicardipine) tend to express a less negative inotropic effect than does verapamil or diltiazem. Additionally, the dihydropyridines have less effect on SA and atrioventricular (AV) nodal function than do the nondihydropyridine agents.

Further Reading

Drugs for stable angina pectoris. Med Lett 36:111–114, 1994.
Yakubov SJ, Bope ET: Cardiovascular disease and arrhythmia: Cardiovascular disease. *In* Rakel RE: Textbook of Family Practice. Philadelphia, WB Saunders, 1995, pp 778, 779.

28. (True or False) True statements regarding the actions of nitrates in angina pectoris include:

A. Nitrates cause peripheral venous dilatation and decrease venous return to the heart.
B. Nitrates prevent coronary artery spasm.
C. Nitrate effectiveness persists with continuous long-term use.
D. Nitrates decrease myocardial oxygen demand.

Answers: A-T, B-T, C-F, D-T

Critique: Nitrates improve angina pectoris through several mechanisms. Peripheral venous dilatation leads to decreased venous return and cardiac preload. Additionally, arterial dilatation decreases cardiac afterload and thus diminishes myocardial oxygen consumption. Nitrate's vasodilatory characteristics serve to inhibit arterial spasm.

Continuous nitrate therapy leads to tolerance; therefore, patients treated with nitrates should experience nitrate-free periods during each 24 hours. Other agents such as β-blockers or calcium channel blockers can be used during these nitrate-free periods to prevent angina.

Further Reading

Drugs for stable angina pectoris. Med Lett 36:111–114, 1994.
Yakubov SJ, Bope ET: Cardiovascular disease and arrhythmia: Cardiovascular disease. *In* Rakel RE: Textbook of Family Practice. Philadelphia, WB Saunders, 1995, p 778.

29. (True or False) True statements regarding the effects of aspirin therapy on cardiovascular effects include which of the following?

A. Reduced MI rate in patients with unstable angina pectoris
B. Reduced rate of coronary reocclusion after thrombolysis
C. Reduced rate of subsequent MI after the first MI
D. Reduced rate of vascular events (i.e., nonfatal stroke and nonfatal MI) in patients with transient cerebral ischemia
E. Reduced rate of first MI in patients with chronic stable angina pectoris

Answers: A-T, B-T, C-T, D-T, E-T

Critique: The antiplatelet effects of aspirin have demonstrated usefulness in a number of contexts. Aspirin has been shown to decrease MI in unstable angina patients and diminishes the rate of coronary reocclusion after thrombolytic therapy. Additionally, aspirin reduces subsequent MI after a first MI. Although controversial, evidence has appeared to indicate that aspirin can reduce vascular events in patients who have experienced transient cerebral ischemic attacks. Additionally, evidence exists to support the use of aspirin in patients who have chronic stable angina pectoris.

Further Reading

Dutch TIA Trial Study Group: A comparison of two doses of aspirin (30 mg vs. 283 mg a day) in patients after a transient ischemic attack or minor ischemic stroke. N Engl J Med 325:1261–1266, 1991.
Juul-Möller S for The Swedish Angina Pectoris Aspirin Trial (SAPAT) Group: Double-blind trial of aspirin in primary prevention of myocardial infarction in patients with stable chronic angina pectoris. Lancet 340:1421–1425, 1992.
SALT Collaborative Group: Swedish aspirin low-dose trial (SALT) of 75 mg aspirin as secondary prophylaxis after cerebrovascular ischaemic events. Lancet 338:1345–1349, 1991.
Yakubov SJ, Bope ET: Cardiovascular disease and arrhythmia: Cardiovascular disease. *In* Rakel RE: Textbook of Family Practice. Philadelphia, WB Saunders, 1995, pp 779, 780.

30. (True or False) Cardiac abnormalities that typically produce elevated ST segments on the electrocardiogram include which of the following?

A. MI
B. Left ventricular hypertrophy
C. Digoxin therapy
D. Pericarditis
E. Coronary vasospasm

Answers: A-T, B-F, C-F, D-T, E-T

Critique: An MI produces ST segment elevation acutely. Pericarditis and coronary vasospasm can also produce elevated ST segments. Left ventricular hypertrophy and digoxin therapy typically produced ST segment depression rather than elevation.

Further Reading

Yakubov SJ, Bope ET: Cardiovascular disease and arrhythmia: Cardiovascular disease. *In* Rakel RE: Textbook of Family Practice. Philadelphia, WB Saunders, 1995, pp 780, 781.

31. (True or False) True statements regarding creatine kinase (CK) or creatine phosphokinase (CPK) in the diagnosis of acute MI include which of the following?

- A. CK levels return to normal within 12 to 18 hours of the onset of infarction.
- B. A normal CK level rules out an acute MI.
- C. The MB fraction of CK demonstrates a higher specificity for myocardial injury than does total CK.
- D. A single CK measurement performs as well as serial measurements in identifying an acute MI.

Answers: A-F, B-F, C-T, D-F

Critique: CK exists in both skeletal and cardiac muscle. The MB fraction is more specific for cardiac muscle than is the total CK, which consists of both MB and MM fractions. The CK returns to normal within 2 to 3 days of the infarction rather than within 12 to 18 hours. A normal CK does not necessarily rule out an MI; an MB fraction as high as 15% and a total CK rise and fall (even though within normal limits) over several days indicates an MI. The MB fraction is more specific for myocardial injury than either total CK or CK-MM. Serial CK and CK-MB measurement over 24 hours performs with much higher sensitivity and specificity than does a single value.

Further Reading

Gibler WB, Lewis LM, Erb RE, et al: Early detection of acute myocardial infarction in patients presenting with chest pain and non-diagnostic ECGs: Serial CK-MB sampling in the emergency department. Ann Emerg Med 9:1359–1366, 1990.
Yakubov SJ, Bope ET: Cardiovascular disease and arrhythmia: Cardiovascular disease. *In* Rakel RE: Textbook of Family Practice. Philadelphia, WB Saunders, 1995, p 781.

32. An acute inferior MI is most frequently associated with which one of the following electrocardiographic patterns?

- A. Deep QRS complexes in leads V_1 to V_3
- B. ST segment elevation in leads I and aVL
- C. ST segment elevation in leads V_1 and V_2
- D. ST segment elevation in leads II, III, and aVF

Answer: D

Critique: An acute infarction isolated to the inferior myocardium demonstrates ST segment elevations in the "inferior" ECG leads II, III, and aVF. Deep QRS complexes in the anterior chest leads (V_1 to V_3) would indi-

cate an old anterior MI. Similarly, ST segment elevation in these leads would be consistent with acute anterior MI. ST segment elevation in leads I and aVL would be most consistent with an anterolateral MI.

Further Reading

Yakubov SJ, Bope ET: Cardiovascular disease and arrhythmia: Cardiovascular disease. *In* Rakel RE: Textbook of Family Practice. Philadelphia, WB Saunders, 1995, pp 780, 781.

33. (True or False) Causes of an acute MI that are NOT associated with atherosclerotic coronary artery stenoses include which of the following?

- A. Kawasaki disease
- B. Vasculitis associated with systemic lupus erythematosus
- C. Cocaine use
- D. Aortic valvular embolic phenomena

Answers: A-T, B-T, C-T, D-T

Critique: Kawasaki disease can lead to an MI in the absence of significant atherosclerotic changes. Additionally, vasculitis associated with systemic lupus erythematosus and polyarteritis nodosa can similarly cause an MI. Intense vasospasm associated with cocaine use can cause an MI, as can emboli from an abnormal aortic valve.

Further Reading

Yakubov SJ, Bope ET: Cardiovascular disease and arrhythmia: Cardiovascular disease. *In* Rakel RE: Textbook of Family Practice. Philadelphia, WB Saunders, 1995, p 782.

34. Clinical signs of cardiogenic shock include all of the following EXCEPT:

- A. Cardiac index of < 1.8 l/min/m^2
- B. Systolic blood pressure > 110 mm Hg
- C. Systemic signs of tissue hypoperfusion
- D. Pulmonary wedge pressure > 18 mm Hg

Answer: B

Critique: Cardiogenic shock occurs as a result of a substantial myocardial insult with resultant impaired cardiac function. Systolic blood pressure is less than 90 mm Hg. Additionally, the patient will demonstrate signs of tissue hypoperfusion, and the cardiac index will be less than 1.8 l/min/m^2. Intravascular monitoring will also reveal elevated pulmonary wedge pressures.

Further Reading

Yakubov SJ, Bope ET: Cardiovascular disease and arrhythmia: Cardiovascular disease. *In* Rakel RE: Textbook of Family Practice. Philadelphia, WB Saunders, 1995, p 782.

35. Pharmacologic agents that should be considered for acute administration for patients with MI and no contraindications include all of the following EXCEPT:

- A. Nitroglycerin (intravenously or sublingually)
- B. β-Adrenergic blocking agents (e.g., metoprolol, atenolol)

C. Aspirin
D. Intramuscular morphine sulfate

Answer: D

Critique: Nitroglycerin acts to improve blood supply to ischemic myocardium and can improve signs of congestive failure by decreasing preload. β-Adrenergic blockers have been demonstrated to improve survival when administered acutely. Additionally, aspirin therapy decreases mortality and subsequent reinfarction. Intramuscular medications should be avoided because of the potential for influencing CK values.

Further Reading

Weston CFM, Penny WJ, Julian DG for the British Heart Foundation Working Group: Guidelines for the early management of patients with myocardial infarction. BMJ 308:767–771, 1994.
Yakubov SJ, Bope ET: Cardiovascular disease and arrhythmia: Cardiovascular disease. *In* Rakel RE: Textbook of Family Practice. Philadelphia, WB Saunders, 1995, p 783.

36. True statements regarding thrombolytic therapy in acute MI include all of the following EXCEPT:

A. Tissue plasminogen activator (tPA), streptokinase, and anisoylated plasminogen streptokinase activator complex (APSAC, anistreplase) all improve survival in MI
B. Thrombolytic agents demonstrate equal survival benefit whether given within 2 hours or within 8 hours of the onset of an MI.
C. Streptokinase and anistreplase demonstrate significant antigenicity and risk of allergic reactions.
D. Acute MIs in all anatomic locations can benefit from acute thrombolytic therapy.

Answer: B

Critique: Thrombolytic therapy represents a major advance in clinicians' ability to reduce mortality from an acute MI. Streptokinase, tPA, and anistreplase have all demonstrated improved survival in clinical studies. Clinical trials have demonstrated that early administration achieves results superior to those obtained with later (e.g., > 6 hours) treatment. Streptokinase and anistreplase demonstrate streptococcal antigenicity and can precipitate allergic reactions. Although anterior MIs appear to benefit most from thrombolytic therapy, all infarction patients demonstrate improved survival with thrombolytic therapy and should therefore receive treatment unless contraindications to thrombolytics exist.

Further Reading

Doorey AJ, Michelson EL, Topol EJ: Thrombolytic therapy of acute myocardial infarction: Keeping the unfulfilled promises. JAMA 268:3108–3114, 1992.
Farkouh ME, Lang JD, Sackett DL: Thrombolytic agents: The science of the art of choosing the better treatment (Editorial). Ann Intern Med 120:886–888, 1994.
Yakubov SJ, Bope ET: Cardiovascular disease and arrhythmia: Cardiovascular disease. *In* Rakel RE: Textbook of Family Practice. Philadelphia, WB Saunders, 1995, pp 783, 784.

37. Absolute contraindications to thrombolytic therapy for an acute MI include all of the following EXCEPT:

A. Recent major surgery (e.g., within 2 months)
B. History of cerebrovascular accident (e.g., within several months)
C. Severe uncontrollable hypertension
D. Age greater than 65 years

Answer: D

Critique: Bleeding events represent the major complication of thrombolytic therapy. In order to minimize these complications, patients with a history of recent major surgery should not receive thrombolytics. Likewise, recent cerebrovascular accident and severe uncontrollable hypertension obviate such treatment. The elderly benefit from thrombolytic therapy, and advanced age (>75 years) represents only a relative contraindication.

Further Reading

Doorey AJ, Michelson EL, Topol EJ: Thrombolytic therapy of acute myocardial infarction: Keeping the unfulfilled promises. JAMA 268:3108–3114, 1992.
Krumholz HM, Pasternak RC, Weinstein MC, et al: Cost effectiveness of thrombolytic therapy with streptokinase in elderly patients with suspected acute myocardial infarction. N Engl J Med 327:7–13, 1992.
Yakubov SJ, Bope ET: Cardiovascular disease and arrhythmia: Cardiovascular disease. *In* Rakel RE: Textbook of Family Practice. Philadelphia, WB Saunders, 1995, pp 783, 784.

38. (True or False) Percutaneous transluminal angioplasty (PTCA) and thrombolytic therapy have been investigated as independent therapies and cotherapies in the management of acute MI. True statements regarding the use of PTCA **after** thrombolytic therapy include which of the following?

A. PTCA performed immediately after thrombolysis confers improved ventricular function compared with PTCA performed 18 to 48 hours later.
B. PTCA performed immediately after thrombolysis confers no greater risk of bleeding than that associated with PTCA performed 18 to 48 hours later.
C. PTCA performed immediately after thrombolysis is associated with a higher rate of infarct extension than is PTCA performed later.
D. PTCA performed immediately after thrombolysis is associated with a higher rate of emergency bypass surgery than is PTCA performed later.

Answers: A-F, B-F, C-T, D-T

Critique: The thrombolysis in myocardial infarction (TIMI) and the thrombolysis and angioplasty in myocardial infarction (TAMI) studies provided guidance in selecting immediate or delayed angioplasty in patients treated initially with thrombolytics. In particular, the TIMI-II A report revealed that immediate angioplasty compared with delayed angioplasty conferred no significant ventricular function improvement. Additionally, immediate angioplasty was associated with an increased risk for bleeding, infarct extension, and emergency bypass surgery compared with delayed angioplasty.

Further Reading

TIMI Research Group: Immediate vs delayed catheterization and angioplasty following thrombolytic therapy in acute myocardial infarction: TIMI-IIA Results. JAMA 260:2849–2858, 1988.

Topol EJ, Califf RM, George BS, et al: A randomized trial of immediate versus delayed elective angioplasty after intravenous tissue plasminogen activator in acute myocardial infarction. N Engl J Med 317:581–588, 1987.

Yakubov SJ, Bope ET: Cardiovascular disease and arrhythmia: Cardiovascular disease. *In* Rakel RE: Textbook of Family Practice. Philadelphia, WB Saunders, 1995, p 784.

39. (True or False) True statements regarding management in the post-MI patient include which of the following?

    A. Aspirin therapy has been demonstrated to decrease subsequent reinfarction.

    B. For patients who have no contraindications, β-adrenergic blockers improve long-term survival.

    C. Oral anticoagulant therapy should be instituted in the hospital for all patients with MI and continued for 3 to 6 months after discharge from the hospital.

    D. Calcium channel blockers should be instituted routinely after a Q-wave MI.

Answers: A-T, B-T, C-F, D-F

Critique: Aspirin therapy has been demonstrated to reduce the likelihood of subsequent infarction in patients who have sustained an acute MI. Additionally, in patients who have no contraindications, β-blockers reduce long-term mortality. Oral anticoagulants should be reserved for patients who have sustained large anterior transmural infarctions who are at risk for mural thrombi. Calcium channel blockers have not been demonstrated to improve significantly the outcome of acute MI, except in patients with non–Q wave infarctions.

Further Reading

Gunnar RM, Passamani ER, Bourdillon PD, et al: Guidelines for the early management of patients with acute myocardial infarction: A report of the American College of Cardiology/American Heart Association Task Force on Assessment of Diagnostic and Therapeutic Cardiovascular Procedures (Subcommittee to Develop Guidelines for the Early Management of Patients with Acute Myocardial Infarction). J Am Coll Cardiol 16:249–292, 1990.

Yakubov SJ, Bope ET: Cardiovascular disease and arrhythmia: Cardiovascular disease. *In* Rakel RE: Textbook of Family Practice. Philadelphia, WB Saunders, 1995, p 784.

Yusuf S, Peto R, Lewis J, et al: Beta blockade during and after myocardial infarction: An overview of the randomized trials. Prog Cardiovasc Dis 27:335–371, 1985.

40. Risk stratification in the post-acute MI patient should include all of the following EXCEPT:

    A. Cardiac catheterization in patients who demonstrate postinfarction angina

    B. Electrocardiographic stress testing (in patients who have not received cardiac catheterization)

    C. Cardiac catheterization in patients who demonstrate congestive heart failure

    D. Electrophysiologic testing in all patients to rule out life-threatening ventricular arrhythmias

Answer: D

Critique: Several characteristics identify patients who are at high risk for subsequent cardiac events. Postinfarction angina and congestive heart failure confer high risk and constitute indications for cardiac catheterization. For patients who do not meet criteria for catheterization, electrocardiographic stress testing should be performed to identify patients who harbor significant residual ischemia. Additional imaging procedures such as echocardiography and radionuclide scans can provide further information regarding at-risk myocardium. Determination of the left ventricular ejection fraction has assumed greater importance in view of evidence that demonstrates survival benefit for angiotensin-converting enzyme (ACE) inhibitor therapy in patients with decreased left ventricular function. Electrophysiologic testing should be reserved for patients who demonstrate high-risk patterns on signal-averaged electrocardiograms or Holter monitoring.

Further Reading

Applegate RJ, Dell'Italia LJ, Crawford MH: Usefulness of two-dimensional echocardiography during low-level exercise testing early after uncomplicated myocardial infarction. Am J Cardiol 60:10–14, 1987.

Pfeffer MA, Braunwald E, Moye LA, et al: Effect of captopril on mortality and morbidity in patients with left ventricular dysfunction after myocardial infarction: Results of the Survival and Ventricular Enlargement Trial. N Engl J Med 327:669–677, 1992.

Ryan T, Armstrong WF, O'Donnel JA, et al: Risk stratification after acute myocardial infarction by means of exercise two-dimensional echocardiography. Am Heart J 114:1305, 1985.

Yakubov SJ, Bope ET: Cardiovascular disease and arrhythmia: Cardiovascular disease. *In* Rakel RE: Textbook of Family Practice. Philadelphia, WB Saunders, 1995, pp 784, 785.

41. Post-discharge management of the patient with an MI should include all of the following EXCEPT:

    A. Smoking cessation counseling and advice

    B. Proscription of sexual activity for 6 months

    C. Cholesterol lowering therapy in patients with elevated cholesterol

    D. Initiation of an exercise program in patients who have negative stress test results

Answer: B

Critique: Smoking cessation improves outcomes in patients who have sustained an MI (however, nicotine replacement should be used only cautiously, if at all, after an MI). Therapy for hyperlipidemia should strive for a low-density lipoprotein (LDL)-cholesterol of 100 mg/dl (2.60 mmol/l) or lower. Once the patients have demonstrated exercise tolerance on a stress test, they should begin a program of moderate exercise. Sexual activity can resume as soon as a patient has completed an unremarkable stress test.

Further Reading

Havranek EP: Managing patients with myocardial infarction after hospital discharge. Am Fam Physician 49:1109–1119, 1994.

Yakubov SJ, Bope ET: Cardiovascular disease and arrhythmia: Cardiovascular disease. *In* Rakel RE: Textbook of Family Practice. Philadelphia, WB Saunders, 1995, pp 784, 785.

42. The most common cause of myocarditis in the United States is/are:

    A. Spirochetal infection (e.g., Lyme disease and leptospirosis)

   B. Bacterial infection (e.g., diphtheria and strepto-
      coccal infection)
   C. Protozoan infection (e.g., *Trypanozoma cruzii*)
   D. Viral infection (e.g., Coxsackie A and B)

Answer: D

Critique: Viral infections represent the most common cause of myocarditis in the United States. Coxsackie A and B represent the most common viral types involved in these infections. *T. cruzii* is the most common cause in South America.

Further Reading

Yakubov SJ, Bope ET: Cardiovascular disease and arrhythmia: Cardiovascular disease. *In* Rakel RE: Textbook of Family Practice. Philadelphia, WB Saunders, 1995, pp 785, 786.

43. True statements regarding pharmacotherapy in dilated cardiomyopathy include all of the following EXCEPT:

   A. Afterload reduction and diuretic therapy are useful in supportive therapy.
   B. ACE inhibitors reduce long-term mortality in symptomatic patients who demonstrate poor ventricular function.
   C. Anticoagulant therapy should be used to prevent thromboembolic phenomena.
   D. Digitalis should be withdrawn in patients who have used this drug for extended periods.

Answer: D

Critique: Afterload reduction, diuretic therapy, and fluid restriction constitute useful supportive therapeutic measures for dilated cardiomyopathy. Additionally, ACE inhibitors have been shown to decrease long-term mortality in symptomatic patients who have depressed ventricular function. Anticoagulant therapy reduces the risk of thromboembolism in heart failure. Digitalis should not be withdrawn routinely in these patients unless specifically indicated.

Further Reading

Uretsky BF for the PROVED Investigative Group: Randomized study assessing the effect of digoxin withdrawal in patients with mild to moderate chronic congestive heart failure: Results of the PROVED Trial. J Am Coll Cardiol 22:955–962, 1993.
Yakubov SJ, Bope ET: Cardiovascular disease and arrhythmia: Cardiovascular disease. *In* Rakel RE: Textbook of Family Practice. Philadelphia, WB Saunders, 1995, p 786.

44. Of the following, which physiologic characteristic manifests in obstructive cardiomyopathy?

   A. Impaired systolic function
   B. Improvement in the outflow obstruction with low systolic blood pressure
   C. Impaired diastolic filling
   D. Normal left ventricular relaxation

Answer: C

Critique: Obstructive cardiomyopathy demonstrates impaired left ventricular relaxation and diastolic filling. Low systolic blood pressure and volume depletion worsen the outflow obstruction. Systolic function remains intact.

Further Reading

Yakubov SJ, Bope ET: Cardiovascular disease and arrhythmia: Cardiovascular disease. *In* Rakel RE: Textbook of Family Practice. Philadelphia, WB Saunders, 1995, p 787.

45. (True or False) True statements regarding clinical findings in obstructive cardiomyopathy include which of the following?

   A. Auscultation may demonstrate a crescendo-decrescendo systolic murmur.
   B. Murmur intensity decreases with the Valsalva maneuver.
   C. Murmur intensity increases with handgrip.
   D. Echocardiography reveals left ventricular hypertrophy with disproportionate thickening of the left ventricular septum.

Answers: A-T, B-F, C-F, D-T

Critique: In patients with obstructive cardiomyopathy (asymmetric septal hypertrophy, idiopathic hypertrophic subaortic stenosis), a crescendo-decrescendo murmur may be present. The murmur will increase with the Valsalva maneuver (due to decreased venous return to the heart) and decrease with handgrip (due to increased afterload). Echocardiography will demonstrate left ventricular hypertrophy with disproportionate thickening of the left ventricular septum.

Further Reading

Yakubov SJ, Bope ET: Cardiovascular disease and arrhythmia: Cardiovascular disease. *In* Rakel RE: Textbook of Family Practice. Philadelphia, WB Saunders, 1995, pp 786, 787.

46. Pharmacologic agents that should be considered in the early medical management of obstructive cardiomyopathy include all of the following EXCEPT:

   A. Calcium channel blockers
   B. β-Adrenergic blocking agents
   C. Antibiotic therapy as prophylaxis before dental procedures
   D. Digoxin

Answer: D

Critique: Calcium channel blockers and β-blockers improve diastolic relaxation and the left ventricular outflow gradient. Antibiotic therapy should be prescribed for endocarditis prophylaxis in patients undergoing dental procedures. Digoxin increases myocardial contractility; agents with positive inotropic effects should not be used routinely in the early management of obstructive cardiomyopathy but might have benefit in late stages of the disease as manifested by severely compromised systolic function.

Further Reading

Maron BJ, Bonow RO, Cannon RO, et al: Hypertrophic cardiomyopathy: Interrelations of clinical manifestations, pathophysiology, and therapy, Part II. N Engl J Med 316:844–852, 1987.

Yakubov SJ, Bope ET: Cardiovascular disease and arrhythmia: Cardiovascular disease. *In* Rakel RE: Textbook of Family Practice. Philadelphia, WB Saunders, 1995, p 787.

47. Clinical findings seen commonly with restrictive cardiomyopathy include all of the following EXCEPT:

    A. Muffled heart sounds
    B. Cardiomegaly on x-ray
    C. Low voltage on the electrocardiogram
    D. Elevated jugulovenous pressure

Answer: B

Critique: Restrictive cardiomyopathy produces restrained diastolic left ventricular filling. This leads to elevated jugulovenous pressure, hepatomegaly, and peripheral edema. Additionally, the electrocardiogram can demonstrate diffuse low voltage. Heart sounds can appear muffled. The cardiac silhouette should not demonstrate cardiomegaly.

Further Reading

Yakubov SJ, Bope ET: Cardiovascular disease and arrhythmia: Cardiovascular disease. *In* Rakel RE: Textbook of Family Practice. Philadelphia, WB Saunders, 1995, p 787.

48. Clinical findings observed in acute pericarditis include all of the following EXCEPT:

    A. Sharp or stabbing chest pain
    B. Pericardial friction rub
    C. Diffuse ST segment depression on the electrocardiogram
    D. Fever

Answer: C

Critique: Acute pericarditis presents typically with a sharp or stabbing chest pain and fever. Additionally, a pericardial friction rub is heard in many patients. The electrocardiogram typically reveals ST segment elevation in multiple leads.

Further Reading

Yakubov SJ, Bope ET: Cardiovascular disease and arrhythmia: Cardiovascular disease. *In* Rakel RE: Textbook of Family Practice. Philadelphia, WB Saunders, 1995, p 788.

49. (True or False) Physical findings observed in cardiac tamponade include which of the following?

    A. Pulsus paradoxus
    B. Systemic hypertension
    C. Pericardial friction rub
    D. Bradycardia
    E. Faint heart sounds

Answers: A-T, B-F, C-T, D-F, E-T

Critique: Cardiac tamponade occurs as a result of restricted diastolic filling due to accumulated fluid in the pericardial sac. The restricted diastolic filling restrains cardiac output, which can manifest as hypotension, tachycardia, and elevated venous pressure. A pericardial friction rub may be present, and the heart sounds might be attenuated by the effusion. Pulsus paradoxus can also be seen commonly.

Further Reading

Yakubov SJ, Bope ET: Cardiovascular disease and arrhythmia: Cardiovascular disease. *In* Rakel RE: Textbook of Family Practice. Philadelphia, WB Saunders, 1995, p. 788.

50. (True or False) True statements regarding neurohumoral adaptations in congestive heart failure include which of the following?

    A. The sympathetic nervous system downregulates.
    B. Atrial natriuretic peptide levels increase.
    C. The renin-angiotensin system is activated.

Answers: A-F, B-T, C-T

Critique: The depressed cardiac output characteristic of heart failure leads to a number of neurohumoral responses. The sympathetic nervous system activates in response to depressed myocardial contractility and cardiac output. The renin-angiotensin system activates with resultant increased aldosterone levels. As vascular volume increases, atrial natriuretic peptide levels increase to promote water diuresis.

Further Reading

Cody RJ, Kubo SH, Pickworth KK: Diuretic treatment for the sodium retention of congestive heart failure. Arch Intern Med 154:1905–1914, 1994.
Dec GW, Fuster V: Idiopathic dilated cardiomyopathy. N Engl J Med 331:1564–1575, 1994.
Navas JP, Martinez-Maldonado M: Pathophysiology of edema in congestive heart failure. Heart Dis Stroke 2:325–329, 1993.
Yakubov SJ, Bope ET: Cardiovascular disease and arrhythmia: Cardiovascular disease. *In* Rakel RE: Textbook of Family Practice. Philadelphia, WB Saunders, 1995, p 790.

51. Of the following, which causes *high-output* heart failure?

    A. Disopyramide therapy (Norpace)
    B. Scleroderma
    C. Cobalt intoxication
    D. Thyrotoxicosis

Answer: D

Critique: Disopyramide, scleroderma, and cobalt intoxication produce depressed myocardial function, which leads to congestive heart failure. Thyrotoxicosis leads to high output states that can overwhelm the heart's compensatory mechanisms.

Further Reading

Yakubov SJ, Bope ET: Cardiovascular disease and arrhythmia: Cardiovascular disease. *In* Rakel RE: Textbook of Family Practice. Philadelphia, WB Saunders, 1995, p 791.

52. Under the New York Heart Association classification for heart disease, a patient who exhibits severe limitation of physical activity and dyspnea at rest meets criteria for which functional class?

A. Class I
B. Class II
C. Class III
D. Class IV

Answer: D

Critique: A patient who demonstrates dyspnea at rest and severely limited physical activity fulfills criteria for New York Heart Association class IV.

Further Reading

Yakubov SJ, Bope ET: Cardiovascular disease and arrhythmia: Cardiovascular disease. *In* Rakel RE: Textbook of Family Practice. Philadelphia, WB Saunders, 1995, p 791.

53. Which one of the following best describes the pathogenesis of a third heart sound?

A. Expansion of the mitral annulus
B. Turbulence of blood passing through the aortic valve
C. Atrial contraction with forcing of blood into a noncompliant left ventricle
D. Increased left ventricular end-diastolic volume with resistance to early filling of the left ventricle

Answer: D

Critique: Expansion of the mitral annulus as a result of ventricular dilatation would generate a murmur of mitral insufficiency. Turbulent flow through the aortic valve would produce an ejection quality murmur. Atrial contraction with forcing of blood into a poorly compliant left ventricle generates a fourth heart sound. The third heart sound occurs as a result of resistance to early filling of the left ventricle in the context of elevated end-diastolic pressures seen in heart failure.

Further Reading

Yakubov SJ, Bope ET: Cardiovascular disease and arrhythmia: Cardiovascular disease. *In* Rakel RE: Textbook of Family Practice. Philadelphia, WB Saunders, 1995, p 791.

54. Kerley's B lines on a chest x-ray occur as a result of which of the following?

A. Intra-alveolar fluid
B. Dilated pulmonary vasculature
C. Fluid in the pleural space
D. Interlobular edema

Answer: D

Critique: Kerley's B lines occur as a result of interlobular fluid accumulation.

Further Reading

Yakubov SJ, Bope ET: Cardiovascular disease and arrhythmia: Cardiovascular disease. *In* Rakel RE: Textbook of Family Practice. Philadelphia, WB Saunders, 1995, p 792.

55. General measures used in the initial treatment of congestive heart failure include all of the following EXCEPT:

A. Dietary salt restriction
B. Abstinence from alcohol
C. Control of hypertension
D. A vigorous program of physical activity

Answer: D

Critique: In addition to searching for treatable causes for congestive heart failure, several general measures should be instituted. Dietary salt should be restricted, and the patient should abstain from alcohol. Elevated blood pressure should be controlled. Vigorous, strenuous physical activity should be avoided.

Further Reading

Yakubov SJ, Bope ET: Cardiovascular disease and arrhythmia: Cardiovascular disease. *In* Rakel RE: Textbook of Family Practice. Philadelphia, WB Saunders, 1995, p 792.

56. (True or False) True statements regarding the effects of ACE inhibitors in patients who have asymptomatic left ventricular dysfunction include which of the following?

A. ACE inhibitor therapy produces a statistically significant decrease in mortality risk.
B. ACE inhibitor therapy confers decreased hospitalization risk.
C. ACE inhibitor therapy decreases the frequency of congestive heart failure episodes.
D. ACE inhibitor therapy decreases end-diastolic ventricular volume during long-term treatment.

Answers: A-F, B-T, C-T, D-T

Critique: The SOLVD trial (using the ACE inhibitor enalapril) demonstrated no statistically significant decrease in mortality in asymptomatic patients who had a pretreatment ejection fraction of less than 35%. However, ACE inhibitor therapy did decrease hospitalization rates and episodes of congestive heart failure. Enalapril therapy led to decreased ventricular end-diastolic volumes; this effect was sustained during long-term treatment. In contrast with the results in asymptomatic patients, enalapril produced a significantly decreased mortality risk in *symptomatic* patients.

Further Reading

Konstam MA, for the SOLVD Investigators: Effects of the angiotensin converting enzyme inhibitor enalapril on the long-term progression of left ventricular dilatation in patients with asymptomatic systolic dysfunction. Circulation 88:2277–2783, 1993.
Yakubov SJ, Bope ET: Cardiovascular disease and arrhythmia: Cardiovascular disease. *In* Rakel RE: Textbook of Family Practice. Philadelphia, WB Saunders, 1995, p 792.

57. Vasodilator therapy in congestive heart failure produces improved left ventricular function through all of the following mechanisms EXCEPT:

A. Decrease in systemic arterial pressure
B. Decrease in systemic vascular resistance
C. Decrease in left ventricular wall tension
D. Decrease in venous return to the heart

Answer: A

Critique: Vasodilator therapy produces several physiologic effects that serve to improve left ventricular function. Vasodilatation reduces systemic vascular resistance and systemic pressure, thus lowering the "pressure head" against which the left ventricle must work to eject blood into the systemic circulation. Additionally, vasodilatation can lead to decreased venous return to the heart, which in turn decreases ventricular volume. These mechanisms all contribute to diminished left ventricular wall tension.

Further Reading

Yakubov SJ, Bope ET: Cardiovascular disease and arrhythmia: Cardiovascular disease. *In* Rakel RE: Textbook of Family Practice. Philadelphia, WB Saunders, 1995, p 792.

58. Digoxin therapy confers little benefit, or is contraindicated, in all of the following conditions EXCEPT:

A. Wolff-Parkinson-White syndrome with concomitant atrial fibrillation
B. Right ventricular failure due to cor pulmonale
C. Mitral stenosis (unless accompanied by atrial fibrillation and rapid heart rate)
D. Congestive heart failure associated with atrial fibrillation

Answer: D

Critique: Digoxin improves myocardial contractility via increasing Ca^{2+} ion influx into myocardial cells. Digoxin should not be used in patients who have Wolff-Parkinson-White syndrome and atrial fibrillation; digoxin therapy in this context can decrease refractory periods in the accessory pathway and increase heart rates. Digoxin also confers little benefit in cor pulmonale or mitral stenosis. In patients with heart failure and atrial fibrillation, digoxin therapy improves myocardial contractility and slows heart rate, thus improving myocardial function.

Further Reading

Yakubov SJ, Bope ET: Cardiovascular disease and arrhythmia: Cardiovascular disease. *In* Rakel RE: Textbook of Family Practice. Philadelphia, WB Saunders, 1995, p 793.

59. (True or False) Cardiac manifestations of digoxin toxicity include which of the following?

A. Second-degree AV block
B. Third-degree AV block
C. Paroxysmal atrial tachycardia with AV block
D. Supraventricular premature beats

Answers: A-T, B-T, C-T, D-T

Critique: Digoxin toxicity can manifest with many different cardiac rhythm disturbances. Second- and third-degree blocks, paroxysmal atrial tachycardia with AV block, and supraventricular premature beats can all occur in this context.

Further Reading

Yakubov SJ, Bope ET: Cardiovascular disease and arrhythmia: Cardiovascular disease. *In* Rakel RE: Textbook of Family Practice. Philadelphia, WB Saunders, 1995, p 793.

60. Physiologic effects of dobutamine include all of the following EXCEPT:

A. Vasoconstriction at low doses
B. Vasodilation at high doses
C. Negative chronotropic effects
D. Increased myocardial contractility

Answer: C

Critique: Dobutamine possesses α- and β-stimulating effects. At a low dose, α-stimulation leads to mild vasoconstriction; at higher doses, β-stimulation leads to vasodilatation. Dobutamine has a mildly positive chronotropic effect and increases myocardial contractility.

Further Reading

Yakubov SJ, Bope ET: Cardiovascular disease and arrhythmia: Cardiovascular disease. *In* Rakel RE: Textbook of Family Practice. Philadelphia, WB Saunders, 1995, p 793.

61. Amrinone exerts beneficial effects in heart failure through all of the following mechanisms EXCEPT:

A. Dilatation of venous vasculature
B. Dilatation of arterial vasculature
C. Decreased intracellular cyclic AMP
D. Positive inotropic effects

Answer: C

Critique: Amrinone exerts its effects through phosphodiesterase inhibition. This leads to increased intracellular cyclic AMP, which causes smooth muscle relaxation. This relaxation produces venous and arterial vessel dilatation. Amrinone also exerts positive inotropic effects on the heart.

Further Reading

Yakubov SJ, Bope ET: Cardiovascular disease and arrhythmia: Cardiovascular disease. *In* Rakel RE: Textbook of Family Practice. Philadelphia, WB Saunders, 1995, p 794.

62. Which one of the following is a major Jones criterion for diagnosing rheumatic fever?

A. Fever
B. Prolonged PR interval on the electrocardiogram
C. Arthralgia
D. Carditis
E. Elevated erythrocyte sedimentation rate

Answer: D

Critique: The diagnosis of rheumatic fever depends on the presence of major and minor Jones criteria. The major criteria include carditis, polyarthritis, subcutaneous nodules, erythema marginatum, and chorea. The minor criteria include fever, previous rheumatic fever, arthralgia, prolonged PR interval, and elevated erythrocyte sedimentation or positive C-reactive protein evaluations. The presence of two major, or one major plus two minor, criteria indicate a high probability for rheumatic fever.

Further Reading

Stollerman GH, Markowitz M, Taranter A, et al: Jones criteria (revised) for guidance in the diagnosis of rheumatic fever. Circulation 32:664, 1965
Yakubov SJ, Bope ET: Cardiovascular disease and arrhythmia: Cardiovascular disease. *In* Rakel RE: Textbook of Family Practice. Philadelphia, WB Saunders, 1995, p 794.

63. (True or False) True statements regarding penicillin therapy in rheumatic fever patients include which of the following?

A. Penicillin therapy alters the course of established rheumatic fever.
B. Penicillin prophylaxis can prevent subsequent episodes of rheumatic fever.
C. Penicillin therapy can limit long-term sequelae of rheumatic fever.

Answers: A-F, B-T, C-T

Critique: Penicillin does not alter the course of established rheumatic fever but can limit long-term sequelae by eradicating streptococci. Elimination of the streptococcal organisms limits possible ongoing valvular inflammation that might arise with continued streptococcal presence.

Further Reading

Yakubov SJ, Bope ET: Cardiovascular disease and arrhythmia: Cardiovascular disease. *In* Rakel RE: Textbook of Family Practice. Philadelphia, WB Saunders, 1995, p 794.

64. Match the clinical characteristics with the appropriate valvular abnormality.

A. Bicuspid aortic valves
B. Calcific aortic stenosis
C. Both A and B
D. Neither A nor B

1. Present as a congenital anomaly

2. Usually becomes symptomatic after age 60

3. Can be associated with left ventricular hypertrophy

4. Can be associated with increased myocardial oxygen consumption

Answers: 1-A, 2-B, 3-C, 4-C

Critique: Bicuspid aortic valves occur as a congenital abnormality and generally become symptomatic before a person is 50 years of age. Calcific aortic stenosis generally presents symptoms after age 50. Both entities can lead to significant aortic stenosis, which leads to left ventricular hypertrophy and increased myocardial consumption. These patients can present with angina, despite normal coronary arteries, due to compromised subendocardial perfusion.

Further Reading

Yakubov SJ, Bope ET: Cardiovascular disease and arrhythmia: Cardiovascular disease. *In* Rakel RE: Textbook of Family Practice. Philadelphia, WB Saunders, 1995, p 795.

65. The single most important diagnostic test for the evaluation of aortic stenosis is:

A. Electrocardiography
B. Cardiac catheterization
C. Chest radiograph
D. Echocardiography

Answer: D

Critique: Echocardiography represents the single most important diagnostic tool for evaluating aortic stenosis. This single procedure provides information about valvular and ventricular function, as well as valvular orifice dimensions and pressure gradients (calculated using the modified Bernouilli equation). Cardiac catheterization should be considered in those who are at risk for concomitant coronary artery disease.

Further Reading

Yakubov SJ, Bope ET: Cardiovascular disease and arrhythmia: Cardiovascular disease. *In* Rakel RE: Textbook of Family Practice. Philadelphia, WB Saunders, 1995, p 796.

66. Match the following entities with the appropriate mechanism for inducing aortic regurgitation.

A. Intrinsic valvular abnormality leads to aortic regurgitation.
B. Dilatation of the aortic root leads to aortic regurgitation.
C. Both A and B
D. Neither A nor B

1. Infective endocarditis

2. Systemic hypertension

3. Connective tissue disorders

4. Rheumatic fever

Answers: 1-A, 2-B, 3-B, 4-A

Critique: Aortic regurgitation occurs as a result of a valvular deformity or dilatation of the aortic root. Infective endocarditis and rheumatic fever distort valvular anatomy, leading to aortic regurgitation. Systemic hypertension and connective tissue disorders can result in ascending aortic dilatation with poor valve leaflet coaptation.

Further Reading

Yakubov SJ, Bope ET: Cardiovascular disease and arrhythmia: Cardiovascular disease. *In* Rakel RE: Textbook of Family Practice. Philadelphia, WB Saunders, 1995, p 796.

67. Clinical characteristics observed in patients with significant aortic regurgitation include all of the following EXCEPT:

A. "Water hammer" pulse (rapid upstroke and collapse of the pulse)
B. Widened pulse pressure

C. Low diastolic blood pressures

D. Crescendo murmur in late diastole

Answer: D

Critique: Aortic regurgitation can manifest a "water hammer" pulse and wide pulse pressures. The diastolic systemic blood pressure tends to be low. The murmur of aortic regurgitation occurs in early diastole and demonstrates a decrescendo profile.

Further Reading

Yakubov SJ, Bope ET: Cardiovascular disease and arrhythmia: Cardiovascular disease. *In* Rakel RE: Textbook of Family Practice. Philadelphia, WB Saunders, 1995, p 796.

68. (True or False) Mitral valve characteristics that suggest that a patient with mitral valve stenosis can be treated with percutaneous balloon valvuloplasty include which of the following?

A. Minimal mitral regurgitation

B. Absence of left atrial appendage thrombi

C. Heavy mitral valve calcification

Answers: A-T, B-T, C-F

Critique: Percutaneous balloon valvuloplasty represents an alternative to open surgical valve repair. Characteristics that indicate that valvuloplasty represents a viable option include trivial or mild mitral regurgitation, absence of left atrial thrombi, and minimal mitral valvular calcification.

Further Reading

Yakubov SJ, Bope ET: Cardiovascular disease and arrhythmia: Cardiovascular disease. *In* Rakel RE: Textbook of Family Practice. Philadelphia, WB Saunders, 1995, pp 796, 797.

69. (True or False) Abdominal aortic aneurysms represent a prospective management challenge: Immediate surgery exposes to surgical morbidity and mortality those whose aneurysms would remain stable, but delay risks catastrophic outcomes for patients whose lesions represent a high risk for rupture. True statements regarding abdominal aortic aneurysm include:

A. Aneurysms with a diameter greater than 6 cm display a high risk of rupture.

B. The median rate for size increase in an aneurysm is about 0.21 cm/yr.

C. Abdominal aortic radiographs represent the best method for prospective surveillance of the size of an aneurysm.

D. An aortic aneurysm should be considered in elderly patients who complain of abdominal pain or back pain.

Answers: A-T, B-T, C-F, D-T

Critique: Abdominal aortic aneurysms over 5 cm demonstrate a substantial risk for rupture. Population-based studies suggest that lesions less than 5 cm in diameter demonstrate much less risk. Aneurysms evaluated in the Rochester, Minnesota area demonstrated a median rate of 0.21 cm/yr increase in size. Abdominal ultrasound represents the best diagnostic tool for prospective follow-up. Abdominal aneurysm should be considered in any elderly patient who complains of abdominal pain or back pain.

Further Reading

Nevitt MP, Ballard DJ, Hallett JW: Prognosis of abdominal aortic aneurysms: A population-based study. N Engl J Med 321:1009–1114, 1989.

Yakubov SJ, Bope ET: Cardiovascular disease and arrhythmia: Cardiovascular disease. *In* Rakel RE: Textbook of Family Practice. Philadelphia, WB Saunders, 1995, p 798.

70. (True or False) Clinical findings found frequently in acute aortic dissection include which of the following?

A. Severe chest pain

B. Mediastinal widening on chest radiograph

C. Arterial hypotension

D. Aortic regurgitation (in approximately one third of patients)

Answers: A-T, B-T, C-F, D-T

Critique: Acute aortic dissection presents with sharp, severe chest pain. Chest radiography can reveal a widened mediastinum, and cardiac auscultation reveals aortic regurgitation in as many as one third of the patients. Arterial hypertension is usually seen at initial presentation. Initial medical therapy should include β-blockers to lower blood pressure and heart rate.

Further Reading

Yakubov SJ, Bope ET: Cardiovascular disease and arrhythmia: Cardiovascular disease. *In* Rakel RE: Textbook of Family Practice. Philadelphia, WB Saunders, 1995, p 798, 799.

71. The ankle-to-brachial index provides an indication of significant peripheral vascular disease in the lower extremities. Significant peripheral arterial obstruction is indicated at an ankle-to-brachial index less than:

A. 1.4

B. 1.2

C. 1.0

D. 0.8

Answer: D

Critique: The blood pressure measured by Doppler flow is usually higher in the dorsalis pedis compared with the brachial artery. An obstruction in the lower extremity arterial supply results in decreased dorsalis pedis pressures. An ankle-to-brachial index of less than 0.8 suggests significant peripheral arterial disease.

Further Reading

Yakubov SJ, Bope ET: Cardiovascular disease and arrhythmia: Cardiovascular disease. *In* Rakel RE: Textbook of Family Practice. Philadelphia, WB Saunders, 1995, p 799.

72. You are seeing a 45-year-old man for a physical examination. He has no cardiac symptoms. He wishes to begin an exercise program and would like to undergo an electrocardiographic stress test to "make sure" that he has no cardiac disease. You perform the stress test, using a positivity criterion (i.e., point at which you describe the test as abnormal or positive) of a 1 mm or greater ST segment depression. The test reveals a 1.2-mm ST segment depression. On the basis of this result, you tell the patient that his probability for significant coronary artery disease is:

A. <5%
B. 17%
C. 22%
D. 35%
E. 54%

Answer: C

Critique: To interpret a stress test, the evaluator must know the patient's prior probability for the disease in question and the operating characteristics (sensitivity and specificity) of the test (indeed this information should be considered in evaluating any clinical test). An asymptomatic 45-year-old man has an approximately 5.5% probability for significant coronary artery disease; this represents the "prior probability" for this condition. The electrocardiographic stress test performs with less than perfect sensitivity and specificity. The sensitivity, using the positivity criterion of ST segment depression equal to or less than 1mm, is about 44%. The specificity under these conditions is about 91%. These values allow the investigator to calculate the patient's "post-test probability" (the likelihood that the patient has the disease, given the test result and prior probability) using Bayes' theorem. The calculation looks like this:

$$\frac{P[D^+] \times P[T^+|D^+]}{((P[D^+] \times P[T^+|D^+]) + ((1\text{-}P[T^-|D^-]) \times (1\text{-}P[D^+])))}$$

where:

$P[D^+]$ = probability of disease

$P[T^+|D^+]$ = probability of a positive test result, given the presence of the disease
= *sensitivity*

$P[T^-|D^-]$ = probability of a negative test result, given the absence of the disease
= *specificity*

In this situation, the prior probability represents the likelihood that an asymptomatic 45-year-old man harbors significant coronary artery disease. This probability is about 5.5% based on autopsy studies. The sensitivity of the electrocardiographic stress test, given a positivity criterion of equal to or greater than 1-mm ST segment depression, is about 44%. The specificity is about 91%. Using these values, the post-test probability that the patient has significant coronary disease, given the positive test, equals:

$$\frac{0.055 \times 0.44}{([0.055 \times 0.44] + ([1\text{-}0.91] \times [1\text{-}0.055]))}$$
$$= 0.22 \text{ (i.e., 22\%)}$$

Further Reading

Reeves TJ: Use of stress electrocardiography in practice. Heart Dis Stroke January/February:13–18, 1992.

Sox HC: Exercise testing in suspected coronary disease. Dis Mon 31:1–93, 1985.

Sox HC, Littenberg B, Garber AM: The role of exercise testing in screening for coronary artery disease. Ann Intern Med 110:456–469, 1989.

Diagnosis and Treatment of Arrhythmias

1. The heart contains several intrinsic pacemakers that generate transmembrane action potentials at different rates. The AV node, when not first depolarized by potentials from the SA node, demonstrates an intrinsic rate of:

    A. 60–100 beats/min
    B. 40–60 beats/min
    C. 20–40 beats/min
    D. 10–30 beats/min

Answer: B

Critique: The SA node demonstrates an intrinsic pacemaker rate of 60 to 100 beats/min. The AV node discharges at a rate of 40 to 60 beats/min when not overridden by impulses from the SA node. The bundle of His and Purkinje fibers discharge at less than 40 beats/min when not stimulated more rapidly by impulses from the SA and AV nodes.

Further Reading

Yakubov SJ, Bope ET: Cardiovascular disease and arrhythmia: Cardiovascular disease. *In* Rakel RE: Textbook of Family Practice. Philadelphia, WB Saunders, 1995, p 802.

2. In the Vaughan-Williams' antiarrhythmic drug classification system, class IA agents act by:

    A. Decreasing the rate of slow repolarization in phase 4 of the transmembrane action potential (TAP)
    B. Slowing the rate of depolarization in conduction tissue
    C. Slowing the rate of conduction through conduction tissue
    D. Widening the transmembrane action potential and reducing the rate of rise in phase 0 of the TAP

Answer: D

Critique: Class IA agents act by inhibiting fast Na^+ channels in pacemaker tissue, thus reducing the rate of rise in phase 0 of the transmembrane action potential. These agents also widen the TAP.

Further Reading

Yakubov SJ, Bope ET: Cardiovascular disease and arrhythmia: Cardiovascular disease. *In* Rakel RE: Textbook of Family Practice. Philadelphia, WB Saunders, 1995, p 805.

3. Cardiac glycosides exert their antiarrhythmic effects through all of the following mechanisms EXCEPT:

    A. Decrease in vagal tone
    B. Decrease in sympathetic tone
    C. Decrease in atrial and junctional pacemaker automaticity
    D. Prolongation of the AV node refractory period

Answer: A

Critique: The cardiac glycosides (e.g., digoxin) exert their antiarrhythmic effects by *increasing* vagal tone, decreasing sympathetic tone, decreasing atrial and junctional pacemaker automaticity, and prolonging the refractory period in the AV node.

Further Reading

Yakubov SJ, Bope ET: Cardiovascular disease and arrhythmia: Cardiovascular disease. *In* Rakel RE: Textbook of Family Practice. Philadelphia, WB Saunders, 1995, p 805.

4. The rhythm tracing shown in Figure 35–1 demonstrates:

    A. First-degree AV block
    B. Prolonged QT_c
    C. Sinus bradycardia
    D. Prolonged QRS duration

Answer: C

Critique: The tracing demonstrates sinus bradycardia, with a rate in the 40s. The PR interval is normal, ruling out first-degree AV block. The QT interval is approximately 0.46, but the QT_c is normal at about 0.40. The QRS duration is about 0.08 second, which is normal.

Further Reading

Yakubov SJ, Bope ET: Cardiovascular disease and arrhythmia: Cardiovascular disease. *In* Rakel RE: Textbook of Family Practice. Philadelphia, WB Saunders, 1995, p 806.

5. Physiologic causes of sinus tachycardia include all of the following EXCEPT:

    A. Hypothyroidism
    B. Anemia
    C. Fever
    D. Hypotension

Answer: A

Critique: Anemia, fever, and hypotension can all cause sinus tachycardia. Sinus bradycardia would be more likely with hypothyroidism.

Further Reading

Yakubov SJ, Bope ET: Cardiovascular disease and arrhythmia: Cardiovascular disease. *In* Rakel RE: Textbook of Family Practice. Philadelphia, WB Saunders, 1995, p 806.

6. The rhythm shown in Figure 35–2 demonstrates which one of the following phenomena?

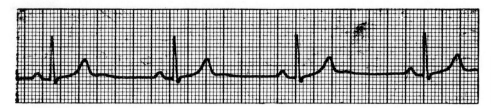

Figure 35-1 (Reproduced with permission from Rakel RE [Ed]: Textbook of Family Practice, 5th ed. Philadelphia, WB Saunders, 1995, p 806.)

Figure 35-2 (Reproduced with permission from Rakel RE [Ed]: Textbook of Family Practice, 5th ed. Philadelphia, WB Saunders, 1995, p 807.)

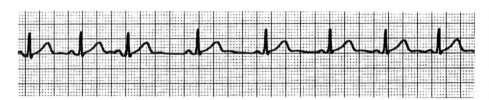

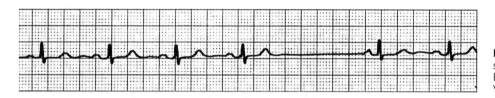

Figure 35-3 (Reproduced with permission from Rakel RE [Ed]: Textbook of Family Practice, 5th ed. Philadelphia, WB Saunders, 1995, p 810.)

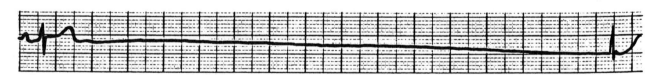

Figure 35-4 Reproduced with permission from Sandoe E, Sigurd B: Arrhythmia: Diagnosis and Management: A Clinical Electrocardiographic Guide. St. Galen, Verlag für Fachmedien, 1984.)

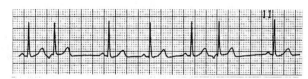

Figure 35-5 (Reproduced with permission from Rakel RE [Ed]: Textbook of Family Practice, 5th ed. Philadelphia, WB Saunders, 1995, p 811.)

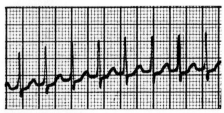

Figure 35-6 (Reproduced with permission from Rakel RE [Ed]: Textbook of Family Practice, 5th ed. Philadelphia, WB Saunders, 1995, p 811.)

A. Sinus tachycardia
B. Second-degree AV block
C. Sinus arrhythmia
D. Prolonged QT_c

Answer: C

Critique: The rhythm strip reveals sinus arrhythmia: the PP and RR intervals vary, but the PP and RR are equal for any one particular complex. This rhythm can occur normally with respiration. The PR interval is about 0.16, ruling out first-degree block. Every P wave is associated with a QRS complex, ruling out second-degree heart block. The QT_c is approximately 0.41, which is normal.

Further Reading

Yakubov SJ, Bope ET: Cardiovascular disease and arrhythmia: Cardiovascular disease. *In* Rakel RE: Textbook of Family Practice. Philadelphia, WB Saunders, 1995, p 807.

7. The rhythm shown in Figure 35–3 demonstrates which one of the following abnormalities?

A. Second-degree AV block
B. Bundle branch block
C. Sinus pause
D. Short QT_c

Answer: C

Critique: The tracing reveals a sinus pause. Each P wave is followed by a QRS complex, which rules out a second-degree block. The QRS duration is normal, which rules out a bundle branch block. The QT_c is about 0.43.

Further Reading

Yakubov SJ, Bope ET: Cardiovascular disease and arrhythmia: Cardiovascular disease. *In* Rakel RE: Textbook of Family Practice. Philadelphia, WB Saunders, 1995, p 807.

8. **(True or False)** The following represent appropriate medical therapies for the tracing shown in Figure 35–4:

A. Propranolol
B. Atropine
C. Atenolol
D. Epinephrine

Answers: A-F, B-T, C-F, D-T

Critique: The tracing demonstrates sinus arrest, which can occur as a result of intrinsic SA node disease or drug intoxications (quinidine or cardiac glycosides). In

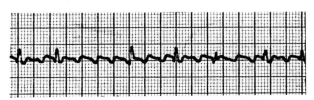

Figure 35–7 (Reproduced with permission from Rakel RE [Ed]: Textbook of Family Practice, 5th ed. Philadelphia, WB Saunders, 1995, p 812.)

this setting, epinephrine and atropine represent appropriate medical interventions. The β-blockers such as propranolol and atenolol should not be used in this setting.

Further Reading

Yakubov SJ, Bope ET: Cardiovascular disease and arrhythmia: Cardiovascular disease. *In* Rakel RE: Textbook of Family Practice. Philadelphia, WB Saunders, 1995, pp 807–810.

9. The tracing in Figure 35–5 demonstrates which one of the following rhythm disturbances?

A. Ventricular premature beats
B. Atrial premature beats
C. Paroxysmal atrial tachycardia
D. First-degree AV block

Answer: B

Critique: The tracing demonstrates atrial premature beats (the second and sixth beats).

Further Reading

Yakubov SJ, Bope ET: Cardiovascular disease and arrhythmia: Cardiovascular disease. *In* Rakel RE: Textbook of Family Practice. Philadelphia, WB Saunders, 1995, pp 810–811.

10. **(True or False)** Potential causes for the rhythm shown in question 8 include the following:

A. Fatigue
B. Alcohol
C. Caffeine
D. Tobacco use

Answers: A-T, B-T, C-T, D-T

Critique: Fatigue, alcohol, caffeine, and tobacco use can all precipitate atrial premature contractions. Treatment

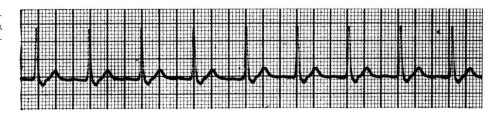

Figure 35–8 (Reproduced with permission from Rakel RE [Ed]: Textbook of Family Practice, 5th ed. Philadelphia, WB Saunders, 1995, p 814.)

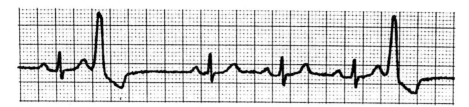

Figure 35–9 (Reproduced with permission from Rakel RE [Ed]: Textbook of Family Practice, 5th ed. Philadelphia, WB Saunders, 1995, p 814.)

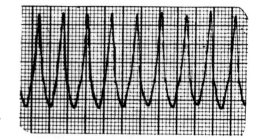

Figure 35–10 (Reproduced with permission from Rakel RE [Ed]: Textbook of Family Practice, 5th ed. Philadelphia, WB Saunders, 1995, p 815.)

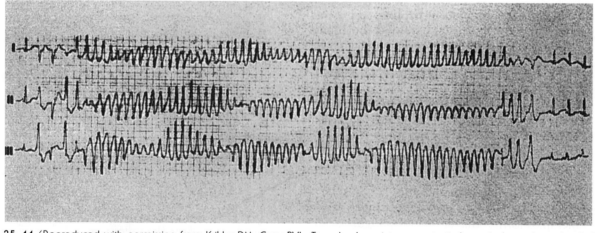

Figure 35–11 (Reproduced with permission from Krikler DM, Curry PVL: Torsade de pointes, an atypical ventricular tachycardia. Br Heart J 38:128, 1976.)

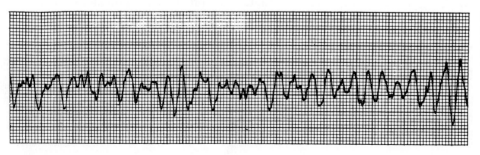

Figure 35–12 (Reproduced with permission from Textbook of Advanced Cardiac Life Support. Dallas, Tx, American Heart Association, 1994. Copyright 1994 American Heart Association.)

involves removal of the offending agent (e.g., smoking cessation, moderate use of or abstinence from alcohol).

Further Reading

Yakubov SJ, Bope ET: Cardiovascular disease and arrhythmia: Cardiovascular disease. *In* Rakel RE: Textbook of Family Practice. Philadelphia, WB Saunders, 1995, p 810.

11. (True or False) Drugs of choice for the arrhythmia shown in Figure 35–6 include:

    A. Adenosine
    B. Encainide
    C. Verapamil
    D. Amiodarone

Answers: A-T, B-F, C-T, D-F

Critique: Drugs of choice for paroxysmal atrial tachycardia include adenosine and the calcium channel blockers such as verapamil and diltiazem (although verapamil should not be used in tachycardias associated with Wolff-Parkinson-White syndrome). Encainide should be used only in life-threatening ventricular arrhythmias. Similarly, amiodarone is indicated for ventricular arrhythmias.

Further Reading

Drugs for cardiac arrhythmias. Med Lett 33(Issue 846):55–60, 1991.
Yakubov SJ, Bope ET: Cardiovascular disease and arrhythmia: Cardiovascular disease. *In* Rakel RE: Textbook of Family Practice. Philadelphia, WB Saunders, 1995, pp 810–812.

12. (True or False) Appropriate pharmacologic agents for treating the rhythm shown in Figure 35–7 include:

    A. Digitalis
    B. Ca^{2+} channel blockers
    C. β-Blockers
    D. Quinidine

Answers: A-T, B-T, C-T, D-T

Critique: The rhythm strip demonstrates atrial flutter; all of the agents listed can be used to treat this arrhythmia.

Further Reading

Yakubov SJ, Bope ET: Cardiovascular disease and arrhythmia: Cardiovascular disease. *In* Rakel RE: Textbook of Family Practice. Philadelphia, WB Saunders, 1995, p 812.

13. The rhythm strip in Figure 35–8 demonstrates which one of the following rhythm disturbances?

    A. Wandering atrial pacemaker

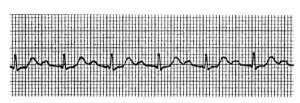

Figure 35–13 (Reproduced with permission from Rakel RE [Ed]: Textbook of Family Practice, 5th ed. Philadelphia, WB Saunders, 1995, p 817.)

    B. Junctional rhythm
    C. Ventricular tachycardia
    D. Second-degree AV block

Answer: B

Critique: The QRS complexes do not demonstrate preceding P waves (retrograde P waves follow the QRS waves), and the rate is consistent with an accelerated junctional rhythm. No P waves precede any of the QRS complexes, indicating that the rhythm does not emanate from the atria; this rules out a wandering atrial pacemaker. The QRS complexes demonstrate normal durations; this rules out a ventricular source for the arrhythmia. The tracing demonstrates no characteristics of second-degree AV block.

Further Reading

Yakubov SJ, Bope ET: Cardiovascular disease and arrhythmia: Cardiovascular disease. *In* Rakel RE: Textbook of Family Practice. Philadelphia, WB Saunders, 1995, pp 813, 814.

14. Figure 35–9 demonstrates which one of the following arrhythmias?

    A. Ventricular tachycardia
    B. Ventricular premature beats
    C. Junctional tachycardia
    D. Atrial premature beats

Answer: B

Critique: The tracing demonstrates ventricular premature beats. The main rhythm is sinus, as demonstrated by the P waves preceding QRS waves in the normal sinus beats. The ventricular premature beats demonstrate a prolonged QRS duration and inverted T waves. These ventricular premature beats are unifocal: they demonstrate identical waveforms.

Further Reading

Yakubov SJ, Bope ET: Cardiovascular disease and arrhythmia: Cardiovascular disease. *In* Rakel RE: Textbook of Family Practice. Philadelphia, WB Saunders, 1995, pp 813–815.

Figure 35–14 (Reproduced with permission from Rakel RE [Ed]: Textbook of Family Practice, 5th ed. Philadelphia, WB Saunders, 1995, p 817.)

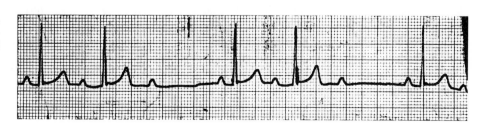

15. Treatment options for the rhythm shown in Figure 35–10 include all of the following EXCEPT:

   A. Intravenous lidocaine
   B. β-Blockers
   C. Electrocardioversion
   D. Verapamil

Answer: D

Critique: The tracing reveals ventricular tachycardia. Appropriate therapeutic interventions include intravenous lidocaine, β-blockers, and electrocardioversion. Verapamil should not be used in this setting, because this agent can cause hypotension and ventricular fibrillation in ventricular tachycardia.

Further Reading

Drugs for cardiac arrhythmias. Med Lett 33(Issue 846):55–60, 1991.
Yakubov SJ, Bope ET: Cardiovascular disease and arrhythmia: Cardiovascular disease. *In* Rakel RE: Textbook of Family Practice. Philadelphia, WB Saunders, 1995, p 815.

16. Of the following options, which agent would be appropriate for treating the rhythm shown in Figure 35–11?

   A. Quinidine
   B. Magnesium sulfate
   C. Procainamide
   D. Disopyramide

Answer: B

Critique: The tracing reveals torsades de pointes. This variant of ventricular tachycardia occurs in association with prolonged QT intervals. Therefore, agents such as the class IA antiarrhythmics that prolong the QT interval are inappropriate in this setting. Of the options, magnesium sulfate would be the agent of choice.

Further Reading

Yakubov SJ, Bope ET: Cardiovascular disease and arrhythmia: Cardiovascular disease. *In* Rakel RE: Textbook of Family Practice. Philadelphia, WB Saunders, 1995, p 815.

17. The tracing shown in Figure 35–12 represents:

   A. Ventricular fibrillation
   B. Atrial fibrillation
   C. Supraventricular tachycardia
   D. Ventricular tachycardia

Answer: A

Critique: The tracing shows coarse ventricular fibrillation. The rhythm appears chaotic with no discrete QRS complexes, P waves, or T waves. The absence of discernible QRS complexes rules out the other three options.

Further Reading

Yakubov SJ, Bope ET: Cardiovascular disease and arrhythmia: Cardiovascular disease. *In* Rakel RE: Textbook of Family Practice. Philadelphia, WB Saunders, 1995, pp 815, 816.

18. The rhythm shown in Figure 35–13 represents:

   A. Sinus bradycardia
   B. Second-degree AV block
   C. First-degree AV block
   D. Junctional rhythm

Answer: C

Critique: The tracing demonstrates first-degree AV block: the PR interval is approximately 0.24. The rate is about 100, which rules out sinus bradycardia. Each QRS complex has an associated preceding P wave, which rules out a junctional rhythm. The tracing reveals only a single P wave associated with each QRS, which is inconsistent with second-degree AV block.

Further Reading

Yakubov SJ, Bope ET: Cardiovascular disease and arrhythmia: Cardiovascular disease. *In* Rakel RE: Textbook of Family Practice. Philadelphia, WB Saunders, 1995, p 817.

19. The tracing shown in Figure 35–14 demonstrates which one of the following rhythm abnormalities?

   A. Third-degree AV block
   B. Mobitz II second-degree AV block
   C. Mobitz I second-degree AV block
   D. Wandering atrial pacemaker

Answer: C

Critique: The tracing reveals a Mobitz I second-degree AV block. The initial PR interval is normal at about 0.18 second; the second PR interval is prolonged at about 0.28 second. The third P wave is not followed by a QRS complex, indicating that the atrial impulse did not propagate through the AV node. This pattern typifies Mobitz I second-degree AV block.

Further Reading

Yakubov SJ, Bope ET: Cardiovascular disease and arrhythmia: Cardiovascular disease. *In* Rakel RE: Textbook of Family Practice. Philadelphia, WB Saunders, 1995, p 817.

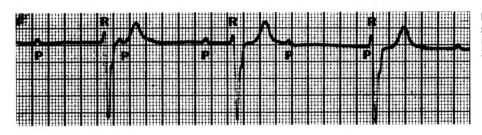

Figure 35–15 (Reproduced with permission from Rakel RE [Ed]: Textbook of Family Practice, 5th ed. Philadelphia, WB Saunders, 1995, p 818.)

20. The tracing shown in Figure 35–15 displays which one of the following arrhythmias?

    A. Sinus bradycardia
    B. Ventricular tachycardia
    C. Second-degree AV block
    D. Third-degree AV block

Answer: D

Critique: The tracing shows third-degree block: the PP interval is constant, with an atrial rate of approximately 60. The RR interval is also constant but with a ventricular rate in the 30s. There appears to be no constant relationship between the P and QRS complexes, which characterizes third-degree block. Option A is incorrect because the tracing does not present a sinus rhythm. The tracing demonstrates bradycardia, which rules out option B. The lack of a consistent relationship between the P and QRS complexes militates against option C.

Further Reading

Yakubov SJ, Bope ET: Cardiovascular disease and arrhythmia: Cardiovascular disease. *In* Rakel RE: Textbook of Family Practice. Philadelphia, WB Saunders, 1995, pp 817, 818.

36

Emergency Medicine

Mary Thoesen Coleman

1. In a patient with cardiopulmonary arrest,

A. The simplest most effective way to maintain a patent airway is through the use of a plastic tongue compressor.

B. With the best external cardiac massage, less than 20% of normal cardiac output can be achieved.

C. Defibrillation is the most important initial treatment for patients with cardiopulmonary arrest secondary to recent or witnessed ventricular fibrillation.

D. The c in the mnemonic ABC stands for color.

E. All of the above

Answer: C

Critique: The American Heart Association's basic cardiac life support/advanced cardiac life support (BCLS/ACLS) system of treatment for cardiopulmonary arrest provides an organized approach. The mnemonic ABC reminds the physician to first assess the airway. The simplest and most effective method is by lifting the jaw of the patient forward. B stands for breathing; if there are no spontaneous breaths, mouth-to-mouth or bag-to-mouth resuscitation is indicated. C reminds the physician to attend to circulation. The best external cardiac compressions achieve only 30% of normal cardiac output. According to ACLS protocols, defibrillation is the most important initial treatment for patients with witnessed or recent ventricular fibrillation.

Page 183

2. Pain may be ineffectively treated in the emergency room because of:

A. Fear of side effects

B. Fear of creating drug dependency

C. Minimal training of physicians

D. Fear of masking an important diagnosis

E. All of the above

Answer: E

Critique: More than 50% of patients in the emergency room present with painful conditions. Studies indicate, however, that pain is treated ineffectively. Reasons include: (1) lack of time devoted to training physicians about effective pain treatment; (2) few studies have addressed treatment of acute pain; (3) fear of masking an important diagnosis; (4) inappropriate fear of side effects due to analgesics; and (5) fear of creating drug dependency.

Page 823

3. Match the method of securing an airway with the injury pattern for which it is indicated:

A. Maxillofacial and cervical spine injuries present

B. Cervical spine injuries likely

C. Midfacial or basilar skull fractures suspected; cervical spine injuries unlikely

1. Blind nasotracheal intubation

2. Orotracheal intubation

3. Cricothyrotomy

Answers: 1-B, 2-C, 3-A

Critique: For the seriously injured patient, a patent airway must be established or maintained while controlling the cervical spine. The method of securing an airway is dependent on the type of injuries. Orotracheal intubation may be used if cervical spine injuries are unlikely or midfacial or basilar skull fractures are suspected. When cervical spine injuries are likely, blind nasotracheal intubation is indicated. Cricothyrotomy is reasonable if maxillofacial and cervical spine injuries are both present.

Pages 824, 825

4. (True or False)

1. Initial sutures of skin wounds should divide a laceration in thirds.

2. Sutures need to be placed every 3 mm to permit approximation without tension.

3. Sutures should be deeper than they are wide to produce eversion of wound edges.

4. Use of a 3-0 suture is indicated for cosmetic repair.

190

5. Silk and cotton sutures are stronger but harder to manipulate than are polypropylene sutures.

Answers: 1-F, 2-F, 3-T, 4-F, 5-F

Critique: Initial sutures should divide a laceration evenly in half and then into quarters. Sutures should enter and exit the wound at equal distances. A distance of 5 mm between sutures usually permits approximation without tension. Sutures that are deeper than they are wide produce eversion of the wound and a better scar. Silk and cotton sutures are not as difficult to manipulate as are synthetic sutures such as polypropylene, which are stronger. For most wound closures, a 4-0 suture is appropriate. Cosmetic closure usually is done with a 6-0 suture. When additional strength is needed, a 3-0 suture may be needed.

Page 833

5. Match the following recommendations for scheduling of suture removal from the list of wound sites:

    A. 3–5 days
    B. 7 days
    C. 10–14 days

1. Face

2. Back

3. Extremity not over the joint

4. Anterior trunk

5. Feet

Answers: 1-A, 2-C, 3-C, 4-B, 5-C

Critique: Suture removal needs to be adjusted according to experience and individual preference. Facial sutures may be removed in 3 to 5 days. At that point, microporous adhesive tape and benzoin tincture may be used for reinforcement. Sutures may be removed from the scalp after 7 to 10 days. Sutures placed over joints or on the feet and back should remain in place for 10 to 14 days. Sutures placed in the anterior trunk and on extremities not near joints may be removed in 7 days.

Page 834

6. Appropriate management of children who have ingested poisons includes which of the following:

    A. 2 oz of syrup of ipecac
    B. Gastric lavage with tap water
    C. 1 g/kg of activated charcoal given as a slurry
    D. All of the above
    E. None of the above

Answer: C

Critique: Gastric decontamination should be undertaken in almost every ingestion of poison. Syrup of ipecac, which induces emesis, is administered in dosages of 5 to 15 ml for small children and 30 to 60 ml for adults. If no vomiting has occurred after 20 to 30 minutes, the dose

may be repeated with 240 ml of water. Vomiting should not be induced if the patient is comatose or stuporous or if the poison ingested is caustic, a low-viscosity hydrocarbon, or a rapid-acting convulsant. Patients seen within 4 to 6 hours of poison ingestion and with incomplete or no vomiting should be lavaged with either tap water or normal saline. Hyponatremia in children may be avoided by the use of normal saline. Activated charcoal in a dose of 1 g/kg may be used to absorb poisons. Usually a slurry flavored or mixed with sorbitol is administered. Sometimes saline cathartics are also given to increase the transit time.

Pages 846, 847

7. (True or False) Answer the following questions regarding iron toxicity:

1. In the United States, 2000 cases of iron toxicity are reported annually in children.

2. Iron toxicity is likely with ingestion of 20 to 30 mg/kg.

3. Charcoal in a dose of 1 g/kg should be given for an overdose of iron.

4. An abdominal flat plate can detect undissolved iron tablets.

5. Deferoxamine should not be used in patients with severe clinical signs of iron ingestion.

Answers: 1-T, 2-T, 3-F, 4-T, 5-F

Critique: Each year about 2000 children in the United States ingest toxic amounts of iron. The most frequent form is that of ferrous sulfate. Toxic levels occur with the ingestion of 20 to 30 mg/kg, with lethal levels occurring at over 60 mg/kg. Gastric lavage with bicarbonate or Fleet Phospho-Soda produces an insoluble carbonate or phosphate iron salt. Use of charcoal is not recommended. An estimate of recent iron ingestion can be made by identifying undissolved tablets on an abdominal flat plate. Deferoxamine increases urinary excretion 100-fold and is indicated in the treatment of iron toxicity with severe clinical signs or history of ingestion of greater than 500 mg.

Pages 850, 851

8. Match the following ingested material to the injuries most likely to be responsible:

    A. Acids
    B. Alkalis
    C. Acids and alkalis

1. Produce coagulation necrosis and eschar formation

2. Result in deep penetration and extensive tissue injury

3. Damage the esophagus more

4. Should not be neutralized

5. Treat with rapid dilution with water, normal saline, or milk

Answers: 1-A, 2-B, 3-B, 4-C, 5-C

Critique: Caustics are either acid or alkali chemicals that injure tissues of the gastrointestinal tract when ingested. Although acids produce coagulation necroses of the gut mucosa, eschar formation usually limits the damage to superficial areas, whereas alkalis produce liquefaction necrosis and tissue saponification leading to deeper, more extensive damage. The stomach is damaged more by acids than by alkalis; the squamous epithelium of the esophagus is relatively resistant to acids and is more readily damaged by alkalis. Treatment of caustic ingestion is the rapid administration of water, normal saline, or milk. Neutralization of either acid or alkali is not recommended because the heat produced by the chemical reaction may be even more damaging to tissues, and gas generated may rupture a viscus.

9.   Tricyclic antidepressants:

   A.   Account for the second highest number of fatal medication ingestions in the United States
   B.   Cause sedation, mood elevation, and peripheral and central anticholinergic actions
   C.   Are metabolized by the kidney
   D.   In overdose should be treated with gastric decontamination and acidification of the blood
   E.   All of the above

Answer: B

Critique: The 1991 report of the American Association of Poison Control Centers found that tricyclic antidepressants accounted for the highest number of fatal medication ingestions in the United States. More than 500,000 overdoses with a 2% mortality were reported. The three pharmacologic activities of tricyclic antidepressants include sedation, elevation of mood, and anticholinergic actions peripherally and centrally. Tricyclics are metabolized by the liver, and most of the circulating drug is bound to protein. The half-life is over 24 hours, at least in part because of lipid solubility and wide volume of distribution of the drugs. Overdoses should be treated with gastric lavage and alkalinization of the blood with sodium bicarbonate.

Pages 855, 856

10. (True or False)

1.   Tetanus is caused by the anaerobic, gram-positive rod *Clostridium tetani.*

2.   Natural immunity to tetanus toxin usually develops after three to five deep wound injuries.

3.   A tetanus booster needs to be given every 5 years for wound management unless a wound is "tetanus-prone," such as a deep puncture, crush injury, or burn that is contaminated with soil or feces, in which case tetanus toxoid should be given no matter when the last dose of tetanus has been given.

4.   Patients who are 7 years of age and older should be immunized with tetanus-diphtheria toxoid to decrease local and systemic reactions and provide enhanced diphtheria protection.

5.   When individuals are not adequately immunized, patients with tetanus-prone wounds should receive 250 to 500 units of human tetanus immune globulin and 0.5 ml of adsorbed toxoid.

Answers: 1-T, 2-F, 3-F, 4-T, 5-T

Critique: Although only approximately 100 cases are reported annually in the United States, a significant reservoir for tetanus remains in the unimmunized (e.g., migrant workers) and the underimmunized (elderly). Tetanus is caused by the anaerobic, gram-positive rod *C. tetani,* the spores of which are ubiquitous in nature and very resistant to destruction. Wounds that are deep, puncture-type, crush, burns, or contaminated with soil or feces are likely to develop tetanus. Because there is no natural immunity to tetanus, appropriate tetanus toxoid injections are necessary. Tetanus toxoids need to be given every 10 years unless a wound is tetanus-prone, in which case a dose should be given if no dose has been administered in the preceding 5 years. Patients who are 7 years of age and older should receive active immunization with tetanus-diphtheria to decrease local and systemic reactions and to enhance diphtheria protection. Tetanus prophylaxis for individuals who are not adequately immunized should include 0.5 ml of adsorbed toxoid for both non–tetanus-prone and tetanus-prone wounds. Tetanus-prone wounds also require 250 to 500 units of human tetanus immune globulin.

11.   Snakebites:

   A.   Occur in approximately 45,000 United States citizens annually
   B.   Are responsible for about 10 to 20 deaths in the United States each year
   C.   Are more likely to be dangerous if snakes have triangle-shaped heads, elliptical pupils, and single rows of subcaudal anal plates
   D.   May cause a metallic taste in the victim's mouth as an early sign of envenomation
   E.   All of the above

Answer: E

Critique: The United States reports 45,000 snakebites each year, with 6000 to 7000 bites from poisonous snakes. About 10 to 20 persons in the United States die each year of snakebites, with 40,000 deaths worldwide. Venomous snakes in the United States consist of two main types: crotalids or pit vipers (e.g., rattlesnakes, cottonmouths, copperheads) and elapids (e.g., coral snakes). Characteristics helpful in identifying venomous snakes from nonvenomous snakes include the following: triangle-shaped heads versus rounded heads, elliptical pupils and fangs versus rounded pupils and no fangs, and single versus a double row of subcaudal anal plates. Snakebite syndromes may be the result of cytolytic and neurotoxic venoms: hemorrhage, hemolysis, drowsiness, hypotension, muscle weakness, trismus, nausea, vomiting, seizures, and cardiorespiratory collapse. A metallic taste may indicate envenomation. Treatment should be immobilization of the bitten part, removal of constrictive rings and other items, application of a venolymphatic tourniquet, and transfer to a site for administration of antivenin.

Pages 868, 869

12. (Matching) Choose one or more answers:

    A. Bee stings
    B. Wasp stings
    C. Fire ant stings
    D. All

1. Lead to evisceration and death of an insect

2. Tetanus prone

3. Venom is 95% alkaloid.

4. Anaphylactic response possible

5. Management includes application of ice.

Answers: 1-A, 2-B, 3-C, 4-D, 5-D

Critique: Anaphylactic reactions from *Hymenoptera* stings kill more Americans than do snakebites. Bee stingers are hooked and remain in the tissue after the sting, leading to death of the insect and spread of the venom. Wasp stings are not hooked, and wasps may sting multiple times. Their stings are prone to tetanus, because wasps feed on excrement. Bites from fire ants are unique in that the venom is 95% alkaloid, which may induce hemolysis, depolarization of cell membranes, activation of the alternate compliment pathway, and general tissue destruction. Bites may be treated with antihistamines, ice, elevation, splinting, and possible antibiotic use. An anaphylactic reaction may require epinephrine, antihistamines, corticosteroids, oxygen, intravenous fluids, and cardiopulmonary resuscitation.

Pages 870, 871

13. Which of the following burns are considered to be major burns, according to the American Burn Association.

    A. Burns involving the hands, face, eyes, ears, feet, or perineum
    B. Second-degree burns covering more than 10% of the body surface area in adults
    C. Any third-degree burns
    D. Superficial sunburns involving more than 95% of the body surface area
    E. All of the above

Answer: A

Critique: The management and triage of a burn patient depend on the extent and gravity of the burn and the age of the patient. The American Burn Association classifies the following as major burns: third-degree burns of greater than 10% of body surface area in adults or children; second-degree burns of greater than 25% of body surface in adults, 20% of body surface in children; burns of the hands, face, eyes, ears, feet, or perineum; and burn patients with inhalation injuries, major trauma, electrical

injuries, or other serious comorbid disease. Most sunburns are first-degree burns and are not considered major burns.

Page 876

14. Management of heat stroke includes:

    A. Administration of oxygen
    B. Application of ice packs to the axilla or groin
    C. Spraying the body with cool water and using fans to facilitate evaporation
    D. Halting cooling procedures when temperatures of 100 to 101° F have been reached
    E. All of the above

Answer: E

Critique: Heat stroke is managed using the techniques of cardiopulmonary resuscitation and rapid cooling. Cooling is most important and can be accomplished by the application of ice packs to the axilla or groin. Cooling blankets may be used; however, spraying the patient with cool water and using fans to blow air over the person to facilitate evaporation is quicker. Oxygen should be administered at 6 to 10 l/min. The body temperature should be monitored, and cooling procedures should be stopped when the temperature reaches 100 to 101° F to avoid hypothermia. Other interventions may be needed, including CVP monitoring, volume expansion, vasopressors, foley catheterization steroids, antibiotics, anticonvulsants, and prophylaxis for gastrointestinal bleeding.

Page 882

15. (True or False)

1. Superficially frostbitten tissue appears white and waxy after thawing.

2. Deep frostbite on thawing may appear either cold and hard or exhibit massive swelling with large hemorrhagic bullae.

3. Attempts to thaw a frostbitten part should always be made as soon as possible, beginning with efforts to rewarm even in a cold environment.

4. Rapid rewarming of a frozen part is best accomplished by use of point sources of heat (e.g., heaters, ovens, and stoves).

5. After thawing, frostbitten parts should be wrapped tightly with a clean, nonabsorbent dressing.

Answers: 1-F, 2-T, 3-F, 4-F, 5-F

Critique: Frostbite injuries that are superficial appear white and waxy until thawed, when the appearance changes to being hyperemic and vesiculated. Deep frostbite also looks white and waxy and is hard until thawed. The appearance is then either cold and hard or massively swollen with large hemorraghic bullae. Eventually, a black eschar forms. Treatment of frostbite should not include rubbing or massage of the affected area because of potential mechanical damage. A frostbitten part should not be rewarmed in a cold environment if there is a chance of refreezing. Rapid rewarming is best accomplished by immersion of the frostbitten part in water at 108 to 112° F for 20 to 30 minutes. Point sources of heat such as heater, ovens, and stoves are not recommended because the rate of heat delivery to the frostbitten part is uneven and unpredictable, and anesthesia in the frostbitten part may predispose to superficial thermal burns. After thawing, the injured part should be wrapped loosely or left open to the air.

Pages 883, 884

37

Sports Medicine

Matthew McHugh

1. Which of the following is the most common symptom associated with exercise-induced asthma?

    A. Wheeze
    B. Cough
    C. Shortness of breath
    D. Chest heaviness
    E. Racing heart

Answer: B

Critique: Cough is the most common symptom associated with exercise-induced asthma. Wheezing, shortness of breath, and chest heaviness are also common. A racing heart is not a frequent complaint in those with exercise-induced asthma.

Pages 900, 901

2. What is the most common reason why young athletes quit sports?

    A. They lack talent.
    B. They are on a losing team.
    C. They are not having fun.
    D. They suffer an injury.

Answer: C

Critique: The most common reason why young athletes quit sports is that they are not having fun.

Pages 898–900

3. (True or False) Athletes tend to be high risk-takers compared with nonathletic peers.

Answer: True

Critique: Studies that compare athletes with nonathletic adolescents show that athletes engage in higher risk activities. Athletes have higher rates of alcohol and drug use, sexual promiscuity, and nonuse of motor vehicle safety equipment such as seatbelts. It is important to discuss these risks during the sports physical examination.

Page 899

4. Acclimatization to heat stress requires an adaptation period of how many weeks?

    A. 0–2
    B. 2–4
    C. 4–6
    D. 6–8
    E. >8

Answer: B

Critique: Acclimatization is an adaptation process that enables the human body to tolerate heat stress. Over 2 to 4 weeks the body becomes more efficient and better able to tolerate heat through cardiovascular, metabolic, and heat loss mechanisms.

Page 911

5. Which of the following is a limited contact/impact sport according to the American Academy of Pediatrics?

    A. Football
    B. Field hockey
    C. Soccer
    D. Lacrosse
    E. Basketball

Answer: E

Critique: The American Academy of Pediatrics Committee on Sports Medicine has classified various sports into groups including contact/collision, limited contact/impact, noncontact/strenuous, noncontact/moderately strenuous, and noncontact/nonstrenuous. Contact sports involve the greatest risk for serious injury. Basketball is considered to have limited contact/impact. Football, field hockey, soccer, and lacrosse all involve high-speed running and the potential for collision and serious injury.

Page 892

6. (True or False) An athlete with only one functioning eye should not participate in any sport with potential to injure that eye.

Answer: False

Critique: An athlete with one impaired organ, including eyes, ears, kidneys, testicles, and ovaries, may participate in sports as long as the part can be protected and the athlete can function. The most significant exceptions include athletes with one kidney, who should not participate in contact/collision sports, and athletes with one eye, who should not box.

Page 895

7. (True or False) The systolic murmur of hypertrophic obstructive cardiomyopathy should decrease with squatting.

Answer: True

Critique: Hypertrophic obstructive cardiomyopathy can cause sudden death, and screening for this condition is part of the preparticipation sports physical examination. The systolic murmur of this condition is decreased with squatting and increased with standing and exercise.

Page 896

8. Which of the following are routinely recommended for children and adolescents during a sports physical examination?

    A. Urinalysis
    B. Blood count
    C. Chest x-ray
    D. Chemistry profiles
    E. None of the above

Answer: E

Critique: There are no routinely recommended screening tests other than the physical for children and adolescent athletes during a sports physical examination. The urinalysis, blood count, chest x-ray, and chemistry profiles may be obtained if indicated.

Page 898

9. (True or False) The extremities are the preferred site of insulin injection in diabetic athletes.

Answer: False

Critique: Diabetic athletes should use the abdomen for the site of injection of insulin. Injecting the limbs can result in an increased rate of insulin absorption and hypoglycemia secondary to vasodilatation.

Pages 901, 902

10. (True or False) To date, there has been no known transmission of human immunodeficiency virus (HIV) in the athletic setting.

Answer: True

Critique: There have been no known transmissions of HIV in the athletic setting. However, universal precautions should be applied in all situations involving exposure to body fluids. Team physicians should educate coaches, trainers, and players on proper and current precautions.

Pages 903, 904

11. Which of the following medicines would be most appropriate in young active athletes with hypertension?

    A. β-Blockers
    B. Calcium channel blockers
    C. Diuretics
    D. Angiotensin-converting enzyme (ACE) inhibitors

Answer: D

Critique: ACE inhibitors and peripheral α-blockers carry few side effects and are recommended as first-line antihypertensive agents in athletes and active individuals. β-Blockers and certain calcium channel blockers blunt the heart rate, and diuretics may lead to hypokalemia and dehydration in active individuals.

Page 903

12. (True or False) All victims of severe hypothermia should be resuscitated until the core temperature is near normal.

Answer: True

Critique: Hypothermia is defined as the lowering of body core temperature below 95° F. With severe hypothermia (core temperature of <90° F), vital organs can remain preserved for prolonged periods of time; therefore, it is recommended that all victims of severe hypothermia be resuscitated until the core temperature is near normal.

Pages 910, 911

13. (True or False) After an athlete suffers a concussion, he or she may return to play even if symptoms persist after an adequate amount of time has elapsed.

Answer: False

Critique: An athlete who has had a concussion should not be allowed to return to that sport until all symptoms have resolved. A player may return to the same game only if it is the athlete's first grade I concussion, and he or she has been asymptomatic for at least 20 minutes. A grade I concussion involves confusion without amnesia or loss of consciousness.

Pages 894, 895

14. (True or False) The three most common causes of sudden death in athletes younger than 30 years of age are hypertrophic obstructive cardiomyopathy, idiopathic left ventricular hypertrophy, and bronchospasm from exercise-induced asthma.

Answer: False

Critique: The three most common causes of sudden death in athletes younger than 30 years of age are hypertrophic cardiomyopathy, idiopathic left ventricular hypertrophy, and coronary artery anomalies. Exercise-induced asthma is common; however, it is not a common cause of sudden death.

Pages 896, 897

15. Which one of the following is the most common injury associated with weight training?

    A. Rotator cuff tendinitis
    B. Inguinal hernia

C. Medial epicondylitis
D. Low back strain
E. Chondromalacia patella

Answer: D

Critique: Low back strain is the most common injury associated with weight training. Adolescent athletes should have proper instruction and supervision. Prepubescent athletes should not perform powerlifting exercises such as deadlifts, squats, powercleans, and the clean-and-jerk.

Page 900

16. (True or False) People with arthritis often benefit from applying heat to their joints prior to exercising.

Answer: True

Critique: Heat applied to arthritic joints prior to exercise decreases joint fluid viscosity and increases joint capsule compliance. Routines should include controlled, low-load, low-impact, high-repetition exercises. There should be a balance of isometric, isotonic, and aerobic exercises.

Page 900

17. Exercise-induced asthma is usually noted more often in which of the following environments?

A. Warm and dry
B. Warm and moist
C. Cool and dry
D. Cool and moist

Answer: C

Critique: Cool and dry environments, such as those found in ice hockey or cross-country skiing, seem to exacerbate exercise-induced bronchospasm. Warm and humid environments, such as found in swimming, are typically better tolerated. Also, short bursts of activity are less likely to cause bronchospasm than are prolonged high-intensity sports.

Pages 900, 901

18. (True or False) In diabetic athletes elevated blood glucose or urinary ketones prior to exercise should lead to postponement of exercise.

Answer: True

Critique: Elevated blood glucose or urinary ketones prior to exercise indicates a higher likelihood of developing hyperglycemia, ketosis, and dehydration during exercise. Blood glucose and ketones should be measured prior to activity and, if the levels are elevated, the athlete should postpone the exercise session. If precautions to prevent hypoglycemia and hyperglycemia are taken, diabetic athletes may participate in high-intensity exercise.

Pages 901, 902

19. (True or False) Preterm labor during a prior pregnancy is a contraindication to exercise during pregnancy.

Answer: True

Critique: The American College of Obstetricians and Gynecologists lists the following contraindications to exercise during pregnancy: pregnancy-induced hypertension, premature rupture of membranes, prior or current history of preterm labor, incompetent cervix or cerclage, persistent second- or third-trimester bleeding, and intrauterine growth retardation. Pregnant women who exercise should perform mild to moderate exercises regularly (at least three times a week).

Pages 902–904

38

Orthopedics

Michael D. Hagen

1. Management of dog bites should include all of the following EXCEPT:

    A. Copious irrigation
    B. Excision of wound edges and loose fat
    C. Subcutaneous sutures
    D. Antibiotic therapy

Answer: C

Critique: Dog bites can lead to significant scarring and risk of infection. These injuries should be treated with débridement, excision of wound edges and loose fat, and antibiotic therapy. Subcutaneous sutures should be avoided.

Further Reading

Orthopedics. *In* Rakel RE: Textbook of Family Practice. Philadelphia, WB Saunders, 1995, p 918.

2. Initial management by family physicians of lacerations sustained in water should include all of the following EXCEPT:

    A. Thorough débridement
    B. Cleansing of the wound
    C. Tetanus prophylaxis
    D. Primary wound closure

Answer: D

Critique: Wounds sustained in surface water should not be closed primarily due to the risk of contamination. These wounds should be débrided and cleansed thoroughly, and appropriate tetanus prophylaxis should be administered.

Further Reading

Orthopedics. *In* Rakel RE: Textbook of Family Practice. Philadelphia, WB Saunders, 1995, p 918.

3. (True or False) In mass casualty situations, appropriate management of wounds includes:

    1. Primary closure of wounds

198

    2. Débridement of damaged muscle and connective tissue
    3. Copious irrigation with antibiotic solutions

Answers: 1-F, 2-T, 3-T

Critique: To avoid gas gangrene in mass casualty situations, wound management should focus on copious irrigation and débridement of nonviable muscle and connective tissue. Wounds should be dressed but not closed primarily.

Further Reading

Orthopedics. *In* Rakel RE: Textbook of Family Practice. Philadelphia, WB Saunders, 1995, pp 918, 919.

4. (True or False) Injuries that are potentially associated with damage to major arteries include which of the following?

    1. Supracondylar humeral fractures
    2. Shoulder dislocations
    3. Deep lacerations about the knee or elbow
    4. Dislocations of the knee

Answers: 1-T, 2-T, 3-T, 4-T

Critique: All of the noted injuries can potentially indicate damage to major neurovascular structures. Injuries in these areas should prompt the physician to confirm the integrity of the arterial blood supply to the potentially affected areas.

Further Reading

Orthopedics. *In* Rakel RE: Textbook of Family Practice. Philadelphia, WB Saunders, 1995, p 920.

5. (True or False) Characteristics of low-velocity (<1000 ft/sec) gunshot wounds include:

    1. Cavitation around the bullet tract
    2. An exit wound much larger than the entrance wound
    3. Minimal damage along the bullet tract

Answers: 1-F, 2-F, 3-T

Critique: Low-velocity bullet injuries produce an exit wound approximately the same size as the entrance wound and demonstrate minimal damage along the projectile's tract. Cavitation is associated with higher-energy gunshot wounds.

Further Reading

Orthopedics. *In* Rakel RE: Textbook of Family Practice. Philadelphia, WB Saunders, 1995, p 920.

6. Gunshot wounds that require open management and débridement include all of the following EXCEPT:

  A. Wounds involving a joint
  B. Wounds that penetrate close to major blood vessels
  C. Low-velocity, low-caliber wounds with entrance and exit sites
  D. Shotgun wounds

Answer: C

Critique: Low-velocity, low-caliber wounds with clear entrance and exit wounds can be managed with local wound care and irrigation. All of the other options require surgical intervention.

Further Reading

Orthopedics. *In* Rakel RE: Textbook of Family Practice. Philadelphia, WB Saunders, 1995, pp 920, 921.

7. (True or False) Techniques that limit the complications associated with crush injuries of the hand include:

  1. Splinting of the metacarpophalangeal joint in full extension
  2. Maintenance of a snugly fitting plaster case irrespective of swelling
  3. Elevation of the hand
  4. Compression dressing applied to the hand

Answers: 1-F, 2-F, 3-T, 4-T

Critique: Crush injuries of the hand can precipitate swelling sufficient to compromise perfusion of the musculature of the hand. To minimize swelling, a compression dressing should be applied and the hand should be elevated. The hand should be immobilized with the metacarpophalangeal joints at approximately 80 degrees, and the interphalangeal joints should be flexed slightly. A plaster cast should be removed in the face of significant swelling; continued casting in such circumstances can lead to intrinsic muscular ischemia and permanent contractures.

Further Reading

Orthopedics. *In* Rakel RE: Textbook of Family Practice. Philadelphia, WB Saunders, 1995, p 921.

8. True statements regarding compartment syndromes include all of the following EXCEPT:

  A. The overlying skin is not usually pallorous.
  B. Passive stretch of the affected area generates extreme pain.

  C. The presence of pulses distal to the area of involvement rules out compartment syndrome.
  D. Intracompartmental pressures higher than 30 mm Hg indicate significant compartment syndrome.

Answer: C

Critique: In compartment syndrome, the overlying skin does not appear pallorous. Passive stretching of the affected musculature induces extreme discomfort. Intracompartmental measurements greater than 30 mm Hg indicate significant compromise. Pulses might remain intact distal to an affected compartment; thus, the presence of pulses does not rule out compartment syndrome.

Further Reading

Orthopedics. *In* Rakel RE: Textbook of Family Practice. Philadelphia, WB Saunders, 1995, pp 923, 924.

9. (True or False) Symptoms and signs associated with anterior compartment syndrome of the leg include:

  1. Weakness of toe flexion and foot inversion
  2. Pain on passive toe flexion and foot plantar flexion
  3. Hypoesthesia in the dorsal first web space
  4. Hypoesthesia of the plantar aspect of the foot

Answers: 1-F, 2-T, 3-T, 4-F

Critique: Anterior compartmental syndrome of the leg produces weakness of toe extension and foot dorsiflexion. Passive toe flexion and foot inversion produce pain. Nerve compression produces hypoesthesia in the dorsal first web space. Plantar hypoesthesia would be expected with posterior compartment syndrome.

Further Reading

Orthopedics. *In* Rakel RE: Textbook of Family Practice. Philadelphia, WB Saunders, 1995, pp 922–924.

10. (True or False) The initial management of gangrene in a warm lower extremity in a diabetic patient should include:

  1. Prompt correction of bony deformities and claw toes
  2. Prompt drainage of infection
  3. Below-the-knee amputation
  4. Protection of the foot with shoe inserts

Answers: 1-T, 2-T, 3-F, 4-T

Critique: Gangrene in a diabetic patient's warm lower extremity should be managed conservatively to preserve maximum function. Bony deformities and claw toes should be corrected promptly, and local infection should also be drained quickly. Below-the-knee amputation should not be performed initially in a warm lower extremity; preserved tissue temperature indicates preservation of at least some tissue perfusion. In this setting, limited ray resections preserve tissue and optimize function. A cold lower extremity indicates major vessel disease; gangrene in this case necessitates below-the-knee amputation.

Further Reading

Orthopedics. *In* Rakel RE: Textbook of Family Practice. Philadelphia, WB Saunders, 1995, pp 924–927.

11. Circumstances that militate toward reimplantation procedures after traumatic amputation include all of the following EXCEPT:

    A. Thumb amputations proximal to the interphalangeal joint
    B. Lower extremity amputations in adults
    C. Proximal upper extremity amputations in children
    D. Loss of multiple digits

Answer: B

Critique: All of the circumstances listed, except lower extremity amputations in adults, are considered reasonable indications for attempting reimplantation procedures.

Further Reading

Orthopedics. *In* Rakel RE: Textbook of Family Practice. Philadelphia, WB Saunders, 1995, p 927.

12. (True or False) Preparation for transport of a severed body part should include:

    1. Packing with a saline-soaked dressing
    2. Maintaining the part at body temperature for transport
    3. Sealing the part in a plastic bag

Answers: 1-T, 2-F, 3-T

Critique: Severed body parts should be prepared for transport by dressing the member with a saline-soaked bandage and packing the part in a plastic bag. The part(s) should be cooled on ice but should not be allowed to freeze.

Further Reading

Orthopedics. *In* Rakel RE: Textbook of Family Practice. Philadelphia, WB Saunders, 1995, p 927.

13. True statements regarding a sprained ankle include all of the following EXCEPT:

    A. The majority of these injuries represent minor anterior talofibular ligament disruptions.
    B. Approximately one quarter of ankle sprains result in recurrent ankle instability.
    C. The patient's degree of pain correlates closely with the severity of the ligamentous injury.
    D. Most ankle sprains result from inversion injuries.

Answer: C

Critique: The amount of pain that the patient experiences does not correlate closely with the severity of the ligamentous injury. Most ankle sprains represent minor injuries to the anterior talofibular ligament; only about one quarter of ankle sprains result in residual joint instability. Most ankle sprains result from inversion injuries.

Further Reading

Orthopedics. *In* Rakel RE: Textbook of Family Practice. Philadelphia, WB Saunders, 1995, p 928.

14. The Ottawa ankle rules provide guidance for determining which patients who have sustained an ankle injury require x-rays. For a patient who has pain in the malleolar area, all of the following findings indicate the need for x-rays of the ankle EXCEPT:

    A. Bony tenderness anywhere along the lower 6 cm of the posterior edge of the fibula
    B. Inability to bear weight immediately or in the emergency department
    C. Bony tenderness over the posterior edge or tip of the medial malleolus
    D. Bony tenderness over the base of the first metatarsal

Answer: D

Critique: The Ottawa ankle rules provide guidance for selecting patients for whom x-rays should be obtained. If the patient has pain in the malleolar zone, x-rays should be obtained if (1) any bony tenderness exists along the posterior lower 6 cm of the fibula or the tip of the lateral malleolus; (2) any bony tenderness occurs along the posterior edge or tip of the medial malleolus; and (3) the patient is unable to bear weight immediately or in the emergency department. Tenderness of the metatarsals is not included in the ankle x-ray indicators but does appear as an indication for foot films.

Further Reading

Orthopedics. *In* Rakel RE: Textbook of Family Practice. Philadelphia, WB Saunders, 1995, p 928.
Stiell IG, McKnight RD, Greenberg GH, et al: Implementation of the Ottawa ankle rules. JAMA 271:827–832, 1994.

15. (True or False) Appropriate management of acute grade I and II ankle sprains should include:

    1. Plaster or fiberglass casting
    2. Application of ice to the injured area
    3. Elevation of the injured limb
    4. Crutches with non–weight-bearing gait

Answers: 1-F, 2-T, 3-T, 4-F

Critique: Grade I and II ankle sprains should be treated with minimal external support (e.g., Ace wrap and tape). Ice should be applied acutely, and the injured limb should be elevated. Partial weight-bearing should be encouraged, because this minimizes disability from the sprain.

Further Reading

Orthopedics. *In* Rakel RE: Textbook of Family Practice. Philadelphia, WB Saunders, 1995, pp 929, 930.

16. The traumatic abnormality depicted in Figure 38–1 should be managed by:

    A. Expectant observation
    B. Splinting the digit with the interphalangeal joints in partial flexion

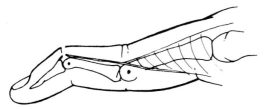

Figure 38–1 (From Connolly JF: DePalma's The Management of Fractures and Dislocations: An Atlas, 3rd ed. Philadelphia, WB Saunders, 1981, p 1148.)

C. Open reduction and internal fixation
D. Splinting of digit with the distal interphalangeal joint fully extended

Answer: D

Critique: The figure reveals a rupture of the extensor tendon with a resultant "mallet finger." Treatment of this injury entails applying a dorsal splint to the injured digit; the splint should allow free motion of the proximal interphalangeal joint and maintenance of the distal interphalangeal joint in full extension. The splint should remain in place for 5 to 6 weeks.

Further Reading

Orthopedics. *In* Rakel RE: Textbook of Family Practice. Philadelphia, WB Saunders, 1995, pp 930, 931.

17. You are called to examine a 15-year-old who fell from his bicycle and landed on his outstretched hand. He has pain on palpation over the radial aspect of the wrist proximal to the first metacarpophalangeal joint. The x-rays of the wrist show no fracture. The most appropriate initial course of treatment should be:

A. Application of an elastic bandage and ice
B. Application of a volar plaster splint
C. Application of a short arm thumb spica cast
D. Application of a sugar tong splint

Answer: C

Critique: The mechanism of injury and physical findings suggest a possible carpal scaphoid fracture. In spite of the normal x-rays, the injury should be treated as a fracture with application of a short arm thumb spica cast. The cast should remain in place for 2 weeks, at which time the cast should be removed and additional x-rays taken. Fractures that did not appear on the initial examination might become evident on the subsequent views. If a fracture does appear, the cast should be reapplied and immobilization should be maintained for 8 to 10 weeks.

Further Reading

Orthopedics. *In* Rakel RE: Textbook of Family Practice. Philadelphia, WB Saunders, 1995, p 932.

18. Clinical findings consistent with carpal tunnel syndrome include all of the following EXCEPT:

A. Paresthesias in the radial three and one-half fingers

B. Night-time pain leading to awakening from sleep
C. Paresthesias in the upper arm
D. Partial relief of symptoms with rest and elevation of the affected hand and wrist

Answer: C

Critique: The paresthesias associated with carpal tunnel syndrome appear in the radial three and one-half fingers and can worsen at night. The symptoms can improve with rest and elevation of the limb. The paresthesias occur distal to the site of compression, rather than in the upper arm.

Further Reading

Katz RT: Carpal tunnel syndrome: A practical review. Am Fam Physician 49:1371–1379, 1994.
Orthopedics. *In* Rakel RE: Textbook of Family Practice. Philadelphia, WB Saunders, 1995, p 933.

19. The mother of a 3-year-old child tells you that, while shopping at the grocery store several hours ago, she had held the child's hand; the child, having seen an item that interested her, attempted to pull away and immediately began crying. The child held her arm in pronation and refused to move the arm. This problem has not occurred previously. An x-ray reveals no bony abnormalities. The most appropriate management for this problem should be:

A. Referral to an orthopedic surgeon for operative repair
B. Gentle but firm supination of the forearm with pressure over the radial head
C. Application of a sugar tong splint to the forearm, with the forearm held in midpronation
D. Full-arm plaster case with the elbow at 90 degrees and the forearm in full pronation

Answer: B

Critique: The scenario represents a fairly typical history for radial head subluxation, or "nursemaid's elbow." The forceful pull on an extended pronated forearm can cause the radial head to slip under the ligamentous investments of the elbow joint, leading to pain and the child's refusal to move the arm. Assuming a normal x-ray, the most appropriate management consists of gentle but firm supination of the forearm with concomitant flexion of the elbow to 90 degrees. The parent should receive instructions not to pull on the child's outstretched arm; immobilization with a sling can also be used for 5 to 7 days.

Further Reading

Orthopedics. *In* Rakel RE: Textbook of Family Practice. Philadelphia, WB Saunders, 1995, p 934.

20. Clinical findings seen in tennis elbow include all of the following EXCEPT:

A. Pain relieved by active wrist extension against resistance
B. Pain radiating down the dorsal forearm

C. Pain worsened by lifting with the elbow in extension
D. Pain radiating toward the shoulder

Answer: A

Critique: The pain associated with tennis elbow can radiate down the dorsal forearm and into the hand. Additionally, the pain can radiate toward the shoulder, and lifting with the elbow in extension can exacerbate the pain. Active wrist extension with the forearm flexed and supinated reproduces, rather than relieves, the pain.

Further Reading

Orthopedics. *In* Rakel RE: Textbook of Family Practice. Philadelphia, WB Saunders, 1995, pp 934, 935.

21. (True or False) Statements regarding supraspinatus tendon tears include:

1. Passive abduction of the shoulder to 30 degrees produces pain.
2. Passive abduction of the shoulder to 90 degrees produces pain.
3. The patient is unable to actively elevate the arm.
4. Magnetic resonance imaging can confirm the diagnosis.

Answers: 1-F, 2-T, 3-T, 4-T

Critique: The supraspinatus tendon constitutes part of the rotator cuff in the shoulder. Tears in this tendon produce pain on passive abduction from about 40 to 100 degrees; passive abduction to 30 degrees would not be expected to produce pain. The patient will be unable to actively elevate the arm or will experience great discomfort doing so. Magnetic resonance imaging can confirm the tendon tear.

Further Reading

Orthopedics. *In* Rakel RE: Textbook of Family Practice. Philadelphia, WB Saunders, 1995, pp 936, 937.

22. (True or False) The initial management for adhesive capsulitis of the shoulder includes which of the following?

1. Referral for surgical adhesiolysis
2. A structured physical therapy program
3. Manipulation of the shoulder under anesthesia
4. A home exercise program utilizing active abduction exercises

Answers: 1-F, 2-T, 3-F, 4-T

Critique: Adhesive capsulitis develops as a result of fibrosis in the shoulder capsule. The initial management should include a structured physical therapy program and home exercises. Manipulation under anesthesia should be reserved for cases that do not improve after 6 weeks of therapy. Surgical intervention becomes necessary very infrequently in this condition.

Further Reading

Orthopedics. *In* Rakel RE: Textbook of Family Practice. Philadelphia, WB Saunders, 1995, pp 937, 938.

Smith DL, Campbell SM: Painful shoulder syndromes: Diagnosis and management. J Gen Intern Med 7:328–329, 1992.
Zuckerman JD, Mirabello SC, Newman D, et al: The painful shoulder. Part II: Intrinsic disorders and impingement syndrome. Am Fam Physician 43:497–512, 1991.

23. Acute anterior glenohumeral dislocations can be reduced with all of the following maneuvers EXCEPT:

A. The Stimson technique
B. The modified Hippocratic maneuver
C. The Kocher maneuver
D. The Hippocratic maneuver

Answer: B

Critique: The Stimson technique and the Kocher and Hippocratic maneuvers are used to reduce anterior glenohumeral dislocations. The modified Hippocratic maneuver is used to treat posterior dislocations.

Further Reading

Orthopedics. *In* Rakel RE: Textbook of Family Practice. Philadelphia, WB Saunders, 1995, pp 938, 939.

24. As the team physician for a local high school football program, you see a 16-year-old young man who sustained a knee injury during a game 1 hour ago. The player relates that he was running to his left and then quickly attempted to change direction to his right. When he planted his left leg and pivoted to his right, he felt a "pop" in his left knee. He has noted swelling in the knee since then and feels as though his knee "gives way." The most likely structure involved in this injury is:

A. The lateral collateral ligament
B. The anterior cruciate ligament
C. The medial collateral ligament
D. The posterior cruciate ligament

Answer: B

Critique: This is a typical history associated with acute anterior cruciate ligament disruption. Ligament injury occurs when the athlete decelerates suddenly and attempts to reverse direction. The injured player frequently reports a "pop" in the joint and that the knee feels unstable. Acute swelling indicates bleeding in the joint. Meniscal tears frequently accompany these injuries.

Further Reading

Orthopedics. *In* Rakel RE: Textbook of Family Practice. Philadelphia, WB Saunders, 1995, pp 939–943.
Roland GC, Beagley MJ: Diagnosing knee injuries: Patient history and physical examination. Fam Pract Recertification 13:35–51, 1991.
Smith BW, Green GA: Acute knee injuries. Part I: History and physical examination. Am Fam Physician 51:615–621, 1995.
Zarins B, Adams M: Knee injuries in sports. N Engl J Med 318:950–960, 1988.

25. Clinical findings associated with patellofemoral pain syndrome include all of the following EXCEPT:

A. Marked swelling
B. Exacerbation of pain on descending stairs
C. Palpable tenderness around the patella

D. Crepitation about the patella on flexion and extension of the knee

Answer: A

Critique: Patellofemoral pain syndrome manifests pain on descending stairs, palpable tenderness around the patella, and crepitation when the knee moves through its range of motion. Swelling, if present at all, is usually only minimal.

Further Reading

Orthopedics. *In* Rakel RE: Textbook of Family Practice. Philadelphia, WB Saunders, 1995, p 943.

26. You are seeing a high-school cross-country runner who has sustained a knee injury. He relates that as he turned a corner while running a cross-country course, he stepped in a shallow hole; his knee was slightly externally rotated. He noted quick swelling in his knee and that the knee seemed to "lock." With the patient supine and his hip and knee flexed, external rotation of the lower leg on the affected side reveals a palpable snap as the knee is flexed and extended. Further examination reveals no drawer sign. The most likely source of this athlete's complaint is:

A. Torn lateral collateral ligament
B. Torn anterior cruciate ligament
C. Torn medial meniscus
D. Torn posterior cruciate ligament

Answer: C

Critique: The history of stepping into a hole with the lower leg externally rotated and associated swelling with a locking sensation suggests meniscal injury. The positive McMurray test with external tibial rotation suggests further that a medial meniscal tear is highly likely. The absence of a drawer sign makes anterior cruciate ligament disruption much less likely. The mechanism of injury militates against posterior cruciate or lateral collateral ligament injuries.

Further Reading

Orthopedics. *In* Rakel RE: Textbook of Family Practice. Philadelphia, WB Saunders, 1995, p 944.
Roland GC, Beagley MJ: Diagnosing knee injuries: Patient history and physical examination. Fam Pract Recertification 13:35–51, 1991.
Smith BW, Green GA: Acute knee injuries. Part I: History and physical examination. Am Fam Physician 51:615–621, 1995.
Zarins B, Adams M: Knee injuries in sports. N Engl J Med 318: 950–960, 1988.

27. The initial management of Osgood-Schlatter disease should include all of the following EXCEPT:

A. Quadriceps strengthening exercises
B. Early referral for surgical correction
C. Hamstring stretching exercises
D. Activity modification

Answer: B

Critique: The initial treatment of Osgood-Schlatter disease includes conservative techniques, such as quadriceps strengthening exercises, hamstring stretching exercises, heel cord stretching exercises, and activity modification. Surgical treatment is needed only rarely.

Further Reading

Orthopedics. *In* Rakel RE: Textbook of Family Practice. Philadelphia, WB Saunders, 1995, pp 944, 945.

28. Which one of the following best describes the third stage of fracture healing?

A. Formation of osteoid matrix around the fracture site
B. Hematoma formation around the fracture site
C. Macrophage and inflammatory cell infiltration into the fracture site
D. Callus remodeling and lamellar bone formation

Answer: D

Critique: Bone healing involves several stages after an acute fracture. The initial response includes inflammatory cell infiltration and hematoma formation. The second stage entails development of an osteoid matrix and callus formation. The final stage involves callus remodeling and lamellar bone formation.

Further Reading

Orthopedics. *In* Rakel RE: Textbook of Family Practice. Philadelphia, WB Saunders, 1995, pp 948, 949.

29. Supracondylar fractures are particularly prone to complications due to injury to all of the following structures EXCEPT:

A. The radial nerve
B. The brachial artery
C. The median nerve
D. The axillary artery

Answer: D

Critique: Supracondylar fractures can compromise nearby neurovascular structures, including the brachial artery and the median and radial nerves. The axillary artery lies proximal to this area.

Further Reading

Orthopedics. *In* Rakel RE: Textbook of Family Practice. Philadelphia, WB Saunders, 1995, pp 949, 950.

30. (True or False) Clinical findings associated with pulmonary fat embolism include which of the following?

1. Mental confusion
2. Petechiae over the chest and in the axillae
3. Arterial $Po_2 > 80$ mm Hg
4. Bradycardia
5. Tachypnea

Answers: 1-T, 2-T, 3-F, 4-F, 5-T

Critique: Fat embolism occurs as a complication of long bone fractures. Clinical findings include mental confusion, petechiae over the upper torso, hypoxemia, tachycardia, tachypnea, and fever. This complication can produce respiratory distress syndrome and death.

Further Reading

Orthopedics. *In* Rakel RE: Textbook of Family Practice. Philadelphia, WB Saunders, 1995, p 950.

31. Under the Gustillo and Anderson classification system, an open fracture with a clean laceration greater than 1 cm in length would be a:

    A. Class I open fracture
    B. Class II open fracture
    C. Class IIIA open fracture
    D. Class IIIB open fracture

Answer: B

Critique: A clean open fracture associated with a laceration greater than 1 cm in length represents a class II open fracture. A class I open fracture involves a clean laceration less than 1 cm in length. A class IIIB open fracture indicates a severe open fracture with loss of tissue overlying the fractured bone. A class IIIA open fracture connotes a crushing injury associated with the open fracture.

Further Reading

Orthopedics. *In* Rakel RE: Textbook of Family Practice. Philadelphia, WB Saunders, 1995, p 950.

32. The acute treatment of open fractures should include all of the following EXCEPT:

    A. Débridement of devitalized tissue
    B. Copious irrigation
    C. Early primary wound closure
    D. Immobilization

Answer: C

Critique: Primary wound closure should not be attempted in the early treatment of open fractures due to the risk of infection. The wound should be débrided and irrigated copiously. The injured body part should be immobilized. Wound closure should not be attempted before 5 to 7 days after the injury.

Further Reading

Orthopedics. *In* Rakel RE: Textbook of Family Practice. Philadelphia, WB Saunders, 1995, p 950.

33. (True or False) True statements regarding "greenstick" forearm fractures include:

    1. Mid-forearm fractures heal well with closed reduction.
    2. "Bayonet" apposition gives satisfactory results.
    3. Angular and rotational deformity do not require correction.

Answers: 1-F, 2-T, 3-F

Critique: Greenstick fractures can be treated with closed reduction and casting, but angular and rotational deformities must be corrected. Bayonet apposition yields satisfactory results. Mid-forearm fractures require open reduction.

Further Reading

Orthopedics. *In* Rakel RE: Textbook of Family Practice Philadelphia, WB Saunders, 1995, p 952.

34. For a patellar fracture, which one of the following clinical findings indicates the probable need for operative intervention?

    A. The patient is able to extend the knee without displacement of the patella.
    B. Pain on flexion of the knee
    C. Pain on extension of the knee
    D. Displacement of the patella with knee flexion

Answer: D

Critique: Displacement of the patella with flexion or inability to extend the knee suggests the need for operative repair. Pain without displacement on flexion or extension indicates that the fracture can be managed with symptomatic therapy and splinting.

Further Reading

Orthopedics. *In* Rakel RE: Textbook of Family Practice Philadelphia, WB Saunders, 1995, p 952.

35. (True or False) True statements regarding management of radial head fractures include:

    1. These fractures should undergo early open reduction and internal fixation.
    2. Aspiration of the associated hemarthrosis relieves greatly the pain associated with the fracture.
    3. The fracture should be immobilized for 4 to 6 weeks.
    4. Limited elbow flexion represents the main motion limitation associated with this fracture.

Answers: 1-F, 2-T, 3-F, 4-F

Critique: Treatment of radial head fractures should stress the return to joint motion rather than anatomic reduction. Aspiration of the associated hemarthrosis relieves greatly the pain associated with the fracture. The elbow should not be immobilized for more than 2 to 3 days. The most common motion limitation is elbow extension. If significant flexion limitation exists, the radial head can be removed surgically.

Further Reading

Orthopedics. *In* Rakel RE: Textbook of Family Practice. Philadelphia, WB Saunders, 1995, p 968.

36. Management of fractures of the surgical neck of the humerus should include all of the following EXCEPT:

    A. Immobilization with a Velpeau dressing for 3 weeks

B. Symptomatic treatment for pain control
C. Range-of-motion exercises, beginning with circumduction, after completion of the immobilization period
D. Emphasis on the return of shoulder function rather than on radiographic evidence of fracture healing

Answer: A

Critique: Prolonged immobilization of a humeral surgical neck fracture promotes atrophy of the supraspinatus muscle and long-term shoulder disability. As soon as the patient's pain allows, range-of-motion exercises should begin. The approach to treatment should emphasize early mobilization of the shoulder rather than radiographic evidence of healing.

Further Reading

Orthopedics. *In* Rakel RE: Textbook of Family Practice. Philadelphia, WB Saunders, 1995, p 969.

37. Intra-articular corticosteroid injections in weight-bearing major joints should be limited to what frequency?

A. No more than once annually
B. No more than twice annually
C. No more than three times annually
D. No more than four times annually

Answer: C

Critique: Intra-articular corticosteroids can provide benefit in the management of osteoarthritis. However, these injections should be limited to no more than three per year to avoid damage to cartilage.

Further Reading

Orthopedics. *In* Rakel RE: *Textbook of Family Practice.* Philadelphia, WB Saunders, 1995, pp 970, 971.
Pfenninger JL: Injections of joints and soft tissue. Part I: General guidelines. Am Fam Physician 44:1196–1202, 1991.

38. (True or False) Patients who are considered to be good candidates for total hip replacement include which of the following?

1. Patients older than 60 years of age
2. Patients who intend to remain vigorously active (e.g., engage in jogging or tennis)
3. Patients who maintain a body weight over 90 kg
4. Patients who have failed therapeutic trials with nonsteroidal anti-inflammatory agents

Answers: 1-T, 2-F, 3-F, 4-T

Critique: Total hip replacement can improve symptoms in patients whose hip disease has not responded to more conservative measures. However, hip replacement does not create a normal hip. Patients who intend to maintain vigorous repetitive impact activities represent a substantial risk for early loosening of the appliance. Additionally, patients who maintain excess body weight risk premature prosthetic hip failure. Patients older than 60 years of age represent good candidates because of lower life expec-

tancy and reduced activity demands on the new joint. Patients should have attempted conservative measures, such as nonsteroidal anti-inflammatory drugs, weight reduction, activity modification, and the use of a cane before considering an artificial hip. Patients who have failed such interventions represent good candidates for hip replacement.

Further Reading

Harris WH, Sledge CB: Total hip and knee replacement (first of two parts). N Engl J Med 323:725–731, 1990.
Orthopedics. *In* Rakel RE: Textbook of Family Practice. Philadelphia, WB Saunders, 1995, p 972.

39. A patient who presents with morning stiffness, pain on motion in a wrist, and symmetrical swelling of the proximal interphalangeal joints meets criteria for what American Rheumatism Association (ARA) category for rheumatoid arthritis?

A. Doesn't meet criteria for rheumatoid arthritis
B. Meets criteria for probable rheumatoid arthritis
C. Meets criteria for definite rheumatoid arthritis
D. Meets criteria for classic rheumatoid arthritis

Answer: B

Critique: The scenario provides three of the 11 ARA criteria for rheumatoid arthritis. This qualifies for "probable" rheumatoid arthritis according to these criteria. The reader should note that the American College of Rheumatology has developed revised criteria based on the following characteristics: (1) morning stiffness, (2) arthritis in three or more joint areas, (3) arthritis of the hand joints, (4) symmetrical arthritis, (5) rheumatoid nodules, (6) the presence of rheumatoid factor, and (7) radiologic changes. If at least four of the criteria are present, rheumatoid arthritis can be diagnosed. Clinical characteristics 1 to 4 must have been present for at least 6 weeks to satisfy the criteria. Arnett has also published a proposed algorithm for implementing these criteria.

Further Reading

Arnett FC: Revised criteria for the classification of rheumatoid arthritis. Bull Rheum Dis 38(5):1–6, 1989.
Orthopedics. *In* Rakel RE: Textbook of Family Practice. Philadelphia, WB Saunders, 1995, p 973.
Smith CA, Arnett FC: Diagnosing rheumatoid arthritis: Current criteria. Am Fam Physician 44:863–870, 1991.

40. According to the ARA functional classification system, a patient whose activity is limited to few or none of the duties of usual occupation or self-care represents what functional class?

A. Class I
B. Class II
C. Class III
D. Class IV

Answer: C

Critique: A patient whose activities are limited to few or none of those associated with his or her usual occupation or self-care manifests class III function in the ARA functional classification system.

Further Reading

Orthopedics. *In* Rakel RE: Textbook of Family Practice. Philadelphia, WB Saunders, 1995, p 973.

41. According to the ARA staging criteria, a patient who demonstrates x-ray evidence of osteoporosis and limited joint mobility without joint deformity harbors what stage of rheumatoid arthritis?

    A. Stage I
    B. Stage II
    C. Stage III
    D. Stage IV

Answer: B

Critique: A patient who has rheumatoid arthritis, characterized by x-ray evidence of osteoporosis and limited joint mobility without joint deformity, has stage II disease by ARA criteria.

Further Reading

Orthopedics. *In* Rakel RE: Textbook of Family Practice. Philadelphia, WB Saunders, 1995, pp 973–975.

42. For a patient with early stage II rheumatoid arthritis, the initial management should include all of the following modalities EXCEPT:

    A. Physical therapy
    B. Salicylate therapy
    C. Occupational therapy
    D. Azathioprine therapy

Answer: D

Critique: Early stage II disease should be managed initially with patient education about the course of rheumatoid arthritis, physical therapy, occupational therapy, salicylates or other nonsteroidal anti-inflammatory agents, and appropriate modifications of activity and exercise. Although some authors now recommend disease-remitting agents such as gold, penicillamine, or methotrexate fairly early in the disease course, initial management would not include these agents. If the initial treatment has yielded little or no benefit in 1 month or so, some authors would recommend adding disease-remitting drugs. At least one randomized trial has shown azathioprine to be inferior to methotrexate.

Further Reading

Harris ED: Rheumatoid arthritis: Pathophysiology and implications for therapy. N Engl J Med 322:1277–1289, 1990.
Jeurissen MEC, Boerbooms AMTh, P LBA, et al: Influence of methotrexate and azathioprine on radiologic progression in rheumatoid arthritis: A randomized, double-blind study. Ann Intern Med 114:999–1004, 1991.
Orthopedics. *In* Rakel RE: Textbook of Family Practice. Philadelphia, WB Saunders, 1995, p 974.

43. Clinical manifestations that support adding second-line disease-remitting drugs to the regimen for a patient with rheumatoid arthritis include all of the following EXCEPT:

    A. Hypersensitivity reactions to nonsteroidal anti-inflammatory drugs
    B. The presence of rheumatoid nodules
    C. A negative rheumatoid factor titer
    D. Periarticular osteopenia on x-ray

Answer: C

Critique: Several clinical characteristics provide guidance regarding the selection of second-line agents. Patients who have demonstrated hypersensitivity to or poor tolerance of nonsteroidal anti-inflammatory drugs should be considered candidates. The presence of periarticular osteopenia and rheumatoid nodules might indicate a tendency toward rapid progression of the disease. A high titer, rather than absent, rheumatoid factor level suggests that the disease might behave aggressively.

Further Reading

Borenstein DG, Silver G, Jenkins E: Approach to initial medical treatment of rheumatoid arthritis. Arch Fam Med 2:545–551, 1993.

44. (True or False) Appropriate initial management of an acute, monoarticular arthritis should include which of the following?

    1. Arthrocentesis with microscopic examination of joint fluid
    2. Blood cultures
    3. Synovial fluid cultures
    4. Initiate intravenous penicillin G while awaiting the results of a culture

Answers: 1-T, 2-T, 3-T, 4-F

Critique: Acute monoarticular arthritis should suggest an infectious etiology; other possible causes include crystal-induced arthritis, trauma, inflamed osteoarthritis, tumor, and other miscellaneous disorders such as the rheumatoid diseases. Blood cultures should be obtained, and joint fluid should be cultured and examined microscopically. If the clinical setting suggests an infectious etiology, intravenous antibiotic therapy should be initiated. However, due to penicillin resistance among *Staphylococcus aureus* and *Neisseria* species, initial therapy should consist of a cephalosporin such as cefotaxime. Further therapy should be guided by culture-demonstrated antibiotic sensitivity results.

Further Reading

Baker DG, Schumacher HR: Acute monoarthritis. N Engl J Med 329:1013–1020, 1993.
Orthopedics. *In* Rakel RE: Textbook of Family Practice. Philadelphia, WB Saunders, 1995, pp 975, 976.

45. (True or False) Of the following joint infections, which circumstances require surgical drainage of the affected joint?

    1. Gonococcal arthritis of the knee in an adult

2. Septic arthritis of the hip in a young child
3. Bacterial arthritis in a wrist affected by rheumatoid arthritis
4. Bacterial arthritis of the ankle in an otherwise healthy adult

Answers: 1-F, 2-T, 3-T, 4-F

Critique: Monoarticular septic arthritis can be treated initially with antibiotic therapy in patients in whom gonococcal infection is suspected and whose joints are otherwise normal. Septic hip arthritis in a young child represents substantial risk for future hip deformity, and open drainage should be accomplished. Additionally, joints that demonstrate anatomic abnormalities due to other processes such as rheumatoid arthritis should undergo drainage because of poor antibiotic penetration.

Further Reading

Orthopedics. *In* Rakel RE: Textbook of Family Practice. Philadelphia, WB Saunders, 1995, pp 976, 977.

46. Match the associated clinical finding(s) with the appropriate low back pain syndrome.

    A. Lumbago
    B. Sciatica
    C. Both A and B
    D. Neither A nor B

1. Result from dural stretching caused by vertebral disk herniation

2. Characterized by radicular pain, usually in L5 and S1 dermatome distributions

3. Characterized by central vertebral disk herniation

4. Pain can occur anywhere from the waist down.

Answers: 1-C, 2-B, 3-A, 4-A

Critique: Sciatica results from peripheral extrusion of herniated vertebral disk, with resultant pressure on nerve roots. This causes a radicular quality pain, usually in the L5 or S1 nerve distributions. Lumbago results from central herniation and can produce pain anywhere from the waist down. Vertebral disk herniation and lumbago should be considered in the differential diagnosis of abdominal pain as well as back and leg pain.

Further Reading

Orthopedics. *In* Rakel RE: Textbook of Family Practice. Philadelphia, WB Saunders, 1995, pp 977, 978.

47. (True or False) True statements regarding the straight leg raising test in evaluation of low back pain include which of the following?

    1. The test result is considered to be positive if radicular pain occurs with a 60-degree (or less) elevation of the leg.
    2. The test performs with high sensitivity (>80%) for a herniated vertebral disk.

    3. The test performs with high specificity (>80%) for a herniated vertebral disk.
    4. The crossed-leg straight leg raising test performs with similar sensitivity and specificity.

Answers: 1-T, 2-T, 3-F, 4-F

Critique: The straight leg raising test is performed by lifting the extended lower leg and noting the elevation at which radicular symptoms occur. The test performs with approximately 95% sensitivity but has very poor specificity (between 10 and 20%). The crossed-leg straight leg raising test performs with much lower sensitivity, but higher specificity, than that observed with the straight leg raising test.

Further Reading

Deyo RA, Loeser JD, Bigos SJ: Herniated lumbar intervertebral disk. Ann Intern Med 112:598–603, 1990.
Orthopedics. *In* Rakel RE: Textbook of Family Practice. Philadelphia, WB Saunders, 1995, p 981.

48. Match the clinical symptoms with the appropriate syndrome.

    A. Spinal claudication
    B. Vascular claudication
    C. Both A and B
    D. Neither A nor B

1. Pain in the back or legs

2. Relieved by rest in any position

3. Relieved only in supine position

Answers: 1-C, 2-B, 3-A

Critique: "Spinal claudication" occurs as a result of spinal canal narrowing in association with disk disease. Patients will experience pain with any movement that stretches the dura in the narrowed canal. This pain is relieved only by assuming the supine position. Pain associated with vascular claudication occurs as a result of exercise-induced ischemia and resolves with rest of the affected limb in any position.

Further Reading

Orthopedics. *In* Rakel RE: Textbook of Family Practice. Philadelphia, WB Saunders, 1995, p 979.

49. Weakness of the great toe extensor indicates nerve dysfunction at what nerve level?

    A. L2–L3
    B. L3–L4
    C. L4–L5
    D. L5–S1

Answer: C

Critique: Weakness of the great toe extensor indicates an ipsilateral L4–L5 nerve lesion.

Further Reading

Deyo RA, Loeser JD, Bigos SJ: Herniated lumbar intervertebral disk. Ann Intern Med 112:598–603, 1990.
Orthopedics. *In* Rakel RE: Textbook of Family Practice. Philadelphia, WB Saunders, 1995, pp 980, 981.

50. Weakness of toe walking and plantar flexion indicate a lesion in which nerve root?

- A. L2
- B. L3
- C. L4
- D. L5
- E. S1

Answer: E

Critique: Weakness of plantar flexion and toe walking indicate an S1 lesion. This motor deficit can accompany sensory changes on the posterior calf and lateral foot.

Further Reading

Deyo RA, Loeser JD, Bigos SJ: Herniated lumbar intervertebral disk. Ann Intern Med 112:598–603, 1990.
Orthopedics. *In* Rakel RE: Textbook of Family Practice. Philadelphia, WB Saunders, 1995, pp 980, 981.

51. (True or False) Appropriate indications for computerized tomographic (CT) scanning in the evaluation of low back pain include:

1. To rule out disk herniation during the initial evaluation
2. For further evaluation of a patient who has not responded to initial treatment
3. To evaluate suspected metastatic involvement of the vertebra
4. To identify suspected congenital anomalies

Answers: 1-F, 2-T, 3-T, 4-T

Critique: CT scanning should not be performed as part of the initial evaluation of low back pain, unless the initial history and physical examination suggest conditions that would not be expected to improve with conservative management (e.g., metastatic disease, extradural infections, and congenital anomalies). The initial evaluation and management should rely on the history and physical examination; if conservative treatment produces inadequate results, then evaluation with CT scanning should be considered.

Further Reading

Orthopedics. *In* Rakel RE: Textbook of Family Practice. Philadelphia, WB Saunders, 1995, pp 981, 982.

52. The initial management of a patient with back pain and no signs of cauda equina syndrome (loss of sphincter control, bilateral weakness and numbness) should include all of the following EXCEPT:

- A. Systemic analgesics and anti-inflammatory medications
- B. 7–10 days of bed rest

- C. Education regarding proper lifting and posture
- D. Instruction in exercises for low back pain

Answer: B

Critique: The management of low back pain has evolved away from traditional emphasis on bed rest. Bed rest should be limited to no more than 2 or 3 days because of deconditioning associated with prolonged rest. Analgesics and anti-inflammatory agents can provide symptomatic relief during the initial painful period. The patient should receive instruction in proper lifting techniques and posture in order to prevent recurrences. The patient should also receive instruction in appropriate back exercises as a means of preventing recurrences. The clinician might want to involve a physical therapist in this aspect of the patient's care. One study has demonstrated that continuing normal daily activities yields results that are just as good as, or better than those obtained with bed rest and exercises.

Further Reading

Deyo RA, Loeser JD, Bigos SJ: Herniated lumbar intervertebral disk. Ann Intern Med 112:598–603, 1990.
Malmivaara A, Häkkinen U, Aro T, et al: The treatment of acute low back pain—bed rest, exercises, or ordinary activity? N Engl J Med 332:351–355, 1995.
Orthopedics. *In* Rakel RE: Textbook of Family Practice. Philadelphia, WB Saunders, 1995, pp 982–984.

53. Indications for laminectomy include all of the following EXCEPT:

- A. Severe, unremitting back pain
- B. Severe, unremitting leg pain
- C. Loss of bowel or bladder control
- D. Moderate foot weakness after 2 weeks of conservative therapy

Answer: D

Critique: Recognized indications for surgical intervention include unremitting back or leg pain and bowel or bladder incontinence. Conservative therapy should be continued for 4 to 6 weeks before considering laminectomy for a nonprogressive motor deficit.

Further Reading

Deyo RA, Loeser JD, Bigos SJ: Herniated lumbar intervertebral disk. Ann Intern Med 112:598–603, 1990.
Orthopedics. *In* Rakel RE: Textbook of Family Practice. Philadelphia, WB Saunders, 1995, pp 984, 985.

54. A 64-year-old white woman presents with pain in her mid-upper back. She relates that this pain began suddenly while she was carrying groceries from her car. Conditions that should be included in the differential diagnosis of this condition include all of the following EXCEPT:

- A. Metastatic cancer (e.g., breast, kidney, gastrointestinal)
- B. Mutliple myeloma
- C. Osteoporotic compression fracture
- D. Myxedema

Answer: D

Critique: The patient presents a history and symptoms consistent with a vertebral compression fracture. The differential diagnosis should include metastases, myeloma, osteoporosis associated with Graves' disease (rather than hypothyroidism), and Cushing's disease syndrome.

Further Reading

Orthopedics. *In* Rakel RE: Textbook of Family Practice. Philadelphia, WB Saunders, 1995, pp 986–988.

55. Which one of the following laboratory findings is normally found in osteoporosis?

    A. Elevated alkaline phosphatase level
    B. Low serum calcium level
    C. Normal parathyroid hormone level
    D. Low serum phosphate level

Answer: C

Critique: The alkaline phosphatase, calcium, and parathyroid hormone levels should be normal in osteoporosis. The serum phosphate level should be in the normal range.

Further Reading

Orthopedics. *In* Rakel RE: Textbook of Family Practice. Philadelphia, WB Saunders, 1995, p 987.

56. Therapeutic modalities that should be incorporated in the treatment of back pain associated with osteoporotic vertebral fractures include all of the following EXCEPT:

    A. Prolonged bed rest to promote compression fracture healing
    B. Discontinuation of smoking
    C. Regular exercise against gravity once the acute pain has resolved
    D. Estrogen replacement (in postmenopausal women) and calcium supplementation

Answer: A

Critique: The patient with a vertebral compression fracture should minimize immobilization and resume activity as soon as the pain allows. The patient should also be encouraged to discontinue smoking and modify alcohol intake. Regular weight-bearing exercise can prevent further bone loss. Calcium supplementation (1500 mg/day in postmenopausal women) should be undertaken, and the postmenopausal woman should consider estrogen-replacement therapy.

Further Reading

Aloia JF, Vaswani A, Yeh JK, et al: Calcium supplementation with and without hormone replacement therapy to prevent postmenopausal bone loss. Ann Intern Med 120:97–103, 1994.
Cauley JA, Seeley DG, Ensrud K, et al: Estrogen replacement therapy and fractures in older women. Ann Intern Med 122:9–16, 1995.
Consensus Development Conference: Diagnosis, prophylaxis, and treatment of osteoporosis. Am J Med 94:646–650, 1993.
Orthopedics. *In* Rakel RE: Textbook of Family Practice. Philadelphia, WB Saunders, 1995, pp 988, 989.

Riggs BL, Melton LJ: The prevention and treatment of osteoporosis. N Engl J Med 327: 620–627, 1990.

57. Neck pain with numbness in the thumb and index finger suggest a nerve root lesion at what level?

    A. C2
    B. C3
    C. C4
    D. C5
    E. C6

Answer: E

Critique: Numbness over the thumb and index finger suggests a lesion at C6.

Further Reading

Orthopedics. *In* Rakel RE: Textbook of Family Practice. Philadelphia, WB Saunders, 1995, p 991.

58. (True or False) Clinical findings which suggest congenital hip dislocation include:

    1. A palpable "clunk" on flexion and abduction of the hip
    2. Asymmetrical hip abduction
    3. Hip stiffness

Answers: 1-T, 2-T, 3-T

Critique: Stiffness is an abnormal finding in a newborn or an infant. A palpable "clunk" on flexion and abduction of the hip suggests an unstable hip. Additionally, both hips should demonstrate symmetrical abduction, and unilateral limitation of abduction to less than 50 degrees is considered diagnostic for dislocation on the affected side.

Further Reading

Churgay CA, Caruthers BS: Diagnosis and treatment of congenital dislocation of the hip. Am Fam Physician 45:1217–1228, 1992.
Orthopedics. *In* Rakel RE: Textbook of Family Practice. Philadelphia, WB Saunders, 1995, p 993.

59. (True or False) A 5-year-old boy presents with a 2-month history of limping and pain in the left knee. An evaluation of this patient's symptoms should include:

    1. Examination of the knee
    2. Reassurance that this probably represents a "growing pain
    3. Examination of the left hip, including internal and external rotation, and abduction and adduction
    4. Frog-leg anteroposterior radiographs if the hip examination is abnormal

Answers: 1-T, 2-F, 3-T, 4-T

Critique: Knee pain and a limp in a child in this age group should suggest Legg-Calvé-Perthes disease. The knee should be examined to rule out problems with that joint, but the examiner should also evaluate the ipsilateral hip. The examination should include internal and external hip rotation and the range of adduction and abduction. If the clinical examination suggests hip dysfunction, anteroposterior frog leg radiographs should be obtained.

Further Reading

Orthopedics. *In* Rakel RE: Textbook of Family Practice. Philadelphia, WB Saunders, 1995, p 996.

60. (True or False) A 15-year-old boy presents for an evaluation of pain in the right knee. The pain apparently began after he jumped off a trampoline. He has no fever or other symptoms. You note that his growth chart indicates that he is overweight for his age and height. You ask him to lie on the examination table; he assumes the position in Figure 38–2. Diagnostic considerations for this patient should include:

1. Femoral neck fracture
2. Slipped capital femoral epiphysis
3. Legg-Calvé-Perthes disease
4. Septic arthritis

Answers: 1-T, 2-T, 3-F, 4-F

Critique: The history is typical for a slipped capital femoral epiphysis, although these patients can also present without a history of recent trauma. Femoral neck fracture should also be considered due to the hip and leg posture shown in Figure 38–2. The patient is older than the usual patient with Legg-Calvé-Perthes disease; additionally, the marked external rotation that the patient demonstrates would be unlikely with Legg-Calvé-Perthes disease. The lack of other symptoms or signs militates against monoarticular septic arthritis.

Further Reading

Orthopedics. *In* Rakel RE: Textbook of Family Practice. Philadelphia, WB Saunders, 1995, pp 997, 998.

61. Causes of in-toeing include all of the following EXCEPT:

A. Tibial torsion
B. Femoral anteversion
C. Metatarsus adductus
D. Femoral retroversion

Answer: D

Critique: Several musculoskeletal conditions can present as in-toeing. Tibial torsion, femoral anteversion, and metatarsus adductus all represent potential causes of this abnormality. Femoral retroversion causes abduction of the feet rather than in-toeing.

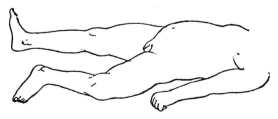

Figure 38–2 (Reproduced with permission from Rakel RE [Ed]: Textbook of Family Practice, 5th ed. Philadelphia, WB Saunders, 1995, p 997.)

Further Reading

Dietz FR: Intoeing-fact: Fiction and opinion. Am Fam Physician 50:1249–1259, 1994.
Orthopedics. *In* Rakel RE: Textbook of Family Practice. Philadelphia, WB Saunders, 1995, pp 998–1000.

62. (True or False) True statements regarding metatarsus adductus include which of the following?

1. Of these children, 80% will require serial casting to correct the deformity.
2. Flexibility (as demonstrated by spontaneous straightening upon stroking the lateral foot) indicates the high likelihood of spontaneous resolution.
3. Spontaneous resolution cannot be expected before 5 to 6 years of age.
4. The parents should be advised to put a right shoe on the left foot and vice versa to correct the deformity.

Answers: 1-F, 2-T, 3-F, 4-F

Critique: Metatarsus adductus represents one of the causes of in-toeing, or "pigeon toes." Most of these cases will resolve spontaneously by 2 to 3 years of age. The foot should be examined for flexibility, as demonstrated by correction of the deformity as a response to stroking the lateral border of the foot. This action stimulates the peroneal musculature; ability to correct the deformity via this maneuver indicates a high likelihood of spontaneous resolution. The parents should not switch shoes from right to left or vice versa, because this can affect the foot's longitudinal arch. The parents can be instructed to perform stretching exercises, although the effectiveness of this maneuver has not been established.

Further Reading

Dietz FR: Intoeing: Fact, fiction and opinion. Am Fam Physician 50:1249–1259, 1994.
Orthopedics. *In* Rakel RE: Textbook of Family Practice. Philadelphia, WB Saunders, 1995, pp 998–1000.

63. Clinical findings consistent with tibial torsion include all of the following EXCEPT:

A. Intoeing
B. Inward foot progression angle
C. Forward-pointing patellas
D. Medial malleoli 20 degrees anterior to the lateral malleoli

Answer: D

Critique: Tibial torsion presents with in-toeing, an inward foot progression angle, and forward-pointing patellas. The medial malleolar position of 20 degrees anterior to the lateral malleoli represents the normal angle in adults. Tibial torsion creates an angle much less than this; indeed, the lateral malleoli might lay anterior to the medial malleoli in this condition.

Further Reading

Dietz FR: Intoeing: Fact, fiction and opinion. Am Fam Physician 50:1249–1259, 1994.

Orthopedics. *In* Rakel RE: Textbook of Family Practice. Philadelphia, WB Saunders, 1995, pp 998–1000.

64. (True or False) True statements regarding femoral anteversion include which of the following?

1. Femoral anteversion represents the most common cause of in-toeing.
2. The femoral neck axis lies 15 to 125 degrees posterior to the axis of the femoral condyles.
3. The hips exhibit increased internal rotation with the patient supine and the hips flexed.
4. Radiographic imaging is necessary to make the diagnosis.

Answers: 1-T, 2-F, 3-T, 4-F

Critique: Femoral anteversion is the most common cause for in-toeing or pigeon toes. In this condition, the femoral neck axis is anteverted with respect to the axis of the femoral condyles. The hips will exhibit expanded internal rotation ability, with restriction of external rotation. The diagnosis is made clinically; radiographic imaging is not necessary in this condition.

Further Reading

Dietz FR: Intoeing: Fact, fiction and opinion. Am Fam Physician 50:1249–1259, 1994.
Orthopedics. *In* Rakel RE: Textbook of Family Practice. Philadelphia, WB Saunders, 1995, pp 998–1000.

65. Which one of the following statements about femoral anteversion is correct?

A. Femoral anteversion will increase with age.
B. Radiographic anteversion correlates closely with the clinical examination.
C. Twisting cables and shoe wedges represent effective treatment for femoral anteversion.
D. Femoral anteversion averages 16 to 24 degrees in normal adolescents aged 14 to 16 years.

Answer: D

Critique: Femoral anteversion is almost 40 degrees in infants and declines by 1 or 2 degrees per year until early adolescence. Radiographic anteversion correlates poorly with the clinical presentation and course. Twisting cables and shoe wedges have not been shown to alter femoral anteversion significantly. By ages 14 to 16, the normal hip demonstrates 16 to 24 degrees of femoral anteversion.

Further Reading

Dietz FR: Intoeing: Fact, fiction and opinion. Am Fam Physician 50:1249–1259, 1994.
Orthopedics. *In* Rakel RE: Textbook of Family Practice. Philadelphia, WB Saunders, 1995, pp 998–1000.

66. True statements regarding rigid flat feet include all of the following EXCEPT:

A. Rigid flat feet represent the majority of cases of flat feet.
B. Rigid flat feet require orthopedic correction.
C. Rigid flat feet remain flat, with or without weight-bearing.

D. Accessory navicular bones and congenital vertical talus represent common causes of rigid flat feet.

Answer: A

Critique: Flexible flat feet represent the majority of flat feet. Rigid flat feet can be caused by congenital bone abnormalities, such as accessory navicular bones, vertical talus, talonavicular dislocation, and congenital bone coalitions. The rigid flat foot remains flat with or without weight-bearing. These abnormalities require surgical correction.

Further Reading

Orthopedics. *In* Rakel RE: Textbook of Family Practice. Philadelphia, WB Saunders, 1995, pp 1000, 1001.

67. (True or False) True statements regarding flexible flat feet include which of the following?

1. The flat foot results from varus positioning of the calcaneus.
2. Flexible flat feet should be treated with corrective shoes.
3. Most infants demonstrate flat feet when they first begin to walk.
4. The medial border of the foot demonstrates a convex configuration.

Answers: 1-F, 2-F, 3-T, 4-T

Critique: Flexible flat feet result from valgus positioning of the calcaneus with subsequent loss of support for the talus. Most flexible flat feet require no corrective treatment. Most infants demonstrate some degree of flat feet when they begin walking. The flat foot demonstrates a convex medial border and concave lateral border.

Further Reading

Orthopedics. *In* Rakel RE: Textbook of Family Practice. Philadelphia, WB Saunders, 1995, pp 1001, 1002.

68. "Rocker-bottom" feet are caused by which one of the following?

A. Congenital talus-calcaneal coalition
B. Congenital vertical talus
C. Congenital navicular-calcaneal coalition
D. Congenital accessory navicular

Answer: B

Critique: Congenital vertical talus causes rocker-bottom foot appearance. Congenital tarsal coalitions, such as between the talus and the calcaneus and between the navicular and the calcaneus, cause a rigid flat foot that demonstrates limited inversion and eversion. Accessory navicular bones can present a bony prominence on the medial aspect of the foot and can cause pain with prolonged standing.

Further Reading

Orthopedics. *In* Rakel RE: Textbook of Family Practice. Philadelphia, WB Saunders, 1995, pp 1002–1004.

69. (True or False) Risk factors for hip fracture in the elderly include which of the following?

1. Poor balance
2. Impaired reflexes and mentation
3. Current use of anticonvulsants
4. Walking for exercise

Answers: 1-T, 2-T, 3-T, 4-F

Critique: Osteoporosis increases the risk for hip fractures in the elderly. However, other risk factors have been shown to contribute independently to this risk. Poor balance and also impaired reflexes and mentation can increase the risk for fractures. Current use of anticonvulsants has also demonstrated an independent risk. Walking for exercise actually confers some protection against hip fracture.

Further Reading

Cummings SR, Nevitt MC, Browner WS, et al: Risk factors for hip fracture in white women. N Engl J Med 332:767–773, 1995.
Orthopedics. *In* Rakel RE: Textbook of Family Practice. Philadelphia, WB Saunders, 1995, p 1004.

39

Rheumatic Disease

Carolyn Frymoyer

1. Which one of the following is most likely to present as an asymmetric oligoarthritis?

    A. Rheumatoid arthritis
    B. Gout
    C. Psoriatic arthritis
    D. Avascular necrosis
    E. Septic arthritis

Answer: C

Critique: Joint pain, swelling, or stiffness may be caused by many different conditions. A thorough evaluation of all joints for swelling, redness, and limitation of movement provides information regarding the number and symmetry of joints involved. This information is important when formulating a differential diagnosis. Monoarticular involvement is seen in septic arthritis, gout, pseudogout, trauma, hemarthrosis, avascular necrosis, and tumors. Asymmetric involvement of few joints is seen in ankylosing spondylitis, psoriatic arthritis, and Reiter's syndrome. Polyarticular and symmetric joint involvement is seen in rheumatoid arthritis and systemic lupus erythematosus (SLE). Psoriatic arthritis less commonly presents with polyarticular involvement similar to rheumatoid arthritis. Osteoarthritis may be monoarticular or oligoarticular but lacks systemic features seen in other rheumatic diseases.

Page 1007

Questions 2–3. A 60-year-old man presents with sudden onset of pain, redness, and swelling of his left knee. His past history is positive for two episodes of gout involving the right great toe and an old football injury to his left knee. The most recent gouty attack was 3 years ago. On examination the patient is in moderate distress due to the pain. He has a low-grade temperature. He refuses to bend the left knee, which is swollen, red, and warm. After obtaining radiographs of the knee, you decide to tap the joint.

2. Which of the following characteristics of the aspirate could be found with both septic arthritis and crystal-induced arthritis?

    A. Clear appearance, normal viscosity, low white blood cell count
    B. Turbid appearance, low viscosity, high white blood cell count
    C. Clear appearance, low viscosity, high white blood cell count
    D. Turbid appearance, high viscosity, normal white blood cell count
    E. Slightly turbid appearance, high viscosity, high white blood cell count

Answer: B

Critique: Synovial fluid characteristics including clarity, viscosity, cell count, crystal analysis, Gram stain, and culture can be critical to the diagnosis of certain joint conditions. Noninflammatory synovial fluid with clear appearance, normal viscosity, and low white blood cell count is seen in osteoarthritis, osteonecrosis, polymyalgia rheumatica, scleroderma, trauma, polyarteritis nodosa, and SLE (although SLE joint fluid occasionally appears inflammatory). Purulent fluid with turbid appearance, low viscosity, and high white blood cell count is seen in septic arthritis, gout, and pseudogout. Inflammatory synovial fluid with slightly turbid appearance, fair viscosity, and high white blood cell count is seen in some cases of gout and pseudogout. Other conditions with inflammatory fluid are rheumatoid arthritis, psoriatic arthritis, Reiter's syndrome, viral arthritis, and Behçet's syndrome. The identification of crystals in synovial fluid confirms the diagnosis of gout or pseudogout. The presence of organisms on a Gram stain or culture of synovial fluid confirms the diagnosis of septic arthritis.

Page 1008

3. Fluid analysis is consistent with an inflammatory fluid. The radiographs demonstrate multifocal linear calcifications in the lateral meniscus. Microscopic examination of the fluid would be expected to show:

    A. Gram-positive cocci in clusters
    B. Negatively birefringent needle-shaped crystals
    C. Gram-negative intracellular diplococci

D. Weakly birefringent rhomboid-shaped crystals
E. Predominantly mononuclear white blood cells

Answer: D

Critique: The history is consistent with an acute inflammatory arthritis. The previously injured knee predisposes the patient to osteoarthritis. A previously arthritic joint is susceptible to septic arthritis or pseudogout. The history of gout also makes it a possibility. The inflammatory fluid and chondrocalcinosis on x-ray increase the likelihood of pseudogout, which most commonly affects the knee. Septic arthritis should yield a frankly purulent effusion. Pseudogout is characterized by weakly birefringent rhomboid-shaped crystals of calcium pyrophosphate crystals in the joint fluid. Gout, on the other hand, is caused by negatively birefringent needle-shaped crystals of monosodium urate. Mononuclear white blood cells are found in noninflammatory fluids.

Pages 1008, 1009, 1017–1019

4. Nonsteroidal anti-inflammatory drugs (NSAID) are commonly used in the treatment of rheumatic diseases. Regarding the use of NSAID in patients with rheumatic diseases, which one of the following statements is true?

A. Suppression of prostaglandin synthesis is the only mechanism of action of these drugs in controlling symptoms.
B. In large studies, most NSAID have comparable efficacy.
C. An individual who has not responded to one NSAID is unlikely to respond to an NSAID from a different class.
D. An adequate therapeutic trial for a patient starting on an NSAID is 5 days.
E. Gastrointestinal (GI) bleeding is the only serious side effect of NSAID use.

Answer: B

Critique: The inflammatory reactions seen in rheumatic diseases are complex and vary over time in a given individual, depending on the state or activity of the disease. Prostaglandin production may not be the only factor in these reactions. This may explain why some individuals respond to one NSAID but not to another, although studies of large groups of patients have shown comparable efficacy. A minimum of 2 weeks is necessary to assess the effectiveness of an NSAID on a patient's symptoms. Serious side effects from use of an NSAID are not limited to GI bleeding but also include renal insufficiency, hepatitis, sodium retention, hypertension, skin reactions, cytopenia, and central nervous system symptoms. Patients who take NSAID should be evaluated periodically for side effects.

Pages 1010, 1011

Questions 5–6. A 50-year-old woman who works as a secretary is seen with a 2-month history of joint pain. She has had no history of trauma or illness. Initially, pain was in the metacarpophalangeal (MP) joints of both hands with swelling but no redness. Stiffness and redness in one shoulder and both wrists subsequently developed. She had no joint deformities, fever, skin rashes or nodules, or pulmonary or GI symptoms. X-rays of the hands revealed soft tissue swelling, periarticular osteopenia, and marginal bone erosions. The erythrocyte sedimentation rate (ESR) was elevated.

5. This presentation is most consistent with:

A. Osteoarthritis
B. Psoriatic arthritis
C. Systemic lupus erythematosus
D. Rheumatoid arthritis
E. Polymyalgia rheumatica

Answer: D

Critique: *Rheumatoid arthritis* is a symmetric, polyarticular disease that may involve other organ systems. Joints show a proliferative synovitis. The peak onset is during the fourth and fifth decades with female:male ratio of 3:1. The onset is usually gradual over weeks to months but may be more acute. Swelling, tenderness, and warmth are seen in at least three joints—typically the proximal interphalangeal (PIP), MP, and wrist joints. Deformities including ulnar deviation may appear with progression of the disease. Initial x-ray findings are limited to soft tissue swelling and joint effusions. Typical x-ray findings, including marginal erosions and periarticular osteopenia, appear with progression. Rheumatoid factor (RF) is usually elevated but may be negative, especially in early stages of the disease. *Osteoarthritis* is a monoarticular or oligoarticular disorder of the large weight-bearing joints and hands. Swelling is due to joint effusions or bony proliferation. No specific laboratory tests are available for osteoarthritis. The ESR is usually normal. *Systemic lupus erythematosus* typically affects young women and is a multisystem disease. Joint distribution is similar to rheumatoid arthritis, but joint destruction is less common. The diagnosis is confirmed by typical involvement of other organs, and the majority of patients have a positive antinuclear antibody (ANA) assay and an elevated ESR. Other tests that may be positive include anti–double-stranded DNA, anti-smith (sm) antibodies, Venereal Disease Research Laboratory (VDRL) with negative confirmatory test, anti-cardiolipin antibodies, and lupus anticoagulant test. *Polymyalgia rheumatica* affects elderly patients with a 2:1 female predominance. Stiffness and aching of the neck, shoulders, and hips are not accompanied by inflammatory changes. Systemic symptoms, muscle tenderness, and an elevated ESR are seen.

Pages 1011–1017, 1019–1022, 1024–1027

6. Initial treatment for her condition might include:

A. Low-dose steroids
B. High-dose steroids
C. Salicylates and NSAIDs
D. Sulfasalizine
E. Methotrexate

Answer: C

Critique: Treatment goals for rheumatoid arthritis include control of synovitis and pain and maintenance or restoration of the functional status of the patient. Education, rest, physical therapy, and joint conservation should be part of the treatment plan for all patients. Pharmacologic treatment begins with anti-inflammatory agents, including use of aspirin products or NSAID. Other medications should be reserved for patients whose symptoms are not controlled by NSAID and should be used in consultation with a rheumatologist. Low-dose prednisone may be used in conjunction with disease modifying antirheumatic drugs (DMARD) and then tapered when clinical improvement is seen. DMARD include gold, D-penicillamine, hydroxychloroquine, sulfasalazine, and methotrexate and are considered for patients with recent onset of disease who show radiographic changes, including erosions or joint space narrowing. These drugs may reduce further joint damage but will not reverse existing damage.

Pages 1011–1017, 1019–1022, 1024–1027

7. The management of asymptomatic hyperuricemia should include:

    A. Allopurinol
    B. NSAID
    C. Colchicine
    D. Uricosuric agents
    E. Dietary counseling

Answer: E

Critique: Patients with asymptomatic hyperuricemia require no specific treatment. Dietary changes to avoid high purine foods and to reduce alcohol intake may be helpful. Medications that increase serum uric acid (diuretics) should be avoided when possible. Acute gouty attacks are treated with NSAID or colchicine. Patients with tophaceous gout may benefit from correction of hyperuricemia by increasing renal excretion of uric acid through the use of uricosuric agents or decreasing uric acid production through the use of xanthine oxidase inhibitors. Lowering of serum uric acid should not be attempted during acute gouty attacks.

Pages 1017, 1018

8. The presence of an enthesopathy is characteristic of:

    A. Spondyloarthropathies
    B. Crystal-induced arthropathies
    C. Osteoarthritis
    D. Rheumatoid arthritis
    E. Drug-induced synovitis

Answer: A

Critique: Enthesopathy is an inflammatory process at the site of insertion of a tendon, ligament, or articular capsule. The presence of an enthesopathy is characteristic of spondyloarthropathies. The inflammatory process leads to many of the spinal, articular, and periarticular symptoms common to these disorders. Calcification may occur at these sites and produce the characteristic radiographic changes seen in the spondyloarthropathies.

Page 1019

9. A 35-year-old missionary presents with a low-grade fever, conjunctivitis, low back pain, painful swelling of the right knee, and left heel pain. He recently returned from Africa where he nearly died of dysentery. On examination, his conjunctiva are red with a scant mucoid discharge. The right knee is warm, swollen, and painful to motion. A small effusion is present. The left heel has boggy swelling and moderate tenderness at the insertion of the Achilles tendon. He has discrete, scaly, circinate, plaque-like lesions on his feet. The most likely diagnosis is:

    A. Psoriasis with spondyloarthritis
    B. Lyme disease
    C. Ankylosing spondylitis
    D. Acquired immunodeficiency syndrome (AIDS)
    E. Reiter's syndrome

Answer: E

Critique: This clinical description presented here is typical of Reiter's syndrome. Reiter's syndrome is a spondyloarthropathy that frequently follows an infection of the genitourinary (often nongonococcal urethritis) or GI tracts (i.e., bacillary dysentery). The syndrome is characterized by an asymmetric oligoarthritis, usually involving the lower extremities, and associated conjunctivitis, urethritis, enthesopathy, and skin changes. The typical skin manifestation is keratoderma blennorrhagia, which resembles psoriatic plaques. Psoriatic arthritis is less likely due to the pattern of joint involvement and the lack of generalized skin involvement. Ankylosing spondylitis should have more dominant back symptoms. The eye manifestations are more likely to be anterior uveitis than conjunctivitis. Lyme disease usually has a specific rash, erythema migrans, as part of its initial presentation. Reiter's syndrome can be associated with human immunodeficiency virus (HIV) infection, but there is nothing to suggest a high risk of HIV in this presentation.

Pages 1019–1021, 1023

10. Which of the following rheumatic syndromes is the most common one that is associated with human immunodeficiency virus type I (HIV-1) infection?

    A. Septic arthritis
    B. Sjögren's syndrome
    C. Rheumatoid arthritis
    D. Reiter's syndrome
    E. Polymyalgia rheumatica

Answer: D

Critique: Several rheumatic syndromes have been associated with HIV infection. The most frequently associated conditions are the spondyloarthropathies. Reiter's syndrome is the most common one reported in HIV-positive patients. In at-risk patients, HIV testing should be done in patients presenting with Reiter's syndrome or other spondyloarthropathies. Other rheumatic syndromes that have been associated with HIV infection include septic arthritis, Sjögren's syndrome, vasculitis, and myopathies; however, they are less commonly seen than is Reiter's syndrome.

Pages 1030, 1031

11. A 10-year-female child presents to your office with a 3-week history of a progressive illness characterized by recurrent fever and joint pain. In the last 2 weeks, she has had a painful, red and swollen right knee, followed by swelling and tenderness of her left wrist and elbow, and most recently severe pain in her right hip that limits ambulation. She denies any rashes or tremors. On examination she appears ill. She has a temperature is 100.6° F, a pulse of 120/min, and normal respirations. Auscultation of the heart reveals a systolic murmur that was not previously noted. Joint examination shows pain with motion of the right hip and a tender, warm, and swollen left wrist with overlying erythema. The remainder of the orthopedic examination is negative. An electrocardiogram shows a sinus rhythm with tachycardia and a first-degree atrioventricular (AV) block. Which of the following findings would satisfy the Jones criteria for the diagnosis of acute rheumatic fever (ARF)?

A. A positive throat culture for group A β-hemolytic *Streptococcus*
B. Erythema marginatum
C. A negative serology for rheumatoid factor
D. An elevated ESR
E. Subcutaneous nodules

Answer: A

Critique: ARF is a rare disorder in today's clinical environment; however, one must maintain a high index of suspicion for risk of missing the diagnosis. The Jones criteria are still useful when establishing the diagnosis. The Jones criteria require two major criteria (polyarthritis, carditis, erythema marginatum, chorea, subcutaneous nodules) or one major and two minor criteria (fever, arthralgias, previous history of ARF) and evidence of an antecedent streptococcal infection (ASO serology, positive throat culture, recent scarlet fever). This case meets two major criteria with migratory polyarthritis and evidence of carditis. The remaining criterion necessary is evidence of a recent streptococcal infection.

Page 1032

Questions 12–16 (True or False) Rheumatic diseases that frequently present with monoarticular arthritis include:

12. Pseudogout

13. Systemic lupus erythematosus

14. Osteoarthritis

15. Reiter's syndrome

16. Ankylosing spondylitis

Answers: 12-T, 13-F, 14-T, 15-F, 16-F

Critique: Joint pain, swelling, or stiffness may be caused by many different conditions. A thorough evaluation of all joints for swelling, redness, and limitation of movement provides information regarding the number and symmetry of joints involved, which is important when formulating a differential diagnosis. Monoarticular involvement is seen in septic arthritis, gout, pseudogout, trauma, hemarthrosis, avascular necrosis, and tumors. Asymmetric involvement of a few joints is seen in ankylosing spondylitis, psoriatic arthritis, and Reiter's syndrome. Polyarticular and symmetric joint involvement is seen in rheumatoid arthritis and systemic lupus erythematosus. Psoriatic arthritis less commonly presents with polyarticular involvement similar to rheumatoid arthritis. Osteoarthritis may be monoarticular or oligoarticular but lacks systemic features seen in other rheumatic diseases.

Page 1007

Questions 17–21 (True or False) True statements about Lyme disease include:

17. Most patients recall removing a tick within the past few weeks.

18. The initial manifestations include erythema migrans and constitutional symptoms of malaise, headache, fever, and myalgias.

19. The oligoarticular involvement is limited to arthritis of the hips and knees.

20. Late manifestations include AV blocks.

21. If present, meningitis is usually seen early in the course of the disease.

Answers: 17-F, 18-T, 19-F, 20-T, 21-F

Critique: Lyme disease is a tick-borne disease caused by *Borrelia burgdorferi*. However, most patients do not recall a tick bite. Early manifestations of the illness include the characteristic rash, erythema migrans, which may be accompanied by constitutional symptoms, such as fever, chills, headache, arthralgias, and myalgias. Monoarticular or oligoarticular manifestations occur later and commonly involve the knees; however, other large and small joints may be involved. Late manifestations of Lyme disease include meningitis, facial palsies, and AV blocks.

Page 1023

Questions 22–26 (True or False) The American College of Rheumatology revised criteria for the diagnosis of SLE in 1982. Criteria that can be used to diagnose SLE include:

22. Erosive arthritis involving at least two peripheral joints

23. Pericarditis documented by electrocardiographic changes or a pericardial rub

24. Skin rash as a result of an unusual reaction to sunlight

25. Thrombocytosis greater than 250,000/mm³

26. Psychosis in the absence of offending drugs or metabolic derangement

Answers: 22-F, 23-T, 24-T, 25-F, 26-T

Critique: The American College of Rheumatology revised criteria for the diagnosis of SLE in 1982. An individual is said to have lupus if any four or more of 11 specific criteria are present, either simultaneously or sequentially, during an interval of observation. The criteria include malar rash, discoid lupus skin changes, photosensitivity, oral ulcers, nonerosive arthritis, serositis (pericarditis), renal disorder, neurologic disorder (seizures or psychosis), hematologic disorder, immunologic disorder, and antinuclear antibodies.

Page 1024

Questions 27–31 (True or False) Which of the following vasculitic syndromes commonly involve the kidney?

27. Polymyalgia rheumatica with giant cell arteritis

28. Polyarteritis nodosa

29. Wegener's granulomatosis

30. Churg-Strauss syndrome

31. Behçet's disease

Answers: 27-F, 28-T, 29-T, 30-F, 31-F

Critique: The vasculitic syndromes make up a group of disorders characterized by an inflammatory process involving blood vessels. They may be idiopathic or associated with collagen vascular diseases. Each vasculitic syndrome has a predilection for certain size vessels and tends to have a pattern of organ involvement; however, there may be considerable overlap. Polyarteritis nodosa and Wegener's granulomatosis are the most likely vasculitic processes to affect the kidney. Polymyalgia rheumatica with giant cell arteritis tends to affect the vessels of the neck and head and may cause headache, visual loss, strokes, or jaw claudication. Churg-Strauss syndrome and Behçet's disease are uncommon disorders. Churg-Strauss syndrome primarily involves the lung; whereas, Behçet's disease primarily affects the skin and mucous membranes.

Pages 1027–1030

40

Evaluation of Skin Lesions

Donald E. Nease, Jr.

1. Which one of the following primary dermatologic lesions is characterized by small, well-defined lesions containing deposits of blood or blood products?

    A. Petechiae
    B. Papules
    C. Vesicles
    D. Wheals
    E. Macules

Answer: A

Critique: Primary dermatologic lesions are those that arise without a prior visible lesion. Petechiae are small, well-defined lesions containing deposits of blood or blood products. Macules are flat, nonpalpable areas of skin that differ in color from the surrounding skin. Patches are similar but are larger than macules. Papules are solid, small, elevated lesions that do not contain fluid. In contrast, both pustules and vesicles are elevated lesions that contain fluid. A wheal is an elevated lesion that appears edematous and fades quickly after the insult.

Page 1040

2. Which one of the following primary dermatologic lesions is characterized by a flat, nonpalpable area of skin that differs in color from the surrounding skin?

    A. Pustules
    B. Papules
    C. Macules
    D. Wheals
    E. Vesicles

Answer: C

Critique: Primary dermatologic lesions are those that arise without a prior visible lesion. Macules are flat, non-palpable areas of skin that differ in color from the surrounding skin. Patches are similar but are larger than macules. Papules are solid, small, elevated lesions that do not contain fluid. In contrast, both pustules and vesicles are fluid-containing, elevated lesions. A wheal is an

elevated lesion that appears edematous and fades quickly after the insult.

Page 1040

3. A 6-year-old child is brought to your office by a concerned mother. The child has a 3-day history of a rash involving well-defined areas on his lower legs and arms. The rash is erythematous and vesicular in most areas, but on the left calf the vesicles appear to have become bullae. The rash is intensely pruritic. On questioning the mother denies using any new laundry detergents or soaps but remembers that during the past weekend the family did their annual spring clean-up in the backyard. This rash is most likely an example of which of the following?

    A. Atopic dermatitis
    B. Poison ivy dermatitis
    C. Neurodermatitis
    D. Eosinophilic dermatitis
    E. Eczema

Answer: B

Critique: Contact dermatitis from poison ivy often appears 1 to 3 days after exposure to the oleoresin of poison ivy. The rash appears vesicular or bullous if severe and often shows a streaking pattern. Atopic dermatitis or eczema is a scaly rash associated with excoriations, erythema, and fissuring. Lesions are present on the flexor surfaces. In pediatric cases a history of asthma, hay fever, or allergic rhinitis is often present. Neurodermatitis lesions are poorly circumscribed patches of excoriation and lichenification that are often chronic in nature.

Pages 1045–1047

4. Which of the following is the most appropriate therapy for this child at this time?

    A. Oral antihistamines
    B. Oral antibiotic
    C. Vigorous cleansing with strong soaps

D. Wet dressings or soaks
E. Occlusive dressing with topical triple antibiotic ointment

Answer: A

Critique: Contact dermatitis is treated first by removing the offending agent. If the rash is weeping, wet dressings or soaks may be used. Oral antihistamines can be effective to reduce the itch, particularly at bedtime. Oral antibiotics are not indicated unless the lesion becomes secondarily infected. Similarly, an occlusive dressing with triple antibiotic ointment is not indicated. Triple antibiotic ointment often contains neomycin, which can also cause contact dermatitis. Depending on the severity of the rash, steroids may be employed topically, orally, or parenterally.

Pages 1045–1047

5. Erysipelas:

    A. Is usually caused by *Staphylococcus aureus*
    B. Is more commonly seen in middle-aged adults than in small children
    C. May be fatal in a few cases
    D. Is always associated with an obvious portal of entry
    E. Has an insidious onset with a slowly progressive course

Answer: C

Critique: Erysipelas is a superficial cellulitis caused by group A streptococci. It is most often found in infants, toddlers, and the elderly. The portal of entry may be a site of minor trauma and is often not recognized. The infection evolves rapidly and spreads to the lymphatics and blood. Patients are often quite ill, and the condition can be lethal.

Page 1053

6. Which of the following statements regarding herpes simplex virus-I (HSV-I) and herpes simplex virus-II (HSV-II) are true?

    A. HSV-I tends to occur "above the belt," whereas HSV-II is primarily a genital infection.
    B. After primary infection, the virus lies dormant in squamous epithelial cells.
    C. Transmission of HSV-I frequently occurs by droplet nuclei.
    D. Acyclovir (Zovirax) has been shown to affect viral cultures and the clinical course of facial and oral outbreaks of HSV-I.

Answer: A

Critique: There are two types of herpes simplex virus (HSV-I and II). HSV-I tends to occur "above the belt," whereas HSV-II is primarily a genital infection. After the primary infection, the virus lies dormant in neural cells. Transmission of HSV-I and HSV-II is usually through direct mucocutaneous contact. Topically applied acyclovir is useful for the treatment of primary genital (HSV-II) lesions. Orally administered acyclovir is indicated for the prevention of outbreaks in patients with three or four genital (HSV-II) outbreaks a year.

Pages 1055, 1056

7. A 30-year-old man presents to your office complaining of a problem with tanning. Specifically, he has patches on his chest that fail to tan with exposure to sun and remain quite pale. On questioning, he notes that the areas itch occasionally. Which one of the following fungal infections is most likely to be the cause of this condition?

    A. *Candida albicans*
    B. *Trichophyton* spp.
    C. *Sporothrix schenckii*
    D. *Malassezia furfur*
    E. Tinea rubrum

Answer: D

Critique: Tinea versicolor is caused by *M. furfur*. The organism produces a natural sunscreen that prevents normal tanning in affected areas. The condition can be itchy as well. Scraping of the affected areas and microscopic examination with KOH will show a "spaghetti and meatballs" appearance of spores and hyphae. Treatment is usually accomplished with application of selenium sulfide shampoo for 10- to 20-minute periods of time. Topical clotrimazole and miconazole may also be used. For resistant cases, oral ketoconazole is effective. *Candida* causes diaper rash, intertriginous rashes, and vulvovaginitis. *Trichophyton* species commonly cause tinea barbae. *S. schenckii*, a fungal saprophyte, can cause a cutaneous infection with indurated papules along the course of the lymphatics. Tinea rubrum causes dermatitis of the hands and feet.

Pages 1057–1061

8. Which of the following skin lesions are related to repeated or chronic sun exposure?

    A. Keratoacanthoma
    B. Dermatofibroma
    C. Actinic keratosis
    D. Junctional nevus
    E. Tinea versicolor

Answer: C

Critique: Repeated or chronic exposure to sunlight produces skin damage that can result in actinic keratoses, skin cancers (e.g., basal cell cancer, squamous cell cancer, and melanoma), and dermatohelioses, including solar lentigo, aging, wrinkles, and telangiectasias. Keratoacanthomas are benign and thought to arise from hair follicles. Dermatofibromas are benign nodules that result from abnormal scar formation. Junctional nevi are not related to solar damage. The appearance of tinea versicolor may be enhanced by sun exposure; however, it is caused by *M. furfur*.

Pages 1057, 1058, 1063–1066, 1073

9. Which of the following is characteristic of a basal cell carcinoma?

A. Tendency to metastasize early
B. Tan or brown macule with adherent scales and surrounding erythema
C. Rapid increase in size
D. Sessile nodule with raised edges and an ulcerated center
E. Usually arises from a previous actinic keratosis

Answer: A

Critique: Basal cell carcinomas rarely metastasize, although if they are left untreated their local spread can be quite destructive. They usually begin as a whitish or pinkish papule with telangiectasias and then evolve into a nodule with a raised, translucent, pearly telangiectatic border. Central ulceration usually develops with crusting that bleeds when disturbed. A biopsy should be taken of suspicious lesions, and treatment is usually by local excision if the lesion is small. Squamous cell carcinomas can be confused with basal cell carcinomas, but they tend to grow rapidly. Actinic keratoses are precursors to squamous cell cancers.

Pages 1065, 1066

10. A 72-year-old farmer presents with a lesion in the nasolabial fold that has gradually increased in size over the last several years. The lesion measures 1.5 cm and has a pearly raised border with telangiectasias and an ulcerated center. He has not been able to get it to heal with a variety of home remedies. A punch biopsy confirms your clinical impression. Which of the following is the most appropriate therapy for this lesion?

A. Cryotherapy with liquid nitrogen
B. Topical 5-fluorouracil
C. Mohs micrographic surgery
D. Simple excision with primary closure

Answer: C

Critique: The lesion described is typical of a basal cell cancer, including the appearance and very gradual growth. Lesions larger than 1 cm, those near the eyes, ears, nose, and mouth, or recurrent lesions should be referred for more extensive surgery including Mohs micrographic surgery. Cryotherapy is good for small lesions. Topical 5-fluorouracil is useful in small lesions or multiple actinic keratoses. Simple excision in this area would produce unsightly scarring.

Pages 1065, 1066

11. A 33-year-old woman presents with multiple, irregular plaques with a red base and superimposed silvery white thick scales. She remembers that her mother had a similar skin condition. A punch biopsy shows increased mitotic figures and increased capillary blood supply. Which of the following is the most likely diagnosis?

A. Seborrheic dermatitis
B. Pityriasis rosea
C. Lichen planus
D. Sporotrichosis
E. Psoriasis

Answer: E

Critique: Psoriasis may be confused with tinea corporis, seborrheic dermatitis, pityriasis rosea, secondary syphilis, and lichen planus. The condition is characterized by multiple, irregular plaques with a red base and superimposed silvery white thick scales. The affected areas of skin develop an increased mitotic rate and increased capillary blood supply. A familial predisposition is known to occur with this disease. A biopsy, KOH preparation, serology, or consultation may be necessary to establish a definitive diagnosis.

Pages 1049, 1050, 1061, 1062, 1067, 1068

12. A 25-year-old woman presents to your office complaining of an itchy rash on the trunk. The rash is papulosquamous with tan or fawn-colored plaques covered by fine scales. The lesions seem to have their axes along skin cleavage lines. One distinct lesion is notable for a erythematous appearance with central clearing. The patient states that this was the first lesion to appear. What is the most likely diagnosis?

A. Psoriasis
B. Pityriasis rosea
C. Lichen planus
D. Tinea corporis
E. Secondary syphilis

Answer: B

Critique: Pityriasis rosea is a papulosquamous rash with tan or fawn-colored plaques covered by fine scales. The lesions have their axes along skin cleavage lines. An initial lesion called a herald patch is usually seen days or weeks before the generalized rash. The rash usually resolves within 5 to 6 weeks. Treatment is symptomatic and directed toward the itching. Because of the similarity with secondary syphilis, a serologic evaluation is indicated if a herald patch is not seen.

Page 1068

Questions 13–17 (True or False) Which of the following statements are true with reference to acne vulgaris?

13. May result from occupational exposure to coal tar derivatives

14. Consumption of chocolate is often implicated in the etiology.

15. *Propionibacterium acnes* is found in the skin follicles.

16. May be aggravated by drugs, including phenytoin or lithium

17. Surface dirt on the skin is related to the etiology.

Answers: 13-T, 14-F, 15-T, 16-T, 17-F

Critique: Acne is usually easy to diagnose, but in addition to the usual multifactorial etiology of genetic predisposition and presence of *P. acnes,* occupational exposure to coal tar derivatives and oils, drugs such as corticosteroids, iodides, bromides, isoniazid, phenytoin, and lithium, and cosmetics may be implicated. Diet, surface dirt, and sexual habits have not been shown to be related to the etiology.

Pages 1047, 1048

Questions 18–22 (True or False) True statements regarding seborrheic dermatitis include:

18. It is a more common cause of a facial "butterfly rash" than is systemic lupus erythematosus.

19. Seborrheic dermatitis is common in infants and adults.

20. It is usually unresponsive to topical steroids.

21. Scalp lesions respond to ketoconazole shampoos.

22. Seborrheic dermatitis is usually a progressive disease in infants.

Answers: 18-T, 19-T, 20-F, 21-T, 22-F

Critique: Seborrheic dermatitis is a common condition that may affect all age groups. It is the most common cause of a "butterfly rash" and should be suspected before one considers systemic lupus erythematosus. Scalp seborrhea usually responds to selenium sulfide, tar, or ketoconazole shampoos used two to three times a week. Skin lesions respond to topical steroids; however, topical steroids should be used sparingly. Hydrocortisone should be used for facial lesions. Infant forms are often seen on the scalp and perineal area. These infant forms are usually self-limiting and respond to ordinary shampoo, clean skin, and dry diapers.

Pages 1049, 1050

Questions 23–27 (True or False) A 6-year-old child is brought into your office with a 1-day history of an itchy rash that began on the face. It has now spread to the trunk. On physical examination the patient has a low-grade fever. The rash consists of numerous well-defined, erythematous lesions. The most recent lesions are macular and vesicular, whereas the older ones are beginning to show crusting. Which of the following statements regarding this illness are true?

23. The condition is usually self-limiting in children.

24. The virus that causes the rash is eliminated as the rash resolves.

25. Acyclovir may be used to treat severe cases.

26. The condition is not preventable.

27. Reactivation of the virus may occur in adults.

Answers: 23-T, 24-F, 25-T, 26-F, 27-T

Critique: Varicella zoster presents as chickenpox in children. The rash is characterized by lesions that begin as erythematous macules and progress rapidly through ve-

sicular, pustular, and crusting stages. The condition is self-limiting in children. With resolution of the rash, the virus retreats to sensory ganglia where it remains dormant. Reactivation of the virus in adulthood manifests most commonly as shingles. Recently, the Federal Drug Administration (FDA) has approved a vaccine for varicella immunization.

Pages 1056, 1057

Questions 28–32 (True or False) Syphilis is a systemic sexually transmitted disease that has many manifestations. Manifestations to some extent depend on the stage of the disease. Which of the following are true of both primary and secondary syphilis?

28. Presence of a relatively painless ulcer with raised, indurated borders and a scant serous exudate

29. Appearance of papulosquamous lesions involving the head, neck, and palms

30. Serology is reliably positive for the VDRL Venereal Disease Research Laboratory (VDRL) or rapid plasma reagin antigen (RPR) tests.

31. Lesions contain viable spirochetes.

32. Intramuscular penicillin is the recommended treatment.

Answers: 28-T, 29-F, 30-F, 31-T, 32-T

Critique: Syphilis results from infection with *Treponema pallidum.* Primary syphilis is most commonly characterized by a single, painless ulcer with raised, indurated borders and a serous exudate; however, multiple erosions and ulcers can be seen in the primary stage. The typical chancre of syphilis may still be present when secondary lesions erupt. The VDRL or RPR may be positive in primary syphilis, but this does not rule out the disease in the primary stage. They are reliably positive in secondary syphilis. Secondary syphilis develops 6 weeks to 6 months after the infection and classically shows multiple papulosquamous lesions of the head, neck, palms, and soles. However, the secondary stage may display a variety of appearances from macules to papules and nodules. Chancres and lesions of secondary syphilis contain viable spirochetes. Penicillin is used to treat both stages with two injections of 2.4 million units of benzathine penicillin 1 week apart.

Page 1062

Questions 33–36 (True or False) Which of the following statements are true regarding Kaposi's sarcoma?

33. It is associated with acquired immunodeficiency syndrome (AIDS).

34. The lesions are often quite uncomfortable.

35. The lesions appear as violaceous or reddish-pink macules that develop into nodules or plaque-like tumors.

36. Related tumors may occur in other organs.

Answers: 33-T, 34-F, 35-T, 36-T

Critique: Kaposi's sarcoma is a multifocal neoplasm with vascular tumors in the skin and other organs. It is associated with AIDS and in persons with a Jewish or East European heritage. The lesions appear as violaceous or reddish-pink macules that develop into nodules or plaque-like tumors. Discomfort is uncommon.

Page 1073

Questions 37–41 (True or False) Early recognition of melanoma is vital for early treatment to prevent metastasis. Which of the following findings in a skin lesion should prompt consideration of a melanoma?

37. An irregular lesion with variegation of color

38. A deeply pigmented lesion that has recently grown rapidly

39. An evenly pigmented lesion with smooth borders

40. Loss of skin markings within the lesion

41. A flat tan lesion with adherent scales and surrounding erythema

Answers: 37-T, 38-T, 39-F, 40-T, 41-F

Critique: Pigmented skin lesions that should prompt suspicion of melanoma and biopsy include those with any of the following: variegation of color, irregularity of the tumor border, rapid growth, and loss of skin markings within the lesion.

Page 1067

41

Endocrinology

Steven A. Crawford

1. A 25-year-old man with insulin-dependent diabetes mellitus (IDDM) presents to your office with nausea and abdominal pain. You detect rapid deep breathing and an unusual odor on his breath. On a dipstick urine, you detect a large reaction to ketones. Another feature common to this situation would include a:

    A. Glucose level greater than 1000 mg/dl
    B. Serum osmolality level around 310
    C. Serum sodium of 145 mEq/l
    D. Tendency toward stupor, coma, and convulsions

Answer: B

Critique: Diabetic ketoacidosis (DKA) commonly occurs when a patient with IDDM does not get enough insulin, resulting in a variety of profound metabolic changes. It causes marked dehydration, Kussmaul breathing (rapid and deep respirations), glucose levels averaging 475 mg/dl, serum osmolality of approximately 310, ketosis, acidosis, and mild hyponatremia. It uncommonly results in stupor, coma, or convulsions. Hyperosmolar hyperglycemic nonketotic syndrome usually occurs in elderly patients with noninsulin-dependent diabetes mellitus with long-standing uncontrolled hyperglycemia who have a precipitating event (particularly infection) and who cannot keep up with the resultant osmotic diuresis. It causes marked dehydration, normal to mild hypernatremia, marked hyperglycemia (mean levels of 1166 mg/dl), and hyperosmolality with levels greater than 340. It does not result in ketosis, although mild acidosis may occur. It has a profound tendency to result in coma, stupor, and convulsion.

Pages 1078, 1079

Further Reading

Medical Management of Non-Insulin Dependent (Type II) Diabetes, 3rd ed. Alexandria, VA, American Diabetes Association, 1994, p 79.

2. Diabetic nephropathy is characterized by:

    A. Higher prevalence in type II diabetics
    B. Microalbuminuria early in its course

    C. Glomerular basement membrane attenuation
    D. Increased insulin requirements as the condition worsens

Answer: B

Critique: Type I diabetics are at a much higher risk for the development of diabetic nephropathy than are type II diabetics. Microalbuminuria, or loss of 30 to 300 mg/day of albumin, is an early sign of diabetic nephropathy. Glomerular basement membrane thickening and increased mesangium are early histologic changes. Insulin requirements change as renal failure progresses, and it is not unusual to see more frequent hypoglycemic reactions.

Pages 1080, 1081

3. Characteristics of pregnant diabetics include:

    A. A decreased risk of fetal caudal dysplasia
    B. A decline in the rate of progression of retinopathy
    C. An increased risk of neonatal macrosomia
    D. A decreased incidence of neonatal respiratory distress
    E. A lower risk of ketoacidosis for the mother

Answer: C

Critique: Perinatal mortality rates increase with increasing severity of diabetes, but they have decreased dramatically with improved prenatal care. The infant of a diabetic mother has an increased chance of having anomalies, macrosomia, prematurity, respiratory distress syndrome, and death. One of the most characteristic congenital anomalies of diabetes is sacral agenesis or caudal dysplasia. The mother faces an increased risk of ketoacidosis as well as acceleration of retinopathy and nephropathy.

Pages 1089, 1090

4. Graves' disease is a type of thyrotoxicosis. It is commonly associated with which of the following manifestations:

    A. Excessive thyroid-stimulating hormone (TSH) excretion

B. Infiltrative dermopathy
C. Bradycardia
D. Anorexia

Answer: B

Critique: Infiltrative dermopathy in the pretibial skin or foot areas is pathognomonic of Graves' disease. The combination of suppressed TSH concentration and elevated free thyroxine index confirms the diagnosis of thyrotoxicosis arising from the thyroid gland. Tachycardia, along with a systolic flow murmur, is a common feature of Graves' disease. Loss of weight, despite a good appetite and adequate caloric intake, is an excellent clue.

Pages 1095–1097

5. Which of the following conditions is associated with hypercalcemia?

A. Sarcoidosis
B. Hypothyroidism
C. Hypomagnesemia
D. Pancreatitis
E. Burns

Answer: A

Critique: Sarcoidosis is an uncommon cause of hypercalcemia (0.9% of cases). Malignancy and hyperparathyroidism are the two most common causes. Hypothyroidism causes decreased bone resorption, which results in hypocalcemia. Pancreatitis and burns, along with either hypomagnesemia or hypermagnesemia, may cause hypocalcemia by preventing parathyroid gland function.

Pages 1106–1109

6. Precocious puberty is defined as the onset of increased testosterone and all its sequelae of secondary sexual development and spermatogenesis before age 9 in boys or estrogen production, breast development, or menarche before age 8 in girls. Its parameters include which of the following?

A. Occurs more commonly in boys than in girls
B. About 20% of girls with true isosexual precocity are idiopathic.
C. Can be caused by epilepsy
D. Preferred treatment is by administering progestational agents

Answer: C

Critique: True sexual precocity occurs 10 times more frequently in girls than in boys. About 80% of girls and only 50% of boys with true sexual precocity are found to be idiopathic. The remainder can be caused by neurologic phenomena, including head trauma, meningitis, and epilepsy. The favored endocrinologic therapy has changed from FSH suppression to the prevention of developmental and growth-stimulating effects of estrogen by administering progestation agents (which are also antiandrogenic) to luteinizing hormone-releasing hormone (LHRH) agonism in constant or nonpulsed fashion. The latter has the paradoxic effect, through binding with gonadotropic cells of the pituitary, of suppressing the gonad-

otropins, follicle-stimulating hormone (FSH) and luteinizing hormone (LH).

Pages 1124, 1125

7. A 51-year-old woman presents to your office for evaluation of hot flashes and lack of menses for 14 months. She had a tubal ligation many years ago. Her periods had been decreasing in amount and frequency over the last 2 years until they stopped completely. Which of the following would it be appropriate to inform her about her menopausal state?

A. FSH must be measured to confirm menopause.
B. Estrogen replacement therapy (ERT) will prevent approximately 20% of the coronary heart disease (CHD) deaths in postmenopausal women.
C. Consumption of calcium at 1500 mg/day is as effective as ERT in preventing osteoporosis.
D. There is no danger in waiting more than 3 years to decide whether to be on hormone replacement therapy (HRT) for preventing osteoporosis.
E. Transdermal estrogen lacks the lipid-remediating effect of oral estrogens.

Answer: E

Critique: Clinically acceptable definitions of menopause include typical symptoms in the appropriate setting, such as age, associated vasomotor and emotional symptoms, and cessation of menses, even for only a few months, with the corroborating finding of an elevated FSH level (>40 IU/l), 1 year of amenorrhea in the appropriate clinical setting, or an increased FSH level (>40 IU/l) in the atypical setting. Only if amenorrhea exists for less than 6 months should there be confirmation of FSH; and pregnancy must be ruled out before instituting HRT. It is estimated that HRT or ERT can prevent approximately half of the deaths due to CHD in postmenopausal women. Oral calcium is the most conservative regimen that can be used for long-term prevention of osteoporosis, at dosages that ensure a total intake of 1.5 g/day. This regimen alone is not nearly as potent as ERT for prevention of osteoporosis and obviously has no beneficial effect on the risk for CHD. ERT or HRT should be started as soon as menopause is eminent. The first 3 years appears to be crucial. A disadvantage of transdermal estrogen is that it misses the first pass through the liver and consequently lacks the lipid-remediating effects.

Pages 1133–1136

8. Other names for type I diabetes mellitus include all of the following EXCEPT:

A. Early-onset diabetes mellitus
B. Juvenile onset diabetes mellitus
C. Autoimmune diabetes mellitus
D. Insulin-resistant diabetes mellitus

Answer: D

Critique: Type I diabetes or IDDM has been called early-onset, juvenile, and autoimmune diabetes. It usually occurs at an early age during a person's childhood and has been associated with an autoimmune reaction involving the islet cells. This reaction, which is thought to be triggered by a viral infection in a genetically susceptible individual, leads to progressive loss of insulin-secretory capacity and ultimately to clinical diabetes. Insulin resistance occurs in type II or NIDDM.

Page 1075

9. Common clinical manifestations of hypoglycemia include all of the following EXCEPT:

    A. Bradycardia
    B. Perspiration
    C. Irritability
    D. Hunger
    E. Tremors

Answer: A

Critique: The clinical manifestations of hypoglycemia are explained by the responses to counterregulatory hormones or the consequences of neuroglycopenia. When glucose falls to 40 to 50 mg/dl, epinephrine, growth hormone, glucagon, and cortisol are secreted to counter hypoglycemia. Perspiration, tremors, hunger or nausea, tachycardia, pallor, and irritability occur.

Page 1079

10. Background diabetic retinopathy causes all of the following changes EXCEPT:

    A. Hard exudates
    B. Retinal detachment
    C. Microaneurysms
    D. Intraretinal dot hemorrhages
    E. Cottonwool exudates

Answer: B

Critique: Diabetes is the leading cause of blindness in the United States. There are two types of diabetic retinopathy: background and proliferative retinopathy. Background retinopathy occurs after 5 years and consists of microaneurysms, intraretinal dot hemorrhages, and serous fluid that leaks from abnormal retinal vessels (hard exudates). Cottonwool exudates represent infarctions in the inner retinal layers. Proliferative retinopathy refers to new vessel formation in response to ischemia that extends from the retina into the vitreous cavity. These vessels are fragile, bleed easily, and promote retinal detachment.

Pages 1079, 1080

11. Syndrome X is the name given to the constellation of conditions that includes adult-onset non-autoimmune diabetes as the central focus. Other manifestations of this condition include all of the following EXCEPT:

    A. Hypertension
    B. Accelerated atherosclerosis
    C. Hypoinsulinemia
    D. Dyslipidemia
    E. Truncal obesity

Answer: C

Critique: In syndrome X, insulin levels rise owing to a compensatory response in the face of insulin resistance. This hyperinsulinemia results in higher levels of hypertension than in the general population. It also contributes to an increase in atherosclerotic conditions, including coronary artery disease and cerebrovascular disease. It also causes increased hepatic production of very low density lipoprotein (VLDL) and therefore triglyceride. Obesity, particularly of the truncal type, is associated with insulin resistance.

Pages 1083, 1084

12. Exercise for diabetics has many salutatory effects. Which of the following is **NOT** considered an effect of exercise:

    A. Potentiation of insulin
    B. Lowering of the blood pressure
    C. Reduction in LDL cholesterol
    D. Prevention neuropathy
    E. Increases in circulating insulin levels

Answer: E

Critique: For most diabetics, exercise should be an integral part of any regimen. Exercise potentiates insulin, has an alleviating effect on hyperinsulinemia, reduces blood pressure, reduces total and LDL cholesterol, and elevates HDL cholesterol. It may mitigate the complications of neuropathy, nephropathy, and retinopathy.

Page 1087

13. Signs and symptoms found with hypothyroidism include all of the following EXCEPT:

    A. Increased pulse pressure
    B. Hyponatremia
    C. Mental agitation
    D. Shortness of breath

Answer: A

Critique: The insufficiency of thyroid hormones affects all tissues. The cardiovascular system findings include a narrowed pulse pressure and bradycardia. Hyponatremia occurs by secondary antidiuretic hormone excess, which results in water retention out of proportion to salt retention. Common psychiatric symptoms include paranoia and depression. The extreme state, myxedema madness, is characterized by agitation. Shortness of breath occurs, especially if there is pleural effusion.

Page 1099

14. Pharmacologic agents that can cause hypothyroidism or goiter include all of the following EXCEPT:

    A. Lithium
    B. Indomethacin
    C. Phenylbutazone
    D. Ethionamide
    E. Amiodarone

Answer: B

Critique: Several drugs in the standard armamentarium are antithyroid and hence goitrous in their effects. Lithium, phenylbutazone, and the antituberculous drug ethionamide can cause goiters. Amiodarone can cause either hyperthyroidism or hypothyroidism. Indomethacin does not affect the thyroid gland.

Page 1100

Further Reading

Physicians' Desk Reference, 49th ed. Montvale, NJ, Medical Economics Co., 1995, p 1556.

15. Clinical manifestations of hypopituitarism include all of the following EXCEPT:

    A. Inability to produce breast milk postpartum
    B. Decreased velocity of growth in an infant
    C. Hyperpigmentation
    D. Easy fatigability

Answer: C

Critique: The clinical features of hypopituitarism are dependent on which hormones are affected, the age of the patient, and the anatomic area of involvement. Inability to produce prolactin will result in a mother being unable to nurse her infant. Growth hormone deficiency presenting at birth results in decreased velocity of growth. Lack of adenocorticotropic hormone (ACTH) results in symptoms similar to those of Addison's disease; however, hyperpigmentation is absent. General weakness, fatigue and lack of energy are relatively common complaints.

Page 1110

16. Common symptoms of diabetes insipidus include all of the following EXCEPT:

    A. Dysuria
    B. Polyuria
    C. Nocturia
    D. Thirst

Answer: A

Critique: A deficiency or absence of vasopressin results in polyuria and the inability to adequately concentrate the urine. This problem also results in nocturia and severe thirst. Dysuria is not a symptom of diabetes insipidus.

Page 1112

17. Signs and symptoms of chronic primary adrenal insufficiency include all of the following EXCEPT:

    A. Salt craving
    B. Hypertension
    C. Weight loss
    D. Hyponatremia
    E. Nausea

Answer: B

Critique: Most cases of primary adrenal insufficiency, also called Addison's disease, are insidious in onset and, therefore, become chronic before the diagnosis is made.

The manifestations of this disease are protean; however, aside from hyperpigmentation and vitiligo, are all nonspecific. However, almost 100% of patients will have decreased energy, anorexia, and weight loss. Along with the skin changes, these findings are essential to the diagnosis. Variable gastrointestinal symptoms, including nausea in 86% of patients, are proportionate to the severity and acuteness of the disease. Hypovolemia due to sodium loss as a result of hypoaldosteronemia is the basis for orthostatic lightheadedness and hypotension and occurs before the onset of persistent hypotension. Salt or ice craving is common.

Pages 1116, 1117

Questions 18–21. Match each of the following statements about adrenal hormone production with the appropriate area of the adrenal responsible for the hormone production. Each lettered option may be used once, more than once, or not at all.

    A. Zona glomerulosa
    B. Zona fasciculata
    C. Zona reticularis
    D. Adrenal medulla

18. Produces the minor adrenal androgens

19. Produces aldosterone

20. Comprises 75% of the cortex

21. Produces a hormone that causes negative feedback on the release of corticotropin-releasing hormone

Answers: 18-C, 19-A, 20-B, 21-B

Critique: The adrenal gland is at least two functional endocrine organs that happen to exist within the same capsule—the cortex and the medulla. The cortex consists of three functional units that are related intimately by virtue of their overlapping control mechanisms emanating from the pituitary. The zona fasciculata forms 75% of the cortex. The fasciculata produces the main glucocorticoids, and the zona reticularis synthesizes minor adrenal androgenic steroids and minute amounts of estrone and estradiol. The zona glomerulosa produces aldosterone, which is the main mineralocorticoid.

Page 1115

Questions 22–25. Match each of the following statements with the best choice from the following agents used to treat hyperthyroidism. Each lettered response may be used once, more than once, or not at all.

    A. Radioiodine
    B. Thyroidectomy
    C. Antithyroid drugs
    D. β-Adrenergic blockers
    E. Iodine

22. Therapeutic effect lost with chronic use

23. Risk of hypoparathyroidism

24. Contraindicated in pregnancy

25. Used primarily to control symptoms

Answers: 22-E, 23-B, 24-A, 25-D

Critique: Radioiodine, surgery, and antithyroid drugs have been widely used for many years to treat hyperthyroidism. Each therapy has its benefits and risks. Radioiodine is the most commonly used treatment in adults. It should not be used in pregnant women because it crosses the placenta readily and can be concentrated by the fetal thyroid. Surgical removal of the thyroid is another option for the treatment of thyrotoxicosis. There is a 1% chance of iatrogenic hypoparathyroidism because of total removal of all of the parathyroid glands. Antithyroid drugs, such as propylthiouracil, can also be used. They are in general safe and relatively effective. There is a small risk of agranulocytosis. They are the preferred treatment during pregnancy. β-blockers, primarily propranolol, produces symptomatic relief in almost all patients with thyrotoxicosis. Iodine can be useful for acute treatment, but its therapeutic effect is lost with chronic use.

Pages 1097, 1098

Questions 26–29. Match each of the following statements with one of the following causes of hypoglycemia. Each lettered response may be used once, more than once, or not at all.

    A. Postprandial hypoglycemia
    B. Postabsorptive hypoglycemia
    C. Insulinoma
    D. Ketotic hypoglycemia

26. This is an exceedingly rare cause of hypoglycemia associated with low fasting glucose concentrations.

27. β-Blockers may offer relief of symptoms.

28. A common cause of hypoglycemia associated with acute alcohol intoxication

29. Benign, short-term starvation phenomenon of childhood

Answers: 26-C, 27-A, 28-B, 29D

Critique: Postprandial or reactive hypoglycemia occurs within 4 hours after a meal or glucose load. Preceding meals tend to be rich in carbohydrate (particularly simple carbohydrates) and devoid of protein. The most common complaints are symptoms of sympathetic discharge (tremulousness, inability to concentrate, sweating, and mental irritability) and, therefore, β-blockers may offer symptomatic relief. Postabsorptive hypoglycemia, defined as clinically low plasma glucose levels during the 12-hour postabsorptive period, can be caused by drugs (e.g., alcohol), critical organ failure, hormonal failure, non–β-cell tumors, endogenous hyperinsulinism, sepsis, and disorders peculiar to childhood. Insulinoma is exceedingly rare (1 in 1 million prevalence). A low fasting blood glucose associated with an inappropriately high insulin level establishes the diagnosis. Ketotic hypoglycemia of child-

hood is a usually benign, short-term starvation phenomenon associated with intercurrent illness.

Pages 1092, 1093

Questions 30–33. Match each of the following numbered statements with the correct laboratory test. Each lettered option may be used once, more than once, or not at all.

    A. Thyroid antibodies
    B. Serum thyroglobulin
    C. Serum TSH
    D. Free T4 index
    E. Radioactive iodine uptake test

30. Prudent to order prior to treating thyrotoxicosis with ^{131}I therapy

31. Yields a satisfactory estimate of free thyroxine levels

32. Usually rises early in primary hypothyroidism

33. Used to follow well-differentiated thyroid carcinomas

Answers: 30-E, 31-D, 32-C, 33-B

Critique: Many laboratory tests are available to measure specific aspects of thyroid function. The free T4 index is an estimate of the free thyroid hormone concentration, which is calculated using the measurement of the total serum T4 and thyroid-binding proteins. Serum TSH concentration is a highly sensitive test that can determine thyroid dysfunction, either hyperthyroidism or hypothyroidism, early in the course of the disease. Serum thyroglobulin measurements are of value primarily for the follow-up of people treated for well-differentiated thyroid carcinomas. Thyroid antibodies to thyroglobulin or to thyroid microsomes are useful for diagnosing Hashimoto's thyroiditis.

Page 1095

Questions 34–38. For each of the following numbered statements, select the most appropriate response.

    A. Sulfonylureas
    B. Biguanides
    C. Both A and B
    D. Neither A nor B

34. May cause an increase in glycogenolysis

35. Does not aggravate hyperinsulinemia

36. Increases insulin receptors

37. Increases intestinal absorption of glucose

38. Not associated with hypoglycemic reactions

Answers: 34-D, 35-B, 36-A, 37-B, 38-B

Critique: Two classes of oral agents are available to help in treating patients with NIDDM. The sulfonylureas act by stimulating the β cells and increasing insulin receptors.

Some second-generation agents may cause a decrease in glycogenolysis as well. Biguanides are represented by the newly released agent, metformin (Glucophage). Its action is not on the β islet cells; therefore, it does not aggravate hyperinsulinemia. It functions to reduce intestinal absorption and hepatic glucose output (gluconeogenesis) and to increase use of glucose in the peripheral tissues. It does not cause hypoglycemic reactions.

Pages 1085, 1086

Further Reading

Medical Management of Non-Insulin Dependent (Type II) Diabetes, 3rd ed. Alexandria, VA, American Diabetes Association, 1994, pp 40, 41.

Questions 39–42. For each of the following numbered statements, select the most appropriate response.

    A. Impaired glucose tolerance
    B. Potential abnormality of glucose tolerance
    C. Both A and B
    D. Neither A nor B

39. Exists when glucose concentrations are above normal but do not meet the criteria for the diagnosis of diabetes.

40. Increased likelihood for becoming a diabetic

41. Nondiabetic mother of a 10-lb infant

42. Individual with fasting serum glucose of 110 mg/dl on two separate occasions and an oral glucose tolerance test with the following glucose values:

Time (min)	mg/dl
Fasting	135
30	190
60	160
90	175
120	150

Answers: 39-A, 40-C, 41-B, 42-D

Critique: Besides diabetes of types I and II, several "near" diabetic conditions are recognized by the World Health Organization. *Impaired glucose tolerance* occurs when fasting glucose levels are consistently between 115 and 139 in otherwise healthy nonpregnant individuals and when a glucose tolerance test shows elevated but nondiagnostic levels of glucose. Approximately 25% of individuals with impaired glucose tolerance eventually develop diabetes. A *potential abnormality of glucose tolerance* occurs when an individual may be at risk for the development of diabetes but has no current evidence of the disease or impaired glucose tolerance. Examples include a homozygous twin of a patient with type II diabetes or a nondiabetic mother of an infant weighing more than 9 lb at birth.

Page 1075

Further Reading

Medical Management of Non-Insulin Dependent (Type II) Diabetes, 3rd ed. Alexandria, VA, American Diabetes Association, 1994, pp 5–11.

Questions 43–46 (True or False) Features of NIDDM include:

43. Age of onset less than 30 years of age

44. Rapid rate of onset

45. Ketosis is uncommon.

46. Prevalence is higher IDDM.

Answers: 43-F, 44-F, 45-T, 46-T

Criteria: The distinction between type I and II diabetes is sometimes difficult to make. According to the American Diabetes Association, a history of ketoacidosis or the detection of moderate to strong urine ketones in the presence of hyperglycemia is the most useful indicator of type I diabetes mellitus. In most cases, the age of onset of type II or NIDDM is over 40 years of age, the rate of onset is slow, and the prevalence is higher than 2% (compared with <0.5% for IDDM).

Pages 1075, 1077

Further Reading

Medical Management of Non-Insulin Dependent (Type II) Diabetes, 3rd ed. Alexandria, VA, American Diabetes Association, 1994, p 11.

Questions 47–51 (True or False) Common manifestations of diabetic neuropathy include:

47. Foot ulcers

48. Constipation

49. Bradycardia

50. Paresthesias

51. Urge urinary incontinence

Answers: 47-T, 48-F, 49-F, 50-T, 51-T

Critique: Diabetic neuropathy is common in both type I and type II diabetics. Three general types occur: (1) peripheral polyneuropathy, (2) mononeuropathy, and (3) autonomic neuropathy. Peripheral polyneuropathy primarily affects sensory fibers. Paresthesias, expressed as burning feet, tingling, and numbness, are characteristic manifestations. Insensitivity to mild trauma or compressive shoes may result in a foot ulcer, most commonly on the plantar aspect of the distal metatarsal. Autonomic neuropathy can be extensive. Besides causing diarrhea and tachycardia, it can cause hypotonicity of the bladder.

Page 1081

Questions 52–56 (True or False) In choosing appropriate antihypertensive agents for diabetics, the following factors should be considered:

52. Thiazide diuretics lower glucose levels.

53. β-Adrenergic blockers aggravate cholesterol levels.

54. α-Adrenergic blockers increase triglycerides.

55. ACE inhibitors have no adverse effect on carbohydrate metabolism.

56. Calcium channel blockers are considered to be a good first-line therapy.

Answers: 52-F, 53-T, 54-F, 55-T, 56-T

Critique: Thiazide diuretics elevate blood glucose and triglycerides and can result in frank diabetes. β-Adrenergic blockers aggravate cholesterol dyslipidemia and may cause hyperglycemia. They also blunt the gluconeogenic response to hypoglycemia and may mask the symptoms of hypoglycemia, depriving insulin-dependent diabetics of important protection. α-Blockers do not affect carbohydrate metabolism and may have a slight beneficial effect on serum lipids. Angiotensin-converting enzyme (ACE) inhibitors do not affect carbohydrate metabolism and may improve glucose tolerance. They may also have a beneficial effect on the development or progression of diabetic nephropathy. Calcium channel blockers have a neutral effect on glucose; thus, along with ACE inhibitors and α-blockers, they are considered reasonable first-step drugs for treating hypertension in diabetics.

Page 1088

Questions 57–61 (True or False) Acromegaly due to growth hormone excess causes striking clinical manifestations. These include:

57. Prognathism

58. Visual field defects

59. Anhidrosis

60. Diabetes insipidus

61. Nerve entrapment syndromes

Answers: 57-T, 58-T, 59-F, 60-F, 61-T

Critique: Clinical manifestations of acromegaly appear gradually, and they are striking. Headaches and visual field defects can occur if the pituitary tumor is large. Other features include prognathism, separation of the front teeth, coarse facial features, an increase in glove and foot size, deepening of the voice, nerve entrapment syndromes, and increased sweating or hyperhidrosis. Growth hormone causes insulin resistance, and about one fourth of acromegalic patients also develop diabetes mellitus. Diabetes insipidus is not related to growth hormone excess.

Page 1113

Questions 62–66 (True or False) Craniopharyngioma, a tumor arising from the cell rests of the craniopharyngeal canal, is characterized by:

62. Accelerated growth

63. Headaches

64. Delayed puberty

65. Visual symptoms

66. Composed of pituitary-type cells

Answers: 62-F, 63-T, 64-F, 65-T, 66-F

Critique: Craniopharyngioma is not a tumor arising from pituitary cells. It is an embryonic Rathke's pouch tumor derived from cell rests of the craniopharyngeal canal. In addition to growth failure, symptoms arise from increased intracranial pressure with headaches and visual symptoms. It is an infrequent cause of sexual precocity during childhood.

Page 1114

Questions 67–71 (True or False) Pheochromocytomas are tumors of chromaffin cells in the adrenal medulla that produce epinephrine or norepinephrine. Parameters of this condition include:

67. Most secrete epinephrine.

68. Paradoxic recumbent hypertension can occur.

69. Very few occur outside of the adrenal medulla.

70. Can be associated with neurofibromatosis

71. Should be suspected if hypertension is present with a family history of diabetes

Answers: 67-F, 68-F, 69-T, 70-T, 71-F

Critique: Most pheochromocytomas secrete norepinephrine despite the fact that 85% of the catecholamine of the normal adrenal is epinephrine. Orthostatic hypotension or paradoxic recumbent hypotension occurs as a manifestation of hypovolemia, refractoriness of overstimulated α₁-receptors, or vasodilatation caused by α₂-stimulation. Of pheochromocytomas, 90% occur in the adrenal medulla. Pheochromocytoma can be associated with neurofibromatosis and with retinal cerebellar hemangioblastosis, Von Hippel Lindau disease. Pheochromocytoma should be considered but not necessarily screened for whenever hypertension is first diagnosed. Suspicion is heightened if hypertension is present in a setting atypical for essential hypertension, such as young age of onset, lack of a family or personal history of hypertension, or diabetes.

Page 1123

Questions 72–76 (True or False) True statements about the evaluation of infertility include:

72. The cause lies in the male partner as frequently as it does in the female partner.

73. Hyperprolactinemia is a major cause of infertility in women.

74. Most women who are found to have tubal disease give a history of previous infections.

75. Ovulation can be confirmed by a basal body temperature (BBT) rise of 0.4° F in midcycle.

76. A positive result on a postcoital test would be finding at least 100 motile sperm per high-power field in an aspirated cervical specimen of mucus 8 hours after coitus.

Answers: 72-T, 73-F, 74-F, 75-T, 76-F

Critique: Infertility is the inability to conceive despite attempts to do so for 1 year. The causes in males and females are approximately equal. Prior to putting a woman through an expensive and potentially uncomfortable evaluation, a semen specimen should be obtained. Failure to ovulate and tubal abnormalities are the major causes of infertility in women. Many women who are found to have tubal disease or adhesion give no history of previous infections. Verification of ovulation can be documented by a BBT rise of 0.4° F in midcycle. A postcoital test is considered to be normal if at least five motile sperm per high-power field are seen.

Page 1131

42

Nutrition and Family Medicine

Donald E. Nease, Jr., and Emily R. Nease

1. A 30-year-old man recently moved to the area and comes to your office to establish his care. His history is significant for a generalized seizure disorder that has been well controlled on phenytoin (Dilantin). He is otherwise healthy. Which of the following nutritional supplements should you recommend?

    A. Ferrous sulfate (iron)
    B. Ascorbic acid
    C. Folic acid
    D. Niacin
    E. Riboflavin

Answer: C

Critique: Patients on phenytoin should receive vitamin supplementation. All patients should receive 0.4 to 1 mg/day of folic acid. If demineralization is present, vitamin D should be added. Pregnant women should receive vitamin D during pregnancy and vitamin K prior to delivery. Ascorbic acid and iron supplementation are indicated for chronic anti-inflammatory therapy. Niacin should be provided to patients taking rifampin. Riboflavin is recommended for patients on major tranquilizers.

Page 1140

2. A 75-year-old man is admitted to the hospital for resection of a carcinoma of the cecum. He appears malnourished and cachectic. Efforts to improve his nutritional status should be implemented to decrease the risk of postoperative complications. Vitamin C and zinc should be included in his nutritional support to:

    A. Improve postoperative wound healing
    B. Prevent high-output heart failure
    C. Decrease the risk of peripheral neuropathy
    D. Increase serum calcium levels
    E. Avoid hyperkalemia

Answer: A

Critique: Vitamin C and zinc deficiencies are associated with poor wound healing. Malnourished patients under-

going surgery should have supplementation with these nutrients as well as vigorous management of their caloric and protein requirements. Thiamine deficiency can cause heart failure. Deficiencies of chromium, B_{12}, B_6, and thiamine may be associated with neuropathy. Magnesium supplementation may be necessary to maintain serum calcium and protect against hypokalemia.

Pages 1143, 1144

3. Pellagra, a syndrome characterized by photosensitive dermatitis, diarrhea, tongue and mucosal inflammation, and dementia, results from a deficiency of:

    A. Thiamine (Vitamin B_1)
    B. Vitamin A
    C. Vitamin C
    D. Vitamin D
    E. Niacin

Answer: E

Critique: Diets seriously deficient in meat, poultry, or fish; legumes or grains; or dairy products may result in niacin deficiency. Niacin deficiency is the cause of pellagra. Scurvy is associated with vitamin C deficiency. Vitamin D deficiency can lead to rickets or osteomalacia. Thiamine deficiency causes beriberi. In alcoholics, neurologic manifestations including Wernicke's encephalopathy are seen in the United States. Vitamin A deficiency is associated with visual and skin problems.

Page 1143

4. A deficiency of folic acid may lead to:

    A. Megaloblastic anemia
    B. Seborrheic dermatitis
    C. Hemorrhagic problems
    D. Heart failure
    E. Peripheral neuropathy

Answer: A

Critique: Folic acid deficiency may result from diets low in green leafy vegetables, legumes, and whole grains. Clinical manifestations include megaloblastic anemia and glossitis. Vitamin B$_{12}$ deficiency also produces megaloblastic anemia and neurologic deficits of combined system disease. Vitamin K deficiency is associated with hemorrhagic problems; seborrheic dermatitis is seen with vitamin B$_6$ deficiency; and heart failure may occur with thiamine deficiency.

Page 1143

5. Which one of the following foods contains the most cholesterol?

    A. Peanut butter
    B. Yogurt
    C. Coconut oil
    D. Avocados
    E. Cashews

Answer: B

Critique: Cholesterol is a fat-like substance found only in animal products (meat, fish, poultry, milk products, and eggs). Of the foods listed, yogurt is the only animal product. The vegetable products listed contain various levels of fats but do not contain cholesterol.

Page 1152

6. The main reason to recommend limiting consumption of foods high in sugar is to prevent:

    A. Diabetes mellitus
    B. Undesirable weight gain
    C. Hyperactivity
    D. Dental caries

Answer: D

Critique: Reducing sugar intake, regular oral hygiene, and adequate fluoride intake are important to prevent dental caries. Sugars, especially sucrose, is a substrate for acid-producing bacteria that are responsible for tooth decay. Dietary fat is more important in controlling weight than sugars. There is no substantial evidence that sugar intake is related to hyperactivity. Diabetes mellitus is related to dietary factors, but simple sugars alone are not causative.

Pages 1153, 1154

7. Which nutrient do Americans routinely take in excess of the minimum requirement?

    A. Sodium
    B. Potassium
    C. Calcium
    D. Zinc
    E. Iron

Answer: A

Critique: The average sodium intake for adults in the United States is 4 to 6 g/day, which is at least eight times the minimum recommended intake. The average potassium intake barely exceeds minimum recommendations.

A proper balance of sodium and potassium intake may reduce the incidence of hypertension. Calcium, zinc, and iron are rarely taken in excess in otherwise healthy persons.

Pages 1154, 1155

8. Which of the following groups has a high risk of developing an iron deficiency?

    A. Breast-fed babies
    B. Toddlers
    C. Vegetarians
    D. Adult males

Answer: B

Critique: The prevalence of iron deficiency is highest in children 1 to 2 years of age, followed by adolescents, and then women of child-bearing years. Breast-feeding or use of iron-fortified formulas is an important safeguard against iron deficiency. Vegetarians get adequate iron from green leafy vegetables and other plant sources. Iron absorption from plant sources is enhanced by vitamin C. Adult males are not at significant risk of iron deficiency.

Pages 1154, 1167, 1168

9. Guidelines to reduce the incidence of spina bifida recommend that the diet should be supplemented with:

    A. Folic acid
    B. Vitamin C
    C. Vitamin E
    D. Niacin
    E. Riboflavin

Answer: A

Critique: Studies suggest that periconceptual supplementation with folic acid will reduce the incidence of spina bifida and other neural tube defects (NTD). All women, with a previous birth with an NTD, who are contemplating pregnancy should take an additional 4 mg/day of folic acid; otherwise, 0.4 to 1 mg/day of folic acid in the preconception period will reduce the risk of NTD in women contemplating pregnancy.

Pages 1157, 1158

10. Which of the following methods can be recommended to lactating mothers to increase milk production?

    A. Increase fluid intake over the demands of thirst.
    B. Drink a glass of wine before nursing to promote milk let-down.
    C. Increase the frequency and duration of nursing.
    D. Omit highly seasoned foods from the mother's diet.

Answer: C

Critique: Nutritional needs during lactation are important for the nursing mother and the breast-feeding infant. The mother's intake must be adequate to ensure an adequate quantity of nutritionally complete milk. Maintaining prenatal dietary recommendations is usually adequate for a woman to support lactation. Alcohol should be avoided, especially near times of nursing, because alcohol may inhibit the milk ejection reflex. Although weak evidence supports omitting foods from the maternal diet that may have untoward effects on the infant, such foods do not affect the production of milk. Adequate fluids are important to lactation; however, exceeding the demands of thirst will not increase milk production. Adequate maternal rest and nutrition combined with increased frequency and duration of nursing will usually increase milk production within 48 hours.

Pages 1159, 1160

11. Data on specific nutritional requirements of the elderly are limited; however, recent surveys and biochemical tests indicate that up to 20% of elderly persons may have deficiencies of:

A. Potassium
B. Vitamin E
C. Magnesium
D. Folate
E. Saturated fats

Answer: D

Critique: Data on specific nutritional requirements of the elderly are limited. Most recommendations are extrapolated from younger age groups. There is some indication that elderly individuals have increased needs for protein and vitamins B_6, B_{12}, and D. Recent surveys indicate that the elderly may have a low dietary intake of calcium and vitamin D. Biochemical tests indicate that up to 20% of elderly persons may have deficiencies of thiamine, riboflavin, iron, and folate.

Pages 1163–1165

12. A 25-year-old man presents for nutritional advice while training for a triathlon (cross-country running and long-distance swimming and biking). Appropriate recommendations for this athlete include:

A. A low-carbohydrate, high-protein diet while training
B. Modified carbohydrate loading (75 to 80% of calories from carbohydrates) for 4 days prior to competition
C. Daily protein supplements to ensure a positive nitrogen balance
D. Loading with rapidly absorbed sugars 30 minutes prior to competition
E. Superhydration 90 minutes prior to prolonged work-outs and competition

Answer: B

Critique: Nutritional requirements for athletes follow similar guidelines as for general health with some modifications based on the type of athletic training and competition. Endurance athletes require increased protein in the diet. A normally balanced diet with 10 to 15% of calories from protein will supply the necessary protein through increased intake to meet caloric needs. Endurance sports that require repeated bursts of maximal effort may benefit from a higher carbohydrate diet. Modified carbohydrate

loading is recommended for endurance sports starting 4 days prior to competition while gradually decreasing training time and resting the day prior to competition. Loading with rapidly absorbed sugars may stimulate insulin release, induce hypoglycemia, and impair performance. Superhydration can induce diuresis.

Page 1168

13. The foundation of any treatment plan for most non-insulin-dependent diabetics is to:

A. Achieve regular meals, consistency of intake, and close coordination of meals with oral hypoglycemics
B. Establish a diet program that results in weight reduction
C. Initiate a diet with at least 60% of calories derived from complex carbohydrate
D. Restrict foods to those with a low glycemic index
E. Coordinate a physical exercise program with dietary intake and administration of oral hypoglycemics or insulin

Answer: B

Critique: The foundation of any treatment plan for the 80 to 90% of noninsulin-dependent diabetics who are obese is weight reduction. Even a modest loss of weight will improve glycemic control. Improved glucose levels can be seen in patients on a hypocaloric diet even before weight loss occurs. Regular meals, consistency of dietary intake, and regular exercise are important in coordinating medications, developing good eating habits, and facilitating weight loss. The balance of carbohydrates, protein, and fat, including saturated versus unsaturated fats, must be individualized. In susceptible individuals, high carbohydrate diets may induce hypertriglyceridemia and lower high-density lipoprotein (HDL) cholesterol. The use of the glycemic index of foods has not proved helpful in most circumstances.

Pages 1173–1175

14. Weight loss and malnutrition frequently accompany many cancers. Which of the following agents may effectively promote weight gain in cachectic cancer patients?

A. Fluoxetine (Prozac)
B. Folic acid
C. Ascorbic acid
D. Megestrol (Megace)

Answer: D

Critique: Nutritional problems in patients with cancer and patients undergoing treatment for cancer present significant challenges for physicians providing care for these patients. Several studies have shown that the use of megestrol acetate (Megace) can produce weight gain in cachectic cancer patients by stimulating appetite and food intake and by decreasing nausea and vomiting. Specific nutrient deficiencies can also occur as a course of cancer therapy. For example, folic acid deficiency is common in patients being treated with methotrexate. Vitamin K deficiency may occur in patients with malabsorption or obstructive jaundice or after prolonged antibiotic therapy. Ascorbic acid may help with absorption of iron and other nutrients but is unlikely to produce significant improvement in weight and caloric intake in cancer patients.

Page 1181

Questions 15–18 (True or False)   Risk factors for poor nutritional status include:

15.   Recent weight loss of 5% or more of body weight

16.   Taking vitamin supplements

17.   Following a restrictive diet

18.   Recently starting a strict vegetarian diet

Answers: 15-T, 16-T, 17-T, 18-T

Critique: Risk factors are those characteristics that increase the likelihood of poor nutritional status developing over time. These risk factors include significant weight loss, which is defined as greater than or equal to 5% of body weight. Rapid weight loss such as this can be an indication of poor intake or poor utilization of nutrients. Vitamin supplements can cause problems if excessive intake occurs, especially of fat-soluble vitamins. The use of vitamin and mineral supplements is not necessary for most healthy persons who consume adequate, balanced diets. The most basic dietary guideline recommends eating a nutritionally adequate diet from a variety of foods. Self-imposed diet restrictions and even therapeutic diet restrictions can be modified to allow for adequate intake of all nutrients and non-nutrients in the diet. Generally, the more restrictive the vegetarian's diet is, the more likely it is to be deficient in one or more major nutrients. Adequate education is the key to reducing the risk of nutritional deficits.

Pages 1139, 1146, 1147, 1165, 1167, 1168, 1185

Further Reading

Stanfield PS: Nutrition and Diet Therapy, 2nd ed. Boston, MA, Jones and Bartlett Publishers, 1992, pp 4, 62.

Questions 19–23 (True or False)   To effectively promote adequate and appropriate nutritional intake, the family physician must understand the role of nutrition in health maintenance. Which of the following are points to consider when reviewing nutrition with patients?

19.   Five of the 10 leading causes of death are associated with dietary factors.

20.   Vitamin supplementation should be recommended for a healthy person whose diet meets the minimum recommended dietary allowances (RDAs) of most nutrients.

21.   Reducing total fat has been shown to facilitate a reduction in cholesterol as well as assisting with maintaining a desirable body weight.

22.   Hypervitaminosis usually occurs as a result of oversupplementation with water-soluble vitamins.

23.   Weight loss diets with less than 1200 kcal/day can meet RDAs for essential nutrients without supplementation.

Answers: 19-T, 20-F, 21-T, 22-F, 23-F

Critique: Five of the 10 leading causes of death (e.g., coronary artery disease; certain cancers, such as colon; stroke; diabetes mellitus; and atherosclerosis) are associated with dietary factors. Supplements are not routinely recommended for individuals whose diet meets minimum levels of RDAs for vitamins and minerals; however, diets restricted to less than 1200 calories may lead to deficiencies over time. In this case, supplementation is reasonable. Reducing total fat benefits cholesterol levels and avoids obesity. Although hypervitaminosis is uncommon, it is most likely to occur with oversupplementation with fat-soluble vitamins. Excessive water-soluble vitamins are readily excreted.

Pages 1147–1150, 1165

Questions 24–26 (True or False)   Several organizations have published dietary guidelines intended to promote a healthy lifestyle. The recommendations are remarkably similar and all recommend that individuals should "eat more food containing complex carbohydrates and fiber." Which of the following statements support this guideline?

24.   Fiber acts to dilute potential carcinogens and reduces travel time through the large intestine, thus decreasing the risk of colon cancer.

25.   Certain fiber components, characterized as soluble fiber, decrease blood glucose levels by delaying gastric emptying and reducing glucose absorption.

26.   Fiber-rich foods decrease stool bulk by assisting with the management of constipation and the prevention of diverticulosis.

Answers: 24-T, 25-T, 26-F

Critique: Food containing complex carbohydrates and fiber include whole grains, legumes, vegetables, fruits, nuts, and seeds. These foods are naturally lower in saturated fats. Fiber adds bulk to the stool, dilutes potential carcinogens, and decreases luminal pressure in the colon. These factors decrease constipation and protect the colon from diverticular changes and carcinogenesis. Components known as soluble fiber tend to reduce postprandial glucose and insulin levels.

Page 1153

Questions 27–30 (True or False)   Which of the following statements, as they relate to an infant's readiness to have solids introduced into the diet, are true?

27.   Solid food can be started when the infant has at least four teeth.

28.   Infants who demonstrate slow growth, particularly those younger than 4 months of age, should have solid food introduced to increase caloric intake.

29. Sufficient control of the head and neck to indicate refusal of food should be present prior to the introduction of solid food.

30. Infants who have a decreased extrusion reflex are ready for solid foods.

Answers: 27-F, 28-F, 29-T, 30-T

Critique: The timing of the introduction of solid foods to an infant's diet is always a concern for parents and physicians. The ability to properly consume solids is a developmental process. Developmental signs of readiness for solid food include sufficient control of the head and neck to indicate refusal of food, ability to sit up with little support, and a decreased extrusion reflex. For infants who demonstrate slow growth, particularly those younger than 4 months of age, increase the frequency and duration of milk feedings, not solid supplementation of their diet, to increase caloric intake.

Pages 1160, 1161

Questions 31–35 (True or False) Candidates for dietary intervention and counseling in order to reduce serum cholesterol include:

31. A 45-year-old man with a total cholesterol of 190 mg/dl and well-controlled hypertension on a calcium channel blocker

32. A 62-year-old woman, recently recovered from a nontransmural myocardial infarction, with a low-density lipoprotein (LDL) cholesterol of 110 mg/dl and no other risk factors for coronary artery disease

33. An asymptomatic 30-year-old woman who has no other risk factors for coronary artery disease but who had an LDL cholesterol level of 155 mg/dl that was discovered at a recent health fair at her place of employment

34. An obese 40-year-old man with recently diagnosed type II diabetes mellitus, well-controlled hypertension on an angiotensin-converting enzyme (ACE) inhibitor, and whose LDL cholesterol is 150 mg/dl

35. An asymptomatic 60-year-old woman with an LDL cholesterol of 190 mg/dl and no other risk factors for coronary artery disease

Answers: 31-F, 32-T, 33-F, 34-T, 35-T

Critique: The National Cholesterol Education Program recommends dietary interventions, combined with counseling and exercise, as the first line of treatment for hypercholesterolemia. Patients with high LDL cholesterol (>160 mg/dl); patients with moderate LDL cholesterol (130 to 160 mg/dl) and two additional risk factors for coronary artery disease; and patients with established coronary artery disease whose LDL cholesterol exceeds 100 mg/dl are candidates for dietary interventions. Patients with borderline total cholesterol or borderline LDL levels, but with fewer than two other risk factors for coronary artery disease, should be instructed in dietary modifications and exercise and re-evaluated in 1 year.

Page 1169

Questions 36–39 (True or False) A 17-year-old female presents to your office concerned about amenorrhea. She has not had a period in 8 months, denies recent sexual activity, but agrees to a pregnancy test that is negative. You note that she is very thin, bradycardiac, and mildly hypotensive. You suspect anorexia nervosa. True statements about this condition include:

36. Anorexia and other eating disorders are more common in dancers and athletes.

37. Treatment is almost always successful with tricyclic antidepressants.

38. As many as 50% of individuals with anorexia engage in behaviors associated with bulimia.

39. Anorexia is much more common than is bulimia.

Answers: 36-T, 37-F, 38-T, 39-F

Critique: Anorexia nervosa and bulimia are problems characterized by grossly disturbed eating behaviors with serious, and potentially fatal, consequences. Anorexia occurs in approximately 1% of the population; bulimia occurs in up to 9% of the population depending on the criteria for diagnosis; but the incidence of eating disorders in dancers and athletes may be as high as 30%. Anorectics divide about evenly between "restrictors" and "bulimics." Eating disorders are very challenging to treat. Pharmacologic therapy is not well established for anorexia; however, antidepressants may be of some benefit in depressed and nondepressed patients but are not curative.

Page 1180

Questions 40–44 (True or False) Chronic renal insufficiency is associated with a number of nutritional complications. In an effort to prevent nutritional complications associated with chronic renal insufficiency, which of the following recommendations are appropriate?

40. Modest protein restriction to 60 g/day of protein

41. Increased phosphorous intake to more than 800 mg/day

42. Potassium supplementation of 20 to 40 mEq/day

43. Calcium supplementation to achieve 1200 to 1600 mg/day

44. Buffers to correct metabolic acidosis associated with chronic renal insufficiency

Answers: 40-T, 41-F, 42-F, 43-T, 44-T

Critique: The goal of nutritional support in patients with chronic renal insufficiency is to slow the progression of kidney disease and to delay the need for dialysis while maintaining an adequate nutritional state. Patients with chronic renal insufficiency, especially in the predialysis phase, usually need buffers to correct metabolic acidosis, protein restriction, and careful monitoring of sodium and potassium balance. Restriction of potassium and cautious restriction of sodium are dependent upon serum values. Chronic renal insufficiency decreases phosphorous excretion and can lead to secondary hyperparathyroidism. Patients with chronic renal insufficiency often need to reduce their phosphorus intake and take phosphate binders such as calcium carbonate. Diets should be supplemented with calcium to maintain normal calcium balance.

Page 1182

Questions 45–48 (True or False) Patients who are unable to ingest adequate nutrition by mouth, but who otherwise have a functioning gastrointestinal tract, can receive adequate nutrition by tube feeding. Which of the following statements about enteral nutrition are true?

45. A nasogastric tube is the preferred route for patients requiring short-term feeding (less than 6 weeks).

46. Diabetic patients with gastroparesis can safely be nourished with nasogastric feedings.

47. Fiber-containing formulas consistently relieve the constipation that some patients experience on long-term enteral feedings.

48. Aspiration is one of the most serious complications of enteral feedings.

Answers: 45-T, 46-F, 47-F, 48-T

Critique: Patients who are unable to tolerate oral feedings can frequently achieve adequate nutrition through enteral alimentation. The two common methods are through nasogastric tubes or percutaneous feeding tubes, usually through a gastroenterostomy. Safe and effective use of enteral nutrition requires a relatively normally functioning gut. Conditions such as gastroparesis may preclude nasogastric feedings in certain patients. Patients requiring short-term feeding can usually be managed with a nasogastric tube or a nasoenteric tube. Patients who require long-term enteral nutrition (for more than 8 weeks) are better managed by an enterostomy tube. Nau-

sea, vomiting, constipation, and diarrhea are the most common complications or side effects associated with enteral feedings. Nausea and vomiting are frequently caused by rapid infusion of the nutrients. Constipation occurs in about 15% of patients. There is no clear evidence that fiber-containing formulas consistently relieve this problem. Aspiration is the most serious complication of enteral feedings but only occurs in approximately 1% of patients.

Pages 1185, 1186

Questions 49–52 (True or False) Metabolic complications associated with total parenteral nutrition, attributable to the large amounts of dextrose in these solutions, include:

49. Reactive hypoglycemia

50. Fatty infiltration of the liver

51. Thiamine deficiency

52. Azotemia

Answers: 49-F, 50-T, 51-T, 52-F

Critique: Patients requiring nutritional support, but who are unable to take nutrition orally and who have a nonfunctioning gut, frequently require parenteral or total parenteral nutrition (TPN). Parenteral nutrition includes dextrose, amino acids, lipids, electrolytes, vitamins, and trace minerals. The large amount of dextrose in TPN fluids is associated with hyperglycemia and may require insulin therapy. Fatty infiltration of the liver also occurs and may cause elevated enzymes. The requirements for thiamine are increased with the use of highly concentrated glucose solutions A relative thiamine deficiency may occur and result in lactic acidosis and peripheral neuropathy. Azotemia, seen with parenteral nutrition, is usually the result of excessive protein administration; however, it is frequently complicated by underlying problems, including dehydration and low cardiac output.

Pages 1186–1188

43

Gastroenterology

Richard Neill

1. (True or False) Which of the following conditions is present in more than 50% of patients aged 65 and over?
1. Diverticulosis
2. Hiatal hernia
3. Constipation
4. Colonic polyps

Answers: 1-T, 2-T, 3-T, 4-F

Critique: Surveys and autopsy studies confirm an incidence of more than 50% for diverticulosis, hiatal hernia, and constipation in persons older than 65 years of age. Colonic polyps, although more common in the elderly, do not approach this prevalence.

Page 1192

2. A previously healthy 16-year-old male presents to your office after 10 hours of severe abdominal pain. Which ONE of the following statements is true regarding the likelihood of a surgical condition as a cause for this patient's pain?

A. A normal white blood cell (WBC) count would rule out a surgical condition.
B. Duration of severe pain longer than 6 hours implies a surgical condition.
C. Increased bowel sounds imply a surgical condition.
D. Normal bowel movements make a surgical condition unlikely.

Answer: B

Critique: Sir Zachary Cope's *Early Diagnosis of the Acute Abdomen* suggests "The general rule can be laid down that the majority of severe abdominal pain which ensues in patients who have been previously fairly well, and which lasts as long as 6 hours, is caused by conditions of surgical import." Normal WBC counts and normal bowel movements do not rule out surgical conditions, although increased bowel sounds can be found in many nonsurgical conditions affecting the abdomen, such as viral gastroenteritis.

Page 1192

3. (True or False) Which of the following conditions are associated with high-fat, low-fiber diets?
1. Appendicitis
2. Irritable bowel syndrome
3. Hiatal hernia
4. Diverticulosis

Answers: 1-T, 2-T, 3-T, 4-T

Critique: Each of the aforementioned has been associated with high-fat, low-fiber diets and thus these diseases are often referred to as diseases of the Western civilization.

Page 1193

4. Which ONE of the following statements is true regarding appendicitis?

A. It is most common in the 5 to 10-year-old age group.
B. A temperature above 103°F is common early in the course.
C. Right lower quadrant ultrasound can rule out appendicitis.
D. Infertility is a complication of a perforated appendix in women.
E. The finding of red blood cells in the urine suggests appendicitis.

Answer: D

Critique: Women who survive a ruptured appendix have a fivefold increased risk of infertility. Appendicitis is most common in the 10- to 30-year-old age group. A mild elevation in temperature is common in appendicitis, but a temperature over 101°F makes other conditions more likely. Red blood cells in the urine suggest a urinary tract pathology such as nephrolithiasis, rather than appendicitis.

Pages 1193–1195

5. All of the following are true regarding cholelithiasis EXCEPT:

A. The presence of stones as seen on ultrasound defines cholelithiasis.
B. Most gallstones dissolve on their own if left alone.
C. Most gallstones are radiolucent.
D. Impaction of a gallstone in the common bile duct results in biliary colic.
E. Most patients with gallstones are asymptomatic.

Answer: B

Critique: Although most patients with gallstones are asymptomatic, gallstones do not dissolve on their own; rather, they tend to grow slowly and only rarely dissolve spontaneously. Because most gallstones consist of cholesterol, they are radiolucent. Impaction of stones in the cystic or common bile ducts is thought to be the cause of episodes of biliary colic.

Page 1195

Questions 6–12. Match each numbered question with the correct letter:

A. Right upper quadrant ultrasound
B. Technetium scintigraphy of the gallbladder
C. Both A and B
D. Neither A nor B

6. Assesses the excretory function of the liver and gallbladder

7. Assesses the patency of the cystic bile duct

8. Test of choice in determining the presence of gallstones

9. Alcoholic liver disease causes a high false-positive rate

Answers: 6-B, 7-C, 8-A, 9-B

Critique: Ultrasound allows for visualization of the structure of the gallbladder, cystic and common bile ducts, and the presence of gallstones but does not assess the function of the liver or gallbladder. Technetium scintigraphy requires hepatic excretion of technetium-labeled iminodiacetic acid into bile, which is concentrated in the gallbladder and then excreted into the duodenum. Failure to visualize the gallbladder after the injection of the technetium label implies a nonpatent cystic duct, regardless of whether stones are present. Alcoholism or other hepatic dysfunction can interfere with technetium label excretion into bile and, therefore, results in a false-positive test (i.e., nonvisualized gallbladder).

Page 1196

Further Reading

Green RA, Griner PF: Cholelithiasis and acute cholecystitis. *In Diagnostic Strategies for Common Medical Problems.* Philadelphia, American College of Physicians, 1991, pp 121–130.

10. All of the following statements are true regarding laparoscopic cholecystectomy EXCEPT:

A. Previous abdominal surgery is a relative contraindication.

B. The risk of bile duct injury is higher than with a conventional open cholecystectomy.
C. The hospital stay is typically 24 to 48 hours.
D. Intraoperative cholangiograms cannot be performed with a laparoscopic cholecystectomy.
E. The cost per patient for laparoscopic cholecystectomy is less than for open cholecystectomy.

Answer: D

Critique: Intraoperative cholangiograms can be performed with open and laparoscopic cholecystectomy. Previous abdominal surgery is a relative contraindication to laparoscopic cholecystectomy. The hospital stay is shorter; costs per patient are lower; and complication rates are lower for laparoscopic cholecystectomy, with the exception that bile duct injury may be slightly higher with laparoscopic cholecystectomy. This is may be due either to the steep learning curve for the procedure or to dissection of the duct with a laser versus an electrocautery.

Pages 1196, 1197

Further Reading

Roslyn JJ, Zinner MJ: Gallbladder and extrahepatic biliary surgery. *In* Schwartz SI, Shires GT, Spencer FC, Husser WC: *Principles of Surgery,* 6th ed. New York, McGraw-Hill, 1994, pp 1379–1380.

11. Colonic diverticuli are found in what percentage of patients older than 60 years of age?

A. Less than 10%
B. Between 10 and 30%
C. Between 30 and 60%
D. Between 60 and 80%
E. Over 80%

Answer: D

Critique: Over 60% of patients aged 60 and over have autopsy confirmed diverticuli.

Page 1197

Questions 12–15 (True or False). Evaluate the statements regarding diverticuli as true or false:
12. Most diverticuli remain asymptomatic.
13. Diverticuli are less common in vegetarians.
14. Hemorrhage from diverticuli typically occurs in the presence of acute diverticulitis.
15. The incidence of operative intervention in diverticulitis is less than 1%.

Answers: 12-T, 13-T, 14-F, 15-T

Critique: It is estimated that fewer than 25% of patients with diverticuli ever develop symptoms related to them. As with many other gastrointestinal (GI) disorders, diverticuli are associated with a high-fat, low-fiber diet. At least one study has confirmed a lower incidence in vegetarians. Hemorrhage from diverticuli typically occurs in the otherwise asymptomatic patient. Indeed, diverticular bleeding is a probable cause in 20 to 40% of patients who present with lower GI bleeding. The incidence of surgical intervention in diverticulitis is estimated to be approximately 0.4%.

Pages 1197, 1198

16. All of the following findings suggest diverticulitis EXCEPT:

    A. An elevated temperature
    B. Left lower quadrant abdominal pain
    C. A history of irritable bowel syndrome
    D. A tender mass in the left lower quadrant

Answer: C

Critique: Diverticulitis is characterized by left lower quadrant pain. The likelihood of diverticulitis rises with the presence of fever and a tender left lower quadrant mass. There is no association beteween diverticulitis and irritable bowel syndrome.

Page 1198

17. The test of choice in establishing the diagnosis of acute diverticulitis is which ONE of the following?

    A. Computed tomography (CT) scan of the abdomen
    B. Flexible sigmoidoscopy
    C. Colonoscopy
    D. Barium enema

Answer: A

Critique: A CT scan is the test of choice in establishing the diagnosis of acute diverticulitis. Sigmoidoscopy, colonoscopy, and barium enema are relatively contraindicated due to the risk of perforation with instrumentation.

Page 1198

18. All of the following are etiologies for pancreatitis EXCEPT:

    A. Hyperlipidemia
    B. Acetaminophen
    C. Alcoholism
    D. Trauma
    E. Cholelithiasis

Answer: B

Critique: Gallstones and alcoholism account for most episodes of acute pancreatitis; hyperlipidemia, trauma, neoplasm, hypercalcemia, and viral infection account for many of the remaining cases. Although many drugs can cause pancreatitis (e.g., thiazide diuretics, DDI), acetaminophen is not associated with pancreatitis.

Page 1200

19. A 43-year-old alcoholic male presents to your emergency room with a 3-day history of mid-upper back pain, which is relieved by lying down; nausea; vomiting; and light-colored, foul smelling stools. Of these findings, which is NOT consistent with the diagnosis of pancreatitis?

    A. Mid-upper back pain
    B. Pain relieved by lying down

    C. Nausea and vomiting
    D. Light-colored, foul-smelling stools
    E. History of alcoholism

Answer: B

Critique: Each of the findings except relief in the supine position is consistent with the diagnosis of pancreatitis. The pain of acute pancreatitis is typically improved by sitting and leaning forward.

Page 1200

20. All of the following are complications of acute pancreatitis EXCEPT:

    A. Diabetes mellitus
    B. Acute respiratory distress syndrome (ARDS)
    C. Pancreatic pseudocyst
    D. Intravascular volume depletion
    E. Parotitis

Answer: E

Critique: Parotitis is a common cause of elevated serum amylase but is not a complication of pancreatitis. Diabetes can result from islet cell damage from pancreatitis. Hypovolemia likely occurs due both to decreased intake and third space accumulation of fluids, putting patients at risk for other complications such as renal failure and shock. ARDS is a well-known complication of pancreatitis. Pseudocysts are late complications of pancreatitis, which often requires surgical intervention.

Page 1200

21. In children as in adults, the most common cause of **mechanical** bowel obstruction (in patients who have not experienced prior abdominal surgery) is which ONE of the following?

    A. Intussusception
    B. Adhesions
    C. Hernia
    D. Volvulus
    E. Cancer

Answer: C

Critique: Hernia is the most common cause of mechanical bowel obstruction in both children and adults. The remaining choices are possible, but less prevalent causes of mechanical obstruction.

Page 1202, Table 43–7

22. All of the following conditions are known to cause adynamic ileus EXCEPT:

    A. Opiates
    B. Hypothyroidism
    C. Diabetes
    D. Hypertension
    E. Appendicitis

Answer: D

Critique: Many conditions can cause adynamic ileus, as shown in Table 43–5. Uncomplicated hypertension alone is not known to cause ileus.

Page 1202, Table 43–5

Questions 23–26 (Matching). For the following questions, indicate the most appropriate lettered response:

    A. Inflammatory diarrhea
    B. Noninflammatory diarrhea
    C. A and B
    D. Neither A nor B

23. Rotavirus infection

24. More than five leukocytes per high-powered field on microscopic examination of stool

25. Lactose intolerance

26. Salmonella

Answers: 23-B, 24-A, 25-B, 26-A

Critique: The etiology of acute diarrheal syndromes can be classified as inflammatory or noninflammatory according to the presence or absence of WBCs on microscopic examination of the stool. More than five WBCs per high-powered field is indicative of an inflammatory process. Viral illnesses are typically noninflammatory (e.g., rotavirus), whereas many bacterial etiologies are inflammatory (e.g., salmonella). Lactose intolerance is a cause of noninflammatory diarrhea.

Page 1203, Table 43–8

27. Which ONE of the following is the most common complication of viral gastroenteritis in children?

    A. GI bleeding
    B. Dehydration
    C. Peritonitis
    D. Bacterial sepsis

Answer: B

Critique: Dehydration is the most common complication of acute diarrheal illness in children. When severe, dehydration can lead to cardiovascular collapse and death. GI bleeding is uncommon, although possible in viral gastroenteritis. Peritonitis and bacterial sepsis suggest other causes for diarrhea.

Page 1204

28. A 25-year-old single man presents to your office with a 2-day history of low-grade fever accompanied by nausea, vomiting, diarrhea (one to two watery stools every hour for the past day), and generalized abdominal cramps. He has had no contact with young children and has not changed his eating habits recently. The most likely cause of his acute diarrheal syndrome is which one of the following?

    A. Rotavirus
    B. Norwalk virus

    C. Staphylococcal food poisoning
    D. Adenovirus
    E. Crohn's disease

Answer: B

Critique: Norwalk virus is the most common cause of diarrheal illness in adults, whereas rotavirus affects mainly infants and young children. Adenovirus is a less common cause of diarrheal illness in children and adults. Staphylococcal food poisoning can cause similar symptoms but is less likely given the lack of exposure in the patient's history. Crohn's disease would not be a likely cause for watery diarrhea.

Page 1204

29. Metronidazole is an appropriate treatment for all of the following causes of diarrheal illness EXCEPT:

    A. *Clostridium difficile*
    B. Giardiasis
    C. Amebiasis
    D. Salmonella

Answer: D

Critique: Metronidazole can be used to treat each of these conditions except salmonella, which typically requires no antibiotic treatment. Indeed, antibiotics can increase the likelihood of a carrier state in patients with salmonella.

Page 1206, Table 43–10

30. Which of ONE the following statements regarding traveler's diarrhea is true?

    A. Prescribing penicillin V to be taken each day as prophylaxis will prevent traveler's diarrhea.
    B. Encouraging travelers to drink freely from native water supplies will enhance resistance to water-borne diarrheal illness.
    C. Antimotility agents are safe for use in dysenteric illness.
    D. Compounds such as kaolin-pectin (Kaopectate) and bismuth subsalicylate (Pepto-Bismol) are generally safe to take for traveler's diarrhea.

Answer: D

Critique: Symptomatic use of Kaolin-pectin or bismuth subsalicylate is generally safe in diarrheal illness. Although traveler's diarrhea is a common reason to use empirical antibiotics, prophylactic antibiotics are not recommended. Travelers should use bottled water rather than drink from native water supplies. Antimotility agents have been associated with toxic megacolon when used in dysenteric illness.

Page 1206

31. Upper GI bleeding is suggested by all of the following EXCEPT:

    A. Bright red blood on the toilet tissue or in the bowl after a bowel movement
    B. Melenic stools

C. Hematemesis

D. A positive test for occult blood on gastric aspirate

Answer: A

Critique: Bright red blood on the toilet tissue or in the toilet bowl after a bowel movement suggests bleeding from hemorrhoids and other anorectal sources rather than an upper GI hemorrhage. All of the other responses are common with upper GI hemorrhages of varying severity.

Page 1206

32. A 40-year-old man admitted yesterday to the hospital for hematemesis has been kept with nothing by mouth (NPO) overnight with a nasogastric tube to low wall suction. His hematocrit has remained stable, and he has had no further episodes of hematemesis. Which ONE of the following tests would be most helpful when establishing a diagnosis?

A. Barium swallow

B. CT scan of the abdomen with contrast

C. Colonoscopy

D. Esophagogastroduodenoscopy

E. Nasopharyngoscopy

Answer: D

Critique: Most patients who exhibit evidence of upper GI bleeding eventually receive upper endoscopy for diagnostic purposes. Although barium imaging can also reveal causes for bleeding, the ability to combine therapeutic maneuvers with a diagnosis accounts for endoscopy being the test of choice for evaluation of upper GI bleeding. A CT scan of the abdomen and colonoscopy are more helpful for evaluation of lower GI bleeding. Nasopharyngeal bleeding is an uncommon cause of hematemesis in the absence of nasal bleeding.

Page 1207

33. Among the following, the LEAST likely cause of massive lower GI bleeding is:

A. Diverticuli

B. Angiodysplasia of colonic vessels

C. Ischemic colitis

D. Colon cancer

E. Ulcerative colitis

Answer: E

Critique: Answers A through D are among the most common causes of massive lower GI bleeding. Ulcerative colitis tends to cause slow lower GI blood loss in the midst of exacerbations of the colitis.

Page 1208

34. A 65-year-old woman is brought to the emergency room complaining of lightheadedness since her episode of hematochezia earlier in the day. Her blood pressure is 80/60, and her pulse is 110. She is otherwise alert. Which ONE of the following should you do first in your management plan?

A. Colonoscopy

B. Flexible sigmoidoscopy

C. Establishment of an airway

D. Insertion of two large-bore intravenous catheters

E. Placement of a nasogastric tube

Answer: D

Critique: In this patient with an established airway, fluids for support of her blood pressure should be the first management step. Diagnostic testing such as endoscopy should be performed once the patient is more stable.

Page 1208

Questions 35–38. Match each numbered question with the correct letter:

A. Internal hemorrhoids

B. External hemorrhoids

C. Both A and B

D. Neither A nor B

35. Originate proximal to the dentate line

36. Drain into the iliac veins

37. Present with blood-streaked stool or toilet tissue

38. Treated by some physicians with ligation (banding)

Answers: 35-A, 36-B, 37-C, 38-A

Critique: Internal hemorrhoids lie proximal to the dentate line, are less likely to cause pain than external hemorrhoids, and are sometimes treated with ligation, although this treatment has declined over the last 10 years due to reports of death from ligation of internal hemorrhoids. Both internal and external hemorrhoids can present with blood-streaked stool or toilet tissue. External hemorrhoids drain into the iliac veins, whereas internal hemorrhoids drain into the inferior mesenteric plexus.

Pages 1208, 1209

Questions 39–43 (True or False). Which of the following tests does the American Cancer Society recommend for screening for colon cancer in asymptomatic individuals at average risk?

39. Digital rectal examination annually after 40 years of age

40. Flexible sigmoidoscopy every 3 to 5 years after 50 years of age

41. Colonoscopy every 3 to 5 years after 50 years of age

42. Stool blood test annually after 50 years of age

43. Serum carcinoembryonic antigen (CEA) every 5 years after 60 years of age

Answers: 39-T, 40-T, 41-F, 42-T, 43-F

Critique: The American Cancer Society recommends three tests for the early detection of colon and rectal cancer in the asymptomatic individual who is at an average risk. A digital rectal examination by a physician during an office visit should be performed every year after the age of 40; the stool blood test is recommended every year after 50 years of age; and sigmoidoscopy, preferably flexible, should be performed every 3 to 5 years after 50 years of age. Colonoscopy is used in the evaluation of positive screening tests but is not recommended for screening itself. Serum CEA is a tumor marker in some colon cancers. It is not recommended by any organization for screening.

Page 1210

Further Reading

American Cancer Society Early Detection Guidelines, as published on the internet 1996 <http://www.cancer.org/detect.html>. (The reader should check this World Wide Web site for updates and changes.)

44. Which ONE of the following suggests an abnormal cause for neonatal jaundice in a term infant?

    A. An increase in bilirubin of less than 5 mg/dl/day
    B. A direct bilirubin of 0.8 mg/dl
    C. Total bilirubin of 6 mg/dl on day 2 of life
    D. Total bilirubin of 10 mg/dl at 12 hours of age

Answer: D

Critique: With "physiologic" jaundice, the bilirubin level rarely rises more than 5 mg/dl/day, is usually associated with a direct bilirubin level of less than 2 mg/dl, and gives initial bilirubin levels typically less than 6 in the first 24 hours of life for a term infant.

Page 1211

45. Which ONE of the following is NOT a cause for abnormal neonatal jaundice?

    A. Cephalohematoma
    B. Polycythemia
    C. Sepsis
    D. Cryptorchidism
    E. Isoimmunization

Answer: D

Critique: When neonatal jaundice exhibits unusual characteristics, a working differential diagnosis should include hemorrhage, isoimmunization, infection, polycythemia, and congenital liver damage. Cryptorchidism (failure of descent of one of both testes) is not associated with hyperbilirubinemia.

Page 1211

Questions 46–50. Match each numbered question with the appropriate lettered response:

    A. Hepatitis A
    B. Hepatitis B
    C. Cytomegalovirus hepatitis
    D. Drug-induced hepatitis
    E. Mononucleosis-associated hepatitis

46. Epstein-Barr virus

47. Immunocompromised patients

48. Passive immunization with immune globulin used to reduce spread among contacts

49. Lacks serum antibody markers

50. Active immunization with virus specific vaccine

Answers: 46-E, 47-C, 48-A, 49-D, 50-B

Critique: Epstein-Barr virus is the etiologic agent of mononucleosis-induced hepatitis. Drug-induced hepatitis generates no serum specific antibody response. Hepatitis A contacts may be passively immunized with immune globulin, while patients wanting to prevent spread of hepatitis B can be immunized with hepatitis B specific vaccine (Heptavax). Cytomegalovirus hepatitis is more common among immune compromised individuals.

Pages 1212–1214

51. Which of the following serum markers for hepatitis B always reflects active infection?

    A. Hepatitis B core antigen immunoglobulin (Ig)G
    B. Hepatitis B e antigen IgG antibody
    C. Hepatitis B surface antigen IgG antibody
    D. Hepatitis B e antigen
    E. Hepatitis B core antigen IgM antibody

Answer: D

Critique: Hepatitis B e antigen suggests current active infection. Persistence of this antigen defines the carrier state. Each of the others is present to varying degrees during the resolution of active hepatitis.

Page 1213

52. Which of the following is useful in the treatment of chronic hepatitis B?

    A. Interferon
    B. Acyclovir
    C. Zidovudine
    D. Acetaminophen

Answer: A

Critique: Interferon has demonstrated benefit in treatment of chronic hepatitis caused by both hepatitis A and B viruses. Although acyclovir and zidovudine are both antiviral agents, they, like acetaminophen, can be hepatotoxic and have no use in the treatment of chronic hepatitis.

Page 1213

Further Reading

Wong DKH, Cheung AM, O'Rourke K, et al: Effect of alpha-interferon in patients with hepatitis B e antigen-positive chronic hepatitis B: A meta-analysis. N Engl J Med 119:312–323, 1993.
Wong JB, Koff RS, Tinè F, Pauker SG: Cost-effectiveness of interferon$_{\alpha 2b}$ treatment for hepatitis B e antigen-positive chronic hepatitis B. N Engl J Med 122:664–675, 1995.

Questions 53–57. Match the one lettered response that best describes the condition:

A. Odynophagia
B. Achalasia
C. Dysphagia
D. Globus hystericus
E. Schatzki's ring

53. Failure of normal relaxation of the lower esophageal sphincter

54. Painful swallowing

55. Difficulty swallowing

56. Anatomic band of tissue at the lower esophageal sphincter

57. Fullness in the throat without difficulty swallowing

Answers: 53-B, 54-A, 55-C, 56-E, 57-D

Critique: Odynophagia describes painful swallowing, whereas dysphagia indicates difficulty swallowing. Patients with globus hystericus complain of fullness in the throat without difficulty swallowing. Achalasia describes a rare abnormal condition of the lower esophageal sphincter in which the sphincter fails to relax normally, resulting in a dilated lower esophagus with few contractions. Schatzki's ring describes a circumferential band of tissue located at the squamocolumnar junction in the esophagus.

Page 1215

58. Which ONE of the following is NOT a complication of dysphagia in the poststroke patient?

A. Dental caries
B. Weight loss
C. Aspiration pneumonia
D. Malnutrition
E. Death

Answer: A

Critique: Weight loss, aspiration pneumonia, malnutrition, and death are all reported complications of dysphagia in the poststroke patient. Dental caries is not a complication of dysphagia, although it is prevalent in elderly patients. Indeed, dental caries can interfere with proper chewing mechanics and thus cause dysphagia.

Page 1215

Questions 59–62 (True or False). Which of the following statements is/are true with respect to Barrett's esophagus?

59. Described histologically by columnar epithelium extending into the lower esophagus

60. Associated with an increased risk of cancer of the esophagus

61. Caused by overuse of aluminum-containing antacids

62. An initial negative biopsy allows subsequent management with medication alone.

Answers: 59-T, 60-T, 61-F, 62-F

Critique: Barrett's esophagus describes the finding of columnar epithelium extending up into the esophagus, displacing the normal squamous epithelial covering. It results frequently from chronic GI reflux, not antacid use. Management includes repeated biopsy every 1 to 2 years to identify dysplasia, which represents a precursor for carcinoma.

Page 1215

63. Which ONE of the following is LEAST useful in the evaluation of dysphagia?

A. Cine-esophagram (swallowing study)
B. Nasopharyngoscopy
C. Esophagoscopy
D. Esophageal manometry

Answer: B

Critique: The usual diagnostic sequence for evaluation of dysphagia would include esophagoscopy followed, if necessary, by a swallowing study and manometry. Of the choices provided, nasopharyngoscopy is least likely to yield clues to the diagnosis.

Page 1216

64. (True or False) Which of the following medicines are associated with non-ulcer dyspepsia?

A. Theophylline
B. Nitrates
C. Atropine
D. Acetaminophen

Answers: 1-T, 2-T, 3-T, 4-F

Critique: Any medications that lower the pressure at the lower esophageal sphincter are likely to cause non-ulcer dyspepsia. Methylxanthines, β-adrenergics, and anticholinergics act through this mechanism. Nonsteroidal anti-inflammatory drugs (NSAIDs) can produce dyspepsia through prostaglandin-mediated mucosal injury. Acetaminophen is not associated with non-ulcer dyspepsia.

Page 1217

65. All of the following place a patient at increased risk for gastric malignancy as a cause for dyspepsia EXCEPT:

A. Female gender
B. Age over 70
C. Vomiting
D. Previous ulcer
E. Hiatal hernia present

Answer: A

Critique: Increasing age, vomiting, male sex, smoking, and the presence of hiatal hernia or history of previous ulcer are all part of a scoring system for predicting the risk for malignancy.

Page 1217, Table 43–16

Questions 66–70 (True or False). A 45-year-old man presents to your office complaining of epigastric pain and bloating that occur 30 minutes after meals and are relieved by eating. He denies any radiation of the pain, nausea, vomiting, or heartburn. He has been awakened by the pain during the last few nights and has taken over-the-counter antacids, which have provided him with some relief. Which of the following initial management plans would be appropriate?

66. Cimetidine (Tagamet) 400 mg twice daily for 6 weeks

67. Omeprazole (Prilosec) 20 mg/day for 2 weeks

68. Misoprostol (Cytotec) 100 mg after meals and at bedtime for 6 weeks

69. Amoxicillin 500 mg four times daily for 6 weeks

70. Famotidine (Pepcid) 40 mg/day for 6 weeks

Answers: 66-T, 67-F, 68-F, 69-F, 70-T

Critique: Appropriate initial empirical therapy for presumed peptic ulcer disease includes H_2-antagonists, including cimetidine, ranitidine, famotidine, and nizatidine, as well as proton pump blockers such as omeprazole. Assuming that the patient responds satisfactorily, therapy should be continued for 6 to 8 weeks. Misoprostol is indicated for treatment of NSAID-induced ulcer disease. Amoxicillin, like metronidazole, tetracycline, and bismuth subsalicylate, treats *Helicobacter pylori.* However, none of these agents is indicated for sole use as treatment for *H. pylori*–associated peptic ulcer disease.

Page 1218, Table 12–17

71. Which ONE of the following does not carry a Federal Drug Administration (FDA)-approved indication for maintenance therapy in patients with peptic ulcer disease?

  A. Cimetidine
  B. Ranitidine
  C. Omeprazole
  D. Sucralfate
  E. Famotidine

Answer: C

Critique: While effective in the initial treatment of ulcer disease, omeprazole does not carry an indication for maintenance therapy, as do the H_2-blockers and sucralfate.

Pages 1218, 1219

72. Endoscopy for gastroesophageal reflux disease (GERD) has a sensitivity of approximately 50% and a specificity of 100%. Which ONE of the following is the most common finding on endoscopy for GERD?

  A. Schatzki's ring
  B. Barrett's esophagus
  C. No abnormal findings
  D. Erosive esophagitis
  E. Hiatal hernia

Answer: C

Critique: While hiatal hernia is a common finding when erosive esophagitis is present, most patients with reflux esophagitis do not have visible findings on endoscopy. Schatzki's ring and Barrett's esophagus tend to develop only after years of reflux, and even then occur in only a few patients with GERD.

Page 1219

73. Medications with FDA-approved indications for GERD include all of the following EXCEPT:

  A. Metoclopromide
  B. Cisapride
  C. Omeprazole
  D. Sucralfate
  E. H_2-blockers

Answer: D

Critique: Motility-enhancing agents such as metoclopromide and cisapride carry indications for GERD, as do H_2-blockers and omeprazole. Sucralfate, although often used as a slurry for GERD, carries no indication for this use.

Page 1219

Further Reading

Gastrointestinal drugs. *In* Drug Facts and Comparisons. St. Louis, MO, Wolters Kluwer, 1995, pp 1746, 1770, 1782, 1791, 1798

74. A 25-year-old man treated by you for GERD with metoclopromide (Reglan) presents to the emergency room complaining of severe neck spasm. Of the following initial treatment options, which ONE would be most appropriate?

  A. Cisapride (Propulsid)
  B. Diphenhydramine (Benadryl)
  C. Epinephrine (Adrenalin)
  D. Diazepam (Valium)
  E. Ibuprofen (Motrin)

Answer: B

Critique: This patient has symptoms of torticollis, a common extrapyramidal reaction due to metoclopromide. Extrapyramidal symptoms are seen in 10 to 30% of patients treated with metoclopromide. Diphenhydramine is used as an appropriate initial treatment. Diazepam therapy is reserved for more refractory cases. Epinephrine is rarely used for extrapyramidal symptoms. Cisapride is another agent for use in GERD but not for treatment of its complications. NSAIDs such as ibuprofen are not indicated for treatment of extrapyramidal symptoms.

Page 1220

75. Which ONE of the following describes the pathologic features of ulcerative colitis?

  A. Skip areas
  B. Full-thickness involvement of the colonic wall

C. Perianal fistulas with burrowing and abscesses
D. Well-defined etiologic agent
E. Involves the rectum in more than 95% of cases

Answer: E

Critique: Ulcerative colitis is characterized by a single continuous area of mucosal inflammation (sparing the full thickness of the bowel wall) that involves the rectum in more than 95% of cases and spreads proximally, but never further than the cecal valve. Choices A and C describe Crohn's disease. The etiologies of both Crohn's disease and ulcerative colitis are unknown.

Page 1221

76. All of the following are extraintestinal manifestations of inflammatory bowel disease EXCEPT:

A. Ankylosing spondylitis
B. Iritis
C. Nondeforming arthritis
D. Erythema nodosum
E. Café au lait spots

Answer: E

Critique: Extraintestinal manifestations of inflammatory bowel disease occur in up to 5% of patients and often assist in differentiating inflammatory from irritable bowel disease. Ankylosing spondylitis, iritis, nondeforming arthritis, pyoderma gangrenosum, and erythema nodosum are common extraintestinal manifestations. Café au lait spots are associated with neurofibromatosis.

Page 1221

Questions 77–80. Match each numbered question with the correct letter:

A. Irritable bowel disease
B. Inflammatory bowel disease
C. Both A and B
D. Neither A nor B

77. Presents with constitutional symptoms in addition to abdominal pain

78. Polymorphonuclear leukocyte infiltration of mucosa on biopsy

79. Normal barium enema

80. Treated with NSAIDs such as ibuprofen

Answers: 77-B, 78-B, 79-A, 80-D

Critique: Inflammatory bowel disease is more likely to present with constitutional symptoms such as weight loss, anemia, and fever. A biopsy of involved mucosa in inflammatory bowel disease shows infiltration of polymorphonuclear WBCs, whereas there are no abnormal findings on endoscopy or barium enema with irritable bowel syndrome. NSAIDs are not indicated in the treatment of either inflammatory bowel disease or irritable bowel disease.

Page 1222

81. A 19-year-old female college student presents to your office complaining of abdominal pain that she has had for 3 weeks and that is associated with alternating constipation and diarrhea. The patient's symptoms began around the time of her final examination. Her physical examination is unremarkable. Appropriate treatment modalities for this patient include all of the following EXCEPT:

A. Psyllium (Metamucil)
B. Dicyclomine (Bentyl)
C. Reassurance
D. Sulfasalazine (Azulfidine)
E. Stress reduction techniques

Answer: D

Critique: Irritable bowel syndrome can be treated with a number of agents for symptomatic relief, including bulk agents such as psyllium, and antispasmodics like dicyclomine. Stress reduction techniques and reassurance can also help the patient to reduce the bowel's response to stress. Sulfasalazine is used for treatment of inflammatory bowel disease and has no place in the treatment of irritable bowel disease.

Pages 1223, 1224, Table 43–18

44

Oncology

Francis P. Kohrs

Questions 1–4. Match items 1 through 4 to the group of carcinogenic agents listed below:

    A. Mutagens
    B. Mitogens
    C. Both A and B
    D. Neither A nor B

1. Cause damage to deoxyribonucleic acid (DNA)

2. Induce cell proliferation and growth

3. Oxyradicals

4. Cytochrome P-450 system

Answers: 1-A, 2-B, 3-A, 4-D

Critique: Carcinogenic agents may be categorized as genotoxic agents or as nongenotoxic agents. Genotoxic agents act by causing DNA damage. Mitogens are nongenotoxic agents and act by causing proliferation and growth of cells rather than DNA damage. The mechanism of action of oxyradicals is to bind to DNA and cause chromosomal damage, not induction of cell proliferation and growth. The cytochrome P-450 system is neither a mutagen nor a mitogen but is rather an enzyme system that metabolizes and detoxifies compounds. The cytochrome P-450 system is also a common mechanism for activating chemical compounds into mutagenic carcinogens.

Page 1228

5. (True or False) Oxyradicals are characterized by which of the following?

    1. They are formed during normal cellular pathways.
    2. Inflammatory processes may cause a decrease in production.
    3. They may be induced by other carcinogens such as asbestos and cigarette smoke.
    4. Their mechanism of action is to bind to DNA.
    5. They are produced by ionizing radiation that interacts with cellular contents.

Answers: 1-T, 2-F, 3-T, 4-T, 5-T

Critique: Oxyradicals are activated oxygen species that are becoming increasingly recognized as mediators of cell damage, including carcinogenesis. They act by binding to and altering DNA. They may be formed during normal cellular metabolic processes, such as lipid metabolism, and their rate of production may be increased by inflammatory processes or by certain other carcinogens, including asbestos, cigarette smoke, and ionizing radiation. Ionizing radiation generates oxyradicals by interaction with cellular contents such as water.

Page 1228

Questions 6–10. Match each of the following viral agents to the cancer with which it is associated:

    A. Human T-cell lymphotropic virus type I (HTLV-I)
    B. Epstein-Barr virus
    C. Human papillomavirus
    D. Hepatitis B virus

6. Hepatocellular carcinoma

7. Cervical cancer

8. Nasopharyngeal cancer

9. T-cell leukemia

10. Burkitt's lymphoma

Answers: 6-D, 7-C, 8-B, 9-A, 10-B

Critique: Viral agents are implicated as being the cause of several cancers. The hepatitis B virus has been associated with hepatocellular carcinoma; Epstein-Barr virus has been associated with both Burkitt's lymphoma and nasopharyngeal carcinoma; human papillomavirus and herpes simplex virus type 2 are associated with cervical cancer, and HTLV-I is associated with human T-cell leukemia and lymphoma.

Page 1229

11. (True or False) A 2-year-old male is brought to the office for well child care. The child has had normal growth and development previously. Strabismus is noted on the physical examination. An examination of the eye is difficult to accomplish, and although a red reflex is seen in the right eye, none can be elicited from the left eye. You consider that these findings might represent retinoblastoma. Which of the following are correct:

1. The median age of diagnosis of retinoblastoma is 2 years of age.
2. Retinoblastoma occurs as a result of mutations in tumor suppressor genes.
3. There are two copies of the retinoblastoma tumor suppressor gene, both of which must be inactivated to allow for the tumor to develop.
4. The sporadic form of retinoblastoma is more common than is the hereditary form.

Answers: 1-T, 2-T, 3-T, 4-F

Critique: Retinoblastoma is a congenital malignancy of embryonic retinal cells. The median age at diagnosis is 2 years of age, and 80% are diagnosed before 4 years of age. Leukocoria (a whiteness in the pupillary area) is the most common presenting sign, and lack of a normal red reflex may indicate retinoblastoma. Strabismus is the second most common presenting clinical sign. Retinoblastoma is the prototype for understanding tumor suppressor genes. Both of two copies of the retinoblastoma gene (Rb) must be damaged in order for the tumor to manifest itself. The hereditary form is much more common than is the sporadic form. Patients with a family history of retinoblastoma should be screened under anesthesia by an ophthalmologist every 2 to 3 months during early childhood.

Page 1230

Further Reading

Schwartz C: Cancers in childhood. *In* Hockelman RA, Friedman SB, Nelson NM, Seidel HM (Eds): Primary Pediatric Care, 2nd ed. St. Louis, MO, Mosby-Year Book, 1992, pp 1161–1162.

12. Considering dysplastic lesions, which of the following statements is *not* correct?

A. They are confined to the epithelial surface.
B. They exhibit histologic dysplastic features.
C. They extend beyond the basement membrane.
D. They may regress spontaneously, remain stable, or advance to invasive cancer.

Answer: C

Critique: Dysplastic lesions are preneoplastic lesions that are confined to the epithelial surface and exhibit dysplastic features on histologic examination. They may regress, remain stable, or advance to become an invasive cancer. Since dysplastic lesions are preneoplastic, they do not extend beyond the basement membrane. Breach of the basement membrane signals the transition from a premalignant to a malignant lesion.

Page 1232

Questions 13–16. For each of the following cancers, select the sites where metastasis most commonly occurs:

A. Liver and lungs
B. Bone
C. Brain and adrenal glands

13. Breast cancer

14. Lung cancer

15. Prostate cancer

16. Colorectal cancer

Answers: 13-B, 14-C, 15-B, 16-A

Critique: Fewer than 0.01% of circulating tumor cells form metastases. Some cancers exhibit tropisms for various body sites and tissues. Breast and prostate cancer commonly metastasize to bone. Lung cancer commonly metastasizes to the brain and the adrenal glands. Colorectal cancers commonly metastasize to the liver and lungs.

Page 1233

17. A 35-year-old man presents to your office for a cancer check-up. His family history is significant for colon cancer in his mother and brother. His mother died of colon cancer at the age of 65, and his brother was diagnosed with cancer of the colon at 40 years of age. The patient's review of body systems, past medical history, other family history, and social history are otherwise unrevealing. According to the American Cancer Society guidelines, the patient should have which of the following screening services performed for a complete cancer screening?

A. Examination of the testicles and skin
B. Examination of the testicles, skin, and thyroid
C. Examination of the testicles, skin, thyroid, oral region, and lymph nodes
D. Examination of the testicles, skin, thyroid, oral region, lymph nodes, and colonoscopy

Answer: D

Critique: According to the American Cancer Society guidelines, a complete cancer screening for an asymptomatic male between 20 and 40 years of age includes an examination of the testicles, skin, thyroid, oral region, and lymph nodes. However, this individual is at high risk for colon cancer because of his family history of colon cancer in two first-degree relatives. Individuals at high risk for colon cancer should receive a colonoscopy beginning at least 5 years before the earliest familial cancer.

Pages 1233, 1234

18. Chemotherapy administered prior to irradiation or surgery may improve local control of the tumor and can be used to assess tumor response to the chemotherapeutic agent. This type of chemotherapy is:

A. Adjuvant
B. Neoadjuvant
C. Brachytherapy
D. Unable to treat metastatic disease

Answer: B

Critique: Neoadjuvant chemotherapy is administered prior to a definitive local procedure at the primary site of the carcinoma. The purpose of the neoadjuvant chemotherapy is to improve local control so that a more conservative procedure can be performed in order to assess the tumor's response to the chemotherapeutic agent and to provide for early control of systemic (metastatic) disease. Adjuvant chemotherapy is administered after removal of the primary tumor when there is no gross evidence of residual disease. Brachytherapy refers to the implantation of a radiation source into or near a tumor. One aim of both adjuvant and neoadjuvant chemotherapy is treatment of clinically inapparent metastatic disease.

Page 1235

19. All of the following factors are associated with increased risk of breast cancer EXCEPT:

    A. Family history of breast cancer
    B. Early age at menarche
    C. Nulliparity
    D. Early onset of menopause
    E. Excessive alcohol intake

Answer: D

Critique: Multiple factors are associated with an increased risk of breast cancer, including a family history of breast cancer in a first- or second-degree relative, early menarche, few or no pregnancies, delayed menopause, obesity, radiation, and excessive alcohol usage. However, 70% of women with breast cancer have no identifiable risk factor.

Page 1237

20. A 58-year-old woman comes to the office for an annual health maintenance examination. She is fit and healthy and has no significant medical problems. She is not taking medication at this time. On physical examination, palpation of the breast reveals a 1- to 2-cm mass in the left breast. There is no asymmetry of the breast or lymphadenopathy. She has no evidence of metastatic disease. Two weeks prior to her visit, she had a negative screening mammogram. Which of the following statements regarding this patient is true?

    A. A negative diagnostic mammogram would exclude breast cancer as a cause for the mass in this patient.
    B. Benign cysts are common in postmenopausal women.
    C. Fine needle aspiration or an incisional biopsy will be required for a work-up of the mass in this patient.
    D. Fine needle aspiration or an excisional biopsy will be required for a work-up of the mass in this patient.

Answer: D

Critique: Benign breast masses are uncommon in postmenopausal women. A negative result on a screening or diagnostic mammogram would not exclude breast carcinoma as a cause of the mass. The appropriate next step

in the work-up of a breast mass palpated on physical examination in a woman older than 35 years of age is a diagnostic mammogram. Either fine needle aspiration by an experienced cytologist or an excisional biopsy would then be done. An incisional biopsy should be done only if the mass is too large to be removed or if there is evidence of metastatic disease.

Page 1237

21. A 23-year-old woman presents with a palpable breast mass. She is otherwise fit and healthy. Her only medication includes an oral contraceptive agent. She tells you that the mass has been present for the last 6 weeks. On physical examination you palpate a 1-cm mass in the right breast. The examination is otherwise negative. The next step in the management of this patient is:

    A. Attempt to aspirate the mass.
    B. Recommend a screening mammogram.
    C. Recommend an excisional biopsy.
    D. Observe the patient for two menstrual cycles.

Answer: A

Critique: A premenopausal woman with a breast mass that is present throughout the menstrual cycle should have aspiration of the mass attempted to determine whether it is solid or cystic. Fluid should be sent for cytologic examination. Screening mammography would not be appropriate in a patient with a palpable breast mass, while a recommendation for excisional biopsy prior to determining whether the lesion was cystic or solid would be premature. Observation of a mass for a menstrual cycle would be reasonable, but this patient relates a history of the mass being present for the last 6 weeks, and observation for two additional menstrual cycles may be excessive.

Page 1237

22. Of the following, which is the most important prognostic variable for individuals with breast cancer?

    A. The size of the primary tumor
    B. The number of axillary lymph nodes involved with metastatic disease
    C. The status of estrogen and progesterone receptors
    D. The histologic grade

Answer: B

Critique: The number of axillary lymph nodes involved with metastatic disease is the most important postsurgical prognostic variable in patients with breast cancer. Survival is markedly decreased in individuals with four or more positive nodes. Large tumor size, negative estrogen and progesterone status, and a high histologic grade are also poor prognostic indicators.

Page 1238

23. For which of the following subgroups of patients with breast cancer is the indication for adjuvant chemotherapy controversial?

A. Premenopausal women with positive axillary lymph nodes and positive estrogen and progesterone receptor status
B. Premenopausal women with positive axillary nodes and negative estrogen and progesterone receptor status
C. Premenopausal women with positive axillary nodes and mixed estrogen and progesterone receptor status
D. Premenopausal women with negative axillary nodes and positive estrogen and progesterone receptor status

Answer: D

Critique: Premenopausal women with positive axillary nodes should receive adjuvant chemotherapy regardless of the hormone receptor status of the tumor. The use of adjuvant therapy in node-negative women is controversial since their prognosis is good; however, studies indicate that breast cancer recurs in 10 to 40% of these women. Therefore, these patients might benefit from adjuvant chemotherapy.

Page 1240

24. A 63-year-old woman presents to the office complaining of severe pain in the right shoulder, which has become progressively worse during the last week. The pain radiates down the medial aspect of her upper arm and has an insidious onset. The physical examination reveals wasting in the interosseous muscles of the right hand. There is drooping of the right eyelid. The right pupil is smaller than the left pupil. You recognize this as:

A. Klumpke's paralysis
B. Horner's syndrome
C. Pancoast's syndrome
D. Brachial neuritis

Answer: C

Critique: This patient presents with symptoms that include pain radiating down the medial aspect of the upper arm (T1 distribution), Horner's syndrome, and evidence of damage to the T1 nerve root as indicated by the wasting of the interosseous muscles of the hand. This constellation is known as Pancoast's syndrome. Klumpke's paralysis is a birth injury to the brachial plexus, which involves the C8 and T1 nerve roots and may also have an associated Horner syndrome if the nerve roots are avulsed. Brachial neuritis may involve any nerve root in the brachial plexus but is not associated with Horner's syndrome. Brachial neuritis has a viral etiology and is associated with the sudden onset of pain.

Page 1240

Further Reading

Gilroy J, Holliday PL: The peripheral neuropathies. *In* Basic Neurology. New York, Macmillan, 1992, pp 315–317.

25. For the patient described in question 24, possible causes of this condition include:

A. Lung cancer
B. Breast cancer
C. Both A and B
D. Neither A nor B

Answer: C

Critique: Both lung cancer occurring at the apex of the lung and direct extension of breast carcinoma into the axilla may cause Pancoast's syndrome, which is described in question 24.

Further Reading

Gilroy J, Holliday PL: The peripheral neuropathies. *In* Basic Neurology. New York, Macmillan, 1992, pp 315–317.

Questions 26–29. Match each of the numbered descriptions below to one of the following lettered choices:

A. Non–small cell cancer of the lung
B. Small cell cancer of the lung
C. Both A and B
D. Neither A nor B

26. Risk factors include tobacco use, radon exposure, and asbestos exposure.

27. Is an aggressive tumor with early metastasis

28. Frequently associated with paraneoplastic syndromes

29. Surgical resection with curative intent indicated for limited (stages I and II) disease

Answers: 26-C, 27-B, 28-B, 29-A

Critique: Tobacco use, radon exposure, and asbestos exposure are all risk factors for bronchogenic carcinoma of the small cell and non–small cell types. Small cell cancer is a more aggressive tumor with early metastasis and is more frequently associated with paraneoplastic syndromes. Frequently, ectopic hormone production is documented in small cell cancers, including antidiuretic hormone, adrenocorticotropic hormone, melanocyte-stimulating hormone, and calcitonin. Electron microscopy of small cell cancers often reveals neurosecretory granules. Surgical resection is indicated for early stage (I and II) non–small cell cancers. A combination of chemotherapy and radiation therapy is most often used for small cell cancers of the lung.

Pages 1240–1243

Further Reading

Portlock CS, Goffinet DR: Small-cell carcinoma of the lung—primary or regional. *In* Portlock C, Goffinet D (Eds): Manual of Clinical Problems in Oncology. Boston, Little, Brown, 1986, p 111.

30. Which ONE of the following is *not* a risk factor for colon cancer?

A. High-fat, low-fiber diet
B. Peutz-Jeghers syndrome

C. Advancing age
D. Crohn's disease
E. Turcot's syndrome

Answer: B

Critique: Peutz-Jeghers syndrome consists of multiple hamartomatous polyps throughout the gastrointestinal tract. Patients with this syndrome are not at risk for malignant change of the polyps. Environmental factors that increase the risk for colon cancer include diets rich in fats and low in fiber, calcium, and folate. Increasing age is a well-recognized risk factor for colon cancer with a progressive increase in risk from 20 to 80 years of age. Inflammatory bowel disease is a risk factor for colon cancer, and patients with both Crohn's disease and ulcerative colitis are at increased risk, although the risk is higher in ulcerative colitis. Turcot's syndrome is an autosomal recessive disease that is characterized by central nervous system (CNS) tumors (ependymoma, glioblastoma, and medulloblastoma) and adenomatous polyposis.

Pages 1240–1243

Further Reading

Levin B: Neoplasms of the large and small intestine. *In* Wyngaarden JB, Smith LH, Bennett JC (Eds): Cecil Textbook of Medicine, 19th ed. Philadelphia, WB Saunders, 1992, pp 716–717.

31. A 67-year-old woman presents to your office to follow up on stool samples that were positive for occult blood. Of the following options, the most appropriate work-up consists of:

A. Anoscopy and digital rectal examination for hemorrhoids
B. Air contrast barium enema and flexible sigmoidoscopy
C. Repetition of the guaiac test on three stool samples
D. Flexible sigmoidoscopy

Answer: B

Critique: The only appropriate choice among these options in this patient is an air contrast barium enema and flexible sigmoidoscopy. Another appropriate diagnostic strategy would be a colonoscopy. In this vignette, the patient's screening test result (guaiac test of the stool for occult blood) is positive. The next step is to search for adenomas and carcinoma. A flexible sigmoidoscopy alone would be inappropriate, because 30 to 50% of patients with an adenoma have a synchronous polyp at another site in the colon and, therefore, the entire colon must be visualized to identify a possible lesion and any synchronous lesions. Since the screening test result is positive, repetition of the test is inappropriate.

Page 1243

32. The patient in question 31 is examined and is found to have a polyp. All of the following are true regarding this patient EXCEPT:

A. All adenomatous polyps contain some dysplasia or glandular atypia.

B. If the polyp is larger than 2 cm, there is an increased risk of a malignancy developing from the polyp.
C. The risk of developing a malignancy is proportional to the percentage of the polyp that has a villous component.
D. If the dysplastic portion of the polyp involves the submucosa, then colonoscopic polypectomy is adequate.

Answer: D

Critique: All adenomatous polyps contain some dysplasia or glandular atypia; however, they do not invade the muscularis mucosa or submucosa. When these structures are breached, the diagnosis is invasive cancer and polypectomy alone is inadequate: A colectomy would be appropriate. The risk of a malignancy developing from an adenomatous polyp is related to the percentage of the polyp that has a villous component on histopathologic examination. Although carcinoma can develop in polyps of any size, polyps that are larger than 2 cm have higher rates of malignancy.

Page 1243

33. A 65-year-old patient undergoes a colectomy for adenocarcinoma of the colon. The tumor has involved one regional lymph node, which is seen in the colectomy specimen. A staging work-up and laparotomy reveal no evidence of distant metastasis. Which of the following is true concerning this patient:

A. This is a Dukes D lesion.
B. The risk of tumor recurrence in this patient is 25%.
C. This patient should be treated with 5-fluorouracil and levamisole for 1 year.
D. This patient should now undergo radiation therapy.

Answer: C

Critique: The lesion described in this patient is a Dukes C lesion (stage III). Treatment with 5-fluorouracil and levamisole for 1 year has been shown to decrease the risk of cancer recurrence (by 41%) and the overall death rate (by 33%) in stage III patients. There is no indication for radiation therapy in this patient. Dukes staging definitions for colon cancer and the risk of tumor recurrence are:

Staging		Recurrence Rate
Dukes A	Limited to mucosa	—
Dukes B	Involvement of the muscularis propria or serosa, or into other organs, but no nodal involvement	25%
Dukes C	Positive regional nodes	50%
Dukes D	Metastatic disease	—

Pages 1244, 1245

34. (True or False) Which of the following are true regarding rectal carcinomas?

1. They are more likely to be asymptomatic than are colon cancers.
2. In general, they have a poorer prognosis than do colon cancers.
3. Rectal cancers may not be visualized on air contrast barium enema.
4. An endoscopic procedure should be performed to visualize the rectum.

Answers: 1-F, 2-T, 3-T, 4-T

Critique: Rectal cancers are more likely to be symptomatic than are colon cancers. Symptoms may include pain, bleeding, tenesmus, and changes in stool caliber. Because of the larger caliber of the more proximal (right) colon and the more liquid nature of the stool, proximal cancers are less likely to produce symptoms. Rectal cancers demonstrate a worse prognosis, stage for stage, compared with colon cancers. Rectal cancers might not be visualized on air contrast barium enema, and an endoscopic procedure, preferably with a flexible endoscope that is retroflexed to visualize the rectal vault, should be performed.

Page 1245

35. According to the American Cancer Society, prostate cancer screening should:

A. Consist of digital rectal examination beginning at age 40
B. Include a blood test for prostate specific antigen beginning at age 50
C. Both A and B
D. Neither A nor B

Answer: C

Critique: American Cancer Society guidelines recommend that a digital rectal examination be offered to all men 40 years of age or older and a prostate-specific antigen test to all men 50 years of age or older. The United States Preventive Services Task Force does not recommend for or against a digital rectal examination. The National Cancer Institute, the American Academy of Family Physicians, the United State Preventative Services Task Force, and the American College of Physicians make no recommendation for routine screening of prostate-specific antigen.

Further Reading

Hayward RS, Steinberg EP, Ford DE, et al: Preventive care guidelines: 1991. Ann Intern Med 114:758–783, 1991.
Sox HC: Preventive health services in adults. N Engl J Med 330:1589–1595, 1994.
U.S. Public Health Service: Cancer detection in adults by physical examination. Am Fam Physician 51:871–885, 1995.
Woolf SH: Screening for prostate cancer with prostate-specific antigen: An examination of the evidence. N Engl J Med 333:1401–1405, 1995.

36. A prostatic nodule palpated on digital rectal examination should initially be evaluated by:

A. A prostate-specific antigen test
B. Ultrasound examination of the prostate
C. Prostatic acid phosphatase test
D. Bone scan

Answer: B

Critique: Once a prostatic nodule is noted on a digital rectal examination, further prostate screening is not warranted and a definitive procedure should be done. The next step in the work-up of this patient is an ultrasound scan of the prostate. If hyperechoic regions are identified, they should be biopsied. A digital rectal examination may also provide guidance for biopsies. Although a positive prostate-specific antigen test result may increase the confidence that a further work-up (ultrasound scan and biopsy) is needed, a negative prostate-specific antigen test result would not change decision-making. Prostatic acid phosphatase is elevated in advanced disease and is not helpful in decision-making in this case. A bone scan is indicated in staging of prostate cancer, but until such a diagnosis is obtained, staging is premature.

Pages 1238, 1246

37. (True or False) The "flare" phenomenon that occurs in patients treated for prostate cancer:

1. Is characterized by increased bone pain
2. Is caused by increased testosterone levels
3. May result in neurologic deterioration in patients with large metastases to the spine
4. May be blocked by the use of antiandrogens

Answers: 1-T, 2-T, 3-T, 4-T

Critique: The use of luteinizing hormone–releasing hormone (LH-RH) agonists, such as leuprolide and goserelin, may result in increased testosterone levels during the initial phase of therapy and the "flare" phenomenon that is characterized by increased pain at the site of bony metastases of prostatic carcinoma. In patients with large metastases to the spine, monotherapy with LH-RH antagonists is contraindicated because acute neurologic deterioration may result secondary to this phenomenon. "Flare" can be reduced or eliminated by the use of concomitant antiandrogens for the first 2 to 4 weeks of LH-RH agonist therapy.

Pages 1238, 1247

38. All of the following are true regarding testicular cancer EXCEPT:

A. It is the most common cancer in the 15- to 35-year age group.
B. Individuals with cryptorchidism are at increased risk.
C. Individuals with a history of orchiopexy are at decreased risk.
D. Individuals with testicular atrophy are at increased risk.
E. Individuals with Klinefelter's syndrome are at increased risk.

Answer: C

Critique: Testicular cancers are the most common malignancy in males who are 15 to 35 years of age and the second most common malignancy in the 35- to 39-year-old age group. Major risk factors for testicular cancer are a history of cryptorchidism, orchiopexy, or testicular atrophy. Individuals with Klinefelter's syndrome, XY gonadal dysgenesis, and isochromosome 12p are also at increased risk for testicular cancers.

Pages 1247, 1248

Further Reading

Henderson BE, Brenton B, Jing J, et al: Risk factors for cancer of the testes in young men. Cancer 23:598–602, 1979.

39. (True or False) A 32-year-old man presents to your office for evaluation of a scrotal mass. The mass has been increasing in size during the last 4 weeks. It is not painful, and there has been no associated fever. On physical examination there is a marked asymmetry with regard to the size of the testis. The mass is nontender and does not transilluminate. There is no regional lymph adenopathy. Bilateral gynecomastia is present. Regarding this patient:
   1. The next step in this patient's work-up is tumor marker analysis and bilateral ultrasound examination of the testis.
   2. Luteinizing hormone may cause a falsely elevated β-hCG level.
   3. Patients with pure seminoma have elevated α_1-fetoprotein (AFP) levels.
   4. Because of the patient's age, transcrotal biopsy would be indicated for definitive diagnosis.
   5. Gynecomastia may be secondary to the testicular tumor.

Answers: 1-T, 2-T, 3-F, 4-F, 5-T

Critique: Testicular cancer is the most common cancer in this patient's group of 15 to 35 years. A testicular carcinoma must be excluded. The first step would be to examine the testis with an ultrasound study and to order tumor markers, including β-hCG, AFP, and lactate dehydrogenase (LDH). Luteinizing hormone (LH) may cross-react with a β-hCG in some assays and, therefore, suppression of LH with 200 mg of testosterone, and a repeated β-hCG within 48 hours may be done to exclude a falsely elevated β-hCG. AFP levels are elevated in more than 50% of testicular cancers. However, patients with pure seminoma and choriocarcinoma do not have elevated AFP levels. The definitive diagnosis of testicular carcinoma is made by radical inguinal orchiectomy, and transcrotal procedures that may increase local recurrences and seed the inguinal nodes are not indicated. Lastly, gynecomastia may be a presenting sign associated with testicular cancer.

Pages 1247–1249

40. (True or False) Risk factors for ovarian cancers include:
   1. Increasing age
   2. Nulliparity or late first pregnancy
   3. Early menopause
   4. Family history of ovarian cancer
   5. Oral contraceptive

Answers: 1-T, 2-T, 3-F, 4-T, 5-F

Critique: Increasing age, nulliparity or late first pregnancy, late menopause, and a positive family history are all risk factors for ovarian cancer. Ovarian cancer is hereditary in only about 5% of cases. Oral contraceptives are protective against ovarian cancer with risk reduction directly proportional to the duration of use of oral contraceptive agents.

Pages 1247–1249

Further Reading

Screening for Ovarian Cancer. *In* Fisher M, Eckhart C (Eds): Guide to Clinical Preventive Services. Baltimore, Williams & Wilkins, 1989, p 81.

41. A 42-year-old premenopausal woman (G0P0) presents to your office for an annual Papanicolaou smear and pelvic examination. On examination, a mass of approximately 6 cm is palpated in the right adnexa. Subsequently, an ultrasonographic examination indicates that it is a simple cystic structure in the right ovary. Indications for surgery include all of the following EXCEPT:

   A. No regression in the mass after three menstrual cycles
   B. Regression after the use of oral contraceptive agents
   C. A mass larger than 8 cm
   D. Ascites present with any ovarian mass
   E. A complex cyst with septations on ultrasonography

Answer: B

Critique: Any mass that is larger than 8 cm, does not regress after three menstrual cycles, has a solid or complex cystic structure (i.e., septations), is associated with ascites, or is fixed should be considered as an indication for surgery. Oral contraceptive agents are commonly used to induce regression of functional cysts. Regression after use of oral contraceptive agents is not an indication for surgery. Adnexal masses in premenopausal and postmenopausal women should be regarded to be suspicious for carcinoma and usually indicate the need for surgical exploration.

Page 1251

42. (True or False) With regard to ovarian cancers:
   1. Epithelial tumors are more common in children and young women.
   2. Germ cell tumors are more common in the elderly.
   3. Tumors are usually asymptomatic until they invade adjacent structures, ascites develops, or clinical evidence of metastasis appears.
   4. The most reliable method of assessing the response to chemotherapy is a second-look laparotomy.
   5. The majority of women with ovarian cancer have advanced disease at the time of diagnosis.

Answers: 1-F, 2-F, 3-T, 4-T, 5-T

Critique: The incidence of epithelial tumors increases with age, and germ cell tumors are more common among children and young women. Because tumors are usually asymptomatic in the early stages, more than two thirds of women with ovarian cancer have advanced disease when diagnosed. The most reliable method when assessing the response to chemotherapy is the second-look laparotomy, which allows for the discontinuation of therapy if no residual disease remains. The second-look laparotomy also facilitates planning of salvage therapy if residual tumor remains.

Pages 1250–1252

43. Risk factors for cervical dysplasia include all of the following EXCEPT:

    A. Onset of sexual activity at an early age
    B. Smoking tobacco products
    C. Diets low in folate
    D. High socioeconomic status
    E. Multiple sexual partners

Answer: D

Critique: Risk factors for cervical dysplasia and cancer include early onset of sexual activity, multiple sexual partners, exposure to herpes simplex virus type 2 (HSV-2) or human papillomavirus (HPV) types 16, 18, 31, 33, 34, or 35. In addition, diets low in folate have been found to increase the risk for cervical dysplasia. Low socioeconomic status is associated with increased risk for cervical dysplasia.

Page 1253

Further Reading

Butterworth CE, Hatch KD, Macaluso M, et al: Folate deficiency and cervical dysplasia. JAMA 267:528–533, 1992.

44. A 4-year-old male presents to your office with a temperature of 102.3° F (oral), petechiae, and splenomegaly. He has not been eating well and complains of pain in his legs. There are no significant infectious contacts. A laboratory work-up reveals a white blood cell count of 50,000 and a platelet count of 25,000. The patient is subsequently diagnosed with acute lymphoblastic leukemia (ALL). In relationship to this patient's diagnosis of ALL, which ONE of the following is correct?

    A. Thrombocytosis is a poor prognostic sign.
    B. The CNS is a major sanctuary site and is the site of relapse in most patients who do not receive prophylactic therapy.
    C. Most children with ALL are not cured with conventional chemotherapy.
    D. The peak incidence of the disease is between 9 and 15 years of age.

Answer: B

Critique: The peak incidence of ALL is between 2 and 6 years of age with a male predominance. It is the most common malignancy in children. Most children with ALL are cured with conventional chemotherapy. Poor prognostic signs include thrombocytopenia, high white blood cell counts, male sex, very young or older age at presenta-

tion, CNS leukemia, lymphadenopathy, organomegaly, and T-cell disease. The CNS is a major sanctuary site for patients not receiving prophylactic therapy: either irradiation with or without methotrexate or triple-drug intrathecal chemotherapy.

Page 1253

45. Which of the following congenital abnormalities are associated with Wilms' tumor?

    A. Hemihypertrophy
    B. Aniridia
    C. Both A and B
    D. Neither A nor B

Answer: C

Critique: Hemihypertrophy and aniridia are both associated with Wilms' tumor.

Page 1256

46. The most common presentation of Wilms' tumor is:

    A. Gross hematuria
    B. Unilateral flank mass or abdominal enlargement
    C. Abdominal pain
    D. Bilateral flank masses

Answer: B

Critique: Abdominal enlargement or a unilateral flank mass is the most common presentation for Wilms' tumor. Only 5% of cases are bilateral. The tumor distorts, but it does not invade, the caliceal system, and therefore gross hematuria is uncommon.

Page 1256

Questions 47–51. For each of the findings in questions 47 to 51, select the type of tumor that is most frequently associated with the finding.

    A. Ewing's sarcoma
    B. Osteosarcoma
    C. Both A and B
    D. Neither A nor B

47. A radiogram reveals osteoid at the site of the lesion, which may extend into the soft tissue.

48. The radiogram reveals a moth-eaten pattern of bony destruction at the diaphysis and elevation of the periosteum.

49. Lesions are more common in the distal femur or proximal tibia or humerus.

50. Lesions are more common at the midshaft of the bone.

51. Characteristically it presents with painful lesions.

Answers: 47-B, 48-A, 49-B, 50-A, 51-C

Critique: Osteosarcoma presents with lesions in the distal femur, proximal tibia, or humerus. The radiogram of the lesion has a characteristic appearance and includes osteoid production, which may extend into the adjacent soft tissues. Ewing's sarcoma typically presents at the midshaft of the bone and frequently involves the femur, tibia, fibula, and pelvis. The radiogram of the lesions reveals a patchy, moth-eaten pattern at the diaphysis with elevation of the periosteum and an "onion-skin" appearance. Both tumors characteristically are painful.

Pages 1256, 1257

52. A 67-year-old white woman with a diagnosis of metastatic breast carcinoma is admitted to the hospital for a fracture of the left hip. Radiograms reveal a large lytic lesion at the fracture site. During the course of the day she becomes progressively more lethargic. The patient responds to a person's voice, but then she lapses back into unconsciousness. The results of a room air blood gas (ABG) are normal. The physical examination, including a neurologic examination, is nonfocal. It is remarkable only for the mental status changes and decreased, but symmetric, deep tendon reflexes. The most appropriate next step is:

    A. Computed tomography (CT) scan of the head
    B. Repeat ABG on 2 liters of oxygen
    C. Determination of serum calcium
    D. Magnetic resonance imaging (MRI) of the head

Answer: C

Critique: The patient's history of breast cancer, a large lytic lesion at the site of the fracture, and the global deterioration in her mental status suggest the diagnosis of hypercalcemia. The normal blood gas essentially rules out problems with oxygenation. Her neurologic examination is also nonfocal. The combination of a global decrease in mental status and a nonfocal neurologic examination in this setting further suggest a metabolic problem over a mass lesion affecting both hemispheres of the brain. Imaging the head as part of the work-up for her mental status change may be reasonable; however, a determination of serum calcium would be the most appropriate next step in the work-up of this patient.

Page 1260

53. For patients with spinal cord compression syndrome, the first step in treatment to prevent further neurologic deterioration is:

    A. Emergency radiotherapy
    B. Decompression laminectomy
    C. Intravenous dexamethasone
    D. Myelogram

Answer: C

Critique: Spinal cord compression most frequently occurs with metastatic cancers of breast, lung, and prostate origin. Once the diganosis is made, therapy with intravenous dexamethasone should be given to prevent further neurologic deterioration. Radiotherapy and decompression laminectomy are definitive but require longer to effect a result and may be planned urgently after administration of the corticosteroid. A myelogram might be needed to plan therapy but will not prevent neurologic deterioration.

Page 1260

45

Hematology

Francis P. Kohrs

1. All of the following are true regarding iron deficiency anemia EXCEPT:

    A. It may occur in up to 25% of infants.
    B. It may occur in up to 50% of menstruating women.
    C. It may occur in up to 30% of pregnant women.
    D. It is more common than folate deficiency in patients with alcoholism.

Answer: D

Critique: Estimates of the incidence of anemia indicate that it may occur in up to 25% of infants, 6% of children, 50% of menstruating women, 30% of pregnant women, and 50% of patients with alcoholism. However, folate deficiency in alcoholic patients is more common: 90% are deficient in folate secondary to poor nutrition.

Page 1263

2. Which one of the following statements is true regarding red blood cell (RBC) production?

    A. Erythropoietin decreases RBC production.
    B. The average life span of an RBC is 120 days.
    C. A reticulocyte is a hypermature RBC.
    D. RBCs are produced from the megakaryocyte progenitor cell.

Answer: B

Critique: The average life span of an RBC is 120 days. Erythropoietin, a protein hormone produced primarily in the kidneys, increases the production and differentiation of RBCs. Reticulocytes are immature RBCs. The megakaryocyte progenitor cell gives rise to platelets, not RBCs, which arise from the erythroid progenitor cell.

Pages 1264, 1265

3. (True or False) True statements regarding hemoglobin and hematocrit determinations include which of the following?

    1. Blacks may have mean hemoglobin levels 0.5 to 1 g/dl lower than do age- and sex-matched whites.
    2. The mean hematocrit at birth is 61%.

    3. The hemoglobin value decreases during the first 6 weeks of life to a mean of 12 g/dl.
    4. There is up to a 4% variation in spun hematocrit from fingerstick specimens.

Answers: 1-T, 2-T, 3-T, 4-T

Critique: All of the statements concerning normal values for hemoglobins and hematocrits are true. Blacks have hemoglobin levels 0.5 to 1 g/dl less than age- and sex-matched whites. The hemoglobin at birth has a mean of 19 g/dl (hematocrit of 61%), which decreases to a mean of 12 g/dl in the first 6 weeks of life and remains relatively constant for the next 2 years. Centrifuged hematocrits from fingerstick capillary tubes may have as much as a 4% variation from one determination to another in the same patient. Electronic determinations of hematocrits are more accurate with only a 1% error.

Page 1266

Questions 4–8. For each of the following blood smear findings, match them with the best corresponding clinical syndrome:

    A. Target cells
    B. Hypersegmentation
    C. Howell-Jolly bodies
    D. Heinz bodies
    E. Toxic granulations

4. The presence of this finding indicates decreased enzyme-reducing power of the RBC.

5. Seen in patients after a surgical or functional splenectomy

6. Indicates infection if present in neutrophils

7. Associated with thalassemia and other hemoglobinopathies

8. Seen in neutrophils of patients with vitamin B_{12} deficiency anemia

Answers: 4-D, 5-C, 6-E, 7-A, 8-B

Critique: Each of these questions relates to abnormalities that may be seen on examination of the peripheral blood smear. Heinz bodies may be seen in the peripheral blood smear of patients with glucose-6-phosphate dehydrogenase (G-6-PD) deficiency. Howell-Jolly bodies are seen in patients with splenectomy, either surgical or functional (as occurs in patients with sickle cell disease). Target cells are characteristically associated with thalassemias or hemoglobinopathies (e.g., hemoglobin C or sickle cell disease) but may also be seen in patients with hepatic disease. Both hypersegmentation and toxic granulations are abnormalities of neutrophils. The former is associated with vitamin B_{12} deficiency anemias, and the latter is associated with infectious processes.

Page 1267

9. (True or False) Clinically, reticulocytes may be characterized by which of the following?

1. They are generally larger in size than are mature RBCs.
2. They circulate for approximately 120 days.
3. The absolute reticulocyte count takes into account the degree of anemia.
4. The reticulocyte percentage takes into account the degree of anemia.

Answers: 1-T, 2-F, 3-F, 4-F

Critique: A blood smear stained with methylene blue is used to direct reticulocytes. Reticulocytes are approximately 1.5 to 2 times larger than are mature RBCs. The circulating life span of reticulocytes is 1 day, after which they lose their residual ribonucleic acid (RNA) and become mature RBCs. Neither the absolute reticulocyte count nor the reticulocyte percentage takes into account the degree of anemia. Because of this, both may inaccurately reflect the appropriateness of the degree of reticulocytosis. The corrected reticulocyte count takes into consideration the degree of anemia and must be calculated based on the hematocrit or hemoglobin value.

Pages 1267, 1268

10. The red blood cell distribution width (RDW) is elevated in all of the following EXCEPT:

A. Early iron deficiency anemia
B. Anemia of chronic disease
C. Patients with mechanical cardiac valves
D. After transfusion with multiple units of packed RBCs

Answer: B

Critique: The RDW is not elevated in the anemia of chronic disease, which is a normocytic or microcytic anemia. Early iron deficiency anemia is characterized by a heterogeneous population of normal-sized older RBCs and newer microcytic cells. Patients with mechanical cardiac valves produce fragmented cells that elevate the RDW. After multiple transfusions with RBCs, the RDW will reflect the various RBC sizes of donors and may be elevated.

Page 1268

11. (True or False) A 67-year-old patient is admitted to the hospital with abdominal pain, hematemesis, and bright red blood per rectum. A complete blood count is obtained, and the result is normal. The patient has chest pain, and her electrocardiogram (ECG) reveals sinus tachycardia with 2 mm of ST segment depression in leads II, III, and aVF. True statements concerning this patient include:

1. Tachycardia may be an early sign of significant blood loss.
2. The normal values for hemoglobin and hematocrit indicate that blood loss is minimal.
3. The patient should be transfused now.
4. The patient is experiencing an inferior myocardial infarction and should undergo thrombolytic therapy.

Answers: 1-T, 2-F, 3-T, 4-F

Critique: This patient presents with symptoms consistent with an upper gastrointestinal (UGI) hemorrhage. Since this patient has hematochezia, this indicates brisk bleeding. Tachycardia and orthostasis are early signs of significant volume loss. Since both volume and RBCs are lost proportionately in acute blood loss, hemoglobin and hematocrit may remain normal early on and are unreliable indicators of acute blood loss early in the bleeding episode. The patient is experiencing angina and has ECG findings consistent with ischemia and should receive a transfusion. Thrombolytic agents would be contraindicated in an acute UGI hemorrhage. Volume replacement may correct the tachycardia and rate-dependent ischemia.

Page 1270

12. Concerning patients with Fanconi's anemia, all of the following are true EXCEPT:

A. RBC production is depressed.
B. White blood cell (WBC) production is depressed.
C. Platelet production is depressed.
D. This is a congenital form of aplastic anemia.
E. Patients most often have associated skeletal abnormalities.

Answer: E

Critique: Fanconi's anemia is a congenital aplastic anemia; however, it may not manifest until adulthood. Aplastic anemias involve depressed production of all cellular elements: RBCs, WBCs, and platelets. Although originally described as an aplastic anemia of childhood with associated abnormalities of the bones and urogenital system, Fanconi's anemia is now defined by a chromosomal abnormality. Studies indicate that most patients with Fanconi's anemia lack any associated abnormality.

Page 1270

Further Reading

Young NS: Aplastic anemia and related bone marrow failure syndromes. *In* Wyngaarden JB, Smith LH, Bennett JC (Eds): Cecil Textbook of Medicine, 19th ed. Philadelphia, WB Saunders, 1992, p 831.

13. The following viral infections may cause aplastic anemia EXCEPT:

    A. Parvovirus
    B. Group B coxsackievirus
    C. Epstein-Barr virus
    D. Hepatitis

Answer: B

Critique: Parvovirus, Epstein-Barr virus, and hepatitis may cause aplastic anemia. Acute non-A non-B hepatitis viral infections, some of which presumably are hepatitis C, may also be complicated by aplastic anemia, especially in the convalescent stage. Group B coxsackievirus is not associated with aplastic anemia but can cause myocarditis and pericarditis.

Page 1271

14. (True or False) A 36-year-old man presents with complaints of fatigue, easy bruising, and bleeding from the gums. His physical examination reveals subconjunctival hemorrhage, ecchymoses over the trunk and limbs, and lymphadenopathy and splenomegaly. The complete blood count (CBC) reveals a hemoglobin of 6 g/dl, a WBC count of 500/mm³, and a platelet count of 23,000. True statements concerning this patient include:

    1. Bleeding is due to poor platelet function.
    2. Lymphadenopathy or splenomegaly are usually seen in patients with aplastic anemia.
    3. The patient is at increased risk for infections.
    4. The work-up should include a reticulocyte count.

Answers: 1-T, 2-F, 3-T, 4-T

Critique: This patient's platelet count is sufficiently high (greater than 20,000) to suggest that the bleeding is more likely to be secondary to poor platelet function than the absolute number of platelets. Lymphadenopathy and splenomegaly are not characteristically associated with aplastic anemia, and other diagnostic possibilities should be considered in patients with these findings. Because of the severe neutropenia associated with a WBC count of 500, the patient is at increased risk for infection. This patient may have an aplastic anemia, and a reticulocyte count should be performed.

Page 1271

15. All of the following medications are associated with aplastic anemia EXCEPT:

    A. Auranofin
    B. Diclofenac sodium
    C. Chlorpromazine
    D. Metronidazole
    E. Isoniazid

Answer: D

Critique: Although metronidazole has been associated with reversible neutropenia and thrombocytopenia, it has not been associated with aplastic anemia. All of the other medications, including a gold compound (auranofin), a nonsteroidal anti-inflammatory drug (NSAID) (diclo-

fenac), an antipsychotic (chlorpromazine), and an antibiotic (isoniazid) are associated with aplastic anemia.

Page 1271

Further Reading

Physicians' Desk Reference, 49th ed. Montvale, NJ, Medical Economics Data Production Co., 1995, pp 1064, 1424, 2398, 2409.

16. A 47-year-old man presents with a complaint of fatigue of recent onset. He is taking no medications and does not have any significant environmental or infectious exposures. His past medical history is noncontributory; he has always been fit and healthy. On physical examination, he is pale; his conjunctiva are not injected; and a new onset systolic ejection murmur (grade III or IV) is heard over the right upper sternal border. Results of a CBC and reticulocyte count indicate a hemoglobin of 5 and no reticulocyte response, but the results are otherwise unrevealing. A bone marrow aspirate reveals essentially no erythoid precursors. As part of this patient's work-up, which one of the following examinations should be included?

    A. A computed tomography (CT) scan of the chest
    B. A CT scan of the abdomen
    C. A CT scan of the brain
    D. A CT scan of the long bones

Answer: A

Critique: The patient described in question 16 has findings most consistent with the acquired adult form of red cell aplasia. For patients with pure red cell aplasia, 30 to 50% will be associated with a thymoma; therefore, as part of the evaluation, a CT scan of the chest is necessary.

Page 1272

Questions 17–21. For questions 17 through 21 use the following answers.

    A. Folic acid only
    B. Vitamin B$_{12}$ only
    C. Both folic acid and vitamin B$_{12}$
    D. Neither folic acid nor vitamin B$_{12}$

17. Is heat labile and cooking destroys the majority of the vitamin present in foods

18. A deficiency causes a macrocytic anemia.

19. Intestinal absorption is blocked by phenytoin.

20. A deficiency is associated with dorsal column findings on physical examination.

21. In pregnant women, a deficiency may result in neural tube defects.

Answers: 17-A, 18-C, 19-A, 20-B, 21-A

Critique: Folic acid is heat labile and cooking destroys 50 to 90% of the available folic acid. The heat used in cooking does not reduce the content of vitamin B$_{12}$

in the food significantly. Intestinal absorption of folic acid is blocked by both ethanol and phenytoin. Vitamin B_{12} deficiency is associated with decreased vibration and position sense, both of which are carried in the dorsal columns of the spinal cord. Lastly, maternal folic acid deficiency is associated with an increase in fetal neural tube defects.

Page 1273

22. Causes of macrocytosis include all of the following EXCEPT:

    A. Zidovudine
    B. Anticonvulsant therapy
    C. Liver disease
    D. Thalassemia
    E. Alcoholism

Answer: D

Critique: Treatment with zidovudine (formerly AZT), anticonvulsant therapy (e.g., phenytoin), excessive ethanol intake, and liver disease are all associated with macrocytosis. Thalassemias are inherited abnormalities in globin chain production and produce microcytic erythrocytes.

Page 1273

23. (True or False) Which of the following represent true statements regarding iron metabolism?

    1. Ascorbic acid, tea, and coffee all tend to increase absorption of nonheme iron.
    2. Transferrin is an iron transport protein in the plasma.
    3. Ferritin is the storage form of iron.
    4. Increased iron-binding capacity and a low transferrin saturation are consistent with a deficiency in iron.

Answers: 1-F, 2-T, 3-T, 4-T

Critique: Ascorbic acid does increase the absorption of nonheme iron; however, tea and coffee reduce the absorption. Transferrin, measured as iron-binding capacity, is an iron transport protein that is found in the plasma. Ferritin is the major storage form of iron. Iron deficiency is classically associated with an increased iron-binding capacity and a low transferrin saturation.

Page 1274

24. All of the following are associated with microcytic indices EXCEPT:

    A. Thalassemia
    B. Iron deficiency anemia
    C. Hypothyroidism
    D. Sideroblastic anemia

Answer: C

Critique: All of the conditions listed except for hypothyroidism are associated with microcytic anemias. Anemias secondary to hypothyroidism usually demonstrate nor-

mocytic indices, although the indices may occasionally be macrocytic.

Page 1275

Questions 25–28. Match the clinical syndromes below with the laboratory findings in questions 25 to 28.

    A. Early iron deficiency anemia
    B. Late iron deficiency anemia
    C. Anemia of chronic disease
    D. Pernicious anemia

25. Decreased hemoglobin, decreased total iron-binding capacity (TIBC), elevated serum ferritin, normal RDW, and normal mean corpuscular volume (MCV)

26. Reduced hemoglobin, normal TIBC, decreased serum ferritin, decreased transferrin saturation, elevated RDW, and normal MCV

27. Markedly reduced hemoglobin, increased TIBC, decreased serum ferritin, decreased transferrin saturation, and reduced MCV

28. Reduced hemoglobin, increased RDW, increased MCV, and hypersegmentation of neutrophils

Answers: 25-C, 26-A, 27-B, 28-D

Critique: Anemia of chronic disease is associated with a decreased TIBC, a normal RDW, and normochromic, normocytic, or normochromic-microcytic indices. In addition, the transferrin saturation is decreased, and the serum ferritin is elevated. Iron deficiency anemia goes through several stages. In the first stage of early depletion, the bone marrow does not stain for iron and the serum ferritin is depressed. In the second stage of early iron deficiency anemia, the transferrin saturation is reduced and two populations of RBCs (the new microcytic cells as well as the older normocytic cells) cause an increase in the RDW. In the early stage, the MCV may be normal or slightly reduced. In the later stages or iron deficiency, the TIBC becomes increased and the MCV is reduced, thus giving the characteristic microcytic and hypochromic smear. The RDW may be elevated and will normalize as only one population of cells dominates. Pernicious anemia (vitamin B_{12} deficiency anemia) is characterized by macrocytic indices, an increased RDW, and neutrophil hypersegmentation.

Pages 1268, 1273, 1275–1277

29. Findings consistent with intravascular hemolysis include all the following EXCEPT:

    A. Jaundice
    B. Increased unbound haptoglobin
    C. Hemoglobinuria
    D. Elevated liver function tests

Answer: B

Critique: When intravascular hemolysis occurs jaundice may ensue; hemoglobin may be excreted in the urine, and liver function tests may be elevated owing to increases in hemoglobin and bilirubin metabolism. Haptoglobin scavenges hemoglobin dimers. During hemolysis, bound haptoglobin (i.e., the haptoglobin associated with hemoglobin dimers) will increase, and unbound haptoglobin will suffer a corresponding decrease.

Page 1277

30. Of the following intracorpuscular mechanisms for hemolytic anemia, the syndrome that is due to a somatic mutation and is not inherited is:

    A. Spherocytosis
    B. Paroxysmal nocturnal hemoglobinuria
    C. G-6-PD
    D. Thalassemia

Answer: B

Critique: Defects producing hemolytic anemias may be categorized as intracorpuscular or extracorpuscular. Of the intracorpuscular mechanisms for hemolytic anemias, only paroxysmal nocturnal hemoglobinuria is not inherited. Instead, a defect of a marrow stem cell leads to a line of RBCs that are highly susceptible to complement-mediated cell lysis. Spherocytosis, G-6-PD deficiency, and thalassemia are all inherited disorders.

Page 1278

31. Complications of hereditary spherocytosis (HS) include all of the following EXCEPT:

    A. Splenic rupture
    B. Cholethiasis
    C. Renal calculi
    D. Aplastic anemia

Answer: C

Critique: HS is an inherited defect in the RBC membrane. Patients with HS exhibit spherocytes on a peripheral smear, an increased mean corpuscular hemoglobin concentration (MCHC), increased reticulocytosis, and a negative result on a Coombs' antibody test. Increased indirect bilirubin also occurs in most patients, and there is frequently a positive family history. On physical examination, splenomegaly is common. Splenic rupture, cholelithiasis, and aplastic anemia are all complications of the syndrome. Renal calculi are not associated with HS.

Page 1278

32. Treatment of patients with paroxysmal nocturnal hemoglobinuria include all of the following EXCEPT:

    A. Transfusion of packed RBCs
    B. Androgens
    C. Heparin for thromboembolic complications
    D. High-dose iron therapy

Answer: D

Critique: A transfusion with RBCs to maintain a hematocrit of 30% or greater is a common practice in the treatment of paroxysmal nocturnal hemoglobinuria. Leukocyte-poor units of packed RBCs are desirable to decrease the risk of sensitization and transfusion reac-

tions. Androgens (e.g., fluoxymesterone) are used to increase RBC production. Anticoagulants such as heparin are used to treat thromboembolic complications. Iron therapy should be used sparingly, because supplementation with iron only provides new RBCs for hemolysis. High-dose iron therapy should be avoided. Most iron is provided by transfusions of RBCs.

Page 1279

33. G-6-PD deficiency:

    A. Is most common in Americans of Mediterranean ancestry
    B. Is most common in African-American males
    C. Is associated with Howell-Jolly bodies on the peripheral smear
    D. Has a higher incidence in females than in males

Answer: B

Critique: Although G-6-PD deficiency is frequently associated with Mediterranean ancestry and favism; in the United States it is most common in African-American males. The gene for the enzyme is X-linked, and there is a higher incidence in males than in females. Males will either have the enzyme defect or they will not, but females may be heterozygous or homozygous for the defective gene. Howell-Jolly bodies are associated with splenectomy. A decrease in the reducing power of the RBC, as seen in G-6-PD deficiency, is associated with Heinz bodies.

Page 1279

34. All of the following drugs may precipitate a hemolytic episode in an individual with G-6-PD deficiency EXCEPT:

    A. Nitrofurantoin
    B. Sulfamethoxazole
    C. Vitamin E
    D. Quinine
    E. Chloroquine

Answer: C

Critique: Several drug categories have oxidative properties and can lead to a hemolytic episode in individuals with G-6-PD deficiency. Nitrofurantoin, chloramphenicol, sulfamethoxazole, quinine, and antimalarials such as chloroquine may cause oxidative stress leading to a hemolytic crisis. Vitamin E is an antioxidant and is not associated with hemolytic episodes in G-6-PD–deficient individuals. Vitamin E has been suggested as a RBC membrane stabilizer in G-6-PD–deficient patients.

Page 1280

35. Concerning the management of children with sickle cell anemia, all of the following are true EXCEPT:

    A. Penicillin prophylaxis should be begun by 2 months of age.
    B. Patients should receive hepatitis B vaccine.
    C. *Haemophilus influenzae* vaccine should be administered, beginning at 2 months of age.

D. 23-Valent pneumococcal vaccine should be administered at 2 years of age, and a booster should be given in 2 to 3 years.

E. *Streptococcus pneumoniae* is most frequently associated with osteomyelitis.

Answer: E

Critique: The most serious infections and complications in sickle cell anemia are sepsis and meningitis caused by *S. pneumoniae*. Mortality is approximately 25% in these circumstances. Current recommendations include starting penicillin prophylaxis by 2 months of age in infants suspected of having sickle cell anemia, regardless of whether the diagnosis has been definitively established or not. Furthermore, the 23-valent pneumococcal vaccine should be administered as soon as possible at or after 2 years of age, and a booster should be given in 2 to 3 years. Since children with sickle cell anemia are likely to require transfusions and are, therefore, at increased risk for hepatitis B, hepatitis B immunization for these individuals is important. *H. influenzae* is another cause of significant morbidity and mortality in children with sickle cell anemia, and compliance with immunization guidelines beginning at 2 months is particularly important. *Salmonella* is the organism that is most frequently associated with osteomyelitis in patients with sickle cell anemia.

Page 1281

Further Reading

Sickle Cell Disease Guideline Panel: Sickle Cell Disease: Screening, Diagnosis, Management, and Counseling in Newborns and Infants. Clinical Guideline No. 6. AHCPR Pub. No. 93-0562. Rockville, MD, Agency for Health Care Policy and Research, Public Health Service, U.S. Department of Health and Human Services, April 1993.

36. Which one of the following statements is true regarding patients with β-thalassemia major (Cooley's anemia)?

A. Patients are unable to produce α-globulin chains in an appropriate amount.

B. It presents in early childhood.

C. It is treated routinely with azactidine to increase Hb F in RBCs.

D. It is treated best with early prescription of low-dose iron therapy.

Answer: B

Critique: Thalassemias are caused by abnormalities in the production of either the α or β chain of hemoglobin. The designation of the type of thalassemia indicates which chain is defective or is not produced in an appropriate amount. Therefore, a β-thalassemia is associated with a defect in or an underproduction of the β chain. Since the fundamental problem is not associated with iron metabolism, iron replacement is not appropriate. In fact, for some forms of β-thalassemia major the cause of death is a cardiomyopathy secondary to iron overload. Azactidine can increase the proportion of hemoglobin F in RBCs, but it is associated with toxicities that are too great a

risk to make routine prescription a workable therapy. β-Thalassemia major usually presents in the first year of life.

Page 1282

Questions 37–42. Match the clinical syndrome with the type of hemolytic anemia that is most associated with that syndrome.

A. Microangiopathic
B. Autoimmune
C. Immune
D. Infectious

37. Parvovirus

38. Procainamide

39. Cyclosporine

40. Ulcerative colitis

41. ABO incompatibility

42. Starr-Edwards valve

Answers: 37-D, 38-B, 39-A, 40-B, 41-C, 42-A

Critique: Microangiographic hemolytic anemias are secondary to stretching or shearing forces and are associated with mechanical cardiac valve replacements (e.g., the Starr-Edwards valve) and certain drugs such as cyclosporine. Autoimmune hemolytic anemias may be drug related or related to other underlying disorders: these autoimmune phenomena are usually mediated by IgG, which attaches to RBCs. Drugs associated with autoimmune hemolytic anemia include procainamide, methyldopa, levodopa, and some NSAIDs. Clinical disorders associated with autoimmune hemolytic anemias include ulcerative colitis, Hodgkin's and non-Hodgkin's lymphoma, and lupus erythematosus. Immune hemolysis may be IgG (removal by the reticuloendothelial system) or IgM mediated (complement mediated destruction). Examples of immune-mediated hemolysis include ABO and Rh incompatibility. Lastly, several infectious agents are associated with hemolysis. Parvovirus, *H. influenzae*, *M. pneumoniae*, *Clostridium* spp., and *Plasmodium* spp. may all cause hemolytic anemias.

Pages 1283–1286

43. Drug therapy for an autoimmune hemolytic anemia includes all of the following EXCEPT:

A. Corticosteroids
B. Azathioprine
C. Mitomycin
D. Cyclophosphamide
E. Folic acid

Answer: C

Critique: Patients with an autoimmune hemolytic anemia should have the underlying disorder treated. Some patients require low-dose alternate-day steroids. In addition, some patients require a splenectomy. Patients who do not respond adequately to corticosteroid therapy and splenectomy are candidates for immunosuppressive drug therapy, including azathioprine (Imuran) and cyclophosphamide (Cytoxan). Almost all patients will require folic acid and iron supplementation. Mitomycin is a chemotherapeutic agent that may cause a hemolytic uremic syndrome, which has a microangiopathic hemolytic anemia as a component. Mitomycin is not indicated for the treatment of autoimmune hemolytic anemias.

Pages 1284, 1285

44. Secondary polycythemia is most commonly due to:

   A. Abnormality of the RBC stem cell
   B. Cellular hypoxemia
   C. High-affinity hemoglobin
   D. Renal failure

Answer: B

Critique: Secondary polycythemia is most commonly caused by cellular hypoxemia. Polycythemia vera is due to an abnormality in a stem cell leading to an absolute increase in the RBC circulating mass. High-affinity hemoglobin may not readily unload oxygen and may lead to increased RBC levels but is classified as a primary form of polycythemia (i.e., familial). Renal failure is associated with a decrease (not an increase) in the RBC mass owing to decreased erythropoietin levels.

Pages 1286, 1287

45. A 48-year-old man presents to the office with a complaint of fatigue. His past medical history is remarkable for hypertension and obesity. He smokes one to two packs of cigarettes each day and has "several" mixed drinks daily. His physical examination is remarkable for a blood pressure of 160/90 and obesity. Results of a CBC reveal a hemoglobin of 17 g/dl and a hematocrit of 51%. The WBC and platelet counts are within normal limits, and the indices are normal. All of the following are true regarding this patient EXCEPT:

   A. This most likely represents spurious polycythemia.
   B. Smoking may increase the RBC mass.
   C. A ^{51}Cr RBC mass determination should be made.
   D. Treatment includes weight reduction and elimination of smoking.

Answer: C

Critique: This patient most likely has spurious polycythemia (also called Gaisböck's syndrome). The syndrome usually occurs in obese, middle-aged men with hypertension and is frequently associated with tobacco and alcohol use. The cause of the syndrome is unknown. In its pure form, it is not associated with an increase in the RBC mass but is related to a decrease in plasma volume. Smoking, however, may increase the RBC mass secondary to increased carboxyhemoglobin levels. Treatment of the syndrome includes weight reduction, elimination of smoking, reduced alcohol consumption, and blood pressure control. A ^{51}Cr RBC mass determination is not indicated at this time. The ^{51}Cr RBC mass determination should be

considered in nonsmoking men with a hematocrit greater than 51% and in nonsmoking women with a hematocrit greater than 48%.

Page 1287

46. Laboratory abnormalities associated with polycythemia vera include all of the following EXCEPT:

   A. Thrombocytosis
   B. Leukocytosis
   C. Elevated leukocyte alkaline phosphatase
   D. Abnormal chromosome studies
   E. Decreased erythropoietin levels

Answer: D

Critique: Polycythemia vera is associated with all of the aforementioned laboratory abnormalities except for abnormal chromosome studies. There are no characteristic chromosome abnormalities associated with polycythemia vera.

Page 1288

47. Lymphadenopathy, which does not have characteristics associated with malignancy, may be observed for several weeks. Often if a bacterial infection is suspected as an etiology, antibiotics are prescribed. When making a determination regarding the significance of an enlarged lymph node, the most important features of the presentation include all of the following EXCEPT:

   A. Patient's age
   B. Family history
   C. Location of the node
   D. Physical characteristics of the node

Answer: B

Critique: The most significant determinants of lymphadenopathy are age, location of the node, node characteristics, and the clinical setting. In general, the patient's family history is not as helpful in decision-making regarding an enlarged lymph node. Patients who are younger than 30 years of age are most likely (80%) to have a benign etiology for the enlargement. Cervical, axillary, and epitrochlear nodes are more likely to be benign. Rubbery, soft, mobile, and tender nodes are more likely to be benign than hard, nontender, fixed nodes.

Pages 1288, 1289

48. All of the following are true regarding WBCs EXCEPT:

   A. Eosinophils are predominantly located in the tissues.
   B. After entering the circulation, neutrophils survive for approximately 10 days.
   C. Once neutrophils leave the circulation, they do not return to the marginating pool.
   D. Monocytes and macrophages are phagocytic cells.

Answer: B

Critique: Circulating neutrophils survive for about 10 hours. Once neutrophils have left the circulation, they do not return to either the circulation or marginating pools. Eosinophils are located mainly in the tissues: The ratio of tissue to blood eosinophils is 100:1. Monocytes, macrophages, and neutrophils are all phagocytic cells.

Page 1290

49. Neutropenia is defined as any absolute neutrophil count of less than:

   A. 500/mm³
   B. 1000/mm³
   C. 1300/mm³
   D. 1800/mm³
   E. 2000/mm³

Answer: D

Critique: An absolute neutrophil count of less than 1800 is defined as neutropenia.

Page 1290

50. Felty's syndrome is:

   A. A triad of neutropenia, chronic rheumatoid arthritis, and thrombocytopenia
   B. A triad of anemia, chronic rheumatoid arthritis, and thrombocytopenia
   C. A trial of neutropenia, chronic rheumatoid arthritis, and splenomegaly
   D. A triad of anemia, chronic rheumatoid arthritis, and thrombocytopenia

Answer: C

Critique: Felty's syndrome is a triad of neutropenia, chronic rheumatoid arthritis, and splenomegaly. Neutropenia may be caused by at least two mechanisms: (1) T-cell–mediated bone marrow failure, and (2) the development of antineutrophil antibodies. Anemia, weight loss, and recurrent fever may be associated with Felty's syndrome.

Pages 1291, 1292

51. All of the following medications may cause neutropenia EXCEPT:

   A. Ranitidine
   B. Phenytoin
   C. Lithium
   D. Methotrexate

Answer: C

Critique: Adverse reactions to many drugs may cause neutropenia. These include histamine-blocking agents (e.g., ranitidine), anticonvulsants (e.g., phenytoin), and chemotherapeutic agents (e.g., methotrexate). Lithium is not associated with neutropenia and may be used to shorten the duration of neutropenia caused by many medications.

Pages 1291, 1292

52. All of the following syndromes are associated with neutropenia EXCEPT:

   A. Paroxysmal nocturnal hemoglobinuria
   B. Mononucleosis
   C. Bulimia nervosa
   D. Felty's syndrome
   E. Human immunodeficiency virus (HIV)

Answer: C

Critique: Anorexia nervosa (not bulimia nervosa) is associated with neutropenia. While both are eating disorders, anorexia nervosa is characterized by weight 15% below what would be expected for age, and bulimia is characterized by recurrent binge eating syndromes. The starvation component of anorexia nervosa causes the associated neutropenia and leukopenia. Paroxysmal nocturnal hemoglobinuria is associated with neutropenia secondary to increased complement lysis of neutrophils. Both mononucleosis and HIV infections are associated with neutropenia. Neutropenia is part of the triad that is described as Felty's syndrome.

Page 1292

Further Reading

Kaplan HI, Sadock BJ: Pocket Book of Clinical Psychiatry. Baltimore, Williams & Wilkins, 1990, pp 198–200.

53. All of the following are associated with neutrophilia EXCEPT:

   A. Prednisone
   B. Exercise
   C. Lithium
   D. Epinephrine
   E. Trifluoperazine

Answer: E

Critique: Trifluoperazine and other antipsychotics can cause neutropenia. Corticosteroids, lithium, and epinephrine are all associated with neutrophilia. Vigorous exercise can also cause neutrophilia.

Page 1293

54. A reduction in the lymphocyte count to less than 1500/mm³ is associated with which ONE of the following conditions?

   A. Brucellosis
   B. Mononucleosis
   C. HIV
   D. Measles
   E. Chickenpox

Answer: C

Critique: A reduction in the lymphocyte count below 1500/mm³ is associated with HIV, Hodgkin's disease, myelosuppressive agents and disorders, and malnutrition. Brucellosis, young adult measles, chickenpox, and mononucleosis are all associated with lymphocytosis.

Page 1293

55. Which ONE of the following is true for patients undergoing elective splenectomy?

    A. They should be immunized prior to the procedure with 23-valent pneumococcal vaccine.
    B. They require prophylactic penicillin 6 months to 1 year prior to the procedure.
    C. They should be immunized with meningococcal vaccine after the procedure.
    D. They should be immunized with HIB vaccine after the procedure.

Answer: A

Critique: Patients undergoing elective splenectomy should be immunized with pneumococcal vaccine prior to the procedure. If other vaccinations are indicated (e.g., *Haemophilus influenzae* B (HIB) or meningococcal vaccine, they should be administered prior to the procedure. After splenectomy, patients do not respond appropriately to pneumococcal vaccine, HIB, or meningococcal vaccine. Patients should be placed on penicillin prophylaxis for 6 to 12 months after the procedure.

Page 1294

56. Patients with thrombocytopenia who have bone marrow that exhibits an adequate number of megakaryocytes, but with defects in maturation, have findings most consistent with:

    A. Vitamin B_{12} or folic acid deficiency
    B. An adverse reaction to gold therapy
    C. Cytotoxic agents
    D. Irradiation

Answer: A

Critique: Vitamin B_{12} and folic acid may result in thrombocytopenia with an adequate number of precursors, but with defects in the maturation process. Abnormalities in other cell lines may also be observed. Thrombocytopenia secondary to gold therapy is most likely to be associated with a decreased number of megakaryocytes, as are cytotoxic agents and irradiation.

Page 1295

57. Transfusion with six platelet packs should increase the platelet count by:

    A. 10,000 to 20,000/mm^3
    B. 20,000 to 40,000/mm^3
    C. 40,000 to 50,000/mm^3
    D. 70,000 to 90,000/mm^3

Answer: C

Critique: Transfusion with six platelet packs will generally raise the platelet count by 40,000 to 50,000/mm^3. Each platelet pack should raise the platelet count by 10,000/mm^3/m^2 of body surface area. Transfused platelets should last for 24 to 48 hours.

Page 1295

58. Treatment of idiopathic thrombocytopenic purpura (ITP) includes:

    A. Prednisone, aspirin, plasmapheresis, and splenectomy
    B. Prednisone, danazol, plasmapheresis, and splenectomy
    C. Prednisone, aspirin, danazol, and splenectomy
    D. Prednisone, aspirin, danazol, and plasmapheresis

Answer: B

Critique: Prednisone, danazol, plasmapheresis, and splenectomy all have indications in the treatment of ITP. However, the use of aspirin and other platelet inhibitors should be avoided because they are likely to exacerbate bleeding complications.

Pages 1295–1296

Questions 59–63. Match the statements to the following syndromes:

    A. Thrombotic thrombocytopenic purpura (TTP)
    B. TTP
    C. Both A and B
    D. Neither A nor B

59. Immunologic pathway mediates platelet destruction.

60. Severe hemolytic anemia

61. Fever

62. Central nervous system (CNS) abnormalities

63. Gastrointestinal bleeding

Answers: 59-B, 60-A, 61-A, 62-A, 63-C

Critique: ITP is mediated by platelet-associated IgG. The pathophysiology of TTP is mediated by nonimmunologic mechanisms, including damaged endothelial cells that induce platelet aggregation, intravascular coagulation, and platelet-activating factors, and thrombin levels. Hemolytic anemia, fever, and CNS abnormalities (e.g., seizures) are associated with TTP. Patients with both ITP and TTP may have mucosal bleeding complicating their disease.

Pages 1295–1297

64. Thrombocytosis with platelet counts in the range of 500,000 to 1×10^6/mm^3 most commonly:

    A. Is a reaction to another process
    B. Is a toxic effect due to excessive alcohol ingestion
    C. Increases the risk of thromboembolism at a platelet count of 1×10^6/mm^3
    D. Is frequently associated with dysfunctional platelets

Answer: A

Critique: Thrombocytosis is most commonly a reaction to some other process, such as inflammation, infection, or carcinoma. Thrombocytosis can occur when ingestion of ethanol is discontinued; however, ingestion of ethanol does not cause thrombocytosis. Ethanol usually acts as a megakaryocyte toxin. Risks for thromboembolism or hemorrhage are not increased at platelet counts of $1 \times 10^6/mm^3$, and thrombocytosis in this range is not generally associated with problems with platelet function. However, platelet counts in myeloproliferative disorders and essential thrombocythemia range from 1×10^6 to $3 \times 10^6/mm^3$ and are associated with increased risk of thromboembolism and platelet dysfunction.

Page 1297

Questions 65–68. Match the statements in questions 65 through 68 with the following clinical syndromes:

    A. Chronic myelogenous leukemia (CML)
    B. Chronic lymphocytic leukemia (CLL)
    C. Both A and B
    D. Neither A nor B

65. More commonly occurs in patients older than 60 years of age

66. Philadelphia chromosome

67. Overproduction of cells of the granulocytic series

68. Increased incidence with age

Answers: 65-B, 66-A, 67-A, 68-C

Critique: Most patients with CLL are older than 60 years of age. The median age at diagnosis for patients with CML is 45 to 50 years of age. For both CML and CLL, incidence increases with age. The Philadelphia chromosome is associated with 90 to 95% of cases of CML. The essential defect in CML is an overproduction of cells of the granulocytic series, usually the neutrophil. The defect in CLL is an overproduction of cells of the lymphocytic series. In more than 95% of cases, this is a B lymphocyte cell type.

Pages 1299, 1300

Further Reading

Keating MJ: The chronic leukemias. *In* Wyngaarden JB, Smith LH, Bennett JC (Eds): Cecil Textbook of Medicine, 19th ed. Philadelphia, WB Saunders, 1992, pp 933–944.

46

Urinary Tract Disorders

Roger J. Zoorob

1. All of the following urologic disorders typically cause flank pain EXCEPT:

    A. Ureterolithiasis
    B. Pyelonephritis
    C. Vascular occlusion
    D. Renal cyst
    E. Renal cell carcinoma

Answer: D

Critique: Flank pain can result from ureteral obstruction and distention due to ureterolithiasis. Flank pain, fever, chills, and pyuria point to pyelonephritis. Renal cell carcinoma produces flank pain due to a renal thrombus. Renal vein thrombosis results in gross hematuria and flank pain; fever and leukocytosis develop if the obstruction is acute. Oliguric renal failure, massive proteinuria, and lower extremity edema differentiate this condition from infections or stones. Renal cysts are usually asymptomatic.

Pages 1302, 1303

Questions 2–5. Match each numbered entry with the correct lettered heading:

    A. Hesitancy
    B. Urgency
    C. Urinary incontinence
    D. Urinary retention

2. Inability to empty the bladder

3. Intense need to void

4. Waiting for the stream to start

5. Loss of urinary control

Answers: 2-D, 3-B, 4-A, 5-C

Critique: Urgency is the immediate need to void and is caused by inflammation. Incontinence is the loss of urinary control per urethra. When associated with urgency, this symptom indicates urinary infection, neurogenic etiologies, or outflow tract obstruction. Hesitancy indicates bladder outlet obstruction. Urinary retention is found in outlet obstruction, bladder injury, and diabetes mellitus.

Page 1303

6. A 50-year-old male patient presents with a history of gross hematuria and left flank pain of 12 hours' duration. His physical examination shows normal vital signs and +3 pitting edema. The laboratory work-up shows a white blood cell count of 15.4; a urinalysis shows +4 proteinuria and numerous red blood cells; and his creatinine is 4.0. Which ONE of the following test options would be the most appropriate at this point?

    A. Urine culture
    B. Computed tomographic (CT) scan of the kidneys
    C. Renal arteriogram
    D. Intravenous pyelogram (IVP)

Answer: B

Critique: This patient presents a clinical picture highly suggestive of renal vein thrombosis. Findings that differentiate this finding from infection or stones include gross hematuria, massive proteinuria, edema of the lower extremities, and oliguric renal failure. If the venous obstruction is acute and extensive, fever, flank pain, and leukocytosis may develop. Ultrasonography and CT scanning are noninvasive means to establish the diagnosis.

Page 1303

7. (True or False) A 15-year-old male presents to your office after having testicular swelling and pain for 6 hours. He has no history of trauma. On physical examination, there is a firm tender mass in the scrotum. Elevation of the involved testicle does not relieve the pain. You should:

    1. Start the patient on antibiotics.
    2. Consult an oncologist.
    3. Consult a urologist.
    4. Draw an immediate amylase level.

Answers: 1-F, 2-F, 3-T, 4-F

Critique: This patient presents with a history typical for acute testicular torsion. Torsion of the testis usually occurs in patients younger than 20 years of age. The pain develops fairly suddenly, and a firm, tender mass appears in the scrotum. In contrast with epididymitis, elevation of the testicle does not relieve the pain. Management includes immediate identification of the problem and rapid urologic intervention. Testicular tumors are usually painless, and bacterial orchitis is rare in persons younger than 20 years of age. Although mumps orchitis is unilateral, it usually follows parotitis, and the patient usually has symptoms of a systemic viral infection.

Pages 1303, 1320

8. All of the following can present with perineal pain EXCEPT:

    A. Acute prostatitis
    B. Chronic prostatitis
    C. Acute ureteral obstruction
    D. Bladder tumors
    E. Vaginitis

Answer: C

Critique: Perineal pain is often caused by acute or chronic prostatitis, which may also result in low back pain. Women with cystitis or vaginitis may present with perineal pain, although this is a rare complaint. Accompanied by other symptoms, invasive bladder cancer may be associated with perineal pain. The pain due to an acute ureteral obstruction is unilateral, colicky, sudden, and radiates to the costovertebral angle, toward the inguinal ligament, and into the scrotum and labia majora.

Pages 1302, 1304

Questions 9–13. Match each numbered entry with the correct lettered heading:

    A. Hard scrotal mass
    B. Soft scrotal mass
    C. Both A and B
    D. Neither A nor B

9. Indirect inguinal hernia

10. Spermatocele

11. Testicular torsion

12. Testicular tumor

13. Hydrocele

Answers: 9-B, 10-B, 11-A, 12-A, 13-B

Critique: Scrotal masses can have either a hard or a soft consistency. Causes of hard masses include testicular torsion, epididymitis, torsion of the appendix testis, post-traumatic hematocele, and testicular tumors. Soft masses include indirect inguinal hernias, spermatoceles, hydroceles, and varicoceles.

14. (True or False) A 55-year-old man presents to your office with a "left testicular enlargement" that he noted 2 weeks ago. On physical examination, palpation shows a soft, nontender mass that feels like "a bag of worms."

The mass disappears when the patient is supine. The patient does not desire any more children. Management at this time includes:

    1. Referring the patient to a urologist.
    2. Performing a spermiogram.
    3. Evaluating for a renal tumor.
    4. Taking a urine culture.

Answers: 1-F, 2-F, 3-T, 4-F

Critique: Varicoceles occur more commonly on the left side than on the right side because of the angle at which the left spermatic vein joins the renal vein. They are usually nontender and disappear when the patient is supine. Varicoceles are asymptomatic, and no intervention is necessary unless fertility is in question; in this case, a spermiogram is indicated. However, a new-onset varicocele might indicate a renal tumor; thus an evaluation for a renal tumor is required. A referral to a urologist is not indicated at this stage. There is no clinical evidence of an infectious process; therefore, a urine culture should not be ordered.

Page 1305

Further Reading

Thomas AJ, Geisinger MA: Current management of varicoceles. Urol Clin North Am 17:893, 1990.

Questions 15–20. Match each numbered entry with the correct lettered heading:

    A. Spermatocele
    B. Hydrocele
    C. Both A and B
    D. Neither A nor B

15. Soft mass

16. Always transilluminates

17. A distinct mass from the testicle on palpation

18. May indicate a malignancy

19. May resolve spontaneously

20. Treated with antibiotics

Answers: 15-C, 16-B, 17-A, 18-B, 19-B, 20-D

Critique: Both spermatoceles and hydroceles are soft masses on palpation; a hydrocele always transilluminates. A spermatocele is also differentiated from a hydrocele by palpability in the upper portion of the junction between the testes and the epididymis. Hydroceles can be confused with scrotal hernias, and they can resolve spontaneously. Noncommunicating hydroceles can occur secondary to a lymphatic obstruction and thus can indicate a malignancy. Neither a spermatocele nor a varicocele is treated with antibiotics, unless the clinical picture suggests the presence of a secondary infection.

Pages 1304, 1305

21. (True or False) Chancroid is differentiated from syphilis by:

1. Lymphadenopathy
2. Presence of an ulcer
3. Darkfield microscopy
4. Response to penicillin

Answers: 1-F, 2-F, 3-T, 4-F

Critique: Chancroid is a bacterial infection that presents with ulcers and lymphadenopathy. The antibiotics of choice include ceftriaxone, erythromycin, and azithromycin. Syphilis responds well to penicillin. A darkfield examination is essential to differentiate syphilis from chancroid.

Pages 1305, 1306

Further Reading

Drugs for sexually transmitted diseases. Med Lett 36:1–6, 1994.
Sanford JP, Gilbert DN, Sande MA: *The Sanford Guide to Antimicrobial Therapy.* Dallas, Antimicrobial Therapy Inc., 1995, p 14.

22. A urine pH of 6.0 is most consistent with:

A. An infection with a urea-splitting organism
B. A normal urinary pH
C. Metabolic alkalosis
D. Respiratory alkalosis

Answer: B

Critique: A pH of 6.0 represents the normal pH of the urine, which is usually somewhat acidic. Urinary tract infections (UTIs) caused by urea-splitting organisms, such as *Proteus* or *Pseudomonas,* can result in an alkaline urinary pH.

Page 1306

23. Reddish or reddish orange urine may result from all of the following EXCEPT:

A. Bile
B. Rifampicin
C. Phenazopyridine
D. Beets

Answer: A

Critique: Normal fresh-voided urine is transparent. Rifampicin, phenazopyridine, and ingestion of beets can cause reddish or reddish-orange urine. Bile will produce brown urine, whereas blood or myoglobin may produce red or rust-colored urine.

Page 1306

24. (True or False) A 70-year-old poorly nourished man presents with malaise and a low-grade fever. On physical examination, he is afebrile and well oriented and has no costovertebral angle tenderness. A rectal examination reveals a slightly enlarged prostate that is smooth and nontender. A urinalysis shows 10 to 15 white blood cells per high-power field, one or two red blood cells, and no bacteria. His white blood cell count is normal. The differential diagnosis should include:

1. Interstitial nephritis
2. Acute prostatitis
3. Acute pyelonephritis
4. Tuberculosis

Answers: 1-T, 2-F, 3-F, 4-T

Critique: The presence of pyuria without bacteriuria may indicate renal tuberculosis or interstitial nephritis. Acute bacterial prostatitis is diagnosed by urinary frequency and pain as well as a swollen tender prostate. Leukocytosis is often seen. Acute pyelonephritis presents with irritative urinary symptoms, flank pain, and bacteriuria in addition to pyuria and leukocytosis.

Pages 1307, 1312

Questions 25–28. Match each numbered entry with the correct lettered diagnostic imaging modality of the urinary tract:

A. Ultrasonography
B. IVP
C. Voiding cystography
D. Retrograde pyelography

25. Differentiates a cystic mass from a solid testicular mass

26. Used to assess the size of the prostate

27. Displays anatomy and, to some extent, urinary function

28. Demonstrates vesicourethral reflux

Answers: 25-A, 26-A, 27-B, 28-C

Critique: Ultrasonography is important in differentiating solid from cystic masses but helps little in assessing function. It has a major role in assessing prostate size and nodularity and provides direction for a biopsy. An IVP displays the anatomy and, to some extent, the functional integrity of the urinary system. Voiding cystograms facilitate the diagnosis of vesicourethral reflux and urethral abnormalities, such as posterior urethral valves.

Page 1307

Questions 29–32. Match each numbered entry with the most appropriate lettered heading:

A. Gross hematuria
B. Microscopic hematuria
C. Both A and B
D. Neither A nor B

29. Kidney stone

30. Cystitis

31. Benign prostate hyperplasia

32. Testicular tumor

Answers: 29-C, 30-C, 31-C, 32-D

Critique: The presence of more than two red blood cells per high-power field in clean-voided urine of men and nonmenstruating women is a significant finding that requires evaluation. The differential diagnosis of both microscopic and gross hematuria includes kidney stones and tumors, bladder infections and tumors, and benign prostatic hyperplasia. A testicular tumor usually presents as a painless hard mass and would not be expected to demonstrate hematuria.

Pages 1304, 1308

33. A 35-year-old man was brought to the hospital by the emergency squad after a motor vehicle accident. He is alert and oriented, and his vital signs are stable. His physical examination shows bruising over the left costovertebral angle. His urine is grossly bloody. The best diagnostic modality to identify the source of the hematuria at this time is:

    A. Diagnostic ultrasound
    B. A flat x-ray film of the abdomen
    C. A retrograde pyelogram
    D. IVP

Answer: D

Critique: Hematuria associated with trauma to the flank requires prompt evaluation. IVP is a reasonable way to start the evaluation. Nonvisualization of the kidneys on IVP in a patient who has sustained possible trauma to the kidneys, with or without hematuria, requires an immediate referral. The other situation that requires an immediate referral is extravasation of the dye into the perinephric space, which indicates a renal rupture or laceration. Bladder integrity in the patient with suspected trauma to the genitourinary tract can also be evaluated by the IVP.

Pages 1308, 1309

34. A 2-year-old patient presents with painless hematuria. Which ONE of the following differential diagnoses should you consider first?

    A. Glomerular lesion
    B. Polycystic renal disease
    C. Scurvy
    D. Blood dyscrasias

Answer: A

Critique: Painless hematuria in children is considered to be caused by a glomerular lesion until proven otherwise. Other diseases to consider in the differential diagnosis are polycystic kidney disease, sickle cell disease, porphyria, vitamin C deficiency, and blood dyscrasias.

Page 1309

35. A healthy 14-year-old male presents to your office for a preparticipation sports evaluation. His physical examination and growth indices are normal. A routine urinalysis shows +3 protein with no hematuria or bacteriuria. The most likely test to yield the diagnosis is:

    A. Urine culture
    B. IVP

    C. Split urine collection for proteins
    D. Renal biopsy

Answer: C

Critique: With normal growth and no symptoms, this finding most likely represents orthostatic proteinuria. The protein excretion usually increases when the patient is sitting upright. The clinician should obtain a split collection of urine for protein to establish the diagnosis. The patient first provides a supine 12-hour urine collection for protein and then obtains another 12-hour collection while in the upright position. A renal biopsy taken from such patients does not reveal any significant abnormality, and the long-term prognosis is excellent.

Page 1311

36. Each of the following antibiotics is a reasonable choice for the outpatient treatment of uncomplicated lower UTIs EXCEPT:

    A. Amoxicillin
    B. Trimethoprim-sulfamethoxazole
    C. Nitrofurantoin (Macrodantin)
    D. Ceftriaxone

Answer: D

Critique: Sulfa drugs and trimethoprim, or fixed combinations of both, as well as ampicillin, amoxicillin, and nitrofurantoin, are all reasonable and inexpensive options for treating uncomplicated lower UTIs. Ceftriaxone is a third-generation cephalosporin and is reserved for the parenteral treatment of complicated UTIs and pyelonephritis.

Page 1310

37. (True or False) A 25-year-old previously healthy woman presents with urgency, dysuria, and urinary frequency, which she has had for 24 hours. There is no history of nausea or vomiting or of similar symptoms in the past. On physical examination, she is afebrile and has no costovertebral angle tenderness. Which of the following should you do at this time?

    1. Obtain a urinalysis.
    2. Obtain a urine culture.
    3. Start the patient on trimethoprim-sulfamethoxazole.
    4. Start the patient on erythromycin.

Answers: 1-T, 2-F, 3-T, 4-F

Critique: Urinalysis with microscopy is a valuable means to evaluate female patients who present with symptoms of a lower UTI. Urine cultures are usually indicated in infants, male patients, and women with unresolved infection. Since 80% of infections in such patients are caused by *Escherichia coli,* a cure is usually achieved with a course of trimethoprim-sulfamethoxazole. Erythromycin does not provide adequate microbial coverage for the usual causes of a UTI.

Page 1311

Questions 38–41. Match each numbered statement with the correct lettered heading:

    A. Perinephric abscess
    B. Pyelonephritis
    C. Both A and B
    D. Neither A nor B

38. Fever

39. Diagnosis by a CT scan

40. Medical treatment

41. Surgical treatment

Answers: 38-C, 39-A, 40-B, 41-A

Critique: The symptoms of acute pyelonephritis and perinephric abscess are similar; however, the duration of the fever is usually longer in the case of a perinephric abscess. When the symptoms last longer than 5 days despite adequate medical treatment of pyelonephritis, a perinephric abscess should be suspected. A CT scan or an ultrasound is useful in the diagnostic work-up. The treatment of a perinephric abscess is surgical drainage.

Page 1312

Questions 42–46. Match each numbered entry with the correct lettered heading:

    A. Acute bacterial prostatitis
    B. Chronic bacterial prostatitis
    C. Both A and B
    D. Neither A nor B

42. Tender prostate

43. Requires 3 to 4 months of antibiotics

44. Quinolone antibiotics

45. Patient may appear toxic

46. Requires 3 weeks of antibiotics

Answers: 42-A, 43-B, 44-C, 45-A, 46-A

Critique: A patient with acute bacterial prostatitis presents with fever, urinary frequency, and pain. The prostate is swollen and tender. The patient may require hospitalization. Chronic bacterial prostatitis is more difficult to diagnose and to cure. Voiding symptoms are minimal. Mild low back pain and perineal discomfort may be the presenting complaints. The prostate is frequently nontender. Quinolones are used in the treatment of both acute and chronic prostatitis. The duration of treatment is 3 weeks in acute prostatitis, whereas chronic prostatitis might require 3 to 4 months of treatment.

Pages 1312, 1313

47. (True or False) Acceptable treatments for gonococcal urethritis include:

    1. Ciprofloxacin 500 mg in a single dose
    2. Ceftriaxone 125 to 250 mg in a single dose
    3. Cefixime 400 mg in a single dose
    4. Amoxicillin 3 g in a single dose

Answers: 1-T, 2-T, 3-T, 4-F

Critique: Ciprofloxacin, ceftriaxone, and cefixime are all acceptable modes for the single-dose treatment of gonococcal urethritis. Of patients with gonococcal urethritis, 50% have a concomitant *Chlamydia trachomatis* infection, and adequate treatment for chlamydia should be provided as well. Amoxicillin is no longer considered adequate for treatment of gonococcal infections.

Page 1313

Further Reading

Drugs for sexually transmitted diseases. Med Lett 36:1–6, 1994.
Sanford JP, Gilbert DN, Sande MA: *The Sanford Guide to Antimicrobial Therapy.* Dallas, Antimicrobial Therapy, Inc., 1995, p 13.

48. Which ONE of the following is true regarding urinary calculi?

    A. A urinary pH of less than 7 is required for the formation of infected calculi.
    B. Of patients with gouty arthritis, 5% develop nephrolithiasis.
    C. Primary hyperparathyroidism, renal tubular acidosis, and medullary sponge kidney account for more than 90% of metabolic stones.
    D. Purines occur in higher concentrations in green leafy vegetables than are found in meats such as kidney or liver.

Answer: C

Critique: Metabolic stones account for only 10% of patients with recurrent stones. Primary hyperparathyroidism, renal tubular acidosis, and medullary sponge kidney are responsible for 90% of metabolic stones. The most common cause of genetically determined nephrolithiasis is gout. Of patients with gouty arthritis, 25% develop stones. Infected stones are triple phosphate calculi formed around a nidus of other substances in a persistently alkaline urine (pH above 7). Beer, wine, and meats are all foods that have a high purine content.

Page 1314

Questions 49–52. Match each numbered management option with the appropriate kidney stone type:

    A. Cystine stone
    B. Uric acid stone
    C. Both A and B
    D. Neither A nor B

49. Hydration

50. Alkalinization of urine

51. Dietary restriction of tea, chocolate, nuts, and citrus fruits

52. Allopurinol

Answers: 49-C, 50-C, 51-D, 52-B

Critique: Alkalinization of the urine and hydration are essential in the treatment of both uric acid and cystine stones. Allopurinol is used as an adjunct in the treatment of uric acid stones. A dietary restriction of tea, chocolate, green leafy vegetables, and caffeine may be important in the treatment of hyperoxaluria.

53. (True or False) Struvite stones:

1. Occur more often in men
2. Account for 15% of urinary stones
3. Consist of magnesium ammonium phosphate
4. Require alkaline urine for stone formation

Answers: 1-F, 2-T, 3-T, 4-T

Critique: Struvite stones are known as triple phosphate stones. The association of UTIs and stone formation has been long recognized. Struvite stones tend to form in the presence of urea-splitting bacteria. The bacterial action alkalinizes the urine and increases the concentration of the struvite component; this saturates the urine and stimulates stone formation.

Further Reading

Spirnak JP, Resnick MI: Urinary stones. *In* Tanagho EA, McAninch JW (Eds): Smith's General Urology, 13th ed. E. Norwalk, CT, Appleton & Lange, 1992, pp 283, 284.

54. (True or False) Evaluate the following statements regarding the management of urolithiasis:

1. Stones in the kidney less than 5 mm and without evidence of infection require only a periodic follow-up.
2. Staghorn calculi can be managed by extracorporeal wave lithotripsy.
3. Ureteral stones larger than 1 cm are managed by percutaneous manipulation but not by extracorporeal wave lithotripsy.
4. Bladder stones can safely be watched.

Answers: 1-T, 2-F, 3-F, 4-F

Critique: Asymptomatic renal calculi less than 5 mm require a semiannual follow-up with urinalysis and abdominal films. If there is no progress, an annual follow-up is sufficient. Renal stones larger than 1 cm can be managed by lithotripsy; however, staghorn stones require surgical removal by pyelolithotomy. Ureteral stones that are 5 mm or less can be managed medically and expectantly; however, if the size is larger than 1 cm, they rarely pass on their own. Both lithotripsy and percutaneous manipulation are effective. Bladder calculi should be removed through a cystoscope, and underlying predisposing factors, such as high residual urine or prolonged catheter drainage, should be corrected.

Pages 1315, 1316

55. Complications of vasectomy include all of the following EXCEPT:

A. Infection
B. Sperm granuloma
C. Urinary retention
D. Bleeding
E. Congestive epididymitis

Answer: C

Critique: A complication of a vasectomy is bleeding, which shows in the first couple of days, whereas infection manifests in 4 to 5 days. Other complications include: (1) sperm granulomas that occur as a result of spillage of sperm; these rarely cause problems unless they involve the spermatic nerve, in which case they are painful and require excision; and (2) congestive epididymitis, which is simply treated with bed rest and scrotal elevation. Urinary retention is not a known complication of vasectomy.

Page 1317

56. Of the following statements, which ONE is true regarding renal cell carcinoma?

A. The classic triad of hematuria, flank pain, and mass is present in 25% of the patients.
B. Hematuria is the first common sign and should be investigated by a positron emission tomographic (PET) scan.
C. Hematuria is the first common sign and should be investigated by an IVP.
D. Surgical treatment followed by chemotherapy offers a good prognosis.

Answer: C

Critique: There is no pathognomonic early sign for renal cell cancer. The triad mentioned earlier occurs in only 9% of the patients, and half of them present with metastasis. IVP is the preferred test for an initial evaluation of hematuria, followed by a CT scan for further evaluation if the result of the IVP is positive. The treatment of choice is nephrectomy, which, in the absence of metastasis, increases longevity. Renal cell cancer is relatively resistant to chemotherapy.

Page 1317

Further Reading

Wilkinson M: Chemotherapy of urologic tumors. *In* Tanagho EA, McAninch J (Eds): Smith General Urology, 13th ed. E. Norwalk, CT, Appleton & Lange, 1992, pp 451, 452.

57. With regard to prostate cancer:

A. An elevated prostate-specific antigen (PSA) is a specific indicator of prostate cancer.
B. Transrectal ultrasound has not proved to be an important tool in the diagnosis of prostate cancer.
C. The standard surgical treatment for disease confined to the prostate is radical prostatectomy.
D. Pain due to bony metastasis responds better to hormonal therapy than to radiation.

Answer: C

Critique: PSA is an important marker for detection and monitoring the progression of prostate cancer. However,

PSA can also be seen with prostatitis and benign large prostate glands. Transrectal ultrasonography has proved to be an invaluable tool in the diagnosis of prostate cancer. For patients who are candidates, a radical prostatectomy is still the gold standard surgical treatment. Hormonal manipulation is the mainstay of disseminated prostate cancer, but painful bony metastasis responds well to local irradiation.

Pages 1318, 1319

Questions 58–61. Match each numbered entry with the correct lettered heading:

  A. Penile cancer
  B. Testicular cancer
  C. Both A and B
  D. Neither A nor B

58. Is a rare tumor

59. Is the most common tumor in persons who are 18 to 40 years of age

60. Presents as a painless mass

61. Is usually a squamous cell cancer

Answers: 58-C, 59-B, 60-B, 61-A

Critique: Both penile tumors and testicular tumors are rare; however, testicular tumors are the most common solid tumors in persons who are 18 to 40 years of age. Testicular tumors present as a painless mass with the pathology representing seminoma or nonseminoma. Penile tumors usually demonstrate squamous cell carcinoma and are usually treated surgically with partial or total penectomy.

Page 1320

62. A 24-year-old man presents with a painless hard mass on the left testicle. An orchiectomy confirms an embryonal carcinoma. A metastatic work-up shows a stage II tumor progress. Which ONE statement is true regarding treatment for this tumor?

  A. The patient has an 80% chance of a cure with chemotherapy.
  B. Radiation is the treatment of choice.
  C. Surgical intervention is the mainstay treatment.
  D. A bilateral orchiectomy and hormonal replacement are essential for a cure.

Answer: A

Critique: Stage II tumors are treated with combination chemotherapy consisting of cisplatin, vinblastine, and bleomycin, with 80% of patients achieving a cure. Surgical intervention is reserved for patients with a residual mass. Radiation is the mainstay in the treatment of seminoma.

Pages 1320, 1321

Questions 63–67. Match each numbered entry with the correct lettered heading:

  A. Terazosin
  B. Finasteride
  C. Both A and B
  D. Neither A nor B

63. Is an α_1-adrenergic antagonist

64. Used for treatment of benign prostate hyperplasia

65. The dose needs to be titrated.

66. Is a 5α-reductase inhibitor

67. PSA needs to be monitored.

Answers: 63-A, 64-C, 65-A, 66-B, 67-C

Critique: Both terazosin and finasteride are approved for treatment of benign prostate hyperplasia. Terazosin is an α-antagonist that inhibits the α_1-receptors in the smooth muscles of the prostate and bladder. This results in decreased resistance to the flow of urine. The dosage should be titrated to minimize side effects. Finasteride is a 5α-reductase inhibitor, and the optimal dose is 5 mg. It lowers PSA levels up to 50% from pretreatment levels in 6 months; hence the PSA level should be checked prior to starting treatment and 6 months later to monitor the response to therapy.

Page 1322

68. All of the following are true about ureteral trauma EXCEPT:

  A. May result in fever
  B. May manifest a mass
  C. Anemia is a presenting sign
  D. Is most commonly a result of multiple trauma

Answer: D

Critique: Ureteral trauma is mostly iatrogenic, resulting from gynecologic or general surgery. Repair is easier and more successful if ureteral trauma is discovered during the surgery. Fever, mass, and anemia are the manifesting signs and symptoms.

Page 1323

69. Overflow incontinence:

  A. Is helped by anticholinergic agents such as oxybutynin
  B. Is usually due to an inflammatory condition
  C. Exhibits a large amount of residual urine
  D. Decreases with increases in intra-abdominal pressure

Answer: C

Critique: Stress incontinence occurs with varying degrees of increased abdominal pressure (e.g., coughing and laughing). Urgency incontinence is a complaint in which the patient has the urge to void but cannot reach the toilet in time. It results from inflammatory conditions and responds to anticholinergic agents and treatment of the infection. With overflow incontinence, small amounts of urine are released every few minutes during the day and at night. Overflow incontinence occurs in diabetes mellitus, stroke, and spinal cord disease. There is a large amount of residual urine. Increased intra-abdominal pressure will increase the incontinence. Intermittent catheterization is the treatment of choice until the primary cause can be resolved.

Page 1324

70. Which ONE of the following is true regarding impotence?

    A. The incidence is 5% at age 45.
    B. The incidence is 25% at age 65.
    C. Organic causes usually have an abrupt onset.
    D. The incidence is very low in diabetics.

Answer: B

Critique: Impotence is the consistent inability to attain erections sufficiently rigid for vaginal penetration. An estimated 10 million men have erectile dysfunction. The incidence is 1.9% at age 40. Persons with diabetes mellitus may have an incidence up to 50%. Psychogenic causes usually have an abrupt onset, whereas organic causes have a gradual onset.

Pages 1324–1328

71. With regard to undescended testicles, which ONE of the following is true?

    A. Orchiopexy should be performed at puberty.
    B. Orchiopexy is occasionally needed for retractile testicles.
    C. Most undescended testicles descend by the first birthday.
    D. A true undescended testicle cannot be palpated.

Answer: C

Critique: Most undescended testicles descend by the first birthday. Orchiopexy should be performed immediately after the first birthday. Orchiopexy should not be performed on any retractile testicles. True undescended testicles may be palpated, but in contrast to retractile testicles, undescended testicles cannot be manipulated into the scrotum.

Page 1326

72. In patients with enuresis, all of the following statements are true EXCEPT:

    A. A urine culture should be obtained.
    B. A urinalysis should be obtained.
    C. A family history should be obtained.
    D. Fifty percent of patients improve on 1-deamino-(8-D-arginine)-vasopressin (DDAVP).

Answer: D

Critique: In children presenting with enuresis, a history suggestive of UTIs should be obtained as well as a family history of enuresis. A work-up should always include a urinalysis and a urine culture. If the result of the urinalysis or culture is positive, further urologic evaluation is indi-

cated to rule out anatomic abnormalities. Treatment starts by exhibiting a nonjudgmental attitude toward the child, by responsibility enforcement (e.g., the patient keeping a record of enuresis episodes), and by pharmacologic treatment. DDAVP therapy improves symptoms in 75 to 90% of patients.

Pages 1326, 1327

73. A 4-year-old female presents with burning on urination and frequency. There is no history of fever, nausea, vomiting, or flank pain. Microscopic urinalysis shows 10 to 15 white blood cells per high-power field. Which ONE of the following is most appropriate in managing her problem?

    A. Start her on intravenous antibiotic therapy.
    B. Refer the patient for a urologic consultation for cystoscopy.
    C. After successful treatment, administer suppressive therapy.
    D. Schedule an ultrasound of the kidneys.

Answer: D

Critique: Children with uncomplicated UTIs should be treated with oral antibiotics on an outpatient basis. A radiologic examination should be scheduled to rule out reflux and anatomic abnormalities after the first infection. Ultrasound has replaced the IVP in children. Cystoscopy is not routinely indicated in the work-up of a UTI in children. Suppressive therapy is indicated if reinfections occur and are not indicated after one uncomplicated infection.

Pages 1327, 1328

Further Reading

Roth RR, Gonzales ET: Urinary tract infection. *In* Oski FA, Feigin RD, McMillan JA, Warshaw JB (Eds): Principles and Practice of Pediatrics, 2nd ed. Philadelphia, JB Lippincott, 1994, pp 1770–1772.

74. (True or False) Which of the following patients represent good candidates for short-term (i.e., 1 to 3 days) oral antibiotic therapy?

    1. A 25-year-old healthy female bank employee who presents with urgency, frequency, vomiting, and flank pain.
    2. A 25-year-old pregnant woman who presents with urgency and frequency of 24 hours' duration.
    3. A 25-year-old healthy female graduate student who presents with urgency, frequency, and dysuria.
    4. A 25-year-old diabetic female housewife who presents with no flank pain, fever, or vomiting.

Answers: 1-F, 2-F, 3-T, 4-F

Critique: Short-term antibiotic therapy for UTIs is indicated in healthy women with acute lower UTIs. Patients presenting with symptoms and signs suggesting pyelonephritis (such as in the first scenario) should not be considered for short-term antibiotic therapy. Diabetes, pregnancy, immunosuppression, reflux, and urinary calculi are contraindications for short-term therapy.

Page 1328

75. True statements regarding UTIs in female patients include all of the following EXCEPT:

A. Ten to 20% of female patients will ultimately develop a UTI.
B. Reinfections account for approximately 30% of frequent recurrent infections.
C. Persistent infection accounts for 1% of recurrent infections.
D. The pathogenesis of a UTI in women involves the interrelationship between bacterial colonization and host susceptibility.

Answer: B

Critique: Ten to 20% of women will develop a UTI during their lives. Most of these infections involve acute cystitis. They are rarely serious infections, except in diabetics and pregnant patients or when accompanied by an obstruction. The pathogenesis involves a balance between bacterial flora of the vagina and host immunity factors. Infections can be recurrent. Ninety-nine percent of recurrences are reinfections (i.e., the urine is sterile between the initial and subsequent infection). Only 1% of the frequent UTIs represent persistent infection.

Page 1328

76. A 50-year-old female presents with a history of frequency, urgency, dysuria, and pelvic pressure. There is no history of fever or flank pain. Urinalysis shows 1 or 2 white blood cells per high-power field on microscopic examination. The urine culture shows no growth. You should do all of the following EXCEPT:

A. Perform a vaginal examination with potassium hydroxide (KOH) and saline smear preparations.
B. Consider a cystoscopy and a bladder biopsy.
C. Refer to a psychiatrist for an evaluation for obsessive-compulsive disorder.
D. Consider a referral to a urologist for urodynamic studies.

Answer: C

Critique: This patient presents a history consistent with urethral syndrome. In the absence of pyuria and with a negative result on a urine culture, vaginitis should be considered, and testing for *Candida, Trichomonas,* and *Gardnerella* should be performed. Other diagnoses to consider include interstitial cystitis and carcinoma in situ, both of which are diagnosed with cystoscopy and biopsy. Urodynamic studies are indicated to rule out a neurogenic bladder. Psychogenic causes should not be entertained at this point, and spastic bladder is a consideration only after organic causes are ruled out.

Page 1329

77. Which ONE of the following statements is true regarding glomerular filtration rate (GFR) and creatinine clearance?

A. Increase from birth until age 6
B. Normal value for creatinine clearance at age 70 is about 125 ml/min.

C. Direct measurements of GFR can be easily accomplished in clinical practice.
D. GFR is not a good indicator of renal function.

Answer: A

Critique: GFR is the single best indicator of overall renal function. It increases from birth till 4 to 6 years of age. It is not directly measured in clinical practice but rather is estimated by creatinine clearance. The normal creatinine clearance in healthy adults may vary between 80 and 125 ml/min, but it decreases linearly with age. Hence a 70-year-old may have a GFR that is 70% of that seen in younger patients.

Pages 1329, 1330

78. (True or False) Evaluate the following statements regarding oliguria and azotemia:

1. Oliguria is defined as urine output less than 250 ml/day.
2. Normal blood urea nitrogen (BUN):creatinine ratio is less than 20:1.
3. Prerenal azotemia can result from cirrhosis.
4. A urinary sodium level of 60 mEq/l is suggestive of prerenal azotemia.

Answers: 1-F, 2-T, 3-T, 4-F

Critique: Oliguria is defined as a urine output that is less than 400 ml/day. Anuria is the absence of urine output. The normal BUN:creatinine ratio is less than 20:1; values greater than 20 indicate prerenal azotemia in conditions such as hypovolemia, hypotension, or congestive heart failure. Urinary sodium in the absence of diuretic intake is usually less than 20 mEq/l in patients with prerenal azotemia.

Page 1330

Further Reading

Finn WF: Diagnosis and management of acute tubular necrosis. Med Clin North Am 74:873–889, 1990.

Questions 79–82. Match each numbered statement with the correct lettered heading.

A. Acute renal failure (ARF)
B. Chronic renal failure (CRF)
C. Both A and B
D. Neither A nor B

79. Characterized by normal hemoglobin

80. Ultrasound shows small kidneys.

81. Urine sodium of 50 mEq/l

82. Ultrasound may show large kidneys.

Answers: 79-A, 80-B, 81-C, 82-A

Critique: ARF is a clinical syndrome characterized by an abrupt decline in the GFR. Major causes include hypovolemic shock, sepsis, hepatic failure, and nephrotoxic injury such as from radiocontrast material and drugs. ARF is characterized by normal hemoglobin, the inability to concentrate the urine, and a urinary sodium level greater than 30 mEq/l. The kidney size, however, remains normal or large. CRF is caused by intrinsic renal diseases, such as chronic glomerulonephritis and chronic interstitial nephritis, and systemic diseases such as diabetes mellitus. Diabetes represents the most common cause of CRF likely to be encountered in clinical practice. Hypertension and obstructive uropathy also cause CRF. CRF is characterized by high urinary sodium, anemia, and small shrunken kidneys on ultrasound.

Pages 1331, 1332

Further Reading

Finn WF: Diagnosis and management of acute tubular necrosis. Med Clin North Am 74:879–884, 1990.

83. Which ONE of the following is an indication for acute hemodialysis?

    A. Serum potassium of 6.0
    B. Drug overdose with a high-molecular-weight substance
    C. Drug overdose with a low-molecular-weight substance
    D. Advanced cirrhosis with encephalopathy

Answer: C

Critique: Acute hemodialysis is indicated in the treatment of fluid overload resistant to medical therapy in the presence of renal dysfunction, hyperkalemia above or equal to 7.0 with electrocardiogram (ECG) changes, uremic symptoms, and drug overdose with low-molecular-weight drugs. Drugs with high molecular weight or that are tightly protein-bound (e.g., theophylline and phenobarbital) are removed poorly by dialysis. Charcoal hemoperfusion is more effective in the latter circumstances.

Pages 1332, 1333

Further Reading

Jameson MD, Wiegmann TB: Principles, uses, and complications of hemodialysis. Med Clin North Am 74:951, 1990.

84. Of the following conditions, all are associated with hyponatremia and *increased* extracellular fluid volume EXCEPT:

    A. Congestive heart failure
    B. Hepatic cirrhosis
    C. Nephrotic syndrome
    D. Hypothyroidism

Answer: D

Critique: Hyponatremia usually reflects an increase in plasma water but may reflect the presence of hyperlipidemia. Hyponatremia occurs in patients with increased total body sodium content, such as congestive heart failure, cirrhosis, and nephrotic syndrome, because renal clearance of solute-free water is impaired. Severe hypo-

thyroidism can result in hyponatremia with *normal* extracellular fluid volume.

Page 1333, Table 46–12

85. An 80-year-old man is brought in by his son with a history of vomiting and diarrhea and decreased mental status of 24 hours' duration. The neurologic examination is unremarkable except for his mental status. His blood pressure is 100/70. He is afebrile and has dry mucous membranes. The results of the laboratory work-up are negative except for a sodium level of 115 mEq/l. You should do which ONE of the following?

    A. Correct the sodium deficit as fast as possible with intravenous 5% NaCl until a sodium level of 135 mEq/l is achieved.
    B. Perform a PET scan.
    C. Correct the hyponatremia at a rate of 2 mEq/l until a sodium level of 120 mEq/l is achieved.
    D. The goal of therapy is initially to raise the sodium level to 120 mEq/l and to correct the hyponatremia at a rate of 1 mEq/l/l.

Answer: D

Critique: When hyponatremia develops, the rapid correction of sodium is dangerous and can result in central pontine myelinosis. Hypertonic saline should be used only with a patient presenting with neurologic symptoms. This patient's hyponatremia resulted from gastrointestinal loss of sodium, and the initial target for correction is a sodium level of 120 mEq/l. The correction of hyponatremia should be at a rate of 1 mEq/l or less in patients with volume depletion. Normal saline is safer to use and is as effective as hypertonic saline.

Pages 1333, 1334

86. A 70-year-old man with a history of congestive heart failure presents with mild shortness of breath on exertion. His examination shows +2 peripheral edema. The results of the laboratory work-up are normal except for a sodium value of 126. The patient has normal mental status. Of the following options, the best treatment plan is:

    A. Diuretics plus oral sodium chloride
    B. Diuretics plus intravenous normal saline to avoid rapid correction of sodium and neurologic injury
    C. Diuretics plus fluid restriction
    D. Diuretics alone

Answer: C

Critique: The patient has edema secondary to congestive heart failure. Diuretics are essential in the treatment. The patient has increased total body sodium and increased extracellular fluid volume, as evidenced by edema. The ideal treatment is, therefore, administration of diuretics with fluid restriction.

Page 1334

Questions 87–94. Match each numbered entry with the correct lettered heading regarding potassium metabolism.

A. Hyperkalemia
B. Hypokalemia
C. Both A and B
D. Neither A nor B

87. Metabolic acidosis

88. Patients on diuretics

89. Patients on angiotensin-converting enzyme (ACE) inhibitors

90. Patients on insulin

91. Nonsteroidal anti-inflammatory agents

92. Treated with intravenous calcium

93. U wave on an ECG

94. Patients with sarcoidosis

Answers: 87-A, 88-B, 89-A, 90-B, 91-A, 92-A, 93-B, 94-D

Critique: The differential diagnosis of hypokalemia includes a shift of potassium into the intracellular fluid, such as occurs with alkalosis or insulin therapy, and gastrointestinal or renal losses, which occur with diarrhea or diuretics. ECG changes of hypokalemia include the appearance of a U wave. The differential diagnosis of hyperkalemia includes renal failure and use of drugs such as ACE inhibitors and nonsteroidal anti-inflammatory agents. ECG changes include a peaked T wave and various degrees of heart block. In life-threatening situations, treatment with intravenous calcium is indicated.

Pages 1335, 1336; Tables 46–16 and 46–17

95. (True or False) Examine the following statements regarding hypercalcemia:

1. Asymptomatic hypercalcemia appearing on a routine chemistry panel is most often due to a malignancy.
2. The presence of normal or high phosphate in patients with hypercalcemia should raise the suspicion of a destructive bony lesion.
3. The treatment of acute hypercalcemia includes saline diuresis.
4. Calcitonin and diphosphonates should be used in the treatment of acute hypercalcemia.

Answers: 1-F, 2-T, 3-T, 4-F

Critique: Asymptomatic high serum calcium discovered routinely on a chemistry panel does not usually indicate a malignancy. However, hypercalcemia might suggest metastatic or destructive bony lesions, especially if the phosphate level is high or normal. Sarcoidosis and paraneoplastic syndromes are other causes. Treatment starts with intravenous saline plus furosemide to induce a saline

diuresis. Calcitonin and diphosphonates are used in chronic and resistant cases.

Page 1336

96. (True or False) The differential diagnosis of respiratory alkalosis includes:

1. Anxiety
2. Salicylates
3. Fever
4. Shock

Answers: 1-T, 2-T, 3-T, 4-F

Critique: Respiratory alkalosis is caused by hyperventilation as a result of anxiety, or by subtle hyperventilation, such as in patients with cirrhosis. Aspirin overdose results in respiratory alkalosis from central stimulation and as a response to metabolic acidemia secondary to the salicylic acid. Shock states produce increased anion gap metabolic acidosis secondary to lactic acidosis.

Page 1338

97. All of the following conditions are associated with metabolic acidosis with increased anion gap EXCEPT:

A. Salicylate ingestion
B. Methanol ingestion
C. Diabetic ketoacidosis
D. Renal tubular acidosis

Answer: D

Critique: The differential diagnosis of metabolic acidosis with increased anion gap includes ketoacidosis due to diabetes, alcohol, or starvation; lactic acidosis due to shock, seizures, carbon monoxide poisoning, or respiratory failure; and toxic ingestion of methanol, aspirin, or paraldehyde. Renal tubular acidosis produces hyperchloremic metabolic acidosis.

Pages 1338, 1339; Tables 46–21 and 46–22

Questions 98–101. Match each of the following numbered statements with the lettered most appropriate glomerular lesion:

A. Minimal change disease
B. Focal glomerulosclerosis
C. Membranous glomerulonephritis
D. Membranoproliferative glomerulonephritis

98. Uncommon and associated with hypocomplementemia

99. Common in adolescents and patients with human immunodeficiency virus (HIV)

100. Common in middle-aged persons and in patients with hepatitis B

101. The most common nephrotic syndrome encountered in children

Answers: 98-D, 99-B, 100-C, 101-A

Critique: Minimal change disease, also called lipoid nephrosis, is the most common cause of nephrotic syndrome in children. The patient is usually normotensive, has no hematuria, and responds to high doses of corticosteroids. Focal glomerulosclerosis is a lesion that appears in part or in some of the glomeruli. The lesion is common in adolescents and young adults and is associated with HIV. Drug therapy has not been successful in most of those patients. Membranous glomerulonephritis is seen most commonly in middle-aged patients. Patients presenting with edema, mild hypertension, and renal function remain normal. The urinalysis shows minimal hematuria. Membranoproliferative glomerulonephritis is uncommon and is characterized by hypocomplementemia. If left untreated, the disease progresses to renal failure.

Pages 1340, 1341

Questions 102–105. Match each of the numbered statements with the most appropriate lettered heading:

   A. Nephrotic syndrome
   B. Nephritic syndrome

   C. Both A and B
   D. Neither A nor B

102. Most common cause is diabetes mellitus

103. Poststreptococcal glomerulonephritis

104. Immunoglobulin (Ig)A nephropathy

105. Hypercholesterolemia

Answers: 102-A, 103-B, 104-B, 105-A

Critique: Diabetes mellitus is the most common cause of nephrotic syndrome. It is characterized hypoalbuminuria, hypoalbuminemia, hyperlipidemia, and edema. Poststreptococcal glomerulonephritis is the prime example of nephritic syndrome. It is characterized by hematuria, red blood cell casts, and evidence of acute renal dysfunction and edema. IgA nephropathy is the most common form of nephritis encountered in medical practice. Hypercholesterolemia can occur concomitant with nephrotic syndrome.

Page 1341

47

Ophthalmology
Mitchell S. King

1. In evaluating the "red eye," which of the following would have associated abnormalities in pupillary size?

    A. Viral conjunctivitis
    B. Acute angle-closure glaucoma
    C. Bacterial conjunctivitis
    D. Keratitis

Answer: B

Critique: When evaluating the red eye, important signs and symptoms to help distinguish among the various causes include visual changes, presence and character of pain, photophobia, discharge, nature of the conjunctival injection, corneal appearance, pupillary sizes, and intraocular pressures. Acute angle-closure glaucoma is a condition requiring urgent evaluation and treatment with an ophthalmologic referral. It is characterized by a dilated oval pupil, visual blurring, severe pain, rainbow halos around lights, nausea and vomiting, as well as photophobia, corneal clouding, and elevated intraocular pressure. An examination of the affected eye may also reveal a narrowed anterior chamber. Precipitating factors may include emotional or physical stress, or pupillary dilatation by dim lighting or eye drops. Treatment should be provided immediately to prevent visual loss and includes medical lowering of intraocular pressure followed by laser iridectomy. Other causes of red eye that can cause pupillary changes are iritis, in which the affected eye will have a constricted pupil, and ocular trauma, in which the affected eye may have a dilated, irregular pupil. Viral conjunctivitis, bacterial conjunctivitis, and keratitis cause red eyes but without pupillary changes.

Pages 1346, 1347, 1352, 1353, 1355

2. (Matching) Which of the following causes of the "red eye" are associated with visual changes?

    A. 1, 2, and 3
    B. 1 and 3
    C. 2 and 4
    D. 4 only
    E. All of the above

1. Iritis

2. Keratitis

3. Glaucoma

4. Bacterial conjunctivitis

Answer: A

Critique: Blurring of vision is an important sign of a more serious cause of a red eye. Iritis, keratitis, and acute angle-closure glaucoma may all cause visual changes. Iritis is characterized by severe pain, circumcorneal injection of the conjunctiva, a constricted pupil, photophobia, and absence of discharge or corneal clouding. Intraocular pressure may be normal or low in iritis. Keratitis is characterized by sharp pain, photophobia, circumcorneal conjunctival injection, corneal clouding, and possibly minimal discharge with normal intraocular pressures and pupillary sizes. Keratitis, iritis, and acute angle-closure glaucoma all warrant an ophthalmologic referral.

Conjunctivitis is characterized by diffuse conjunctival injection, discharge and absence of visual changes, photophobia, corneal clouding, pupillary changes, or pain. Conjunctivitis can be treated with topical antibiotics, typically sulfacetamide, erythromycin, or aminoglycosides, unless gonococcal or chlamydial conjunctivitis is suspected in which case systemic antibiotics are warranted.

Pages 1346, 1347, 1351, 1352

3. A 3-month-old infant is brought into the office with a history of excessive tearing of the right eye since birth and a history of yellow discharge from the eye. The mother states that she is using antibiotic eye drops and performing massage as directed by your partner. An examination of the eye is within normal limits except for pooling of tears along the lower lid. Which of the following is true regarding management of this condition?

    A. Treatment should include systemic antibiotics.
    B. An immediate ophthalmologic consultation is required.

C. This condition will most likely require surgical intervention to resolve.

D. This condition will likely resolve spontaneously within the next 3 months.

Answer: D

Critique: The condition present in this infant represents chronic dacryocystitis or partial nasolacrimal duct obstruction. Eighty percent of cases spontaneously resolve by 6 months of age. Treatment may include topical antibiotics and massage. In persistent cases, probing of the duct is required. Acute dacryocystitis is a related condition that presents with pain, tearing, and redness along with the discharge. The child may be febrile and will require systemic antibiotics and a more prompt ophthalmologic consultation because probing and irrigation of the nasolacrimal duct may be necessary.

Page 1348

4. Which of the following is a side effect of corticosteroid ophthalmic preparations?

A. Macular degeneration
B. Open-angle glaucoma
C. Strabismus
D. Optic neuritis
E. Hyphema

Answer: B

Critique: Topical steroids should be used cautiously and are indicated for a limited number of ophthalmologic conditions that will likely require consultation. Topical steroids should not be used in conjunction with antibiotics for treating conjunctivitis. Side effects of steroids include worsening of herpetic corneal infections, facilitation of fungal corneal infections, open-angle glaucoma, and with prolonged use, cataracts. Systemic steroids may occasionally have similar effects. Steroids have not been found to cause macular degeneration, strabismus, hyphema, or optic neuritis.

Pages 1351, 1374–1376

5. A 65-year-old man presents with acute loss of vision in his right eye. Upon examination you note a pale optic disc with diffuse retinal pallor and arteriolar narrowing. Appropriate initial treatment while awaiting an ophthalmologic consultation may include which of the following?

A. 1, 2, and 3
B. 1 and 3
C. 2 and 4
D. 4 only
E. All of the above

1. Ocular massage

2. Topical steroid drops

3. Ask the patient to breathe into a paper bag.

4. Administer a carbonic anhydrase inhibitor.

Answer: B

Critique: The patient has central retinal artery occlusion, which can occur secondary to an embolus, atherosclerosis, or arteritis. This represents an emergent situation and prompt treatment may help to restore arterial perfusion. Initial maneuvers that may be helpful involve increasing the inspired carbon dioxide level by rebreathing into a bag and lowering intraocular pressure by ocular massage. An additional procedure, which is sometimes used by ophthalmologists and may restore vision, is the performance of paracentesis, or the removal of aqueous humor, which will rapidly decompress the eye. Topical steroid drops are used for select inflammatory conditions of the eye and would not be indicated or effective for central retinal artery occlusion. Carbonic anhydrase inhibitors are used to treat glaucoma.

Pages 1353, 1378

6. A 10-year-old girl is brought to your office after an upper respiratory infection with a painless left red eye and no visual complaints or discharge. She has had no prior episodes. Her past medical history includes only a tonsillectomy without complications 5 years ago. The examination, including visual acuity, is normal except for what you are confident is a subconjunctival hemorrhage. A true statement regarding the care of this patient is:

A. An immediate ophthalmologic consultation is required.
B. Treatment includes surgical removal of the hematoma.
C. No therapy is needed, and this should resolve in 2 to 3 weeks.
D. A hematologic work-up for bleeding diathesis is needed.
E. A referral to social services for suspected abuse is indicated.

Answer: C

Critique: Subconjunctival hemorrhage, though impressive to look at, is generally a benign condition with no visual symptoms or associated pain. Commonly, patients will present as this patient did with a history of coughing, sneezing, or straining or with no obvious cause. No therapy is indicated, and the condition should resolve in 2 to 3 weeks.

Subconjunctival hemorrhage can be present when trauma occurs, and in this case an ophthalmologic referral may be warranted. Hematologic studies would not be indicated in the presence of an isolated case of subconjunctival hemorrhage but may be warranted with recurrent episodes or other symptoms suggestive of a bleeding diathesis. As noted, trauma can cause subconjunctival hemorrhage, and other signs of bodily injury may warrant consideration of abuse.

Page 1352

7. True statements regarding hyphema include:

A. 1, 2, and 3
B. 1 and 3
C. 2 and 4

D. 4 only

E. All of the above

1. Most occur spontaneously.

2. Secondary hemorrhage is a determinant of the prognosis.

3. The recovery of good visual acuity occurs in fewer than 50% of patients.

4. Complications may include glaucoma, corneal staining, or optic atrophy.

Answer: C

Critique: Hyphema refers to hemorrhage into the anterior chamber of the eye and occurs most commonly in children secondary to trauma. Spontaneous hyphema is rare and occurs secondary to vascular anomalies or neoplasms. The amount of bleeding that occurs is graded 1 through 4, and the grade along with the occurrence of complications or damage to other intraocular structures determines the prognosis for visual recovery. Complications that may occur include secondary hemorrhage, optic atrophy, corneal staining, and glaucoma. Treatment is directed at reducing the incidence of secondary hemorrhage and controlling intraocular pressures. Treatment results in the recovery of acceptable visual acuity in 75% of cases.

Pages 1355, 1356

8. Screening for eye disease in children is currently recommended at what ages?

A. 1, 2, and 3

B. 1 and 3

C. 2 and 4

D. 4 only

E. All of the above

1. Newborn

2. 6 months

3. 3 years

4. 5 years

Answer: E

Critique: In children, ocular examinations and vision screening are recommended in the newborn, at ages 6 months, 3 years, 5 years, then every other year until age 12. Additionally, children with mental retardation, cerebral palsy, or with visual signs or symptoms and learning disabilities should be screened regardless of age. Adults should be screened for glaucoma every 3 years, beginning at 35 years of age, and should have a complete examination every 3 years beginning at age 40 and every 2 years beginning at age 65. Details of the examination are presented in the text.

Pages 1356–1371, 1376

9. (True or False) The following parts of the eye examination are performed to detect strabismus:

1. Funduscopic examination

2. Binocular visual acuity

3. Cover/uncover test

4. Corneal light reflex test

5. Test for color vision

Answers: 1-F, 2-F, 3-T, 4-T, 5-F

Critique: Strabismus is a misalignment of the eye muscles resulting in loss of fusion of the two images from the eyes to the brain. Adults will frequently present with double vision; however, children will learn to suppress one of the images, resulting in loss of central vision in the unused eye. Testing for strabismus using the cover/uncover test, corneal light reflex test, and extraocular rotations can lead to earlier detection and treatment of strabismus, thus possibly preventing amblyopia, or loss of vision. Amblyopia occurs in about 50% of patients with strabismus and is treatable if detected by 3 or 4 years of age. Amblyopia is generally irreversible after age 7.

Funduscopic examination in the patient with strabismus may be normal. Testing binocular vision will not detect strabismus, because there may be no visual loss, or the patient may test normally with binocular vision despite visual loss in one eye. Testing monocular vision may detect some visual loss if amblyopia is present. Similarly, testing color vision would not be useful for detecting strabismus.

Pages 1361–1363

10. Heredity plays an important role in all of the following EXCEPT:

A. Strabismus

B. Cataracts

C. Glaucoma

D. Retinoblastoma

E. Chalazion

Answer: E

Critique: There is a positive family history in 34 to 67% of patients with strabismus and up to 55% of patients with congenital cataracts. Primary open-angle glaucoma, the most common form, is inherited multifactorially or as an autosomal recessive trait. Retinoblastoma is inherited as an autosomal dominant trait, with 6% of patients having positive family history and the remainder being genetic mutations. Thus, the family history is an important element of the ocular history and physical examination.

Pages 1360, 1370, 1375

11. Cataracts in children may be secondary to:

A. 1, 2, and 3

B. 1 and 3

C. 2 and 4

D. 4 only

E. All of the above

1. Intrauterine infections

2. Trauma

3. Heritable disorders

4. Medications

Answer: E

Critique: There are a multitude of causes for pediatric cataracts. Evaluating the patient to determine the etiology should include the time of apparent onset, history of intrauterine infections, trauma, medication exposure, and family history. Trauma accounts for 40% of acquired pediatric cataracts, and an additional one third are inherited. Further evaluation should include an examination for genetic abnormalities or syndromes and may include a metabolic evaluation, chromosomal analysis, *t*oxoplasmosis, *r*ubella, *c*ytomegalovirus, and *h*erpes (TORCH) titers, and ocular imaging. Close ophthalmologic follow-up and evaluation will be necessary to determine the etiology and timing and the need for treatment.

Pages 1367–1370; Table 47–8

12. The most common type of cataract presenting in adults is related to:

    A. Irradiation
    B. Trauma
    C. Diabetes
    D. Aging
    E. Heat

Answer: D

Critique: Cataracts are a common condition, which, in adults, are most commonly caused by the aging process. In this case, cataracts develop slowly, over months or years. Cataracts may also develop secondary to the other processes listed, although less commonly. Treatment will depend on the degree of visual impairment and on limitations in lifestyle and generally involves cataract removal and lens implantation.

Page 1374

13. A true statement regarding glaucoma is:

    A. It is more severe in whites than in blacks.
    B. It accounts for 50% of cases of blindness in the United States.
    C. Central vision is affected initially.
    D. Tonometry is recommended every 3 years, beginning at 35 years of age to screen for glaucoma.

Answer: D

Critique: Glaucoma accounts for about 10% of blindness in the United States and affects blacks more severely than whites. Peripheral vision is usually affected first, followed by progressive visual loss involving the entire visual field. There is a familial tendency to develop primary open-angle glaucoma, the most common form. Glaucoma may also occur secondary to

steroid use, ocular trauma, retinal vein occlusion, intraocular inflammations, diabetes, and carotid vascular disease. As the incidence increases dramatically after age 40, tonometry is recommended every 3 years beginning at age 35.

Pages 1374–1376

14. (Matching) A 70-year-old active man presents to you with difficulty reading and performing close-up work while building models. You are unable to detect any abnormalities but suspect macular degeneration as being the cause of this patient's difficulty. True statements regarding macular degeneration include:

    A. 1, 2, and 3
    B. 1 and 3
    C. 2 and 4
    D. 4 only
    E. All of the above

1. This condition is age-related in 70% of cases.

2. Central vision is spared until late in the course of the disease.

3. Laser surgery may be helpful in treatment.

4. Adequate control of blood glucose has been shown to prevent or slow the progression of macular degeneration.

Answer: B

Critique: Breakdown of the macular region, referred to as macular degeneration, is age-related in 70% of cases. Central vision is affected, generally with sparing of peripheral vision, thus reading and close-up work becomes difficult to accomplish. There is no cure for most people with this problem; however, in a small percentage of cases, laser surgery may be helpful. Macular degeneration may also occur in other forms, including a heritable form and a form secondary to injury, inflammation, or infection. The occurrence of macular degeneration is not related to blood glucose control or to the presence of diabetes.

Page 1377

Questions 15–18. With regard to diabetic retinopathy, match each question with the type of diabetes (type I or type II) that is associated with the listed response:

    A. Type I diabetes
    B. Type II diabetes
    C. Both types of diabetes
    D. Neither type of diabetes

15. Retinopathy often presents at the time of diagnosis of disease.

16. Background retinopathy is characterized by microaneurysms, dot hemorrhages, and hard exudates.

17. Macular edema causes visual loss.

18. Annual ophthalmologic examinations are recommended.

Answers: 15-B, 16-C, 17-B, 18-C

Critique: Diabetic retinopathy is the most common cause of blindness in Americans aged 20 to 74. In type I diabetes, it is uncommon for retinopathy to be present before 5 years into the disease. Type II diabetics, presenting after age 30, commonly have retinopathy at the time of diagnosis. The background retinopathy, consisting of microaneurysms, dot hemorrhages, hard exudates, and intraretinal microvascular abnormalities, is similar in both types of diabetes. Macular edema, which is one of the common causes for visual loss is much more common in type II diabetics. Good control of diabetes can help to prevent or delay the onset of retinopathy, and laser photocoagulation can reduce the rate of severe visual loss and proliferative disease when retinopathy is present. Thus, annual ophthalmologic examinations are recommended for both types of diabetics.

Pages 1377, 1378

48

Neurology in Family Practice

Paul Dusseau

1. (Matching) In your bedside evaluation of a comatose patient, you perform ice water irrigation of the left ear in an effort to localize the lesion. Match the observed response with the lesion:

  A. Left third nerve lesion
  B. Psychogenic coma
  C. Nerves III and VI with pons intact
  D. Pontine destruction

1. Both eyes deviate to the left.

2. No response is observed.

3. The right eye looks to the left; the left eye stays at the midline.

4. Intense right-beating nystagmus occurs.

Answers: 1-C, 2-D, 3-A, 4-B

Critique: Ice water irrigation is a simple way to assess pontine function as well as cranial nerves III and VI. Nystagmus is not observed in the comatose patient—the eyes conjugately look toward the cold water irrigation. If this response is seen, you can conclude that pontine function is intact. If one eye does not deviate, you can suspect compression of the cranial nerve III by a mass lesion. If no response is seen, you can suspect a pontine catastrophe.

Page 1387

2. Vertigo that is present in the morning, lasting 30 to 60 seconds, precipitated by head motion, and severe in its intensity is:

  A. Meniere's disease
  B. Tumor at cranial nerve VIII
  C. Labyrinthitis
  D. Benign positional vertigo

Answer: D

282

Critique: Severe, brief vertiginous attacks that are precipitated by head motion are likely to be of peripheral origin, whereas mild constant vertigo is more likely to be of central origin. Meniere's disease is associated with low-frequency hearing loss, tinnitus, and vertigo that may last for several hours. Labyrinthitis is usually associated with middle ear disease and a protracted course of vertigo that lasts for days. Benign positional vertigo is the most common cause of dizziness seen in a primary care practice. Due to dislodgement of otoconia, the brief, self-limited spells of severe vertigo are precipitated by head motion and decrease in frequency over several weeks.

Page 1391

3. (True or False) The following are characteristics of hemorrhagic stroke:

  1. Stiff neck and headache
  2. Nausea and vomiting
  3. Account for 80% of all cerebrovascular accidents (CVAs)
  4. Rapid progression with loss of consciousness

Answers: 1-T, 2-T, 3-F, 4-T

Critique: Intracerebral hemorrhage constitutes 14% of all CVAs. Subarachnoid hemorrhage accounts for another 6%, and ischemic strokes account for 80% of all CVAs. Hemorrhagic infarcts may appear abruptly with a local lesion associated with headache, nausea, vomiting, and generally rapid progress to obtundation and coma. A CT scan is urgently needed to differentiate this from ischemic stroke and dictates urgent neurosurgical consultation.

Page 1394

4. In a patient with a known embolic stroke, with a negative duplex-Doppler scan of the carotids and normal laboratory studies, which is the most appropriate procedure to evaluate a cardiac source of the emboli?

A. Electrocardiogram (ECG)
B. Left heart catheterization
C. Echocardiogram
D. Stress test
E. Transesophageal echocardiography

Answer: E

Critique: The heart is the source of cerebral emboli in more than 20% of stroke cases. Rhythm disturbances, left atrial enlargement, mitral valve disease, and mural emboli from the left ventricle are the most commonly recognized sources of emboli. Transesophageal echocardiography is the most definitive test to visualize a mural thrombus and the mitral valve apparatus.

Page 1397

5. (Matching) Match the medical condition with the proper anticoagulation strategy:

A. Warfarin (Coumadin)
B. Aspirin 325 mg/day
C. Ticlopidine (Ticlid) 250 mg bid

1. Asymptomatic bruit with 60% stenosis

2. Women with multiple transient ischemic attacks (TIAs)

3. Congestive heart failure (CHF) with very low ejection fraction

4. Status post-carotid endarterectomy

5. Atrial fibrillation

Answers: 1-B, 2-C, 3-A, 4-B, 5-A

Critique: Data are insufficient to recommend endarterectomy in asymptomatic patients with stenosis less than 60%. These patients should receive aspirin prophylaxis. Ticlid has been demonstrated to be superior to aspirin in stroke prophylaxis in women and may be considered appropriate therapy in patients with multiple TIAs. CHF with low ejection fraction has a high risk of mural thrombus and is treated with warfarin. Patients in chronic atrial fibrillation have a fivefold increase in embolism and are usually treated with warfarin.

Page 1398

6. (True or False) Moderate hypertension should be treated vigorously in patients with ischemic stroke.

Answer: False

Critique: Cerebral arteries lose their ability to autoregulate during an acute ischemic attack and must have at least moderate blood pressure to perfuse the local ischemic area. Systemic antihypertensive drugs should be given to those with diastolic pressures higher than 120 mm Hg. Blood pressure often spontaneously drops without treatment several days after a stroke.

Page 1399

7. (Matching) Match the antiepileptic drug with its primary indication:

A. Complex partial seizures
B. Partial, generalized, and absence seizures
C. Generalized seizures
D. Absence spells
E. Myoclonic jerks

1. Phenytoin (Dilantin)

2. Clonazepam (Klonopin)

3. Ethosuximide (Zarontin)

4. Valproic acid

5. Carbamazepine (Tegretol)

Answers: 1-C, 2-E, 3-D, 4-B, 5-A

Critique: Classical childhood absence seizures are best treated with ethosuximide, but valproate is useful if the child has other types of coexisting seizures. Partial seizures may be suppressed by carbamazepine or by valproic acid. Generalized seizures (grand mal) may be controlled by phenytoin, carbamazepine, or valproic acid. Clonazepam is used for myoclonic jerks, drop attacks, and nocturnal myoclonus.

Page 1406

8. (Matching) Match the type of seizure with the following symptoms:

A. Simple partial seizure
B. Complex partial seizure

1. Postictal paralysis

2. Excellent recall of the seizure episode

3. Alteration in size of objects seen for 30 seconds

4. Evolution to generalized seizure

5. Lip smacking, picking, and eye blinking

6. Autonomic symptoms of piloerection, sweating, pupillary dilatation

Answers: 1-B, 2-A, 3-A, 4-B, 5-B, 6-A

Critique: Simple partial seizures are autonomic, psychic, motor, or sensory symptoms that are brief, do not interrupt consciousness, and are remembered by the patient. Complex partial seizures may involve more sophisticated repetitive movements and may evolve into a generalized seizure. After a complex partial seizure, the patient may recall the aura but will not remember the generalized event or the postictal paralysis.

Page 1402

9. (Matching) You immediately diagnose status epilepticus in a patient presenting to the emergency room.

Prioritize your orders in terms of importance on a scale of 1 to 6, with number 1 being the first thing that you would do and number 6 being the last thing in your algorithm.

    A. Draw laboratory values for electrolytes, calcium, magnesium, arterial blood gases, and antiepileptic drug levels.

    B. Consult anesthesiology for general anesthesia and a barbiturate-induced coma.

    C. Administer an intravenous (IV) solution with D10 bolus and thiamine.

    D. Start a phenytoin loading dose at 18 mg/kg.

    E. Have an endotracheal intubation cart ready.

    F. Give IV diazepam, 10 to 20 mg.

Answers: 1-C, 2-E, 3-F, 4-A, 5-D, 6-B

Critique: Status epilepticus is a true medical emergency with a mortality rate of 25%. Medication withdrawal and noncompliance as well as metabolic disorders are frequent causes. Electroencephalogram (EEG) monitoring and an anesthesia consultation are necessary in refractory cases.

Page 1410

10. (True or False) Indicate if the following statements about febrile seizures are true or false:

    1. Febrile seizures mandate a lumbar puncture (LP).

    2. Peak incidence is between 3 months and 5 years of age.

    3. Febrile seizures recur in two thirds of patients.

    4. Complex febrile seizures of long duration, an abnormal neurologic examination, and frequent recurrence puts a child at excess risk of developing epilepsy.

    5. Conservative management with antipyretics is the only treatment necessary for febrile seizures.

Answers: 1-T, 2-T, 3-F, 4-T, 5-F

Critique: Most febrile seizures are not associated with meningitis; but in infants younger than 6 months of age, one must have a higher index of suspicion. An LP is ordered based on clinical judgment. Seizures occurring in patients older than 5 years of age raise concerns of causes other than fever. A second febrile seizure occurs in one third of patients; a third seizure occurs in one of six patients. Fifty percent of children with these features develop long-term nonfebrile seizure disorders. Anticonvulsants are of unproven benefit and have too many side effects to treat febrile seizures.

Page 1411

11. (True or False) The following types of dementia are treatable and can often be reversed:

    1. Alzheimer's disease

    2. Normal pressure hydrocephalus

    3. Parkinson's disease

    4. Multi-infarct dementia

    5. Hypothyroidism

    6. Depressive pseudodementia

Answers: 1-F, 2-T, 3-F, 4-F, 5-T, 6-T

Critique: Normal pressure hydrocephalus (which is a triad of increasing dementia, gait disturbance, and urinary incontinence) may often respond to surgical shunting. Hypothyroidism responds to slowly increasing thyroid replacement therapy. Pseudodementia often has a gratifying response to antidepressants. The dementia of degenerative diseases such as Parkinson's disease, Alzheimer's disease, and poststroke syndromes does not respond to the limited medical treatments available.

Page 1413

12. (Matching) Match the headache remedy with the type of headache:

    A. Steroids

    B. Nadolol

    C. Nonsteroidal anti-inflammatory drugs (NSAIDs)

    D. Valproic acid and NSAIDs

    E. Sumatriptan succinate (Imitrex)

    F. Antidepressants

    G. Carbamazepine

1. Analgesic rebound headache

2. Migraine abortive treatment

3. Tension headache prophylaxis

4. Common migraine or tension headache

5. Migraine prophylaxis

6. Temporal arteritis

7. Tic douloureux

Answers: 1-D, 2-E, 3-F, 4-C, 5-B, 6-A, 7-G

Page 1417

13. Which of the following statements is not typical of a cluster headache?

    A. Unilateral orbital pain lasting from 15 to 180 minutes

    B. Presents at nighttime

    C. Predominance in middle-aged women

    D. Conjunctival injection, sweating, nasal congestion, or increased lacrimation

    E. Seasonal cluster (groups) of attacks

Answer: C

Critique: A cluster headache occurs in middle-aged men, whereas chronic paroxysmal hemicrania occurs more often in women. The headache will cluster many times each day for weeks to months and will then remit for 3- to 18-month periods.

Page 1415

14. (Matching) Match the tremor characteristic with the illness:

    A. Cerebellar lesion

    B. Huntington's chorea

C. Benign essential tumor
D. Parkinson's disease

1. Resting tremor and rigidity

2. Action tremor of arms and head tremor

3. Quick, fluid, dance-like movements

4. Truncal tremor with scanning speech

Answers: 1-D, 2-C, 3-B, 4-A

Critique: A resting tremor associated with rigidity, shuffling gait, and masked facies suggests the diagnosis of parkinsonism. The differential diagnosis includes a history of taking antipsychotic medication, multiple CVAs, Wilson's disease, carbon monoxide or manganese poisoning, normal pressure hydrocephalus, and other rarer neurodegenerative diseases. Benign essential tremor often occurs at a young age, occurs with intention, is provoked by stress or fatigue, and is relieved by alcohol or β-blockers. A positive family history with the onset of exaggerated movements in the 30s suggests Huntington's chorea. Cerebellar pathology is suggested with an intention tremor noted in finger-to-nose testing, truncal ataxia with staggering gait, and uncoordinated speech.

Page 1420

15. (Matching) Match the compressed nerve and its clinical syndrome with the given historical data:

A. Peroneal nerve/footdrop
B. Ulnar nerve/hand intrinsic weakness
C. Lateral femoral cutaneous nerve/meralgia parcsthetica
D. Radial nerve/wristdrop
E. Median nerve/carpal tunnel syndrome

1. Pregnancy

2. Jackhammer operator

3. Crutch ambulation

4. Pipefitter

5. Postoperative paralysis

Answers: 1-C, 2-E, 3-D, 4-B, 5-A

Critique: Entrapment of the lateral femoral cutaneous nerve, a sensory nerve, under the inguinal ligament causes numbness and paresthesias of the anterolateral thigh: It occurs during pregnancy, after weight gain, or with wearing very tight garments. Quadriceps strength and knee jerk reflex are normal. Repetition and heavy lifting along with arthritis and endocine disorders cause hypertrophy of the transverse carpal ligament in the wrist, entrapping the median nerve. Symptoms of carpal tunnel syndrome often present nocturnally and involve motor (opponens) weakness as well as sensory symptoms (e.g., pain, paresthesias, numbness). Compression of the radial nerve over the medial humerus can cause wristdrop. Leaning on the exposed ulnar nerve as it passes through a narrow groove of the elbow causes numbness of the fourth and fifth fingers and intrinsic hand muscle paralysis. Improper positioning of the leg during a surgical procedure, crossing legs, and sitting on a hard surface with pressure against the proximal fibula compresses the peroneal nerve and causes footdrop.

Page 1422

16. (True or False) Which of the following statements are true about myasthenia gravis (MG)?

1. Ocular MG has a better prognosis than does generalized MG.

2. Serum acetylcholine receptor antibody has a poor specificity for generalized MG.

3. A chest x-ray is the best screening device for reversible causes of MG.

4. Respiratory disorders are the most serious complication of MG.

Answers: 1-T, 2-F, 3-F, 4-T

Critique: If ocular symptoms remain as the only manifestation of MG after 2 years, there is a 95% likelihood of nonprogression. Ocular MG does not put the patient at excess risk for respiratory failure or aspiration. The antibody is positive in 80 to 90% of patients with generalized MG; but only 50% positive in patients with ocular disease. Thymomas or thymic hypcrplasia may be missed on plain chest films. A CT scan is warranted. A thymectomy may allow for complete remission of symptoms. Aspiration pneumonia and respiratory failure are the primary causes of morbidity and mortality in patients with MG. Frequent monitoring of vital capacity, especially when the patient is ill, may alert you to begin more intensive therapy.

Page 1429

17. Back pain and leg weakness constitute a neurologic emergency in the cancer patient. Which of the following steps are options for treatment?

A. Ask for a history of bowel, bladder, and sexual dysfunction.
B. Do an immediate magnetic resonance imaging (MRI) scan of the spine.
C. Administer a high dose of steroids.
D. Prescribe radiation treatment.
E. All of the above

Answer: E

Critique: Cord compression may evolve very quickly and gives symptoms of back pain, leg weakness, and bowel and bladder dysfunction. Decompression by surgery, steroids, or radiation treatment may prevent permanent paralysis because cord compression is considered to be a neurosurgical emergency.

Page 1436

49

Sexual Health Care

Juan A. Pérez

1. Which of the following statements regarding the sexual response cycle is not true:

    A. Excitement describes a subjective sense of pleasure.

    B. Appetite involves fantasies about and a desire for sexual activity.

    C. Orgasm is the phase in which only the male partner experiences involuntary pelvic thrusting and only the female partner experiences generalized muscular contractions.

    D. Resolution involves a sense of general muscular relaxation.

Answer: C

Critique: Orgasm is the phase in which humans experience peaking of sexual pleasure with release of sexual tension. Both men and women experience generalized muscular tension, contraction, and involuntary pelvic thrusting.

2. Which of the following best relates to "spectatoring":

    A. Fears concerning family income dominate the sexual relationship.

    B. The sexual partners are spontaneous in experiencing sexual pleasure.

    C. The sexual experience is no longer natural because the partners become observers of their own sexual behavior.

    D. Spectatoring is best treated by advising the couple to have intercourse even if it is not pleasurable.

Answer: C

Critique: "Spectatoring" refers to the lack of spontaneity in the sexual act because fears concerning sexual performance dominate the relationship. The partners become observers of their own sexual behaviors, and the individual becomes unable to focus on pleasurable sensations.

3. All of the following are true regarding excitement disorders in women EXCEPT:

    A. Women who suffer from excitement disorders experience lubrication without experiencing erotic feelings.

    B. Lack of pleasure is the key to the diagnosis.

    C. Women often experience irritation rather than a pleasurable sensation on being touched.

    D. The prognosis is better when the woman has been able to become aroused in the past.

Answer: A

Critique: Excitement disorder in women is a condition in which the patient derives slight or no pleasure over sexual stimulation. Erotic feelings and desires are not experienced, and physiologic signs of arousal, such as lubrication and development of the orgasmic plateau, do not occur.

4. All of the following are true regarding primary erectile dysfunction EXCEPT:

    A. It is very common in the general population.

    B. These patients have never been able to achieve an erection sufficient for intercourse.

    C. Severe sexual anxiety related to religious beliefs may be the cause.

    D. It may occur in conjunction with vaginismus in a sexually anxious couple.

Answer: A

Critique: Primary erectile dysfunction is rare. Such patients have never been able to achieve erection sufficient for intercourse. In the absence of congenital, acquired, physical, or endocrine factors, a psychogenic cause is likely.

5. Which of the following best describes secondary erectile dysfunction:

    A. When a man experiences erectile problems in 10% of coital opportunities

    B. May be secondary to fatigue, preoccupation with work, overeating, or drinking excessively

C. In 75% of the cases, it has a psychological etiology.

D. It is not important to screen for organic causes.

Answer: B

Critique: Secondary erectile dysfunction is much more common than is primary erectile dysfunction. Transient episodes are considered normal. Fatigue, preoccupation with work, overeating, or drinking too much can easily cause a temporary problem. Because society puts enormous value on the man's ability to become erect, a single failure can produce performance anxiety that precipitates recurrences thus establishing a pattern of dysfunction.

6. All of the following are organic causes of secondary erectile dysfunction EXCEPT:

A. Vascular
B. Drugs
C. Diabetes
D. Seizure disorder

Answer: D

Critique: Seizure disorder is not considered to be an organic cause of secondary erectile dysfunction. Vascular etiology accounts for 50% of organic causes, 6 to 45% of endocrine causes, 2 to 20% of diabetes, and 2 to 8% of neurologic causes. All patients with a pure organic cause also have some degree of psychogenic potentiation of the disorder.

7. In treating secondary erectile dysfunction, the family physician should:

A. Focus the treatment on the psychological problems as well as on the organic components of the problem.
B. Encourage the couple to continue to try intercourse until they are successful.
C. Advise the male partner to focus on his partner and not on experiencing pleasurable feelings.
D. Nondemand pleasure exercises should not be recommended because they are not effective.

Answer: A

Critique: Performance anxiety and negative partner response may be a part of organic erectile failure; therefore, treatment may need to focus on the psychological problems as well as on the organic problems. The treatment plan begins with a ban on intercourse. The couple is instructed on nondemand pleasure exercises. The male partner needs to focus on himself and let his partner feel and speak for herself.

8. (True or False) Options for treating organic erectile dysfunction are:

1. Suction devices
2. Yohimbine hydrochloride
3. Large doses of vitamin E
4. Papaverine injections
5. Penile implant devices

Answers: 1-T, 2-T, 3-F, 4-T, 5-T

Critique: Large dosages of vitamin E do not improve organic erectile dysfunction. In addition to the options listed in question 8, various vasoactive drugs, such as papaverine, phentolamine, and prostaglandin E, have been utilized for intracavernous injection of the penis.

9. All of the following are true regarding primary orgasmic dysfunction in women EXCEPT:

A. The physiologic response pattern is underdeveloped or inhibited.
B. These patients may have experienced orgasm through self-stimulation.
C. An effective treatment may be directed at masturbation exercises.
D. A negative body image often accommodates primary anorgasmia.

Answer: B

Critique: In primary orgasmic dysfunction, the woman has never experienced orgasm by any means, including self-stimulation, partner stimulation, fantasy, or dreams. It is very important to explore a woman's sexual history since any experience of orgasm precludes the diagnosis of true primary anorgasmia.

10. Which one of the following is true concerning secondary orgasmic dysfunction:

A. It can be treated easily, even after avoidance patterns have developed.
B. The family physician should immediately refer these patients to a sex therapist.
C. This condition has no relation to courting time.
D. Some of the most common contributing factors are fatigue, the stress of raising young children, and preoccupation with careers.

Answer: D

Critique: Secondary orgasmic dysfunction is easiest to treat if it is discovered and dealt with before frustration, anxiety, and negative feelings have grown and before avoidance patterns have developed. This condition may arise from decreased time and attention to courting as a preliminary to intercourse. Fatigue, the stress of raising young children, preoccupation with careers, and the allocation of too little time for intimacy are the most common contributing factors. The family physician should initiate therapy by helping the couple to discuss the problem openly. If no progress is achieved after several follow-up office visits, a referral is indicated.

11. (True or False) Mr. and Mrs. Garcia, who were married 3 months ago, come to you for advice because Mr. Garcia ejaculates prior to penetration. After taking a sexual history, you diagnose Mr. Garcia with premature ejaculation. Please answer whether the following statements are true or false regarding premature ejaculation:

1. It is typified by the male becoming erect and ejaculating just before intercourse or quickly after insertion.
2. Premature ejaculation is due to hostile feelings toward women.

3. Control of the ejaculatory reflex is largely a matter of conditioning based on learning from early experiences.
4. The best treatment is a retraining process involving both partners.
5. The adolescent boy who learns to masturbate in order to ejaculate develops a rapid response pattern.

Answers: 1-T, 2-F, 3-T, 4-T, 5-T

Critique: In the past, premature ejaculation has been attributed to the presence of psychopathology of hostile feelings toward women. Now it is understood that control of the ejaculatory reflex is largely a matter of conditioning based on learning from early experiences.

12. (True or False) The following describe retarded ejaculation:

1. A number of men experience retarded ejaculation as they grow older.
2. Retarded ejaculation and retrograde ejaculation describe the same syndrome.
3. Some men fake ejaculation in order to stop the sexual interaction.
4. Some of these men can ejaculate with masturbation.
5. The caress activities are employed to heighten the man's awareness of his physical sensation.

Answers: 1-T, 2-F, 3-T, 4-T, 5-T

Critique: It appears that a number of men experience retarded ejaculation or difficulty ejaculating, particularly as they grow older. This problem should not be confused with retrograde ejaculation, which may result from diabetes, medications, or prior surgery. Anxiety about this normal development may cause further difficulty and, in some cases, may lead to erectile dysfunction. Some men report faking ejaculation in order to be able to stop the sexual interaction. When a man continuously pressures himself to ejaculate, performance anxiety tends to interrupt the natural response.

13. (True or False) Answer true or false for the following statements regarding vaginismus:

1. Vaginismus occurs reflexively in response to imagined, anticipated, or real attempts at penetration.
2. Vaginismus refers to voluntary spastic contractions of the muscles of the outer third of the vagina.
3. This condition does not allow the patient to experience orgasm even with masturbation or oral stimulation.
4. This condition can effectively prevent intercourse.

Answers: 1-T, 2-F, 3-F, 4-T

Critique: Vaginismus refers to involuntary, not voluntary, spastic contractions of the muscles of the outer third of the vagina. These contractions occur reflexively in response to imagined, anticipated, or real attempts at penetration. This condition does not preclude an orgasm for the patient. Many women with vaginismus are orgasmic with masturbation or with oral stimulation by their partner. The most common presenting complaint is "no sex life."

14. (True or False) Answer true or false for the following statements concerning secondary vaginismus:

1. The most common cause of secondary vaginismus is the vaginitis-vaginismus syndrome.
2. Secondary vaginismus may be seen following attempted or completed rape.
3. In cases of vaginal infection, the family physician should insist that the couple continue sexual intercourse using a condom.
4. Lack of lubrication, fibrositis in the vaginal wall, and traumatic conditions resulting from childbirth can cause secondary vaginismus.

Answers: 1-T, 2-T, 3-F, 4-T

Critique: The patient and her partner should be given appropriate education and guidance, with a ban on sexual intercourse until the infection is effectively eliminated. If the patient continues to have intercourse while the infection is present, she will experience pain along with sexual activity. Eventually the woman's vaginal muscles may learn to say "no" for her as a result of negative conditioning.

15. (True or False) The role of the family physician in caring for the homosexual patient is:

1. To be understanding of the "coming out" period
2. To immediately refer to a sex therapist for behavioral modification
3. To assist in developing a positive self-image and safer sex practices
4. To advise lesbian patients that they are at higher risk for sexually transmitted diseases

Answers: 1-T, 2-F, 3-T, 4-F

Critique: In dealing with the homosexual patient, the family physician must put aside value judgments and give the patient the opportunity to ventilate his or her ideas. Options 2 and 4 are false. The physician must be especially supportive during the process of acceptance and disclosure or "coming out" with relatives and friends. This can be a stressful time in the life of a homosexual patient. There tends to be a sense of isolation, and support systems are often painfully lacking. Lesbians have much less risk of contracting sexually transmitted diseases than are their homosexual counterparts, and gay men are more likely to have more sexually transmitted diseases than do heterosexuals.

16. All of the following are true statements about rape EXCEPT:

A. The highest incidence of rape and other sexual assault occurs in the adolescent age group.
B. Half of the female rape victims report voluntarily agreeing to go into a car, house, or apartment with a new male acquaintance.

C. The experience of rape produces an acute stress reaction known as the "rape trauma syndrome."
D. Rapes rarely, if ever, occur in the victim's own home, and the rapist is always a stranger.

Answer: D

Critique: All the options are true except for D. Many rapes occur in the victim's own home, resulting in the feeling that "no place is safe." The perpetrator is often known to the victim. The rape trauma syndrome is most severe 6 weeks to 3 months or more after the attack. The victim's initial feeling is gratitude at being alive. The feelings then turn to self-blaming and preoccupation with the event, accompanied by a sense of loss of control over his or her life. Depression is a common sequela, and suicide attempts are frequent.

17. (True or False) Mark true or false for the following statements about sexual abuse of children:

1. Physicians are not mandatory child abuse reporters.
2. Most sexual abuse relationships involve incestuous intercourse and molestation.
3. Most incest involving a father and daughter involves a stepfather or father substitute.
4. The family physician should always be alert to the possibility of abuse when there is vaginal or pelvic discharge, genital trauma, painful urination or defecation, or the presence of infection.
5. Sexual abuse relationships involving a mother and her son are never seen by the primary care physician.

Answers: 1-F, 2-T, 3-T, 4-T, 5-F

Critique: Physicians are mandatory child abuse reporters in all states. A random survey of general practitioners and pediatricians in the state of Washington revealed that most sexual abuse relationships encountered involve incestuous intercourse and molestation. Father-daughter incest accounts for 75% of cases (mostly involving a stepfather or father substitute). Mother-son, father-son, mother-daughter, and brother-sister incest accounts for the remaining 25%.

18. Which of the following main categories of drugs does not alter the sexual cycle?

A. Antihypertensives
B. Antipsychotics
C. First-generation cephalosporins
D. Antihistamines

Answer: C

Critique: Antihypertensives, antipsychotics, and antihistamines are implicated in altering the sexual cycle. First-generation cephalosporins are not responsible for altering the cycle.

19. (True or False) Mark true or false for the following statements about diabetes and sexual dysfunction:

1. Females are found to have vaginal dryness, vaginal infections, and atrophy of the vaginal epithelium.
2. Men commonly experience an organic form of erectile failure.
3. The cause of erectile failure in men is thought to be secondary to autonomic and sensory neuropathy.
4. External suction devices are never used in diabetes.

Answers: 1-T, 2-T, 3-T, 4-F

Critique: Most male diabetics with sexual dysfunction related to erectile failure benefit from sex therapy and improved communication for the reduction of performance anxiety. Erection may be improved by utilizing suction devices (Ved Vacuum Erection Device or the Synergist Erection System).

20. All of the following are true about sexual activity and heart disease EXCEPT:

A. Depression is almost always present after myocardial infarction.
B. If a patient cannot climb five flights of stairs, the capacity to perform during sexual intercourse is absent.
C. The average heart rate during orgasm is 115 to 120 beats/min.
D. Long-acting nitrates may be used prior to intercourse for prophylaxis of angina.

Answer: B

Critique: If a patient can climb two sets of stairs, not five, the capacity to perform during sexual intercourse is present. The average heart rate at orgasm is 115 to 120 beats/min. Most patients do not experience angina until the heart rate reaches a mean of 145 (±20) beats/min. These averages indicate that sexual activity is usually safe. It is wise for the patient to undergo submaximal exercise testing in order to establish the presence of dysrhythmias or the probability of performing at the required energy level.

50

Clinical Genetics and Genetic Counseling

Richard Neill

1. What percentage of infants are born with major birth defects?

    A. 1%
    B. 3%
    C. 5%
    D. 7%
    E. 9%

Answer: B

Critique: Three percent of all infants are born with a major birth defect, whereas 7% of all individuals manifest symptoms of a genetic disorder during childhood or adolescence.

Page 1456

2. When considering causes for birth defects in a newborn infant, the most common identifiable cause is likely to be which ONE of the following?

    A. Chromosomal abnormalities
    B. Single gene defects
    C. Multifactorial inheritance (polygenic and environmental factors)
    D. Environmental factors (maternal conditions and teratogens)

Answer: C

Critique: Approximately 50% of birth defects arise from unknown causes. Multifactorial inheritance accounts for the most common identifiable cause, with chromosomal abnormalities and single gene defects each accounting for between 3 and 10%, and environmental factors alone (maternal conditions and teratogens) accounting for 4 to 5% of identifiable causes.

Page 1456, Table 50–1

Questions 3–6. Match the numbered statement with the appropriate lettered response:

    A. Malformation
    B. Deformation
    C. Disruption

3. Abnormally positioned ears

4. Ventricular septal defect

5. Fetal amputation defects

6. Club feet

Answers: 3-A, 4-A, 5-C, 6-B

Critique: Malformations arise from a primary defect in morphogenesis, whereas deformations and disruptions are caused by extrinsic mechanical forces in utero. The primary distinction between deformations and disruptions is that disruptions involve atrophy, amputation, or breakdown of previously normal body parts, whereas deformations arise via compression, constriction, or immobility of normally developing body parts.

Page 1457

7. Which ONE of the following does NOT carry a known risk of birth defects?

    A. Warfarin
    B. Tetracycline
    C. Erythromycin
    D. Streptomycin
    E. Valproic acid

Answer: C

Critique: Erythromycin carries no known risk of birth defects. Warfarin and valproic acid cause characteristic syndromes; streptomycin causes hearing defects; and tetracycline causes dental abnormalities.

Table 50–2

Questions 8–12 (True or False). For each of the following, indicate whether a genetic evaluation is indicated:

8. Abnormal results on a state-mandated screening test

9. Hypoglycemia in the newborn nursery

10. Familial history of breast cancer

11. Psychomotor retardation in an infant

12. Short stature or other growth disorders

Answers: 8-T, 9-F, 10-T, 11-T, 12-T

Critique: Hypoglycemia in itself does not suggest a genetic problem requiring genetic counseling, whereas each of the other conditions implies the potential for a genetic etiology.

Page 1459, Table 50–3

13. A 37-year-old G1P0 woman is in her fourth month of pregnancy. To date her prenatal course has been unremarkable. During her visit with you she requests to be tested in order to confirm whether or not her unborn child suffers from Down syndrome. Which ONE of the following approaches would be most appropriate?

    A. Chorionic villus sampling for chromosomal analysis
    B. Amniocentesis for chromosomal analysis
    C. Measurement of maternal serum alpha-fetoprotein (MSAFP)
    D. Providing reassurance that the woman's risk of having a child affected with Down syndrome is low
    E. Fetal biopsy

Answer: B

Critique: Because this patient is over 35 years of age, she has a higher risk of having a child affected by a genetic defect such as Down syndrome. Although a low MSAFP level can indicate an elevated risk of Down syndrome, a normal MSAFP cannot exclude the diagnosis. Amniocentesis is an appropriate test for this stage of pregnancy. Chorionic villus sampling is typically performed at 9 to 10 weeks of pregnancy, whereas a fetal biopsy is more invasive. The risk of complications with amniocentesis is approximately 1:2 to 1:4.

Page 1460

14. Which ONE of the following results on a "triple screen" suggests Down syndrome?

    A. Elevated MSAFP, unconjugated estriol, and human chorionic gonadotropin (hCG)
    B. Elevated MSAFP, decreased unconjugated estriol, and decreased hCG
    C. Decreased MSAFP, elevated unconjugated estriol, and elevated hCG
    D. Decreased MSAFP, decreased unconjugated estriol, and elevated hCG
    E. Decreased MSAFP, unconjugated estriol, and hCG

Answer: D

Critique: A low MSAFP and unconjugated estriol combined with an elevated hCG indicate an increased risk for Down syndrome. Elevations of MSAFP are associated with neural tube defects and abdominal wall defects.

Page 1460

Questions 15–20. For each numbered statement, match the appropriate lettered response.

    A. Turner's syndrome
    B. Klinefelter's syndrome
    C. Myotonic dystrophy
    D. Down syndrome
    E. Cystic fibrosis
    F. Hemophilia

15. X-linked recessive disorder

16. Autosomal recessive

17. Palmar creases, mental retardation

18. Hypogonadism, infertility

19. Autosomal dominant

20. Short stature, nuchal webbing

Answers: 15-F, 16-E, 17-D, 18-B, 19-C, 20-A

Critique: Klinefelter's syndrome, Turner's syndrome, and Down syndrome are all examples of chromosomal abnormalities resulting from whole chromosome addition or deletion. Myotonic dystrophy is an example of an autosomal dominant single gene mutation, whereas cystic fibrosis represents an autosomal recessive single gene mutation. Hemophilia represents an X-linked recessive pattern in which a female carrier contributes the affected X gene to a male offspring who demonstrates the genetic phenotype. Other examples of X-linked disorders include Duchenne's muscular dystrophy and fragile X syndrome.

Tables 50–7 and 50–8

21. A live birth is likely in all of the following EXCEPT:

    A. Tetraploidy
    B. Mosaicism
    C. Subchromosomal deletion
    D. Balanced chromosomal inversion
    E. Single gene defect

Answer: A

Critique: Tetraploidy (carrying four, rather than the normal two, copies of genetic material) is generally incompatible with a live birth. Aneuploidy (having an abnormal amount of genetic material) in all its forms accounts for the most common reason for first-trimester spontaneous abortions. Mosaicism (differing chromosomal complements within the cells of the same individual), subchromosomal deletions, balanced chromosomal inversions, and single gene defects are all more likely to result in a live birth.

Pages 1461–1463

22. A female patient carries the gene for an X-linked recessive disorder. What is the probability that any of her offspring will exhibit the genetic disorder?

    A. 100%
    B. 75%
    C. 50%
    D. 25%
    E. 0%

Answer: D

Critique: X-linked recessive disorders typically manifest themselves only in males who carry the affected X chromosome. There is a 50% chance of having a male offspring and a 50% chance of passing the affected chromosome to that affected male offspring, resulting in a 25% chance of having any affected offspring. There is similarly a 25% chance of producing a female carrier offspring.

Page 1464

23. Autosomal dominant conditions such as neurofibromatosis manifest themselves whenever a single gene copy is present. Which ONE of the following can account for the variability of phenotype exhibited by different carriers of this gene?

    A. Incomplete penetrance
    B. Spontaneous remission of disease
    C. Drug therapy
    D. Homozygosity for the condition
    E. Submicrosomal genetic deletion

Answer: A

Critique: Individuals affected by autosomal dominant conditions tend to exhibit an all-or-none phenomenon, with some exhibiting almost no evidence of disease. Penetrance usually refers to the all-or-none expression of a mutant genotype, whereas expressivity describes the extent to which a genetic defect is expressed. Patients inheriting an autosomal dominant trait with 100% penetrance but variable expressivity show variable phenotypes, from mild to severe.

Page 1464

Further Reading

Thompson MW, McInnes RR, Willard HF: Thompson and Thompson Genetics in Medicine, 5th ed. Philadelphia, WB Saunders, 1991.

24. Which of the following does NOT represent an autosomal dominant pattern of inheritance?

    A. Thalassemia
    B. Achondroplasia
    C. Spinocerebellar ataxia
    D. Familial Alzheimer's disease
    E. Familial breast cancer

Answer: A

Critique: Common autosomal dominant conditions include most skeletal dysplasias and disorders of connective tissue, some neurodegenerative disorders (including familial Alzheimer's disease and multiple sclerosis), as well as familial cancers. Thalassemias, other hemoglobinopathies, and enzymatic defects are common autosomal recessive disorders.

Page 1464

Questions 25–29 (True or False). Evaluate each of the following statements regarding mitochondrial DNA mutations:

25. The severity of expression of a mitochondrial DNA mutation depends on the fraction of mitochondrial DNA molecules within the mitochondrion that contain the mutation.

26. The severity of expression of a mitochondrial DNA mutation depends on the fraction of cells within tissue that contains mitochondria bearing the mutation.

27. The severity of expression of a mitochondrial DNA mutation depends on the fraction of mitochondria within the cell that contain mitochondrial DNA with the mutant gene.

28. Mitochondrial DNA is contributed equally by egg and sperm.

29. Mitochondrial DNA mutations affect skeletal muscle, cardiac muscle, brain, and liver more severely than mucosal cells, spleen, and bone marrow.

Answers: 25-T, 26-T, 27-T, 28-F, 29-T

Critique: Mitochondrial DNA mutations are variably expressed depending on each of the first three factors stated earlier. Unlike autosomal gene pairs, mitochondrial DNA is contributed primarily from the egg. Because mitochondria are active in the process of energy metabolism, tissues with the highest rate of energy metabolism are usually affected most severely when mitochondrial DNA mutations are present.

Pages 1464–1465

30. A 25-year-old woman delivers a son with an isolated neural tube defect. Which ONE of the following statements is FALSE regarding this circumstance?

    A. The risk of recurrence in a second child is approximately 3%.
    B. The general population rate of neural tube defects is 0.1%.
    C. Third-degree relatives of this woman have no greater risk of affected offspring than do the general population.
    D. Neural tube defects such as a cleft palate are more common than is spina bifida.
    E. Cardiac or limb defects in association with spina bifida suggest a possible teratogenic cause.

Answer: D

Critique: Cleft palate is not a neural tube defect but is rather a defect of branchial arch formation. Neural tube defects are inherited in a multifactorial pattern. In general, multifactorial traits indicate a slightly higher risk of recurrence in a first-degree relative (3 to 5%) than the general population at large (0.1% in the case of neural tube defects). Cardiac and limb malformations in addition to spina bifidia are seen, along with characteristic facies, and they can be caused by fetal exposure to valproate.

Page 1465

Questions 31–35 (True or False). A 2-year-old with Down syndrome and a benign history visits your office with his mother for the first time. Which of the following procedures are appropriate at this time?

31. Echocardiogram if not performed earlier

32. Barium swallow

33. Auditory testing

34. Thyroid testing

35. Pediatric ophthalmologic examination

Answers: 31-T, 32-F, 33-T, 34-T, 35-T

Critique: The care of a patient with Down syndrome, as with patients with other chronic illness, requires monitoring and evaluation tailored to the condition, in addition to the usual schedule of health maintenance activities appropriate for the patient's age, sex, and risk factors. A patient with Down syndrome is at increased risk of cardiac defects, even in the absence of murmurs, hence the need for an early echocardiogram. While feeding difficulties are common in patients with Down syndrome, a gastrointestinal evaluation may be reserved for patients with symptoms. Auditory testing is recommended yearly for the first 3 years of life, whereas an ophthalmologic examination is recommended at 6 months of age and every 2 years thereafter. Thyroid testing is performed at birth, 6 months, and annually thereafter to check for hypothyroidism, which is more common in patients with Down syndrome.

Page 1466

51

Diagnosis and Treatment of Anxiety Disorders

Michael D. Hagen and Betty Walker

1. Of the following, all represent DSM-III subclasses of anxiety EXCEPT:

    A. Obsessive-compulsive disorder
    B. Panic disorder
    C. Post-traumatic stress disorder
    D. Manic-depressive disorder

Answer: D

Critique: Obsessive-compulsive disorder, panic disorder, and post-traumatic stress disorder all represent subclasses of anxiety in the DSM-III R. Manic-depressive or bipolar disorder does not appear as a subclass of the anxiety disorders.

Page 1470

2. Of the following, all are true of panic disorder EXCEPT:

    A. Persons with this disorder exhibit episodes of intense apprehension.
    B. The disorder might be associated with a sense of chest pain or discomfort.
    C. Persons with this disorder might exhibit feelings of unreality or dizziness.
    D. Persons with this disorder exhibit minimal familial association.
    E. The disorder affects women more frequently than men.

Answer: D

Critique: Studies indicate that panic disorder exhibits strong familial tendencies with studies indicating that 18 to 40% of first-degree relatives also suffer from this disorder. All of the other symptoms represent sensations commonly experienced by patients afflicted with panic disorder.

Page 1470

3. (True or False) Which of the following represent diagnostic criteria for panic disorder according to DSM-III?

    1. The patient must exhibit recurrent unexpected attacks.
    2. At least one of the panic attacks has been followed by at least 1 month of persistent concern about having additional attacks.
    3. The panic attacks can be explained by other medical conditions (e.g., hyperthyroidism).
    4. The panic attacks are explained by another disorder such as social phobia.

Answers: 1-T, 2-T, 3-F, 4-F

Critique: The DSM-III criteria provide fairly specific descriptions for the diagnostic criteria for panic disorder. The patient must experience recurrent unexpected attacks, and the patient must have experienced an attack that was followed by at least 4 weeks of persistent concern about having additional attacks. Additionally, the panic attacks should not be due to other conditions such as obsessive-compulsive disorder, post-traumatic stress disorder, separation anxiety disorder, or social phobia. Furthermore, the attacks should not be due to other medical conditions (e.g., hyperthyroidism) or substance abuse.

Page 1470

4. Of the following statements regarding panic disorder, all are true EXCEPT:

    A. Affected patients exhibit more frequent stressful life events than do unaffected individuals.
    B. Panic disorder can be precipitated by events that the patient perceives as uncontrollable.
    C. Panic disorder has not been associated with rape or physical assault.
    D. Death or severe illness of a loved one can precipitate panic attacks.

Answer: C

Critique: Panic disorder appears to be associated with life stresses: panic attack sufferers have higher reported frequencies of stressful life events that imply danger or threat, uncontrollable circumstances associated with lowered self-esteem, and serious illness or death of loved ones. Panic attacks can be precipitated by emotionally traumatic events such as rape or physical assault.

Page 1470

5. Clinical characteristics associated with the second stage of panic disorder include all of the following EXCEPT:

   A. Agoraphobia
   B. Anticipatory anxiety
   C. Increased frequency of panic attacks
   D. Increased consultation with health professionals for somatic complaints

Answer: A

Critique: Panic disorder can exhibit three stages over time. The first stage consists of the patient's first acute attack or attacks. The patient can then proceed to the second stage, in which he or she experiences increased frequency of panic attacks, anticipatory anxiety (anxiety that another attack will occur), increased use of medical care services, and development of phobias. In the third stage, the patient progresses to agoraphobia and demonstrates increased dependence and chronic somatization.

Page 1471

6. Of patients who present with chest pain and demonstrate normal coronary arteries at angiography, what percentage are ultimately diagnosed with panic disorder?

   A. 20%
   B. 35%
   C. 50%
   D. 70%
   E. 90%

Answer: C.

Critique: Cardiac symptoms represent one of the most commonly identified types of complaints presented by panic disorder patients. Neurologic and gastrointestinal complaints are also reported frequently. Among patients who present with cardiac symptoms but who demonstrate normal coronary arteries, approximately 50% will ultimately prove to have panic disorder.

Page 1471

7. In the second stage of panic disorder, a patient might exhibit all of the following EXCEPT:

   A. Anticipatory anxiety
   B. Avoidance behaviors
   C. Multiple phobias
   D. Agoraphobia

Answer: D

Critique: Panic disorder can exhibit three chronologic stages. In stage I, the patient experiences the first panic attack. Early intervention in this first stage can prevent progression to stages II and III. In the second stage, patients may exhibit anticipatory anxiety, expressing constant fear of another panic attack. During stage II, the patient can also engage in avoidance behaviors as a means of limiting exposure to circumstances that the patient fears might precipitate another attack. In stage II, patients might also demonstrate multiple phobias. Stage III is defined by the development of agoraphobia; this condition is associated with global fear of exposure to possible panic-inducing stimuli and can eventuate in a patient who is afraid to leave his or her own home for fear of exposure to circumstances that might induce panic.

Page 1471

Questions 8–10. Match the following options with the appropriate numbered statements:

   A. Specific phobia
   B. Panic disorder
   C. Both A and B
   D. Neither A nor B

8. The patient becomes overwhelmingly fearful when exposed to the appropriate stimulus.

9. Affected patients can exhibit substantial anticipatory anxiety.

10. Patients experience panic-like symptoms only in response to a particular stimulus.

Answers: 8-C, 9-C, 10-A

Critique: With both panic disorder and specific phobias, patients can develop overwhelming fear when exposed to suitable stimuli. In both disorders, patients can exhibit anticipatory anxiety for circumstances that they associate with panic-like symptoms. Patients who have specific phobias demonstrate panic-like symptoms only in response to circumscribed stimuli. Patients with panic disorder demonstrate symptoms in response to multiple phobias or global fear rather than the circumscribed circumstances implied by specific phobias.

Pages 1471, 1472

11. (True or False) The criteria for definition of generalized anxiety disorder include which of the following?

   1. The patient experiences excessive anxiety and worry occurring on most days for at least 6 months.
   2. The patient expresses difficulty in concentrating.
   3. The patient reports irritability.
   4. The symptoms occur as the result of a medical condition such as hyperthyroidism.

Answers: 1-T, 2-T, 3-T, 4-F

Critique: The diagnosis of generalized anxiety disorder requires that the patient experience symptoms on most days for at least 6 months. Additionally, difficulty in concentrating and irritability appear among the symptoms required for making the diagnosis. In order to support the diagnosis, the symptoms must not be due to a medical disorder such as hyperthyroidism.

Page 1473

12. Post-traumatic stress disorder can be associated with all of the following findings EXCEPT:

   A. Avoidance of stimuli associated with the trauma
   B. Strong feelings of dependency on others
   C. Diminished interest in significant activities
   D. Restricted range of affect

Answer: B

Critique: Post-traumatic stress disorder occurs as a consequence of catastrophic circumstances beyond the scope of those encountered in usual human experience. Patients can exhibit avoidance of stimuli associated with the original traumatic event, diminished interest in activities usually considered significant for the individual, and restricted range of affect. Patients can demonstrate feelings of detachment and alienation, rather than dependency.

Pages 1473, 1474

13. All of the following can present symptoms similar to anxiety EXCEPT:

   A. Caffeine intoxication
   B. Ischemic heart disease
   C. β-Adrenergic blocker drug therapy
   D. Thyrotoxicosis

Answer: C

Critique: Whenever presented with a patient who displays symptoms of anxiety, the clinician should investigate possible medical causes. Intoxication with stimulants such as caffeine and amphetamines can produce symptoms that mimic anxiety disorders. Likewise, patients with ischemic heart disease can present symptoms of anxiety related to fears regarding the implications of their cardiac disorder. The hypermetabolic state associated with thyrotoxicosis can also present symptoms that mimic anxiety. β-Adrenergic blockers tend to produce depressive symptoms rather than anxiety.

Pages 1474, 1475

Further Reading

Drugs for stable angina pectoris. Med Lett 36:113–114, 1994.

14. (True or False) Which of the following statements are true regarding depression and anxiety disorders?

   1. Heavy long-term alcohol use is associated with lowered anxiety levels.
   2. Approximately 60% of patients who exhibit major depression also harbor significant anxiety.

   3. Panic disorder is associated with a high lifetime risk of major depression.
   4. The prevalence of lifetime panic disorder among depressed primary care patients is higher than that found among similar patients seen by mental health professionals.

Answers: 1-F, 2-T, 3-T, 4-F

Critique: Habitual long-term use of alcohol is associated frequently with anxiety disorders. Although alcohol might lower anxiety symptoms temporarily, anxiety symptoms worsen when blood levels decline. Additionally, alcohol's adverse impact on sleep and long-term impact on the sympathetic nervous system serve to augment anxiety symptoms. Several studies have demonstrated a high correlation between depression and the presence of anxiety symptoms. The lifetime prevalence of panic disorder appears to be higher in depressed patients managed by mental health professionals than in those seen by primary care providers.

Page 1475

Further Reading

Sherbourne CD, Jackson CA, Meredith LS, et al: Prevalence of comorbid anxiety disorders in primary care outpatients. Arch Fam Med 5:27–34, 1996.

15. All of the following represent frequently reported anxiety symptoms EXCEPT:

   A. Impaired ability to concentrate
   B. Tachycardia, palpitations, or pain in the chest
   C. Delayed ejaculation
   D. Slowness of thought and speech

Answer: C

Critique: Anxiety can present with a multitude of somatic symptoms. Slowness of thought and speech, impaired ability to concentrate, and cardiac symptoms such as palpitations, tachycardia, and chest pain can all represent anxiety-related complaints. Premature rather than delayed ejaculation appears to be associated with anxiety.

Page 1476

16. The family APGAR assesses all of the following aspects of family function EXCEPT:

   A. Growth
   B. Adaptation
   C. Affection
   D. Sexual abuse
   E. Resolve

Answer: D

Critique: The family APGAR assesses the growth, adaptation, affection, resolve, and partnership dimensions of family function. The APGAR does not assess sexual abuse explicitly.

Page 1477

17. (True or False) The management plans for patients with anxiety disorders should include which of the following components?

1. After a complete history and physical and laboratory evaluation, tell the patient that the symptoms are "all in your head."
2. Base the management plan on the specific psychiatric diagnosis.
3. Involve the patient in developing an agreed-upon set of interventions and schedule a time for a follow-up visit.
4. Instruct the patient in stress reduction techniques such as relaxation therapy and exercise.

Answers: 1-F, 2-T, 3-T, 4-T

Critique: The clinician should approach anxiety manifestations in a manner similar to other medical conditions. The clinician should conduct an appropriately thorough history and physical and laboratory evaluation in order to ascertain possible medical conditions that might explain the symptoms. The clinician should attempt to define the psychiatric disorder as specifically as possible, because this has implications for further therapy. The clinician should to the extent possible involve the patient in developing a plan for treatment and follow-up. Additionally, the patient who exhibits anxiety symptoms can benefit from nonpharmacologic measures, such as relaxation therapy and regular exercise. The clinician should also attempt to explain the biophysiologic substrate for anxiety and not suggest to the patient that his symptoms are "all in your head."

Page 1478

18. (True or False) Family physicians are frequently the first health care professionals to see patients after their first panic attacks. Once the patient begins to exhibit avoidance behaviors and frequent attacks, the physician should initiate which of the following therapeutic options?

1. The clinician should initiate a specific pharmacologic intervention for panic disorder.
2. Once treatment has controlled panic attacks, the patient should be counseled to avoid those situations known to precipitate acute episodes.
3. The patient should be counseled to avoid reading about panic disorder, because contact with such literature might aggravate the patient's condition.
4. Cognitive-behavioral psychotherapy should be considered as an alternative treatment for patients who would prefer nonpharmacologic management.

Answers: 1-T, 2-F, 3-F, 4-T

Critique: Once the patient with panic disorder has begun to demonstrate avoidance behavior and phobia development, specific therapy should be instituted. After the attacks have been controlled, the patient should be encouraged to participate in activities and situations that had previously induced panic. Additionally, the patient should be encouraged to read literature regarding panic as a means to knowing more about the disorder. For those patients who prefer nonpharmacologic therapy, cognitive-behavioral psychotherapy has been shown to be effective for mild to moderate panic disorder.

Pages 1478, 1479

19. Pharmacologic agents that have proved to be effective for panic disorder include all of the following EXCEPT:

A. β-Adrenergic blocking agents (e.g., propranolol)
B. High-potency benzodiazepines (e.g., alprazolam)
C. Tricyclic antidepressants (e.g., imipramine)
D. Serotonin reuptake inhibitors (e.g., fluoxetine)

Answer: A

Critique: Well-done studies have demonstrated the efficacy of high-potency benzodiazepines, tricyclic antidepressants, and serotonin reuptake inhibitors for managing panic disorder. β-Adrenergic agents, while demonstrating some ability to control palpitations, perform no better than do placebos in controlling panic attacks.

Page 1479

Further Reading

Brown CS, Rakel RE, Wells BG, et al: A practical update on anxiety disorders and their pharmacologic treatment. Arch Intern Med 151:873–884, 1991.

20. For a patient who is experiencing marked anticholinergic side effects from imipramine, which of the following heterocyclic antidepressants would be *least likely* to cause similar consequences?

A. Doxepin
B. Amitriptyline
C. Trimipramine
D. Desipramine

Answer: D

Critique: The heterocyclic antidepressants, while effective for panic disorder, exhibit a wide spectrum of side effects. Doxepin and amitriptyline both exhibit high anticholinergic activity and thus would not be good choices for a patient who suffered anticholinergic side effects with desipramine. Trimipramine has somewhat less anticholinergic effect, but, of the list provided, desipramine offers the lowest anticholinergic activity.

Page 1479

Further Reading

Pary R, Lewis S: Identifying and treating patients with panic attacks. Am Fam Physician. 46:841–848, 1992.

21. A number of benzodiazepines have been used for treatment of panic disorder. Of the following which *one* has the United States Food and Drug Administration (FDA) approved for this use?

A. Lorazepam
B. Alprazolam
C. Clonazepam
D. Diazepam

Answer: B

Critique: Although several benzodiazepines have been advocated for panic disorder, only alprazolam has FDA approval for this indication.

Further Reading

Drugs for psychiatric disorders. Med Lett 33:43–44, 1991.
Shader RJ, Greenblatt DJ: Use of benzodiazepines in anxiety disorders. N Engl J Med 328:1398–1405, 1993.

22. (True or False) True statements regarding counseling for generalized anxiety disorder by primary care physicians include which of the following?

1. A brief series of short sessions of supportive psychotherapy yield results similar to those obtained with benzodiazepine therapy.
2. Brief supportive psychotherapy requires more physician time than that required for initiating and monitoring standard therapy with benzodiazepines.
3. Counseling for generalized anxiety can be incorporated successfully into physician visits scheduled for other medical problems.

Answers: 1-T, 2-F, 3-T

Critique: Randomized trials have revealed that structured brief supportive psychotherapy for generalized anxiety disorder can yield results similar to those attained with pharmacotherapy. Additionally, a series of short supportive psychotherapy sessions appear to require no more physician time than that needed for pharmacotherapeutic approaches. Studies have also demonstrated that brief supportive psychotherapy can be incorporated successfully into the context of encounters scheduled for other medical illnesses.

Pages 1480, 1481

23. (True or False) Patient characteristics that correlate with successful counseling for generalized anxiety disorder include which of the following?

1. Lack of awareness regarding how counseling works
2. Highly motivated to change self
3. Awareness that the disorder has a psychological basis
4. Previous unsuccessful experiences with counseling

Answers: 1-F, 2-T, 3-T, 4-F

Critique: Several patient characteristics indicate higher probability for successful counseling experiences. Patient awareness regarding the process of counseling, high level of motivation, awareness of the psychological basis of the disorder, and previous successful counseling experiences all correlate with successful counseling experiences in generalized anxiety disorder.

Page 1481

24. (True or False) Strategies that the clinician can use to lessen the likelihood of rebound anxiety when attempting to taper benzodiazepine therapy include which of the following?

1. Taper the medication dose slowly over a period of weeks (e.g., decrease the dosage by 25% per week).
2. Convert from a short- to a long-acting agent before tapering the dosage.
3. Initiate tricyclic antidepressant therapy prior to tapering the benzodiazepine dose.

Answers: 1-T, 2-T, 3-T

Critique: Several approaches can facilitate tapering benzodiazepine dosage in patients with generalized anxiety disorder. The drug should be tapered slowly over a period of weeks to months; one suggested regimen is to decrease the dose by 25% weekly until the person is off the drug. Additionally, switching from a short-acting agent (e.g., alprazolam) to a long-acting agent (e.g., clonazepam) prior to tapering can facilitate the process. Tricyclic antidepressants begun prior to tapering can facilitate the tapering process; indeed evidence exists to suggest that at least some patients with generalized personality disorder can be managed with tricyclic antidepressants alone.

Page 1481

25. Behavior modification techniques that have been shown to improve specific phobias include all of the following EXCEPT:

A. Desensitization using increasingly intense stimuli
B. In vivo "flooding" in which the patient receives full exposure to the phobic stimulus
C. In vivo exposure to gradually more intense examples of the phobic stimulus
D. Development of strategies for avoiding situations in which the phobic stimulus might occur

Answer: D

Critique: Behavioral modification techniques have demonstrated success in treatment of specific phobias. Desensitization involves exposing the patient to increasingly intense examples of the phobic stimulus while using relaxation techniques (e.g., progressing from a photograph of the stimulus to actual exposure to the agent). In vivo exposure involves either gradual or immediate exposure to the phobic stimulus. The goal of therapy is to help the patient face the phobic stimulus circumstances rather than avoid them.

Page 1482

52

Depression

Marilyn Mehr and Michael D. Hagen

1. All BUT ONE of the following account for the fact that family physicians miss the diagnosis of major depression in as many as 30 to 50% of their patients:

    A. Many depressed patients present with strong somatic symptoms.

    B. Family practice patients have fewer neurovegetative features.

    C. Patients seen by family physicians have higher educational levels and more vegetative symptoms than do those seen by psychiatrists.

    D. Many patients deny that they are depressed even when asked directly.

    E. It may require several patient visits to detect depressive symptoms.

Answer: C

Critique: All of the aforementioned answers are true of family practice patients except C. Depressed patients seen in family practice have a lower educational level than do those seen by psychiatrists and tend to demonstrate fewer vegatative symptoms compared with patients seen by psychiatrists.

Page 1486

2. (True or False) True statements regarding the standard criteria for major depression include:

    1. The Diagnostic and Statistical Manual of Mental Disorders-4th edition (DSM-IV) criteria identify a heterogenous group of patients.

    2. Many patients suffer intermittent symptoms but do not meet DSM-IV criteria for depression.

    3. Depressed family practice patients usually meet all DSM-IV criteria for depression.

    4. A mood disturbance is required for the diagnosis of depression.

Answers: 1-T, 2-T, 3-F, 4-T

Critique: While family practice patients are a heterogenous group, two patients can be depressed without sharing a single symptom. Furthermore, many patients suffer intermittent depressive symptoms chronically or episodically but do not meet the criteria for a specific psychiatric diagnosis. The DSM-IV criteria include nine symptom complexes; a diagnosis requires the presence of at least five of the criteria, one of which must be depressed mood or loss of interest or pleasure in usual daily activities.

Page 1488

3. (Matching) Match the following questionnaires for diagnosing depression with descriptors of their characteristics and use.

    A. Beck Depression Inventory (BDI)

    B. Center for Epidemiologic Studies-Depression Scale (CES-D)

    C. Both A and B

    D. Neither A nor B

1. Useful for screening general or medical care populations

2. Measures subjective experiences and psychological components of depression

Answers: 1-B, 2-A

Critique: A number of questionnaires have been validated for identifying potentially depressed primary care patients. All have strengths and weaknesses and tend to perform with low specificity. According to Schwenk and Coyne, the CES-D is useful for screening general and medical populations. The Beck Depression Inventory is more useful for measuring subjective experiences and psychological components of depression.

Page 1489

4. Dysthymic patients are characterized by ALL BUT ONE of the following features:

A. Long-term personality styles with persistent or cyclical dysphoria, self-pity, and irrational negativity
B. Few or none of the neurovegetative symptoms requiring pharmacologic treatment
C. No evidence of cognitive impairment
D. No response to a supportive physician-patient relationship
E. Evidence of residual or impending major depression in some patients

Answer: D

Critique: Although these patients are often "characterologically depressed" and have a persistent depressive affect and personality style, they often do respond to a supportive, positive, and constructive relationship with a physician. They suffer few or none of the vegetative signs of major depression, and cognitive function remains intact. Some of these patients have impending major depression or less severe forms of other types of depression.

Page 1440

5. Despite the assumption that major depression is a neuroendocrinologic disorder, which of the following research findings question this premise?

A. Only about 60% of severely ill patients demonstrate neurohormonal abnormality.
B. The proportion of depressed patients seen in a family practice with neuroendocrine abnormalities may be as low as 20 to 30%.
C. Both A and B
D. Neither A nor B

Answer: C

Critique: Although an assessment of neuroendocrine function showed initial promise, studies using the dexamethasone suppression test have demonstrated that this line of investigation has little use in primary care practice. Only a small proportion of patients in family practice demonstrate significant neuroendocrine abnormalities. Additionally, the test reveals abnormalities in only 60% of severely ill patients, and thus the test suffers from low sensitivity.

Further Reading

APA Task Force on Laboratory Tests in Psychiatry: The dexamethasone suppression test: An overview of its current status in psychiatry. Am J Psychiatry 144:1253, 1987.

6. Which ONE of the following is the single best indicator of risk for suicide:

A. Presence of physical illness
B. History of prior attempts
C. A direct or indirect statement of intent
D. Coexistent alcoholism or substance abuse
E. Positive family history of a successful suicide

Answer: C

Critique: Although other indicators are strongly correlated with a suicide risk, the single best indicator remains a direct or indirect statement of intent. The physician should respond seriously to any mention of suicide and should not be deterred from a frank discussion of the patient's feelings and intentions.

Page 1495

7. (Matching) Match each psychiatric situation with the therapeutic intervention that is most appropriate for that condition:

A. Psychotherapy
B. Antidepressant medication

1. Patients with major depression

2. Resolving interpersonal problems

3. Alleviating sleep disturbances

4. Women who are pregnant or lactating

5. Improvement of social functioning

Answers: 1-B, 2-A, 3-B, 4-A, 5-A

Critique: Controversy still surrounds the issue of psychotherapy versus pharmacotherapy for depressive disorders. In most circumstances, combined therapy will optimize outcomes. Major depression requires pharmacotherapy; these patients achieve 70% response with or without concurrent psychotherapy. Psychotherapy is most effective for managing interpersonal difficulties and improvement of social functioning. Antidepressant therapy is most effective for relieving a sleep disturbance.

Page 1497

8. (True or False) True statements regarding depression in family practice include which of the following?

1. Depression has an estimated prevalence of 5 to 10%.
2. Depression is the most common psychiatric problem seen by family practitioners.
3. Few clinically significant cases of depression go untreated.
4. Depressive symptoms lead to little functional impairment.

Answers: 1-T, 2-T, 3-F, 4-F

Critique: Depression is the most common psychiatric problem seen by primary care practitioners and affects 5 to 10% of the population. Unfortunately, most clinically important cases go untreated. Additionally, depressive symptoms accrue functional impairment similar to that associated with chronic medical conditions, such as high blood pressure, diabetes, and chronic obstructive lung disease.

Page 1486

9. All of the following represent DSM-IV criteria for major depression EXCEPT:

    A. Depressed mood most of the day, nearly every day
    B. Markedly diminished interest in all, or almost all, activities
    C. Insomnia or hypersomnia nearly every day
    D. Depressive symptoms due to substance abuse or a medical condition
    E. Clinically significant impairment of social function

Answer: D

Critique: To meet the DSM-IV criteria for major depression, the depressive symptoms should not be caused by substance abuse or chronic illness. All of the other characteristics reflect DSM-IV criteria for major depression.

Page 1487

10. (True or False) Many patients who exhibit depressive symptoms do not satisfy criteria for major depression but remain significantly impaired nonetheless. Dysthymia represents an alternative diagnosis for many of these individuals. Criteria for the diagnosis of dysthymia include which of the following?

    1. Symptoms not due to the direct effects of drugs or medication
    2. Major depressive disorder within the first 2 years of symptoms
    3. Low self-esteem or feelings of inadequacy
    4. Social withdrawal
    5. Previous history of a manic episode

Answers: 1-T, 2-F, 3-T, 4-T, 5-F

Critique: To meet criteria for dysthymia, the patient's symptoms should not be due to medications or substances. Additionally, low self-esteem and social withdrawal are among the features contained in the DSM-IV criteria for dysthymia. The criteria indicate that the patient must not have had a major depressive episode within 2 years of the onset of symptoms. Additionally, the patient must not have experienced manic or hypomanic episodes previously.

Page 1488

11. (True or False) Symptoms that support the diagnosis of adjustment disorder with depressed mood include which of the following?

    1. Symptoms lasting longer than 6 months
    2. Intact cognitive function
    3. Preserved psychomotor function

Answers: 1-F, 2-T, 3-T

Critique: Adjustment disorder with depressed mood includes depressive symptoms lasting up to 6 months. Patients should demonstrate intact, or nearly intact, cognitive and psychomotor function.

Page 1490

12. (True or False) Patients who have "masked depression" frequently present with somatic symptoms rather than complaints about mood. Symptoms that such patients might exhibit include which of the following?

    1. Chronic pain, such as headache or abdominal pain
    2. Nausea, diarrhea, indigestion, and excessive flatulence
    3. Fatigue, dizziness, and blurred vision
    4. Dyspnea and palpitations

Answers: 1-T, 2-T, 3-T, 4-T

Critique: Depressed patients can present with symptoms other than mood disturbance. Somatic symptoms such as headache, abdominal pain, nausea, diarrhea, indigestion, flatulence, fatigue, dizziness, blurred vision, dyspnea, and palpitations can all serve as indicators for masked depression.

Pages 1490, 1491

13. The age group in which depression occurs most commonly is:

    A. 16–32 years
    B. 20–36 years
    C. 18–44 years
    D. 40–65 years

Answer: C

Critique: Depression occurs most commonly in the age group 18 to 44 years. Women experience depression two to three times more frequently than do men.

Pages 1491, 1492

14. (True or False) True statements regarding the epidemiology and natural history of major depression include which of the following?

    1. The prevalence appears to be 5 to 10% in medical populations.
    2. The mean age of onset is the mid-forties.
    3. Of those experiencing major depression, 80% will incur only a single episode.
    4. Social support does not affect vulnerability to major depression.

Answers: 1-T, 2-F, 3-F, 4-F

Critique: The prevalence of major depression in medical populations appears to range between 5 and 10%. The mean age of onset of major depression is in the mid-twenties rather than the mid-forties. Only about half of those who experience major depression will have only a single episode. Approximately 50% will have a relapse within 2 years. Low social support appears to increase the vulnerability to major depression.

Pages 1491, 1492

15. (True or False) Major depression is associated with a number of neuroendocrinologic abnormalities. Which of the following represent identified neurobiologic abnormalities seen in major depression?

1. Excess 5-hydroxyindoleacetic acid (5-HIAA)
2. Disordered thyroid-stimulating hormone (TSH) stimulation by thyrotropin-releasing hormone (TRH)
3. Abnormal levels of melatonin and luteinizing hormone
4. Disordered hypothalamopituitary-adrenal axis function

Answers: 1-T, 2-T, 3-T, 4-T

Critique: Major depression demonstrates multiple neuroendocrinologic abnormalities. These patients can have abnormal 5-HIAA levels and disordered thyroid regulation. They can also exhibit abnormal growth hormone, luteinizing hormone, melatonin, and prolactin levels. Major depression can also cause abnormal hypothalamopituitary-adrenal axis function.

Page 1493

16. (True or False) Of the following characteristics, which confer increased risk of suicide in depressed patients?

1. Young patient age
2. Presence of a physical illness associated with chronic pain
3. Coexistent substance or alcohol abuse
4. Communication of a specific plan for suicide

Answers: 1-F, 2-T, 3-T, 4-T

Critique: Increased age confers a higher risk of suicide. Coexistent physical illness, particularly if associated with chronic pain or terminal status, increases the risk of suicide. Coexistent substance abuse also confers higher risk. Contrary to common belief, communication of intent, with a plan for how the patient will complete suicide, represents the single best predictor for suicide.

Page 1495

17. In primary care settings, the pharmacotherapy of major depression can be expected to demonstrate what efficacy?

A. 25–30%
B. 35–40%
C. 55–60%
D. 80–90%

Answer: C

Critique: According to their synthesis of the published primary care experience, the Agency for Health Care Policy and Research Depression Guidelines panel concluded that drug therapy for major depression demonstrates 55 to 60% efficacy in such practices.

Page 1496

18. (True or False) For a 45-year-old woman with major depression who has no cardiac problems but has signifi-

cant anxiety and insomnia, which of the following would be most suitable for initial drug therapy?

1. Fluoxetine
2. Doxepin
3. Amitriptyline
4. Sertraline

Answers: 1-F, 2-T, 3-T, 4-F

Critique: For patients who have prominent anxiety and insomnia, the sedative effects of the older tricyclic antidepressants represent a reasonable choice for initial therapy in major depression. The newer selective serotonin reuptake inhibitors (SSRIs) frequently cause insomnia and agitation and thus represent a less attractive option in this case.

Page 1496

Further Reading

Choice of an antidepressant. Med Lett 35:25–26, 1993.

19. (True or False) The AHCPR Depression Guidelines panel recommended full dose maintenance therapy (longer than one year) for patients who demonstrate which of the following?

1. Previous history of severe or debilitating depression
2. Previous history of suicidal action
3. Strong family history of recurrent depression
4. History of three episodes or more of severe depression

Answers: 1-T, 2-T, 3-T, 4-T

Critique: Continuous pharmacologic treatment for extended periods may be necessary for certain depressed patients. Those who have a history of severe, debilitating depression, or three or more episodes of severe depression, warrant maintenance therapy. Additionally, those patients who have demonstrated previous suicidal intent should be considered for long-term drug treatment. A strong family history of depression also militates toward maintenance therapy.

Page 1496

20. Of the following options, which represents the best time of day for administering SSRI antidepressants (e.g., fluoxetine, paroxetine, sertraline)?

A. 10:30 P.M.
B. 5:30 P.M.
C. 11:30 A.M.
D. 8:30 A.M.

Answer: D

Critique: Because of their tendency to disrupt sleep, the SSRIs should, at least initially, be administered in the morning.

Page 1497

Further Reading

Choice of an antidepressant. Med Lett 35:25–26, 1993.

21. (True or False) Which of the following represent indications to consider psychiatric referral for a patient with major depression?

1. High suicidal risk
2. Psychotic symptoms
3. Satisfactory response to antidepressants
4. Bipolar depression

Answers: 1-T, 2-T, 3-F, 4-T

Critique: A satisfactory response to antidepressants would suggest continued therapy by the primary care physician. If antidepressants are unsuccessful, and the patient demonstrates severe vegetative signs and symptoms, referral should be considered because these patients might be candidates for electroconvulsive therapy. The other identified characteristics represent indications to at least consider psychiatric referral.

Page 1499

53

Crisis Intervention in Office Practice

Marilyn Mehr and Michael D. Hagen

1. Match each of the research scientists with the concept that the individual explained and developed.

    A. Eric Erickson
    B. Thomas Salmon
    C. Gerald Caplan
    D. Thomas Holmes and Robert Rahe
    E. Eric Lindemann

1. Normal developmental crises throughout the life cycle

2. Crisis reactions in survivors of the Coconut Grove fire

3. Treatment of "shell shock" in Allied troops

4. Synthesized crisis theory into a treatment with four possible outcomes

Answers: 1-A, 2-E, 3-B, 4-C

Critique: Eric Erickson described the concept of the life cycle, characterized by a number of developmental stages and crises. Eric Lindemann described the natural history of emotional response to personal tragedy, as experienced by family members of the victims of the Boston Coconut Grove fire. Thomas Salmon described the treatment and outcome of victims of shell shock in World War I. Gerald Caplan synthesized concepts into modern crisis theory and treatment approaches.

Pages 1502–1504

2. (True or False) According to Caplan's description of the consequences of crisis, which of the following represent possible expected outcomes?

    1. Severely impaired but stable functioning
    2. Incompletely restored function and susceptibility to future crises

    3. Function restored to pre-crisis levels
    4. Improved functioning compared with pre-crisis levels

Answers: 1-T, 2-T, 3-T, 4-T

Critique: Caplan's work indicated that most crises resolve in 6 weeks with four potential results: (1) improved function compared with pre-crisis levels; (2) function restored to pre-crisis levels; (3) incomplete restoration of function and concomitant susceptibility to future crises; and (4) severely impaired but stable function.

Pages 1502–1504

3. Holmes and Rahe created a Social Readjustment Scale that ranked events or occurrences likely to precipitate stress in most individuals. Of the following, which one ranks the highest on their scale?

    A. Divorce
    B. The Christmas holiday season
    C. Change of occupation
    D. Death of a spouse

Answer: D

Critique: Of the 43 external stressors described by Holmes and Rahe, death of a spouse ranked number one as a stress precipitator for most people.

Page 1503

4. A man who brought his dead 2-year-old son into the emergency room after a drowning accident appeared completely normal, revealing no emotional response to the tragedy. In order to help this man recognize his feelings and begin the grieving process, the physician should approach the patient with which one of the following interventions?

    A. Explain that every parent makes mistakes and reveal some mistakes that you have made.

B. Prescribe an antianxiety medication presuming that the patient is too "frozen" in his fear to respond appropriately.

C. Take a thorough psychosocial history, allowing the patient time to reflect.

D. Ask the man to describe the specific events of his son's death.

E. Ask a family member to speak for the patient and explain the events surrounding the crisis.

Answer: D

Critique: It is essential for the patient to begin to face the crisis realistically and express his feelings about the event. The physician must, therefore, ask the patient concrete questions about the event and allow time for the patient to respond emotionally. If the patient denies his feelings, he is likely to experience only partial relief and recovery.

Pages 1504, 1505

5. Which one of the following is NOT true of crisis evaluation?

A. An in-depth history of the patient's life will allow the physician to counsel the patient more effectively to move through the crisis.

B. The physician should help the patient to choose and then mobilize the most helpful people in the support network.

C. There is a correlation between a previous personality or psychiatric disorder and one's capacity to deal with a crisis.

D. Those with severe personality disorders and rigid coping styles are more vulnerable to developing a crisis.

E. There are some cases in which a pre-existing psychiatric disorder may cause or influence the development of a crisis.

Answer: A

Critique: All of the aforementioned are true except A. In an acute crisis, the physician should mobilize the patient's resources to cope with the present situation. Therefore, the history should be focused and selective, and the physician should inquire about details that may increase the understanding of the crisis and enable the patient to begin to organize and move through the situation.

Pages 1505, 1506

6. **(True or False)** According to Feinstein and Carey, which of the following should serve as the focus or foci for crisis intervention?

1. Assessment of the patient's support network
2. Precipitants of the current crisis
3. Personal meaning to the patient of the crisis events
4. "Selective" history relevant to the crisis

Answers: 1-T, 2-T, 3-T, 4-T

Critique: According to Feinstein and Carey, several issues should be addressed in crisis intervention. The therapist should assess the patient's social support,

discern the personal meaning that the crisis holds for the patient, take a "selective" history (i.e., focus the history on previous crises and precipitants in those circumstances), explore the crisis state itself, and identify a concurrent psychiatric illness that might affect the crisis intervention.

Page 1506

7. According to Feinstein and Carey, a "time line" of events leading up to a crisis should include all of the following EXCEPT:

A. Events that have occurred over the previous year
B. Possible precipitating events
C. Events that have contributed to the current crisis
D. Selective history appropriate to the crisis

Answer: A

Critique: As described by Feinstein and Carey, the crisis "time line" should include events for the previous 6 weeks leading up to the crisis. The time line should also include precipitants, events that might have contributed to the crisis, and an appropriate selective history.

Page 1506

8. In developing a support network map, all of the following should be included EXCEPT:

A. People in the patient's immediate living environment
B. Religious and social agencies that might provide support
C. The patient's family of origin for at least five generations
D. Close friends who might be called upon to lend support

Answer: C

Critique: As described by Feinstein and Carey, the support network map should include the patient's family of origin for three generations, people in the patient's immediate living environment, religious and social support sources, and close friends. This list could include neighbors and the patient's physician.

Page 1506

9. **(True or False)** Which of the following represent adaptive coping styles as described by Feinstein and Carey?

1. Use of imagination, feelings, and perceptions to solve the problem
2. Use of the threat of suicide as an attempt to solve the problem
3. Use of dishonesty, lying, or cheating to solve the crisis
4. Use of emotion, such as tears or anger, to help solve the problem

Answers: 1-T, 2-F, 3-F, 4-T

Critique: Feinstein and Carey describe a number of coping styles that patients use to cope with crisis. Use of imagination, feelings, and perceptions constitutes an intuitive approach to solving the problem. Additionally, constructive use of emotion, such as tears and anger, represents another adaptive coping style. Use of dishonesty, lying, cheating, and threats of suicide represent pathologic coping styles.

Page 1506

10. All BUT ONE of the following strategies should be used by the family physician to resolve a crisis:

    A. Recognize early warning signs of a crisis for early intervention.

    B. Identify the specific areas of the patient's life that are most affected by the crisis.

    C. Teach patients to evaluate their own support system by using a "network map."

    D. Implement a plan for resolution of one of the causes of the crisis.

    E. Avoid categorizing the patient's coping style to prevent "medicalizing" the crisis.

Answer: E

Critique: Feinstein and Carey outline a 14-step strategy for crisis resolution. The physician should learn about the patient's current coping style and encourage him or her to use other coping styles when needed. Additionally, the physician should educate the patient regarding the warning signs of crisis. The patient should be encouraged to talk over the problem with a trusted friend or family doctor. The patient should be encouraged to discuss painful feelings and emotions and to identify the area of life most affected by the crisis. Also, the patient should identify the stresses and precipitants that have, during the previous 6 weeks, led to the crisis. Patients should learn how to develop support network maps as a means to identify sources of support during crises. Together with the patient, the therapist should help the patient to develop a crisis treatment plan, taking the patient's coping styles into consideration.

Pages 1508, 1509

54

Personality Disorders in Office Practice

Michael Dunaway

1. Roger has always been a "loner" and has few friends. He prefers jobs in which he can work alone. Generally, Roger responds to criticism with indifference. He is not married. People who know Roger note that he never seems very happy. Many years ago Roger worked as a forest ranger but gave it up after being transferred to a national park. "I didn't like the tourists," Roger said. Which of the following conditions is Roger most likely to have?

    A. Schizotypal personality disorder
    B. Avoidant personality disorder
    C. Schizoid personality disorder
    D. Schizoaffective disorder

Answer: C

Critique: Schizoid personality disorder is characterized by a pattern of lack of desire for relationships and difficulty expressing emotions. Individuals with this disorder prefer spending time alone, often don't marry, are disinterested in sex, and appear "cold." Here schizoid personality is distinguished from avoidant personality disorder by a lack of hypersensitivity to criticism. A major feature of schizotypal personality disorder is odd thinking, behavior, language, or dress, of which there is no evidence here. In schizoaffective disorder, there is a period of depression, mania, or mixed episode in combination with two or more ("A") criteria for schizophrenia (e.g., delusions, hallucinations, disorganized speech, disorganized or catatonic behavior, or negative symptoms).

Page 1519

Further Reading

American Psychiatric Association: Diagnostic and Statistical Manual of Mental Disorders, 4th ed. Washington, DC, American Psychiatric Association, 1994, p 638.

2. All of the following are true of personality disorders EXCEPT:

    A. They affect both the patient and the physician.
    B. They lead to significant personal distress.
    C. They contribute to poor quality medical care.
    D. They are clearly evident clinically.

Answer: D

Critique: One source of difficult patient-physician relationships is personality disorders. "Hateful" patients often leave their physician feeling frustrated, exhausted, or angry. The resultant dysfunctional patient-physician relationship may lead to poor quality medical care. Despite being relatively common and causing significant distress for the patient, personality disorders often go unrecognized because the patient does not report to the physician the more typical features of the condition. Sometimes a clearer picture can be obtained from the patient's family or friends.

Page 1510

Questions 3–7. Match the following numbered statements to their appropriate lettered option.

    A. Personality style
    B. Personality disorder
    C. Both A and B
    D. Neither A nor B

3. Unique

4. Maladaptive

5. Enduring

6. Extreme

7. Lifelong

Answers: 3-C, 4-B, 5-C, 6-B, 7-C

Critique: The difference between personality disorders and personality styles is mainly one of degree. Personality styles are a unique, enduring way that one thinks, feels, and behaves. Personality styles become personality disorders when they are rigid, extreme, or maladaptive or "lead to social or occupational impairment."

Page 1510

8. All of the following personality disorders are included in cluster A (odd or eccentric) EXCEPT

    A. Schizoid
    B. Schizotypal
    C. Histrionic
    D. Paranoid

Answers: C

Critique: Histrionic is included in cluster B (dramatic, emotional, or erratic).

Page 1511

9. Tom is a 50-year-old man in your practice. You have followed him for approximately 3 years, primarily for chronic obstructive pulmonary disease. Although Tom has always been pleasant, he never seems very happy. At the beginning of your relationship he seemed suspicious, refusing to divulge personal information or even his current medication regimen. He lives alone and has few friends. He relies mostly on his brother for support. His brother says, "That's the way Tom's always been." His hobbies include collecting bottles and reading. At office visits he usually wears a blue sweatsuit and dark sunglasses. Each time that Tom brings to you a long list of questions, most have little or no relevance to his condition. Which of the following personality types does Tom demonstrate?

    A. Schizoid
    B. Schizotypal
    C. Paranoid
    D. Avoidant

Answer: B

Critique: Persons with schizotypal personality disorder have difficulties with interpersonal relationships, perception (including ideas of reference, magical thinking, "odd thinking," or suspiciousness), and behavioral eccentricities. Like persons with a schizoid personality disorder, these individuals are "loners," but they are differentiated mainly by their odd thinking and behavior. Like paranoid personality disorder there may be an element of suspiciousness, but again the schizotypal personality disorder is differentiated by marked eccentricity. Individuals with avoidant personality disorder can also appear as "loners," but their social isolation is due to fear of rejection.

Page 1518

Further Reading

American Psychiatric Association: Diagnostic and Statistical Manual of Mental Disorders, 4th ed. Washington, DC, American Psychiatric Association, 1994, p 641.

10. All of the following personality disorders are included in cluster B (dramatic, emotional, or erratic) EXCEPT:

    A. Antisocial
    B. Histrionic
    C. Passive aggressive
    D. Self-defeating

Answer: C

Critique: Passive aggressive is included in cluster C (anxious or fearful).

Page 1511

11. Cluster C (anxious or fearful) includes: passive aggressive, obsessive compulsive, avoidant, and which ONE of the following?

    A. Narcissistic
    B. Borderline
    C. Paranoid
    D. Dependent

Answer: D

Critique: Narcissistic and borderline are in cluster B (dramatic, emotional, or erratic), and paranoid is in cluster A (odd or eccentric).

Page 1511

12. Which ONE of the following is true of antisocial personality disorder?

    A. Can be diagnosed at any age
    B. Can appear in adulthood with no prior history of behavioral problems
    C. Becomes worse with age
    D. Is associated with low socioeconomic status

Answer: D

Critique: Antisocial personality disorder is diagnosed in individuals who fail to conform to social norms; violate the rights of others; and are aggressive, impulsive, or lack remorse. The individual must be at least 18 years old and have had evidence of a conduct disorder since at least 13 years of age. Antisocial personality disorder is a chronic problem but may improve as the individual grows older. Antisocial personality disorder is associated with a low socioeconomic status.

Page 1519

Further Reading

American Psychiatric Association: Diagnostic and Statistical Manual of Mental Disorders. 4th ed. Washington, DC, American Psychiatric Association, 1994, p 649.

Questions 13–18. For the following numbered statements choose the appropriate lettered high-level defense mechanism.

    A. Repression
    B. Suppression
    C. Reaction formation

D. Passive aggressive
E. Intellectualization
F. Rationalization

13. Superficial compliance with passively disguised anger

14. Consciously putting a disturbing experience out of one's mind

15. Unconsciously replacing feeling with facts of details

16. Unacceptable impulses expressed as behaviors directly opposite those impulses

17. Involuntarily forgetting a painful experience

18. Creating socially acceptable explanations for behaviors

Answers: 13-D, 14-B, 15-E, 16-C, 17-A, 18-F

Critique: Defenses are unconscious psychological processes used by the patient to help resolve internal conflicts, manage anxiety, or alleviate depression. Patients with a neurotic personality organization typically use high-level defenses of which A through F are examples.

Page 1514

19. Which of the following is *not* a high level (repression-centered) defense?

A. Ambivalence
B. Hypochondriasis
C. Distortion
D. Sexualization

Answer: B

Critique: Hypochondriasis (the irrational fear of having a physical illness) is included in the splitting centered defenses of borderline personality organization.

Page 1514

Questions 20–23. Match the following numbered statements to the most appropriate lettered option.

A. Neurotic personality organization
B. Borderline personality organization
C. Psychotic personality organization

20. Stable view of self

21. Loss of reality testing

22. Primitive defenses

23. Splitting defenses

Answers: 20-A, 21-C, 22-C, 23-B

Critique: Reality testing is generally intact in neurotic and borderline functioning patients but can be lost in borderline functioning patients when under stress. In patients functioning at the psychotic level, reality testing is

characteristically lost. Neurotically functioning patients have a stable view of self, but patients with borderline and psychotic functioning have changing views of self (identity diffusion). Neurotically functioning patients typically have high-level defenses, but patients with borderline function tend to use splitting centered defenses (splitting, omnipotence, devaluation, projection, denial, regression, and hypochondriasis), and psychotic functioning patients tend to use primitive defenses (acting out, incorporation, somatization, and schizoid fantasy).

Page 1512

Questions 24–27. Match the following numbered physician reactions to the appropriate lettered personality disorder. Use each choice only once.

A. Self-defeating
B. Schizoid
C. Antisocial
D. Histrionic

24. Exploited

25. Need to rescue

26. Detached

27. Captivated

Answers: 24-C, 25-A, 26-B, 27-D

Critique: Patients with personality disorders can evoke strong emotions from their physicians. The aforementioned examples represent reactions that can possibly occur in response to specific personality disorders. Clearly other reactions are possible, and many overlap (e.g., a physician might feel fearful of a patient with either paranoid or antisocial personality disorder). However, close attention by the physician to his or her own reactions may be a clue that there is a problem with the patient-physician relationship or even a clue to specific diagnosis.

Pages 1515, 1516

Questions 28–31. For the following personality disorder types select the level of functioning that is most representative of the disorder.

A. Neurotic personality organization
B. Borderline personality organization
C. Psychotic personality organization

28. Paranoid personality disorder

29. Schizotypal personality disorder

30. Antisocial personality disorder

31. Borderline personality disorder

Answers: 28-C, 29-C, 30-B, 31-B

Critique: Individuals with paranoid or schizotypal personality disorder typically function at the psychotic level. Antisocial and borderline patients typically function at the borderline level but, with stress, can function at the psychotic level.

Pages 1518–1520

32. (True or False) Which of the following represent statements concerning antisocial personality disorder?

1. Often demand special treatment
2. Should be referred if malingering is suspected
3. Verification of symptoms with other sources is helpful
4. The physician might wish to punish the patient.

Answers: 1-T, 2-F, 3-T, 4-T

Critique: Patients with antisocial personality disorder often demand special treatment. They can evoke strong emotions in their physician, including a desire to punish the patient. If malingering is suspected, it might help to attempt to confirm the patient's symptoms with other reliable sources. The patient should not be referred if malingering is suspected.

Page 1519

33. (True or False) Which of the following represent true statements concerning persons with a histrionic personality disorder?

1. They are often dramatic and flirtatious.
2. They can function on either the neurotic or borderline level.
3. They may react with regression.
4. They use defenses centered on splitting.

Answers: 1-T, 2-T, 3-T, 4-T

Critique: All of the aforementioned statements are true concerning the histrionic personality disorder. Interestingly, patients with histrionic personality disorder can use defenses centered on splitting, neurotic defenses (sexualization), or primitive defenses (acting out or somatization).

Page 1519

34. (True or False) Of the following, which statements are true concerning borderline personality disorder?

1. Display identity diffusion
2. Have a neurotic personality organization
3. Fear being abandoned
4. Use acting out as a primary defense

Answers: 1-T, 2-F, 3-T, 4-F

Critique: Patients with borderline personality disorder typically function at the level of borderline personality organization, but under stress they may function at the psychotic level. Splitting is one of their main defenses, although they also rely on projection, projective identification, devaluation, and occasionally acting out. Patients with this disorder have an intense fear of abandonment, and the threat of separation may trigger their mental decompensation. For the patient who displays fear of abandonment, frequent, structured visits should be conducted.

Page 1520

Further Reading

Searight HR: Borderline personality disorder: Diagnosis and management in primary care. J Fam Pract 34:605–612, 1992.

35. When dealing with patients who have a self-defeating personality disorder, telling such patients that they are getting better or will soon be cured is likely to:

A. Lead them to realize "it's all in your head"
B. Lead them to feel hopeful for recovery
C. Lead them to feel relieved
D. Lead them to experience worsening symptoms

Answer: D

Critique: It should not be suggested that the patient's symptoms are psychological or that the patient will improve or be cured quickly. Such misstatements may paradoxically increase the patient's symptoms, complaints, telephone calls, and office visits.

Page 1521

55

The Somatic Patient

Arch G. Mainous III

1. Evaluate the following statements regarding the somatic patient:

1. Individuals with mental disorders commonly present with somatic complaints.
2. More than 75% of patients presenting to primary care physicians with somatic symptoms have psychosocial precipitants.
3. Although depression has somatic components, patients tend to seek care because of their dysphoric mood.
4. Older patients with depression commonly focus on somatic symptoms.

Answers: 1-T, 2-F, 3-F, 4-T

Critique: Mental disorders, particularly depression, are common in primary care with presenting symptoms commonly displaying somatic characteristics. Evidence indicates that up to 50% of patients presenting with somatic symptoms have psychosocial precipitants. Individuals with mental disorders are high utilizers of health care and have significant functional disability. Although depression is highly prevalent, it is frequently undiagnosed, possibly because dysphoric mood is an infrequent complaint. Older persons tend to focus on somatic conditions rather than on affective states, possibly because of stigmatization associated with mental disorders.

Page 1523

Further Reading

Katon W, Sullivan MD: Depression and chronic medical illness. J Clin Psychiatry 51 (Suppl 6):3–11, 1990.
Zung WWK, Broadhead WE, Roth ME: Prevalence of depressive symptoms in primary care. J Fam Pract 37:337–344, 1993.

2. (True or False) Which of the following somatic symptoms are characteristically associated with depression?

1. Poor appetite
2. Insomnia
3. Hypersomnia
4. Fatigue

Answers: 1-T, 2-T, 3-T, 4-T

Critique: All of these symptoms are characteristics of a major depressive disorder. Many patients with undiagnosed depression receive aggressive medical treatment and testing for somatic complaints that put them at risk for iatrogenic injury.

Page 1523

3. (True or False) Which of the following statements are true regarding somatoform disorders:

1. Patients with somatoform disorders tend to consciously manufacture symptoms to gain attention.
2. Hypochondriacal patients frequently come from families with other hypochondriacal family members.
3. An important therapeutic strategy in patients with conversion disorder is to confront them early in management with the reality that no organic disease exists.
4. Individuals with somatization disorder tend to have complaints localized to a specific organ system.
5. Conversion disorders are characterized by long-term loss of physical functioning.

Answers: 1-F, 2-T, 3-F, 4-F, 5-F

Critique: Somatoform disorders are characterized by physical symptoms with no demonstrable physical findings of organic disease. The patient does not consciously produce symptoms. Hypochondriacal patients tend to come from alcoholic or dysfunctional families with other hypochondriacal family members. Conversion disorders are precipitated by conflict or stressors and are typically of short duration. Because the patient does not produce the symptoms intentionally, and conflict and stressors precipitate the event, confronting the patient prematurely regarding the cause of the functional loss is not recommended. Somatization disorder is characterized by a multitude of general medical conditions with involvement of multiple organ systems.

Page 1524

4. Palpitations, sweating, trembling or shaking, dyspnea, feelings of choking, chest pain or discomfort, and parasthesias are major manifestations of which one of the following conditions?

    A. Hypochondriasis
    B. Anxiety
    C. Conversion disorder
    D. Somatoform pain disorder

Answer: B

Critique: Although all of the conditions may exhibit one or more of these symptoms, they are particular manifestations of anxiety and panic disorders. Hypochondriasis refers to a fear of having a belief that one has a serious disease based on a misinterpretation of one or more bodily signs. The essential feature of a conversion disorder is a symptom or deficit affecting voluntary motor or sensory functioning. Paralysis and paresthesias are common complaints in conversion disorder. Somatoform pain disorder is characterized by pain that causes clinically significant distress or impairment in functioning but has no demonstrable physical findings.

Pages 1523, 1524

5. A patient who presents with physical complaints of a bizarre or unusual nature (e.g., a complaint that the patient's large intestine is not functioning) is most commonly characterized as suffering from:

    A. A personality disorder
    B. An adjustment disorder
    C. A psychotic disorder
    D. An affective disorder (e.g., depression)

Answer: C

Critique: Individuals with psychotic disorders are characterized by impairments in reality testing as evidenced by delusions and hallucinations. Delusional disorder–somatic type involves delusions of bodily functions or sensations. For individuals with psychotic disorders, a mental health specialist should be consulted for their care.

Page 1525

Questions 6–8. Match the following types of conditioning with the appropriate scenario:

    A. Operant conditioning
    B. Classical conditioning
    C. Modeling

6. A child experiences nausea, vomiting, and severe gastrointestinal distress soon after eating in the school cafeteria. Although the gastrointestinal distress was unrelated to the food in the cafeteria, the child develops debilitating nausea whenever he goes into the cafeteria and later whenever he is at school.

7. A child has severe gastrointestinal distress every weekday before school. When the child is allowed to stay home from school, the nausea and diarrhea tend to dissipate by late morning. Although the mother is frustrated with the child's inability to attend school, the mother acknowledges that she appreciates having company around the house during the day.

8. A child has frequent severe gastrointestinal distress. A family history reveals that the child's father and paternal grandfather both suffer from similar frequent bouts of abdominal pain and gastrointestinal distress.

Answers: 6-B, 7-A, 8-C

Critique: Classical conditioning is characterized by the creation of a conditioned response to a previously neutral stimulus. Although the food in the cafeteria did not cause the boy to become ill, the boy associated his illness with the cafeteria (for the sake of this example, a previously neutral stimulus for nausea). The response was later generalized to a variety of stimuli, including school itself. Operant conditioning involves the altering of behavior based on subsequent consequences (reinforcement). The child whose gastrointestinal distress dissipates once she does not have to go to school gains positive reinforcement from her mother's attention. The mother's current behavior increases the likelihood that the child will remain school-phobic. Modeling is a form of social learning in which individuals learn via vicarious reinforcement attributable to the behaviors of others. The child whose father suffers from abdominal pain sees the attention and comforting that the father receives and models his behavior accordingly.

Pages 1525, 1526

9. (True or False) Increased risk of somatization is associated with which of the following characteristics?

    1. Low socioeconomic status
    2. Japanese immigrant status
    3. Chinese immigrant status
    4. Middle Eastern immigrant status

Answers: 1-T, 2-F, 3-T, 4-T

Critique: The manifestation and presentation of mental distress are shaped by the patient's cultural context. Lower socioeconomic environments tend to de-emphasize expression of emotion, and thus patients from such environments are more likely to somatize. Chinese and Middle Eastern cultures tend to somatize depression. Asian culture is not homogeneous on this issue, and evidence suggests that Japanese are less likely than are Chinese to somatize depression. However, the more westernized that individuals of Chinese and Middle Eastern descent become, the less likely they are to somatize.

Page 1526

Further Reading

Kirmayer LJ, Young A, Robbins JM: Symptom attribution in cultural perspective. Can J Psychiatry 39:584–595, 1994.

10. (True or False) Functional disability in somatic patients may be the result of which of the following?

    1. The underlying mental disorder
    2. A coexistent organic medical problem
    3. Poor compliance with treatment recommendations

Answers: 1-T, 2-T, 3-T

Critique: Many individuals have both chronic medical conditions and psychiatric disorders, particularly depression. Recent evidence indicates that psychiatric disorders are more functionally disabling than are many chronic medical conditions. It is important to address both types of problems in both the diagnosis and treatment. Mental disorders may lead to decreased compliance, poor motivation associated with anhedonia, and feelings of helplessness and hopelessness.

Page 1527

Further Reading

Ormel J, Von Korff M, Ustun TB, et al: Common mental disorders and disability across cultures: Results from the WHO collaborative study on psychological problems in general health care. JAMA 272:1741–1748, 1994.

11. (True or False) In an assessment of the somatic patient, which of the following statements are true?

1. Formal psychological testing is necessary to make a diagnosis.
2. A substance abuse history may indicate an underlying cause for somatic complaints.
3. All organic etiologies should be eliminated prior to making a diagnosis.
4. Symptomatic behavior includes only physiologic symptoms.

Answers: 1-F, 2-T, 3-F, 4-F

Critique: It is not possible to rule out all possible organic etiologies prior to making a diagnosis. An assessment should include an investigation of both biomedical and psychosocial issues. Historical information can be particularly productive. A history of substance abuse could be the primary cause of somatic complaints like sleep disturbance and anorexia. When operationalizing the patient's presenting complaints through a functional analysis, it is important to remember that symptomatic behavior includes physiologic and cognitive symptoms as well as overt behavior. Formal psychological testing is necessary in cases in which the biomedical and psychosocial evaluations are not productive.

Pages 1527, 1528

12. A multidisciplinary treatment approach utilizing physical and vocational therapy, psychological and behavioral therapy, and medical management is frequently required in the treatment of which one of the following conditions?

A. Depression
B. Somatoform pain disorder
C. Conversion disorder
D. Hypochondriasis
E. Somatization disorder

Answer: B

Critique: Treatment of the somatic patient often involves both family physicians and mental health professionals. However, individuals with somatoform pain disorder have a predominant focus on chronic pain. The pain may disrupt various aspects of their daily life. A multidisciplinary treatment approach using physical and vocational therapy as well as family physicians and mental health professionals has shown to be effective.

Page 1529

13. The treatment of choice for depression-related somatization as well as panic attacks is/are:

A. Benzodiazepines
B. Buspirone
C. Antidepressants
D. Phenothiazines

Answer: C

Critique: Both antidepressants and anxiolytics can play a role in the management of the somatic patient, but antidepressants are the treatment of choice for depression-related somatization and panic attacks. Although the recent clinical practice guideline produced by the Agency for Health Care Policy and Research on treatment of depression in primary care did not indicate meaningful differences in efficacy between tricyclic antidepressants and selective serotonin reuptake inhibitors (SSRIs) in treating depression, SSRIs are associated with fewer side effects. Long-term use of benzodiazepines has particular risk for dependency. Buspirone may be useful for the chronically anxious patient. Phenothiazines are used in the treatment of psychotic episodes.

Page 1529

56

Dementia

Michael Dunaway

1. Which ONE of the following is true regarding dementia?

    A. It is exclusively a disease of elderly people.
    B. It results only from aging.
    C. It is decreasing in frequency.
    D. It can intensify pre-existing personality traits.

Answer: D

Critique: Dementia is a state of deteriorated "intellectual and emotional function" that usually, but not exclusively (e.g., dementia in young individuals with human immunodeficiency virus [HIV]), occurs in elderly individuals. Patients with dementia typically have memory impairment (particularly short-term memory) but may lose visuospatial skills or develop other cognitive deficits. Intensification of personality traits may be noticed (e.g., increased suspiciousness in a previously suspicious individual). Like other age-related illnesses, dementia is increasing in frequency.

Page 1531

2. (True or False) Which of the following statements regarding HIV dementia are true?

    1. It is a subcortical dementia.
    2. It results from direct infection of the nerve cell.
    3. It occurs in older individuals as well as in young people.
    4. Central nervous system (CNS) infection occurs in asymptomatic individuals.

Answers: 1-T, 2-F, 3-T, 4-T

Critique: HIV dementia is primarily a disease of young people, but 10% of cases occur in individuals older than 50 years of age, leading to occasional confusion with Alzheimer's disease. In the CNS, the most commonly infected cell is the macrophage (not nerve or glial cells). Along with Jakob-Creutzfeldt disease, HIV dementia is considered to be subcortical. Twenty to 30% of HIV-infected individuals with a normal electroencephalogram (EEG) and psychometric testing will have CNS infection.

Page 1533

3. Which ONE of the following is the most common cause of dementia in the United States?

    A. Multi-infarct dementia
    B. Alzheimer's disease
    C. Pick's disease
    D. Depression

Answer: B

Critique: One half to two thirds of dementia patients will have dementia of the Alzheimer type (DAT). Up to one third will have multi-infarct dementia. Together, DAT and the vascular type (multi-infarct dementia) may represent as many as 85% of cases.

Page 1533

Further Reading

Fleming KC, Adams CA, Peterson RC: Dementia: Diagnosis and evaluation. Mayo Clin Proc 70:1093–1107, 1995.

4. Of the following options, which ONE is the major risk factor for developing DAT?

    A. History of blood dyscrasia
    B. History of vasculitis
    C. Family history
    D. History of anoxia

Answer: C

Critique: The primary risk factor for developing DAT is a family history positive for the disease. All of the other choices are possible mechanisms for developing vascular dementia.

Page 1533

Further Reading

Breitner JCS: Clinical genetics and genetic counseling in Alzheimer disease. Ann Intern Med 115:601–606, 1991.

5. According to the National Institutes of Health, all of the following diagnostic studies are recommended in the work-up of new-onset dementia EXCEPT:

A. Testing for syphilis
B. Thyroid function testing
C. A positron emission tomographic (PET) scan of the head
D. Vitamin B$_{12}$ level

Answer: C

Critique: All of the aforementioned tests are recommended, *except* a PET scan of the head. Other recommended tests are a complete blood count, electrolytes, metabolic screen, urinalysis, ECG, and chest radiograph.

Page 1534

Further Reading

Fleming KC, Adams CA, Peterson RC: Dementia: Diagnosis and evaluation. Mayo Clin Proc 70:1093–1107, 1995.

Questions 6–9. Match the following numbered terms concerning cognitive impairment with the appropriate lettered option.

A. Language disturbance
B. Inability to carry out motor activities
C. Inability to recognize objects
D. Difficulty abstracting

6. Agnosia

7. Aphasia

8. Apraxia

9. Executive function disturbance

Answers: 6-C, 7-A, 8-B, 9-D

Critique: The aforementioned terms and definitions are taken from the diagnostic criteria for DAT.

Page 1534

10. (True or False) Of the following, which represent true statements concerning the diagnosis of DAT?

1. Although there are diagnostic criteria for DAT, it is also a diagnosis of exclusion.
2. The post mortem diagnosis of DAT is characterized by neurofibrillary cords and tufts.
3. DAT is progressive and eventually results in severe impairment.
4. DAT is primarily a subcortical dementia.

Answers: 1-T, 2-F, 3-T, 4-F

Critique: Although there are diagnostic criteria for DAT, three of the six concern ruling out other disorders. DAT is characterized pathologically by neurofibrillary plaques and tangles and by loss of neurons in the cortex. DAT has a gradual onset, is progressive, and eventually results in severe impairment. It is the "classic" cortical type of dementia, although it is known to affect several subcortical structures.

Page 1534

Further Reading

Fleming KC, Adams CA, Peterson RC: Dementia: Diagnosis and evaluation. Mayo Clin Proc 70:1093–1107, 1995.

11. All of the following are true concerning the pharmacologic treatment of dementia EXCEPT:

A. Behavioral problems are the usual focus of pharmacotherapy.
B. All classes of antidepressants can be used for treating associated depression.
C. Low-potency antipsychotics (chlorpromazine or thioridazine) have low cardiovascular effects.
D. Neuroleptics are commonly used to control agitation.

Answer: C

Critique: All the aforementioned options are true concerning the pharmacologic treatment of depression except for option C. Low-potency antipsychotics are more likely to produce cardiovascular effects than are high-potency antipsychotics like haloperidol. High-potency antipsychotics are more likely to produce extrapyramidal symptoms.

Page 1535

12. (True or False) Which of the following statements concerning Pick's disease are true?

1. There are few focal neurologic findings other than dementia.
2. It is characterized by neurofibrillary plaques and tangles like DAT.
3. The cerebral atrophy primarily affects the parietal lobes.
4. It has a similar age distribution to DAT.
5. It is characterized by circumscribed areas of atrophy.

Answers: 1-T, 2-F, 3-F, 4-T, 5-T

Critique: Pick's disease is a chronic, progressive, dementing disease that usually lacks focal neurologic findings. Grasp and sucking reflexes may be seen when the frontal lobes are severely affected. Although fibrillary deposits are seen in the cytoplasm of affected neurons and biochemical changes similar to DAT are seen, there are no neurofibrillary plaques and tangles as seen in DAT. Unlike DAT, which is a diffuse process, Pick's disease is well circumscribed and primarily affects the frontal and temporal lobes. Age distribution is similar for DAT and Pick's disease.

Page 1532

Further Reading

Beal MF, Richardson EP, Martin JB: Alzheimer's disease and other dementias. *In* Isselbacher KJ, Braunwald E, Wilson JD, et al (Eds): Harrison's Principles of Internal Medicine, 13th ed. New York, McGraw-Hill, 1994, p 2272.

13. Which one of the following statements regarding the Mini-Mental State Examination (MMSE) is true?

A. The MMSE performs with high sensitivity and specificity in screening for cognitive impairment.
B. The MMSE's performance does not change with a change in the normal or abnormal cut score for the examination.
C. MMSE scores correlate closely with the rate of progression in Alzheimer's dementia.
D. The MMSE score declines with age in normal subjects.

Answer: D

Critique: The MMSE has gained fairly wide use as a screening tool and as a method for monitoring the progress of Alzheimer's dementia. Unfortunately, the MMSE performs with somewhat poor sensitivity and specificity in unselected populations and, therefore, probably works best as a tool for investigating cognitive function in patients who demonstrate possible symptoms of dementia. The test characteristics (e.g., sensitivity, specificity, predictive value) appear to vary depending on the cut score selected and on the population tested. The MMSE does not demonstrate a linear correlation with the disease progression. Investigators have established norms for different age groups; the normal scores do demonstrate some decline with age.

Further Reading

Fleming KC, Adams CA, Peterson RC: Dementia: Diagnosis and evaluation. Mayo Clinic Proc 70:1093–1107, 1995.
Galasko D, Klauber MR, Hofstetter CR, et al: The Mini-Mental State Examination in the early diagnosis of Alzheimer's disease. Arch Neurol 47:49–52, 1990.

14. (True or False) Several other assessment tools in addition to the MMSE have demonstrated utility in assessing cognitive function. True statements regarding these tools include:

1. The clock drawing test functions with acceptable sensitivity and specificity in screening for cognitive dysfunction.
2. The Mattis Dementia Rating Scale exhibits poor sensitivity and specificity in detecting cognitive dysfunction in dementia patients.
3. The Short Test of Mental Status (developed by Kokmen and colleagues) provides an assessment of cognitive function similar to that provided by the MMSE.

Answers: 1-T, 2-F, 3-T

Critique: A number of relatively short cognitive function assessments have become available. Sunderland and colleagues reported the development of the clock drawing test; this test consists of having the patient draw a clock face reading 2:45. The authors provided a set of criteria for scoring the test. The scoring procedure demonstrates high inter-rater reliability. Wolf-Klein and colleagues reported 87% sensitivity and 93% specificity for the test in a geriatric assessment center. Death and colleagues confirmed good performance more recently. The Mattis Dementia Rating Scale also demonstrates good test operating characteristics: Monsch and associates demon-

strated 98% sensitivity and 97% specificity in an outpatient population. The Short Test of Mental Status developed by Kokmen and colleagues assesses cognitive function dimensions similar to those in the MMSE but with greater depth.

Further Reading

Death J, Douglas D, Kenny RA: Comparison of clock drawing with Mini Mental State Examination as a screening test in elderly acute hospital admissions. Postgrad Med J 69:696–700, 1993.
Fleming KC, Adams CA, Peterson RC: Dementia: Diagnosis and evaluation. Mayo Clinic Proc 70:1093–1107, 1995.
Kokmen E, Naessens JM, Offord KP: A short test of mental status: Description and preliminary results. Mayo Clin Proc 62:281–288, 1987.
Monsch AU, Bondi MW, Salmon DP, et al: Clinical validity of the Mattis Dementia Rating Scale in detecting dementia of the Alzheimer type. A double cross-validation and application to a community-dwelling sample. Arch Neurol 52:899–904, 1995.
Sunderland T, Hill JL, Mellow AM, et al: Clock drawing in Alzheimer's disease: A novel measure of dementia severity. J Am Geriatr Soc 37:725–729, 1989.
Wolf-Klein GP, Silverstone FA, Levy AP, Brod MS: Screening for Alzheimer's disease by clock drawing. J Am Geriat Soc 37:730–734, 1989.

15. (True or False) False statements regarding apolipoprotein E (Apo E) and its association with Alzheimer's disease include:

1. The presence of the ε4 allele identifies patients with Alzheimer's disease with high sensitivity.
2. Approximately 80% of those who have at least one Apo E ε4 allele will develop Alzheimer's disease.
3. Family members of patients with Alzheimer's disease should undergo Apo E screening.

Answers: 1-F, 2-F, 3-F

Critique: Recent evidence indicates an association between Apo E (a plasma protein involved in cholesterol transport) and Alzheimer's disease. Some laboratories have begun offering Apo E screening services. Several characteristics of this association argue for caution in widespread application. The ε4 allele is present with higher frequency in Alzheimer's patients, but the sensitivity of this finding is only about 30% (specificity about 93%). Additionally, only between 25 and 50% of those who possess one or more ε4 alleles will develop Alzheimer's disease. At present, no intervention exists that can alter the disease course in those found to have the marker. In view of the modest predictive value and lack of suitable interventions, the American College of Medical Genetics/ American Society of Human Genetics Work Group on Apo E and Alzheimer's disease recommend against Apo E genotyping for the purpose of establishing the risk of Alzheimer's disease.

Further Reading

American College of Medical Genetics/American Society of Human Genetics Work Group on ApoE and Alzheimer Disease: Statement on use of apolipoprotein E testing for Alzheimer disease. JAMA 274:1627–1629, 1995.

Polvikoski T, Sulkava T, Haltia M, et al: Apolipoprotein E, dementia, and cortical deposition of β-amyloid protein. N Engl J Med 333:1242–1247, 1995.

16. True statements regarding the use of tacrine in Alzheimer's dementia include all of the following EXCEPT:

    A. Tacrine reverses the neuronal degeneration found in Alzheimer's dementia.

    B. As of 1995, tacrine is the only medication approved by the Food and Drug Administration (FDA) specifically for treating Alzheimer's dementia.

    C. Up to 50% of patients taking tacrine will experience increases in serum transaminase.

    D. Nausea, vomiting, diarrhea, and anorexia increase in a dose-related manner.

Answer: A

Critique: Tacrine produces modest improvements in cognitive function in patients with mild to moderate disease. The drug does not affect the neuronal degeneration that occurs in Alzheimer's dementia. Up to 50% of patients will experience increases in their serum transaminases, and adverse side effects such as nausea, vomiting, diarrhea, and anorexia increase with increasing doses of tacrine. As of 1995, tacrine is the only drug approved by the FDA specifically for treating Alzheimer's dementia.

Further Reading

Fleming KC, Evans JM: Pharmacologic therapies in dementia. Mayo Clin Proc 70:1116–1123, 1995.

17. (True or False) Which of the following can ameliorate the behavioral disturbances associated with Alzheimer's dementia?

    1. Provide hearing aids for patients who have impaired hearing.

    2. Develop planned activities that are appropriate for the patient's interests and abilities.

    3. Allow the patient to perform the personal care tasks that he or she can still perform.

    4. Minimize or eliminate daytime naps, and provide opportunities for appropriate exercise.

Answers: 1-T, 2-T, 3-T, 4-T

Critique: Several strategies can be utilized to minimize or control the behavioral disturbances associated with Alzheimer's dementia. Sensory deprivation enhances the patient's sense of disorientation; provision of hearing aids for those with hearing impairment and visual aids for those with vision difficulties can help to minimize behavioral disturbances attributable to these deficits. Planned activities that foster the patient's sense of success and minimize frustration can also limit behavioral disruptions. The patient should be encouraged to carry out those personal care tasks that he or she can still perform. Daytime naps should be minimized, and appropriate exercise encouraged to minimize nighttime sleep disruptions and associated behavioral disturbances.

Further Reading

Carlson DL, Fleming KC, Smith GE, Evans JM: Management of dementia-related behavioral disturbances: A nonpharmacologic approach. Mayo Clin Proc 70:1108–1115, 1995.

57

Alcohol Abuse

Michael D. Hagen and Betty Walker

1. Of the following statements regarding alcohol-related behaviors, which ONE is *false?*

    A. Almost 50% of men experience at some time an alcohol-related "blackout."

    B. Fewer than 50% of women experience an alcohol-related blackout or single driving arrest.

    C. Most men who experience alcohol-related blackouts ultimately develop alcoholism.

    D. Most women who experience alcohol-related blackouts ultimately moderate their drinking habits.

Answer: C

Critique: Nearly 50% of men and a smaller percentage of women experience at some time an alcohol-related blackout in which they have no memory of the events that occurred during an episode of heavy drinking. Fortunately, most of these individuals ultimately moderate their drinking behavior.

Page 1537

2. The lifetime risk for men of developing alcoholism is nearly:

    A. 5%

    B. 15%

    C. 25%

    D. 35%

Answer: B

Critique: Men have a lifetime risk of almost 15% for developing alcoholism. The risk for women is slightly less at approximately 5%.

Page 1537

3. Average middle-class alcoholic patients who agree to enter and ultimately complete a rehabilitation program have what percentage chance of maintaining sobriety for 1 year?

    A. 10–20%

    B. 30–40%

    C. 50–60%

    D. 60–70%

Answer: D

Critique: The average middle-income alcoholic who enters and completes an alcohol rehabilitation program has a 60 to 70% chance of remaining sober for 1 year.

Page 1537

4. The blood alcohol level will rise on average how much per drink consumed in 1 hour?

    A. 10 mg/dl

    B. 20 mg/dl

    C. 30 mg/dl

    D. 40 mg/dl

Answer: B

Critique: The blood alcohol level achieved for a given dose of ethanol depends on several factors, including body weight, percentage of body fat, age, and medications that the consumer might be using. On average, the typical 10-g alcoholic drink will raise the blood alcohol level by 20 mg/dl, and the body requires approximately 1 hour to metabolize this dose.

Page 1574

5. Match items 1, 2, and 3 with options A, B, C, or D.

    A. Pharmacokinetic tolerance

    B. Pharmacodynamic tolerance

    C. Both A and B

    D. Neither A nor B

1. Adaptation of nerve cells to the effects of alcohol

2. Induction of enzymes to increase the rate of metabolism of alcohol

3. Contributes to the ability of the alcoholic to appear awake and alert in the face of consuming large amounts of alcohol

Answers: 1-B, 2-A, 3-C

Critique: The phenomenon of tolerance to alcohol's effects involves pharmacokinetic, pharmacodynamic, and behavioral adaptations. Enzyme induction enhances the metabolism of ethanol, thus allowing the alcoholic to consume larger quantities without exhibiting symptoms expected with such doses in nonhabituated individuals. Nerve cell adaptation also acts to limit the effects of alcohol in the nervous system. Behavioral tolerance develops as alcoholics learn to perform their usual tasks under the influence of the drug. All three mechanisms contribute to the phenomenon of tolerance in habitual drinkers.

Page 1538

6. Several criteria exist for diagnosing alcoholism. One method utilizes evidence of serious alcohol-related adverse events in the patient's social history. Social history events that suggest strongly that the patient has a problem with alcohol include all of the following EXCEPT:

    A. History of marital separation or divorce as a result of alcohol-related behaviors
    B. Evidence of physical harm from alcohol or withdrawal symptoms when the patient discontinues alcohol consumption
    C. Job loss related to drinking behaviors
    D. Patient's history of an occasional glass of wine with dinner

Answer: D

Critique: Schuckit has demonstrated that a social history of any of the following represents strong evidence of alcoholism: a history of marital separation or divorce as a result of alcohol use, evidence of adverse health effects due to alcohol or withdrawal symptoms when alcohol is discontinued, and a history of job loss or layoff as a result of drinking behavior. Schuckit's criteria do not include occasional social use of alcohol.

Page 1539

7. Several screening instruments exist for identifying problem drinkers. The Michigan Alcoholism Screening Test (MAST) consists of 25 items to which the patient responds "yes" or "no." Positive responses on how many items constitutes cause to suspect alcoholism?

    A. 1 item or more
    B. 2 items or more
    C. 3 items or more
    D. 4 items or more
    E. 5 items or more

Answer: E

Critique: The MAST includes 25 questions that explore multiple dimensions of drinking behavior and consequences. The instrument includes a point scoring system in which a score of 5 to 9 indicates an 80% probability of alcohol dependence and a score of 10 or more indicates 100% certainty of alcohol dependence. Additionally, posi-

tive responses to five items or more raises strong suspicion of alcohol dependence.

Pages 1539, 1540

8. Alcoholism can occur as a primary disorder in which the patient has no preceding psychiatric diagnosis or as secondary alcoholism in the context of pre-existing psychopathology. Primary alcoholism constitutes approximately what percentage of patients who present for treatment?

    A. 30%
    B. 55%
    C. 65%
    D. 75%
    E. 95%

Answer: D

Critique: About three fourths of the patients who present for treatment of alcoholism represent cases of primary alcoholism; these individuals do not demonstrate evidence of premorbid psychiatric disorders.

Pages 1539, 1540

9. (True or False) Scientific evidence for a hereditary basis for alcoholism includes:

    1. Identical twin studies
    2. Fraternal twin studies
    3. Studies of first-degree relatives of alcoholics

Answers: 1-T, 2-T, 3-T

Critique: A number of pieces of scientific evidence highlight the genetic basis of alcoholism. Identical twin studies indicate a high degree of concordance in alcohol-related behaviors. Fraternal twin studies demonstrate a lower level of concordance, which is consistent with the lower level of shared heredity seen in these individuals. The risk of alcoholism increases directly with the number of alcoholic first-degree relatives. Additionally, children of alcoholics demonstrate less decrement in motor performance and less change in electrophysiologic measures when exposed to alcohol. All of these characteristics indicate a strong genetic basis for alcoholism.

Pages 1540, 1541

10. Nervous system effects observed with heavy use of alcohol can include all of the following EXCEPT:

    A. Blackouts in which the drinker has no or fragmentary memory for events during a period of heavy drinking
    B. Cerebellar degeneration and motor incoordination
    C. Peripheral neuropathy in the hands and feet
    D. Improved sleep patterns

Answer: D

Critique: Continued heavy consumption of alcohol has multiple ill-effects on the central and peripheral nervous systems. The individual can experience memory blackouts in which he or she has no memory of the events that occurred during an episode of heavy drinking. The alcoholic can experience cerebellar degeneration leading to motor incoordination. Additionally, peripheral neuropathies in the extremities can develop. Although alcohol might help to induce sleep, overall sleep patterns are affected adversely.

Page 1542

11. True statements regarding psychological effects of heavy drinking include all of the following EXCEPT:

    A. Heavy drinking can lead to intense sadness lasting for days.
    B. The intense sadness seen during heavy alcohol use usually requires antidepressant therapy.
    C. Acute withdrawal can be associated with panic attacks and severe anxiety.
    D. Alcohol hallucinosis can be expected to resolve spontaneously.

Answer: B

Critique: Heavy alcohol use can have a number of psychological effects. Heavy use can lead to intense sadness that might persist for days and resemble major depression. However, this deep sadness can usually be expected to clear with abstinence from alcohol and does not usually require antidepressant therapy. Withdrawal from alcohol can lead to panic attacks and severe anxiety, which might persist for many months after the last drink. Alcohol hallucinosis affects 1 to 3% of alcoholics and can be expected to resolve spontaneously.

Page 1542

12. (True or False) Components of the gastrointestinal system that alcohol affects adversely include:

    1. The esophagus
    2. The stomach
    3. The pancreas
    4. The large intestine

Answers: 1-T, 2-T, 3-T, 4-T

Critique: Alcohol has ubiquitous effects on the gastrointestinal tract. Heavy use can precipitate esophagitis and gastritis and is associated with acute and chronic pancreatitis. Additionally, the effects of alcohol on the large intestine can lead to bouts of diarrhea.

Page 1542

13. (True or False) Laboratory abnormalities seen as a consequence of heavy alcohol use include which of the following?

    1. An elevated mean corpuscular volume (MCV)
    2. Low gamma-glutamyl transferase (GGT)
    3. Aspartate aminotransferase (AST)/alanine aminotransferase (ALT) ratio greater than one
    4. Elevated AST

Answers: 1-T, 2-F, 3-T, 4-T

Critique: Chronic alcohol abuse can produce a number of laboratory abnormalities. An elevated MCV, an AST/ALT ratio greater than one, and elevated AST levels can all be seen with heavy alcohol consumption. Heavy alcohol use typically leads to elevated rather than low GGT levels.

Page 1543

Further Reading

Hoeksema HL, de Bock GH: The value of laboratory tests for screening and recognition of alcohol abuse in primary care patients. J Fam Pract 37:268–276, 1993.

14. (True or False) Hematologic effects seen with heavy alcohol use include which of the following?
    1. Diminished granulocyte adherence
    2. Increased production of most white blood cells
    3. Enhanced hypersensitivity responses
    4. Increased granulocyte mobility

Answers: 1-T, 2-F, 3-F, 4-F

Critique: Heavy alcohol use depresses a number of immune system components. Granulocyte adherence is diminished, as is granulocyte mobility. These two effects impair the alcoholic's ability to ward off infection. Diminished white blood cell production also impairs overall immune function. Hypersensitivity responses can be diminished rather than enhanced.

Page 1543

15. Heavy chronic use of alcohol (i.e., more than six drinks per day) is associated with all of the following cardiovascular effects EXCEPT:

    A. Elevated blood pressure
    B. Congestive cardiomyopathy
    C. Cerebrovascular accidents
    D. Decreased incidence of coronary artery disease

Answer: D

Critique: Heavy alcohol use affects multiple aspects of cardiovascular function. Prolonged use is associated with hypertension, congestive cardiomyopathy, and cerebrovascular accidents. Although low alcohol intake (two or fewer drinks per day) may be associated with a lower incidence of coronary artery disease, this benefit disappears with heavy consumption of ethanol.

Page 1543

Further Reading

Klatsky AL, Armstrong MA, Friedman GD: Alcohol and mortality. Ann Intern Med 117:646–654, 1992.
Regan TJ: Alcohol and the cardiovascular system. JAMA 264:377–381, 1990.

16. Features of the fetal alcohol syndrome include all of the following EXCEPT:

    A. Well-formed teeth with uniformly well-developed enamel

B. Epicanthal folds
C. Ventricular septal defects
D. Mental retardation

Answer: A

Critique: Alcohol use during pregnancy has led to a number of reported fetal anomalies (these effects can occur with as little as two drinks per day.) Atrial and ventricular septal defects, mental retardation, and epicanthal folds can all be seen in infants exposed to ethanol in utero. These children would be expected to demonstrate poorly formed teeth with imperfect enamel structure.

Page 1543

Further Reading

Kitchens JM: Does this patient have an alcohol problem? JAMA 272:1782–1787, 1994.

17. (True or False) Clinical findings that should raise the clinician's suspicion regarding possible ethanol abuse include:

1. Consistently low blood pressure readings
2. Repeated infections such as pneumonia
3. Unexplained episodes of pancreatitis
4. Peripheral neuropathies

Answers: 1-F, 2-T, 3-T, 4-T

Critique: The presence of several clinical findings should raise the clinician's suspicion that a patient abuses alcohol. Elevated, fluctuating blood pressure levels can occur as a result of heavy alcohol use. Additionally, the alcohol-abusing patient might experience repeated infections (e.g., pneumonia) and episodes of pancreatitis. Unexplained peripheral neuropathies should also lead the clinician to suspect alcohol abuse.

Pages 1543, 1544

18. Physician approaches to identifying alcohol abuse in a patient should include all of the following EXCEPT:

A. Link the patient's complaints (e.g., insomnia or sexual disturbance) to his or her use of alcohol.
B. Avoid confronting the patient about his or her alcohol use.
C. Explain to the patient how continued heavy alcohol use might affect his or her long-term health.
D. Share information regarding possible treatment approaches.

Answer: B

Critique: When the patient's clinical findings and history suggest alcohol abuse, the clinician should confront the patient with this diagnosis. The clinician can use the patient's chief complaint(s) as a focus for discussing the problem of alcohol use. Additionally, the clinician should attempt to educate the patient regarding potential long-term effects of continued heavy use and explore available options of treatment.

Page 1544

19. (True or False) Symptoms commonly seen with acute alcohol withdrawal include:

1. Tremors
2. Bradycardia
3. Hypersomnolence
4. Panic attacks

Answers: 1-T, 2-F, 3-F, 4-T

Critique: Alcohol withdrawal is characterized by disinhibition of central nervous system functions suppressed by heavy alcohol use. Tremors, autonomic nervous system hyperactivity (tachycardia, elevated temperature), insomnia and anxiety, and panic attacks can all be observed.

Page 1544

20. Among patients experiencing acute alcohol withdrawal, how many might be expected to develop delirium tremens?

A. Fewer than 5%
B. Approximately 15%
C. Approximately 30%
D. More than 40%

Answer: A

Critique: Fewer than 5% of patients who withdraw acutely from alcohol will develop delirium tremens.

Page 1544

21. (True or False) Important steps to include in the management of a patient withdrawing acutely from alcohol include which of the following?

1. Prescribe a central nervous system depressant such as a benzodiazepine over the first several days of withdrawal.
2. Prescribe multiple B vitamins and thiamine.
3. Perform a thorough physical examination to identify the sequelae of long-term ethanol use.
4. Provide routine rehydration with intravenous fluids.

Answers: 1-T, 2-T, 3-T, 4-F

Critique: Treatment for acute alcohol withdrawal should include several components. The clinician should perform a thorough physical examination. Multiple B vitamins and thiamine should be administered because heavy alcohol use impairs vitamin absorption in the small intestine. The patient should receive a central nervous system depressant to limit the hyperactivation that occurs with withdrawal. The benzodiazepines represent a safe option in this situation. Routine intravenous rehydration is not indicated because most alcoholics present in an overhydrated rather than a dehydrated state.

Pages 1544, 1545

22. (True or False) Benzodiazepine use for acute alcohol withdrawal should include:

1. Tapering of the dose daily by about 20% of the initial dose
2. Prescribing the drug on an as-needed basis only

3. Use of short-acting agents such as oxazepam or lorazepam in patients who demonstrate impaired liver function.
4. Addition of carbamazepine for seizure prevention

Answers: 1-T, 2-F, 3-T, 4-F

Critique: Benzodiazepines have demonstrated safety and efficacy in managing central nervous system manifestations of acute alcohol withdrawal. These agents should be prescribed on an around-the-clock basis rather than as necessary. Additionally, short-acting agents should be used in patients who demonstrate impaired liver function. The starting dose should be tapered by about 20% daily during the acute withdrawal period. Commonly used benzodiazepines (e.g., diazepam, chlordiazepoxide, oxazepam, and lorazepam) prescribed at adequate levels have antiseizure activity that obviates the need for carbamazepine.

Page 1545

23. (True or False) Patient characteristics that should suggest inpatient rather than outpatient alcohol rehabilitation include:

1. The patient has medical problems that require intense medical therapy.
2. The patient has significant depression that might impair his or her ability to comply with an outpatient regimen.
3. Previous failures of outpatient management.
4. Great distance from the patient's home to the treatment center

Answers: 1-T, 2-T, 3-T, 4-T

Critique: Although little evidence exists demonstrating superior results for inpatient rather than outpatient rehabilitation, several patient characteristics militate toward inpatient management: Medical problems that require intense therapy, significant psychiatric problems such as depression, history of previous failures in outpatient management programs, and great distance from the patient's home to an outpatient center all suggest the need for inpatient rehabilitation.

Page 1545

24. During the first 3 to 6 months of abstinence, most alcoholics experience some degree of sleep disturbance. Management of insomnia in this setting should include all of the following EXCEPT:

A. Reassurance that improvement will occur with time
B. Encouraging the patient to avoid daytime naps
C. Discouraging the use of caffeinated beverages late in the day
D. Routine use of sleeping pills such as benzodiazepines or barbiturates

Answer: D

Critique: Although most withdrawing alcoholics can be expected to experience sleep disturbance, the clinician should reassure the patient that these phenomena are transient and should improve with time. Additionally, the patient should be encouraged to avoid daytime naps and to refrain from consuming caffeinated beverages in the evening. Routine use of sleeping medications such as benzodiazepines or barbiturates should be avoided.

Page 1546

25. True statements regarding the use of disulfiram (Antabuse) in alcohol rehabilitation include all of the following EXCEPT:

A. Disulfiram can cause neuropathy.
B. Irreversible liver failure has occurred with use of disulfiram.
C. Disulfiram might contribute to increased risk for cardiovascular disease.
D. Disulfiram has repeatedly outperformed placebos in controlled trials of this drug's efficacy in maintaining abstinence.

Answer: D

Critique: Disulfiram has been used in alcohol rehabilitation programs for several years. Unfortunately, no controlled trials demonstrate convincing evidence that disulfiram performs better than does a placebo in maintaining sobriety. Additionally, disulfiram has been associated with neuropathies and liver failure and might also contribute to risk for cardiovascular disease.

Page 1546

26. True statements regarding performance of the CAGE questionnaire in screening for alcohol abuse include all of the following EXCEPT:

A. A CAGE score of 0 performs with good negative predictive value in populations who exhibit low prevalence of alcohol abuse.
B. A score of 4 indicates a high likelihood of alcohol abuse.
C. A score of 1 will reliably distinguish normal from problem alcohol use.
D. The CAGE questionnaire performs with poor sensitivity for identifying hazardous drinking behavior at relatively low problem drinking levels (e.g., four drinks or more per day).

Answer: C

Critique: Several screening instruments exist for identifying problem drinking behaviors. Like all screening tests, however, the test performs variably well depending on the positivity criterion used (e.g., score of 1 or more, 2 or more, etc.) and the prevalence of problem drinking behaviors in the screened population. The CAGE questionnaire consists of four questions: (1) Have you ever felt that you ought to *c*ut down on your drinking?; (2) Have people *a*nnoyed you by criticizing your drinking?; (3) Have you ever felt bad or *g*uilty about your drinking?; and (4) Have you ever had a drink first thing in the morning to steady your nerves or get rid of a hangover (*e*ye opener)? The sensitivity and predictive value depend on whether 1, 2, 3, or 4 positive responses define a positive test. Defining one or more positive response(s) as a positive test result yields high sensitivity but at the cost of low specificity (i.e., high false-positive rate). Alternatively, using three or four positive responses for the cutoff yields high specificity but at the cost of a high false-negative rate. Additionally, the sensitivity of the CAGE questionnaire declines in groups who have problem drinking habits at lower consumption rates such as four drinks or more per day. A CAGE score of 1 performs with a positive predictive value of only 0.14 (i.e., 86% of the positive results will represent false-positive results) in a population with a 10% prevalence for alcohol abuse. On the other hand, a score of 4 indicates a 92% probability that an individual from this same population has a drinking problem.

Further Reading

Kitchens JM: Does this patient have an alcohol problem? JAMA 272:1782–1787, 1994.

58

Nicotine Addiction

Walton Sumner

1. (True or False) Tobacco smoking leads to an addiction to nicotine that:

1. Is distinguishable from other addictions by the absence of intoxication
2. Results in a typical withdrawal syndrome after smoking cessation
3. May be as hard to break as addictions to heroin or cocaine
4. Is adequately treated by tapering doses of transdermal nicotine alone

Answers: 1-F, 2-T, 3-T, 4-F

Critique: Intoxication and addiction are different medical concepts. Nicotine withdrawal syndrome occurs following smoking cessation. The relapse rate for smoking cessation is actually slightly worse than the relapse rate for cocaine and heroin users, although the greater availability of cigarettes may play a role in relapse. Transdermal nicotine is a very useful treatment for nicotine addiction but is only one aspect of the most successful smoking cessation techniques. Behavioral modification, accountability, and support also play important roles in smoking cessation.

Pages 1549, 1558

2. (True or False) In the United States, tobacco smoking:

1. Is the leading cause of preventable death
2. Causes the majority of cancer deaths
3. Has caused more deaths than have occurred in war in the 20th century
4. Causes more cancer deaths in women than does breast cancer
5. Decreases a smoker's life expectancy by about 7 years
6. Is second only to motor vehicle accidents as a cause of disability

Answers: 1-T, 2-F, 3-T, 4-T, 5-T, 6-F

Critique: Smoking is currently the leading preventable cause of death in the United States, contributing to an estimated 400,000 deaths per year. Smoking has caused far more deaths of United States citizens than wars have in this century. For average 32-year-old men, these smoking-related deaths occur about 7 years earlier than do nonsmokers' deaths. Smoking causes 40% of cancer deaths, making smoking the leading preventable cause of cancer deaths but not the cause of most cancer deaths. Smoking-related chronic obstructive pulmonary disease is the leading cause of disability payments.

Page 1549

3. All of the following statements about the demographics of smoking in the United States are correct EXCEPT:

A. Smoking prevalence declined after the Surgeon General's 1964 report on smoking and health.
B. African-American teenagers are at high risk to commence smoking.
C. Ten percent of adult smokers began smoking after reaching age 18 as nonsmokers.
D. A majority of adult smokers state that they would like to stop smoking.
E. About one in four adults smoke.

Answer: B

Critique: The rate of smoking among African-American teenagers is actually at an intriguing all-time low for unknown reasons. The rate of smoking fell from about 42% to 27% from 1964 to 1992. Persons who reach age 18 without smoking are fairly unlikely to ever smoke. Page 1562 of the *Textbook of Family Practice* states that adolescents who reach age 18 without smoking have about a 10% chance of becoming smokers. Other sources state that 90% of smokers start before age 18, so that 18 year olds who do not smoke have only about a 4% chance of ever starting. Twenty-seven percent of adults smoke: four out of five adults state that they would like to stop.

Pages 1549, 1558

Further Reading

McIntosh H: Black teens not smoking in great numbers. J Natl Cancer Inst 87:564, 1995.

Nelson DE, Giovino GA, Shopland DR, et al: Trends in cigarette smoking among U.S. adolescents, 1974 through 1991. Am Public Health 85:34–40, 1995.

Surgeon General: The health consequences of smoking: 25 years of progress: A report of the Surgeon General. Rockville, MD, U.S. Department of Health and Human Services Publication (CDC) 89-8411, 1989.

4. Smoke from burning tobacco contains all of the following components EXCEPT:

    A. ^{210}Po
    B. Carbon monoxide
    C. Asbestos
    D. Nitrosamines
    E. Phenol

Answer: C

Critique: Cigarette smoke contains more than 4000 chemicals and 40 carcinogens. Tobacco plants concentrate many heavy metals from the soil in which they grow; radioactive ^{210}Po is one of these. Carbon monoxide is an important ingredient that directly interferes with oxygen transport. Several carcinogenic nitrosamines are present. Phenol, which denatures most proteins on contact, is another constitutent. Asbestos is not present in smoke from burning tobacco but has been present in cigarettes. The Kent Micronite filter of the 1950s is the most famous example and is the basis of some of the most successful lawsuits ever filed against an American cigarette manufacturer (a large recent award to one plaintiff is being appealed by Lorillard, a Loews subsidiary). The United States Patent Office has reportedly awarded many patents for asbestos-based cigarette components to the cigarette industry.

Pages 1551, 1554

Further Reading

Blum A: When "more doctors smoke Camels": Cigarette advertising in the journal. NY State J Med 83:1347–1352, 1983.

Chiba M, Masironi R: Toxic and trace elements in tobacco and tobacco smoke. Bull World Health Organ 70:269–275, 1992.

5. The strongest available evidence that smoking is hazardous to health comes from this type of study:

    A. Case-control study
    B. Cohort study
    C. Randomized controlled trial
    D. Longitudinal case series

Answer: C

Critique: For 3 decades, the cigarette industry has argued that more data are required to resolve the "controversy" about smoking and health. The evidence that smoking caused cancer and heart disease came from case control studies, which are retrospective in design, and cohort studies, in which nonrandomized groups of people are studied for a period of time. Both study designs are suspect because the lack of randomization may introduce biases and ignore confounding variables; nevertheless, the circumstantial evidence that smoking caused disease was overwhelming—for instance, some diseases occur essentially only in smokers (e.g., Berger's disease).

This situation changed with the results of a 20-year randomized controlled trial published in 1992. Because it was considered unethical to randomize nonsmokers to receive a "start smoking" intervention, this study randomized 1445 English male smokers at high cardiorespiratory risk to receive a stop-smoking intervention, or not, and followed them prospectively. The intervention was simply individual advice about the relationship of smoking to health, followed by an average of four supportive office visits for interested subjects. The results, analyzed on an intention-to-treat basis, confirm all suspicions. The group receiving the intervention smoked fewer cigarettes, suffered fewer lung cancers and heart attacks, and their collective survival improved, compared with the control group. This study proved that smoking cessation advice saves lives. It would be ludicrous to ascribe this benefit to the counseling event rather than to the act of smoking cessation. This study design had weaknesses: Many in the intervention group continued to smoke, and many control group members quit. That a significant effect was seen nevertheless attests to the magnitude of damage done by smoking and to the effectiveness of smoking cessation advice. Smoking is more than a risk factor: Smoking kills.

Further Reading

Rose G, Colwell L: Randomized controlled trial of anti-smoking advice: Final (20 year) results. J Epidemiol Community Health 46:75–77, 1992.

6. Compared with nonsmokers, smokers are many times more likely to develop the following diseases EXCEPT:

    A. Lung cancer
    B. Laryngeal cancer
    C. Coronary artery disease
    D. Cerebrovascular accidents
    E. Diabetes mellitus

Answer: E

Critique: Smokers are 10 to 20 times as likely to develop lung cancer, 20 to 30 times as likely to develop laryngeal cancer, two to three times more likely to develop coronary artery disease, and two to six times more likely to develop strokes. Smokers are slightly more likely to develop diabetes. Diabetic smokers are much more likely to develop diabetic complications but improve with smoking cessation.

Pages 1549–1552

7. Smoking has a detrimental dose-response relationship with all of the following diseases EXCEPT:

    A. Pancreatic cancer
    B. Renal cancer
    C. Graves' disease
    D. Ulcerative colitis
    E. Cervical cancer

Answer: D

Critique: Smokers have several times the risk of developing pancreatic, renal, and cervical cancers, compared with nonsmokers, and the risks are dose related. Graves' disease is a multifactorial illness occurring in genetically predisposed patients. A dose-response relationship exists with smoking. Family members of patients with Graves' disease may reduce their risk with smoking cessation. Smoking is associated with a reduced risk of ulcerative colitis and an increased risk of Crohn's disease. Nicotine from any source has a beneficial effect on active ulcerative colitis but is not useful for maintenance of remission.

Pages 1550–1552

Further Reading

Boyko EJ, Koepsell TD, Perera DR, Inui TS: Risk of ulcerative colitis among former and current cigarette smokers. N Engl J Med 316:707–710, 1987.

Pullan RD, Rhodes J, Ganesh S, et al: Transdermal nicotine for active ulcerative colitis. N Engl J Med 330:811–815, 1994.

Thomas GA, Rhodes J, Mani V, et al: Transdermal nicotine as maintenance therapy for ulcerative colitis. N Engl J Med 332:988–992, 1995.

8. Passive smoking has been shown to affect all of the following conditions EXCEPT:

    A. Laryngeal cancer
    B. Cervical cancer
    C. Lung cancer
    D. Birthweight

Answer: A

Critique: Sidestream smoke is diluted by ambient air before reaching nonsmokers, but the cooler temperature and lack of filtering by the cigarette and its tip leaves high levels of carcinogens in sidestream smoke. Of the problems listed, only laryngeal cancer is not currently thought to be an important concern for those exposed to passive smoke.

Pages 1553–1556

9. The criteria for diagnosing "fetal tobacco syndrome" include all of the following EXCEPT:

    A. No evidence of maternal hypertension
    B. Symmetrical growth retardation in the infant
    C. Maternal smoking of 5 cigarettes or more per day
    D. No other obvious cause of growth retardation
    E. Gestational age at birth less than 36 weeks

Answer: E

Critique: The first four items have been proposed as a definition of "fetal tobacco syndrome." Smoking one pack per day roughly doubles the probability of delivering at or before 32 weeks' gestation but is not part of the proposed syndrome.

Page 1556

10. (True or False) Children born to mothers who smoke one pack per day during pregnancy but not afterwards:

    1. Weigh 7 oz less at birth than do nonsmokers' children

    2. Are more likely than nonsmokers' children to smoke as adolescents
    3. Have normal birthweights if the mother quits before the third trimester
    4. Are at higher than normal risk for spontaneous abortion
    5. Are at higher than normal risk for congenital anomalies

Answers: 1-T, 2-T, 3-T, 4-T, 5-T

Critique: Mass at birth falls about 10 g for each daily cigarette: one pack a day is 20 cigarettes, translating to a decline in birthweight of about 7 oz. This weight loss occurs in the third trimester: Mothers who stop smoking prior to the third trimester deliver children with a normal weight. Maternal smokers run a greater risk of spontaneous abortion and delivering children with congenital anomalies. The risk of a cleft palate increases with cigarette smoking during the 3 months before or after conception. Recent evidence indicates that daughters of maternal smokers, even those who quit post partum, are more likely to smoke and persist in smoking than are the daughters of nonsmokers. This suggests that prepartum smoking renders daughters' brains more susceptible than normal to nicotine addiction—13 years after birth. Pregnancy is an important opportunity to intervene in the familial disease of smoking.

Pages 1555–1557

Further Reading

Kandel DB, Wu P, Davies M: Maternal smoking during pregnancy and smoking by adolescent daughters. Am J Public Health 84:1407–1413, 1994.

Lieberman E, Gremy I, Lang JM, Cohen AP: Low birth weight at term and the timing of fetal exposure to maternal smoking. Am J Public Health 84:1127–1131, 1994.

11. (True or False) Parental smoking is associated with the following childhood disorders:

    1. Teenage smoking
    2. Otitis media
    3. Bronchitis
    4. Pneumonia
    5. Wilms' tumor
    6. Hematopoietic malignancy
    7. Sudden infant death syndrome

Answers: 1-T, 2-T, 3-T, 4-T, 5-F, 6-T, 7-T

Critique: Smoking is associated with all of the aforementioned childhood conditions, except Wilms' tumor. Three fourths of people who take up smoking have at least one parent who smokes. Respiratory infections are six times as likely for children in families who smoke, and hospitalizations for these illnesses are twice as likely. Childhood hematopoietic malignancies are also more common in families who smoke. Sudden infant death syndrome is more common in families who smoke, although sleeping position probably plays a more important role in prevention (infants who sleep on their stomachs are clearly at increased risk of sudden infant death syndrome.)

Page 1555

Questions 12–18. Classify the ideals in items 12 to 18 as one of the following:

  A. Research finding
  B. Popular myth
  C. Advertising theme
  D. Research finding and advertising theme
  E. Popular myth and advertising theme

12. Filtered cigarettes are safer than are unfiltered cigarettes.

13. Filtered cigarettes have lower standardized nicotine yields.

14. Filtered cigarette smokers can obtain high nicotine yields.

15. Smoking is an activity of young adults.

16. Smoking relieves stress.

17. Smoking reduces weight.

18. Menthol cigarette smoke is cooler than regular smoke.

Answers: 12-B, 13-D, 14-A, 15-E, 16-B, 17-B, 18-E

Critique: Cigarette advertising themes typically establish or reinforce popular myths; therefore, answer C is unusual. On the other hand, reinforcing some popular myths could raise liability issues for manufacturers. Filtered and low-yield cigarettes are not safer than are high-yield cigarettes. Although low standardized cigarette yields are a prominent advertising theme, smokers often overcome filters by blocking filters or taking more or deeper inhalations to obtain the desired nicotine dose. Filters do remove some tar, slightly decreasing the risk of lung cancer, but can actually increase yields of carbon monoxide, linked to the risk of heart attacks. The net benefit of a filter is negligible at best. Claims of health benefits from filters are conspicuously absent in smoking advertisements. Smokers portrayed in cigarette advertising are almost invariably young and healthy and engaged in activities that appeal to some segment of the smoking market. The social acceptability of smoking varies dramatically among states and in different social settings. The primary stress that smoking relieves is the stress of withdrawal from nicotine. Smokers weigh a few pounds less than do nonsmokers: Smoking cessation returns a person's weight to normal. Ex-smokers can control fat gain by taking advantage of aerobic exercise capacity, which will also return their weight to normal. Menthol is an anesthetic that merely blunts a smoker's sensation of harshness in the smoke. Coolness and freshness are advertising themes on this sensory deprivation (e.g., Kool, Salem, Alpine.)

Pages 1559–1562

Questions 19–23. Match the adverse effect of smoking to the most pertinent audience.

  A. Monetary cost of smoking.
  B. Change in appearance (e.g., wrinkles, yellowed teeth, breath)
  C. Increased chance of Alzheimer's disease and stroke
  D. Effects of second-hand smoke on children
  E. Reduced exercise capacity

19. A 22-year-old single mother smoking GPCs

20. A 16-year-old male smoking Camel Lights

21. A 17-year-old female cheerleader smoking Misty Lights

22. A young, newly married couple in entry level jobs collecting Marlboro miles

23. 60-year-old new grandparents smoking Winstons

Answers: 19-D, 20-E, 21-B, 22-A, 23-C

Critique: Risk and benefit discussions should be tailored to emphasize the risks pertinent to the individual smoker or family. Discussions should emphasize the benefits of smoking cessation at least as much as the hazards of smoking. A young single mother smoking discount cigarettes will likely be concerned about the cost of smoking, but the effect on her children could be more compelling. Teenage smokers are likely to consider unappealing changes in appearance, reduced exercise tolerance, and possibly cost. The male might consider exercise capacity as being particularly important to employment and sexual function (many believe that Joe Camel implies prowess); the cheerleader might consider changes in appearance as being particularly threatening (the Misty theme is "Slim and Sassy"). A newlywed couple smoking a premium brand on a low income will be keenly aware of costs, including lost work time (Marlboro miles are a "continuity program" offering merchandise in exchange for Marlboro Universal Product Codes). The couple who are close to retirement age might respond to the risk of encumbering one another or missing the growth of their grandchildren (Winston has an aging customer base).

Pages 1559, 1560

24. (True or False) An effective office-based smoking cessation strategy is likely to include which of the following?

  1. Weekly or biweekly office visits during the cessation effort
  2. Behavior modification information
  3. Tapering transdermal nicotine prescription
  4. Unequivocal advice to stop smoking
  5. Setting a quit date within 2 months
  6. Focusing efforts on motivated smokers

Answers: 1-T, 2-T, 3-T, 4-T, 5-F, 6-F

Critique: The chapter in Rakel recommends all of these strategies except the last two. Setting a distant quit date could reinforce excuses to continue smoking. If office interventions are limited to motivated smokers, physicians abrogate their responsibility to help unmotivated smokers and might reinforce the notion that it would be too difficult for them to become nonsmokers. Suitable behavior modification materials are available from local heart, lung, and cancer associations and the National Cancer Institute (*Clearing the Air* pamphlet; 1-800-4CANCER). These materials should be tailored to the individual patient (i.e., by highlighting pertinent ideas). Nicotine replacement is an adjunct to other smoking cessation strategies. Nicotine should be started at 80 to 100% of the smoker's daily intake to maintain comfort. Daily intake can be estimated at 1 mg of nicotine per cigarette when the patient is smoking at will. Nicotine reductions should be done slowly—certainly no faster than recommended in the package instructions.

Pages 1558, 1561

Further Reading

Clearing the air. Office of Cancer Communications, National Cancer Institute, Bethesda, MD. NIH publication no. 92-1647, 1992.
Cooper TM, Clayton MR: Stop smoking program using nicotine reduction therapy and behavior modification for heavy smokers. J Am Dent Assoc 118:47–51, 1989.
Henningfield JE: Nicotine medications for smoking cessation. N Engl J Med 333:1196–1203, 1995.

25. (True or False) Obstacles to office-based smoking cessation include:

1. Lack of insurance reimbursement
2. Lack of cost-effective behavioral interventions
3. Lack of time for counseling
4. Inadequate social support for smoking cessation

Answers: 1-T, 2-F, 3-T, 4-F

Critique: Behavioral interventions are extremely cost-effective when compared with other medical technologies: Even though cessation rates seem discouragingly low, the large benefits of smoking cessation make small improvements in the cessation rate very valuable. Direct insurance coverage for smoking cessation is uncommon; however, physicians may find smoking cessation interventions cost-effective for long-term patients who select capitated health insurance plans. The reduced health care visits and costs of ex-smokers are a tangible benefit to providers in health maintenance organizations. Although social support for smoking is variable, the trend is generally towards decreased acceptability. Spontaneous smoking cessation rates probably reflect the social value of liability attached to smoking.

Pages 1558, 1559

26. Regarding the effect of smoking and nicotine on cognitive task performance, all of the following are true EXCEPT:

A. Nicotine is an antidepressant.
B. Nicotine improves cognitive performance.
C. Nicotine withdrawal impairs cognitive performance.
D. Smokers have more motor vehicle accidents than do nonsmokers.
E. Nicotine is less intoxicating than are most abused substances.

Answer: B

Critique: Early research suggested that smoking improved cognitive performance, because smokers deprived of nicotine performed better after smoking a cigarette. The results of this dubious study design are at odds with more recent observations, including findings that smokers deal poorly with increasingly complex cognitive tasks, that smokers who are temporarily deprived of nicotine do even worse, and that smokers have a 50% higher risk of motor vehicle accidents compared with nonsmokers. One exception to this rule could be among depressed patients for whom nicotine is a cheap, accessible, easily titrated antidepressant. Treatment of underlying depression is, therefore, an important component of smoking cessation efforts. The absence of intoxicating effects is often used by the cigarette industry to justify a more lenient regulatory approach to smoking, taking form in statements such as, "Would you rather fly with a pilot who just had a beer or a cigarette?" As the foregoing illustrates, we should probably prefer a nonsmoking pilot over a smoking pilot, whom we should prefer over a smoking pilot in withdrawal, whom we should possibly prefer over a drinking pilot. However, the cognitive abilities of withdrawing smokers versus light drinkers have not been directly compared.

Pages 1551–1553

Further Reading

Hall SM, Munoz RF, Reus VI, Sees KL: Nicotine, negative affect, and depression. J Consult Clin Psychol 61:761–767, 1993.
Sacks JJ, Nelson DE: Smoking and injuries: An overview. Prev Med 23:515–520, 1994.
Spilich GJ, June L, Renner J: Cigarette smoking and cognitive performance. Br J Addiction 87:1313–1326, 1992.

59

Abuse of Controlled Substances

Roger J. Zoorob

1. (True or False) Examine the following epidemiologic data regarding drug addiction:

1. Heroin addiction prevalence has stabilized between 500,000 and 800,000 Americans.
2. It is estimated that 5 million Americans use cocaine regularly.
3. High-school surveys have demonstrated a continuous increase in cocaine use.
4. Marihuana use has remained stable.

Answers: 1-T, 2-T, 3-F, 4-T

Critique: All the aforementioned statements are true except that high-school student surveys showed a continuing decline in the use of cocaine. Trends during the early 1990s showed an escalation in the use of amphetamines.

Page 1565

2. Which one of the following most closely implies pharmacologic dependence?

A. The heavy continuous use of a chemical substance
B. The genetic predisposition to drug abuse
C. Physiologic withdrawal syndrome in the absence of the drug
D. Euphoria due to the drug use

Answer: C

Critique: Dependence implies an abstinence syndrome or physiologic withdrawal syndrome. The presence of the drug prevents the appearance of withdrawal symptoms characteristic of each drug.

Page 1566

Questions 3–6. Match each numbered withdrawal symptom with the lettered drug class that corresponds best with it.

A. Sedative/hypnotic
B. Opiate
C. Alcohol
D. D-lysergic acid diethylamide (LSD)

3. Lacrimation, piloerection, gastrointestinal disturbances, and cough

4. No withdrawal symptoms

5. Mimics delayed alcohol withdrawal

6. Tremors and autonomic nervous system dysfunction

Answers: 3-B, 4-D, 5-A, 6-C

Critique: Opiate withdrawal is characterized by lacrimation, frequent yawning, gastrointestinal disturbances, rhinorrhea, and piloerection. Sedative hypnotic and depressant drugs mimic delayed alcohol withdrawal. LSD is a very potent drug; however, abrupt abstinence following continued use does not produce withdrawal signs or symptoms.

Page 1567

Further Reading

Mendelson JH, Mello NK: Cocaine and other commonly abused drugs. *In* Isselbacher KJ, Braunwald E, Wilson JD, et al (Eds): Harrison's Principles of Internal Medicine, 13th ed. New York, McGraw-Hill, 1994, pp 2429–2433.

Questions 7–10. Match each numbered statement with a lettered heading:

A. Opiate overdose
B. Cocaine overdose
C. Benzodiazepine overdose
D. Amphetamine overdose

7. Respiratory, central nervous system (CNS) depression, meiotic pupils

8. Hypertensive crisis, seizures, and vomiting

9. Anxiety, hallucination, and seizures

10. Blurring of vision, nystagmus, and ataxia

Answers: 7-A, 8-B, 9-D, 10-C

Critique: Cocaine toxicity manifests as nausea, vomiting, seizures, tachyarrhythmias, hypertensive crisis, and extreme anxiety. Opiate overdose produces CNS and respiratory depression with meiotic pupils. An overdose of benzodiazepines may result in blurring of vision, ataxia, and nystagmus, whereas an amphetamine overdose results in anxiety, agitation, hallucinations, and seizures.

Page 1567

11. LSD:

    A. Is an alkaloid
    B. Is known as angel dust
    C. Ingestion results in a sense of slowing of time.
    D. Has anesthetic properties

Answer: C

Critique: LSD is an acid, whereas cocaine is an alkaloid extracted from the South American shrub erythroxylon, coca. Ingestion of LSD results in distorted stimuli and sounds, and smells may be altered. The sense of the passage of time may be slowed. Phencyclidine hydrochloride (PCP) is known as "angel dust" and has anesthetic properties.

12. Cocaine results in all of the following EXCEPT:

    A. Powerful euphoria
    B. Meiosis
    C. Hypertensive crisis
    D. Extreme anxiety

Answer: B

Critique: Cocaine is a powerful euphoric and stimulant, and it also has constrictive and anesthetic properties. The effects of cocaine use include mydriasis, hypertension, anxiety, tachyarrhythmias, strokes, and seizures. Opiates, on the other hand, cause meiosis.

Page 1567

13. (True or False) Examine the following statements regarding marihuana:

    1. Conjunctival injection and a dreamy state are the objective findings.
    2. Acute CNS effects include delirium, euphoria, confusion, ataxia, and dysarthria.
    3. Toxic doses may alter body image and produce depersonalization and paranoia.
    4. Use of marihuana may produce alertness, lessened fatigue, a sense of well-being, and improved motor skills.

Answers: 1-T, 2-F, 3-T, 4-F

Critique: Marihuana results in conjunctival injection and a dreamy state. Euphoric enhanced perceptions and an altered sense of time are frequent effects. Toxic doses may alter body image and result in paranoia. Acute CNS effects such as delirium, euphoria, confusion, and ataxia result from inhalation of chlorinated volatile solvents or propellants. Amphetamines in small doses manifest in increased alertness and improved motor skills.

Questions 14–17. Match each of the numbered clinical findings with the controlled substance associated with each finding:

    A. Chronic cocaine use
    B. Chronic stimulant use
    C. Chronic inhalant use
    D. Chronic opiate use

14. Chronic rhinorrhea

15. Weight loss and insomnia

16. Maternal use during pregnancy results in placental abruption.

17. Neurotoxicity and direct lung injury

Answers: 14-A, 15-B, 16-A, 17-C

Critique: Chronic effects of cocaine dependence include rhinorrhea and nasal septum atrophy and perforation. Use during pregnancy can result in fetal brain infarcts, prune belly syndrome, intrauterine growth retardation, and abruptio placentae. Chronic inhalant use results in peripheral neuropathy, direct lung injury, and non-anion gap acidosis. Chronic stimulant use results in weight loss, insomnia, anxiety, depression, and paranoid states.

Page 1568

Questions 18–21. Match the numbered detoxification drug with the most appropriate lettered controlled substance:

    A. Cocaine
    B. Opiates
    C. Alprazolam
    D. Stimulants

18. Bromocriptine

19. Clonidine

20. Methadone

21. Long-acting benzodiazepine

Answers: 18-A, 19-B, 20-B, 21-C

Critique: Detoxification can be done on an inpatient or outpatient basis. Detoxification regimens are specific to the abused agent. The most frequently used are desipramine or bromocriptine for cocaine; substitution of a long-acting benzodiazepine for a short-acting one; clonidine or methadone for opiates; and minor tranquilizers for stimulants. No detoxification drug is available for hallucinogens.

Page 1570

22. The last personal characteristic to demonstrate deterioration in the chemically dependent physician is:

    A. Personal hygiene
    B. Job performance
    C. Personality
    D. Speech

Answer: B

Critique: Physician impairment is an increasingly recognized issue. Physicians have a higher rate of physical dependency. Personality changes appear early in the chemically dependent physician. These changes include sarcasm, isolation, depression, and angry outbursts. Physical changes include tired appearance, poor personal hygiene, drowsiness, slurred speech, or weight changes. Job performance is last to be affected and is exhibited in dosage errors, late medical records, procedural errors, and missed appointments for meetings.

Page 1571

60

Interpreting
Laboratory Tests

Douglas J. Knutson and Stephen E. Markovich

1. The likelihood that the result of a laboratory test will be negative in a patient without disease is referred to as:

    A. Sensitivity
    B. Specificity
    C. Positive predictive value
    D. Negative predictive value
    E. None of the above

Answer: B

Critique: The sensitivity of a test is the likelihood that the result of the test will be positive in a patient with disease. Specificity refers to the likelihood that the result of a test will be negative in patients without disease. Physicians can confuse these concepts with positive and negative predictive values. The positive predictive value of a test refers to the number of true positive tests as a percentage of all positive test results. Similarly, the negative predictive value refers to the number of true negative tests as a percentage of all negative test results. When evaluating laboratory tests, it is important to know the test reliability through an understanding of these concepts.

Page 1573

2. To diagnose a urinary tract infection in a symptomatic woman, the urine culture must grow at least:

    A. 100,000 colonies/ml of urine
    B. 50,000 colonies/ml of urine
    C. 10,000 colonies/ml of urine
    D. 5000 colonies/ml of urine
    E. None of the above

Answer: E

Critique: Recent studies have indicated that colony counts as low as 100/ml of urine may indicate an infection in symptomatic female patients. In fact, there is no level of bacteria that is used as a gold standard in diagnosing an infection. Therefore, physicians must continue to interpret these results using their knowledge of reference

ranges, gold standards, and most important, common sense.

Page 1574

3. A 60-year-old female patient presents with painless jaundice. You suspect a biliary obstruction. Which of the following laboratory values, if elevated, would best support your suspicion?

    A. Alkaline phosphatase
    B. Gamma-glutamyltransferase (GGT)
    C. Transaminase (aspartate aminotransferase [AST]/alanine aminotransferase [ALT])
    D. Amylase
    E. None of the above

Answer: E

Critique: Alkaline phosphatase is usually elevated with biliary obstruction, advanced cirrhosis, and severe hepatitis. Disorders of osteoblastic activity also increase alkaline phosphatase. The GGT is less specific for an obstruction, and the transaminases are more specific for hepatocellular damage.

Page 1576

4. A 35-year-old man presents with an ALT of 2500 U/l and an AST of 1200 U/l. Your next step in the work-up should be:

    A. Review the patient's chart for a history of alcohol use. These abnormalities are classic for alcoholic hepatitis.
    B. Ask about postprandial right upper quadrant pain with fatty meals.
    C. Review the patient's sexual history.
    D. Order GGT, alkaline phosphatase, amylase, and lipase tests.

Answer: C

Critique: Transaminases that are elevated to this extent usually indicate hepatitis. Alcoholic hepatitis is unlikely,

332

because AST is usually elevated higher than ALT in that case. In gallbladder disease, transaminases are usually not elevated to this extent. Further laboratory evaluation may be necessary, but not until a sexual, drug abuse, and transfusion history are obtained.

Pages 1575–1578, 1592

5. Which of the following is true regarding amylase levels?

    A. A normal level generally rules out pancreatitis.
    B. Large elevations can be seen in patients with chronic renal failure.
    C. The degree of elevation usually correlates with the severity of pancreatic injury.
    D. In addition to elevated amylase, elevated lipase is necessary to confirm the diagnosis of pancreatitis.
    E. None of the above

Answer: A

Critique: In most cases, a normal amylase rules out pancreatitis. The exception may be with chronic disease or a long duration of disease prior to the diagnosis. Usually only modest elevations of amylase are seen with chronic renal failure. The degree of elevation does not always correlate with the severity of the injury, and severe pain and symptoms can be seen with modest elevations. Lipase can be used as an adjunct to amylase if the diagnosis is in question.

Page 1578

6. What is the most common cause of hypercalcemia in the inpatient setting?

    A. Hypoalbuminemia
    B. Hyperparathyroidism
    C. Diuretic use
    D. Malignancy
    E. None of the above

Answer: D

Critique: Breast, lung, and kidney cancers are the most common cancers causing an increase in calcium. In the inpatient setting, malignancy is the most common cause of hypercalcemia. While hyperparathyroidism is the most common cause of elevated calcium in the outpatient setting, it is usually asymptomatic. Other causes of hypercalcemia are thiazide diuretics, multiple myeloma, sarcoidosis, and thyrotoxicosis.

Pages 1579, 1580

7. A patient presents for a routine history and physical examination. Screening laboratory tests (non-fasting) show a cholesterol level of 250. Your next step should be:

    A. Calculate the low-density lipoprotein (LDL) value and treat the patient if the LDL is greater than 160.
    B. Order a fasting lipoprotein profile.

    C. Teach the patient about a low cholesterol diet, and repeat the cholesterol test in 6 months.
    D. Evaluate the patient's coronary artery disease risk by taking a more extensive history.

Answer: B

Critique: Calculating lipoprotein levels based on a nonfasting serum sample is not beneficial. Accurate levels can be obtained after a 12-hour fast and 24-hour abstinence from alcohol. Repeat cholesterol levels are beneficial only to monitor the patient's response to therapy and to screen for future disease. The decision of when to treat for hypercholesterolemia is part of a thorough evaluation of coronary artery disease risk and is not based solely on an elevated level.

Page 1581

8. Why is it difficult to use creatinine to measure renal function?

    A. It is nonspecific.
    B. It is insensitive.
    C. Creatinine normally rises with age.
    D. Creatinine falls in response to certain illnesses.

Answer: B

Critique: Creatinine is the best of the common tests for measuring renal insufficiency. As the glomerular filtration rate (GFR) falls, creatinine rises. Because creatinine is slow to react to changes in renal function, and it is measured logarithmically, creatinine is a relatively insensitive screening test. Normally, creatinine falls with age owing to decreased muscle mass. A low creatinine is clinically insignificant.

Page 1582

9. Which of the following is not consistent with digoxin toxicity?

    A. Nausea and vomiting
    B. Cardiac disturbances
    C. Blurred vision
    D. A serum digoxin level of 3 ng/dl at least 6 hours after dosing
    E. All of the above

Answer: E

Critique: The most common mistake when following serum drug levels is "treating the level" instead of the patient. One third of patients with digoxin toxicity have levels within the normal range, and higher than normal levels are required in some clinical situations. However, an elevated serum level with symptoms such as nausea, vomiting, blurred vision, and cardiac disturbances supports the diagnosis of digitalis toxicity.

Pages 1584, 1585

10. Which of the following is not associated with an elevated sedimentation rate?

    A. Anemia
    B. Sepsis

C. Steroid use
D. Macrocytosis
E. Viral hepatitis

Answer: C

Critique: Although the sedimentation rate is not useful as a screening test, it has limited use in evaluating vague complaints. It is very useful if you suspect temporal arteritis or polymyalgia rheumatica. The most common cause of an elevated sedimentation rate is anemia. Any inflammatory condition, including sepsis or hepatitis, can also increase the sedimentation rate. Owing to laboratory methods, any disorder of red blood cell (RBC) size or shape can result in an abnormal sedimentation rate. The sedimentation rate can be helpful in following connective tissue diseases. Use of steroids will decrease the sedimentation rate rather than elevate it.

Page 1586

11. What is the most sensitive test for detecting iron deficiency?

A. Ferritin
B. Serum iron
C. RBC folate
D. Total iron-binding capacity (TIBC)
E. Mean corpuscular volume (MCV)

Answer: A

Critique: In iron-deficient states, ferritin often decreases before anemia or microcytosis occur. Ferritin also decreases before serum iron decreases or iron-binding capacity increases. Ferritin levels return to normal within days of initiating oral iron therapy.

Pages 1586, 1587

12. A 40-year-old obese woman complains of weight loss, polydipsia, and polyuria. A serum glucose at that time (non-fasting) is 190 mg/dl. A follow-up fasting glucose test is 121 mg/dl. What should your next step be?

A. Follow the patient closely, because she is likely to develop diabetes in the future.
B. Begin an oral hypoglycemic agent.
C. Repeat a fasting serum glucose test to confirm the diagnosis.
D. Order a glucose tolerance test.

Answer: D

Critique: According to the American Diabetic Association Guidelines, a fasting glucose greater than 140 on two occasions is diagnostic for diabetes. Fasting levels from 115 to 140 require a confirmatory glucose tolerance test to diagnose diabetes.

Page 1588

13. Screening hemoglobin and hematocrit tests are appropriate in which of the following?

A. Pregnant women
B. Infants
C. Elderly patients in extended care facilities

D. All of the above
E. None of the above

Answer: D

Critique: Screening hemoglobins in the general population is of little benefit. However, in high-risk populations, including infants, menstruating women, pregnant women, or institutionalized elderly, screening is justified. If patients are symptomatic, testing is appropriate and may require further evaluation to define the type of anemia.

Page 1590

14. What is the false-negative rate of Papanicolaou smears?

A. 1%
B. 10%
C. 30%
D. 50%
E. 66%

Answer: C

Critique: Normal Papanicolaou smears should be interpreted with caution, because the false-negative rate is approximately 30%. After an abnormal Papanicolaou smear, the physician cannot be reassured with a single, normal follow-up smear.

Page 1594

15. Which is true regarding serum potassium?

A. Screening is useful in the outpatient population.
B. Hemolysis is an unlikely cause of hyperkalemia.
C. Patients on digoxin therapy with hyperkalemia should be treated owing to the increased risk of digoxin toxicity with even mild hyperkalemia.
D. It is helpful to check the potassium level in a patient complaining of weakness.
E. None of the above

Answer: D

Critique: Potassium levels are routinely useful in renal or cardiac patients, patients on diuretics, or patients complaining of weakness. Because of the frequent use of intravenous fluids and nasogastric suction, potassium levels should be followed in hospitalized patients. It is not useful to screen healthy outpatients. The most common cause of hyperkalemia is hemolysis. The risk of digoxin toxicity increases with hypokalemia, and even mildly low levels should be corrected in this setting.

Page 1596

16. Prostate-specific antigen (PSA) should be used in all of the following EXCEPT:

A. Screening elderly men for prostate cancer
B. Staging patients with known prostate cancer
C. Detecting a recurrence of prostate cancer
D. Confirming the response to therapy for prostate cancer

Answer: A

Critique: PSA is produced by normal, hyperplastic, and cancerous prostate tissue. The screening of asymptomatic men has received much acclaim, but no studies have shown that treatment of those cancers detected provides benefit to the patient. Therefore, there is currently no agreement that PSA should be used as a screening tool. The level of PSA increases with higher stages of cancer, and PSA can be used to stage prostate cancer.

Pages 1596, 1597

17. The reticulocyte count serves as a measure of bone marrow responsiveness to anemia. Which of the following would be the expected reticulocyte count in the given clinical situations?

    A. A reticulocyte count of 1.5% in a newborn
    B. A reticulocyte count of 2% in a patient with aplastic anemia
    C. A reticulocyte count of 1.6% in a patient with rheumatoid arthritis and a hematocrit of 33%
    D. A reticulocyte count of 3% in a patient after treatment of a bleeding peptic ulcer
    E. A reticulocyte count of 2% in a nutritionally depleted homeless person

Answer: D

Critique: A normal reticulocyte count in a healthy person is approximately 1%. Nutritional anemia will cause a drop in reticulocyte count, which will not increase until nutritional defects are corrected. Lower than normal reticulocyte counts are also seen in anemias of chronic disease, septicemia, aplastic anemia, and infiltrative marrow diseases. Newborns and patients with hemolytic anemia or hemorrhage have an elevated count.

Page 1599

18. Which of the following decreases theophylline levels?

    A. Liver disease
    B. Heart failure
    C. Smoking
    D. Cimetidine
    E. Erythromycin

Answer: C

Critique: Most diseases and many medications interfere with theophylline metabolism and increase its blood levels. On the other hand, smoking actually accelerates theophylline metabolism and decreases the level.

Page 1600

19. A 23-year-old type I diabetic presents in ketoacidosis with a sodium level of 128 and a glucose level of 714. With regard to the patient's hyponatremia, you should:

    A. Check laboratory studies to rule out syndrome of inappropriate antidiuretic hormone (SIADH), a common complication of diabetic ketoacidosis.
    B. Ask the patient about recent water intake, because psychogenic polydipsia can precipitate ketoacidosis.
    C. Infuse 3% hypertonic saline to correct the sodium level and prevent cerebral edema.
    D. Monitor serial sodium levels.

Answer: D

Critique: In the face of hyperglycemia, serum sodium levels are falsely low. To calculate the corrected sodium level, multiply 1.6 by the glucose elevation above normal (in hundreds) and add that to the measured serum sodium. In the aforementioned example:

$$1.6 \times 6 \text{ (hundred)}* = 9.6 + 128$$
$$= 137.8 \text{ (normal sodium)}$$
$$*714 \text{ (measured glucose)} - 100 \text{ (normal glucose)} = 600$$

Page 1600

20. A 25-year-old woman presents with palpitations and anxiety. Your laboratory evaluation shows a normal thyroid-stimulating hormone (TSH) level but an elevated thyroxine (T_4) level. Your next step should be:

    A. Order exogenous triiodothyronine (T_3) to correct for the patient's peripheral conversion disorder.
    B. Administer propylthiouracil to inhibit thyroid hormone synthesis.
    C. Follow serial T_4 and TSH levels, because the patient will likely develop a clinical hyperthyroidism.
    D. Treat the patient for panic attacks.
    E. Take a detailed medication history.

Answer: E

Critique: Further evaluation of this patient's history may reveal causes of increased thyroid-binding globulin (e.g., oral contraceptives, pregnancy, exogenous estrogens), which elevates T_4 measurements. Other medications also affect thyroxine levels. The single best test to monitor hypothyroidism or hyperthyroidism is the TSH.

Pages 1602, 1603

Part V

Management of
the Practice

61

The Problem-Oriented Medical Record

Kent E. Anthony

1. Regarding the medical record, the following are true EXCEPT:

    A. The medical record should be organized in a systematic, logical, and consistent manner.

    B. The record should be kept as simple as possible.

    C. The medical record is a diary of everything that happens to the patient in the practice of medicine at that respective office.

    D. The chart should be organized according to the individual physician's preferences.

Answer: C

Critique: A diary is a passive document. Rakel emphasizes that the medical record should not be thoughtlessly accumulated data but should be information that is anticipated to be needed—thought is required when adding information to the record.

Page 1609

2. The problem-oriented medical record (POMR):

    A. Differs from the patient-oriented medical record in that the problem orientation is organized by the diagnosis

    B. Was developed by Lawrence Weed for busy primary care physicians who needed better record systems

    C. Works better for the initial patient visit but becomes confusing for continuing patient care or for care of chronic diseases

    D. Permits other health care personnel to understand the patient's management and communicates all elements that are important to the patient's care

Answer: D

Critique: The medical record is an important vehicle of communication between various health care workers who take care of the patient. The difference between the problem-oriented approach and the patient oriented approach is a semantic one and is not a formal distinction. The POMR, which was developed by Weed, was a hospital record. It required modification to become useful in outpatient care. The POMR is designed to simplify records and to make ongoing care and chronic disease management more efficient.

Page 1610

3. Through the Federal Privacy Act of 1974, patients legally have access to the physician's patient record. Which one of the following statements is true?

    A. Most physicians believe that patients should not be permitted to see their records, unless legal channels are followed.

    B. Because non-health professionals are frequently given access to the medical record, the physician should be careful about how confidential information is included in the record.

    C. Patients who read their records subsequently worry about medical matters that they are not adequately educated to understand, thus producing more harm than good.

    D. Allowing a patient to read his or her record puts the physician at great risk of being sued for malpractice.

Answer: B

Critique: Rakel states, "Access to medical records for management purposes is being given to more and more non-health professionals who are neither sensitive to patients' concerns about confidentiality nor bound by strong ethical or professional codes of conduct regarding the use of such information." Subsequently, it is advisable that issues of violation of law or issues that may bridge social taboos be left out of the record or alluded to obliquely. For example, a minister's wife might now be very sensitive about the abortion that she had as a teenager. The physician could refer to it as an "incomplete gestation." Such unusual terminology could remind

339

the recording physician of the subject without allowing utilization reviewers to have knowledge of a very sensitive matter. Michael and Bordley are cited as finding that 80% of physicians believe that patients should be allowed to see physicians' records about them. Tufo and associates report giving patients copies of their medical records, contending that "it is what patients do not know, but vaguely suspect, that causes them corrosive worry." Schade's practice of allowing patients to keep their medical record is described. Schade believes that if a patient has a better understanding of his or her medical problems, he or she is less likely to file a malpractice suit.

Pages 1610, 1611

4. Conversion from the traditional source-oriented record to the POMR involves a reassessment and reorganization of records. Which one of the following statements most closely reflects this process?

A. Because the POMR is very valuable in managing multiple problems, patients with chronic and several comorbid conditions should be transferred to the new record system initially.
B. Progress notes from other physicians are important to patient care and require easy access in the chart.
C. Temporary helpers can be hired to transfer record contents to new jackets, but the physician should prepare the problem list.
D. The POMR is set up uniquely to the physican's preference. This record is not particularly helpful for physicians in other specialties when consulting a patient's chart.

Answer: C

Critique: The POMR is an active tool that is intended to improve the care of the patient. It cannot be effective in medical support without the input of the physician, who best understands the patient's medical condition. Most active patients should be transferred first. Other patients may never present for further care. Progress notes are seldom found to be useful to other physicians when transferring records. The positioning in the chart is an extrapolation of that finding: if they are not useful, they do not need to be accessed readily. A well-organized record system allows other health workers ready access to information that is important to their work.

Pages 1611, 1612

5. Which one of the following statements about the POMR is correct?

A. The display and organization of the POMR make the logic behind clinical decisions apparent.
B. The POMR requires attention to carry through on the functions that it is designed to deliver.
C. Progress notes are required to number problems consistently with corresponding numbers on the problem list; otherwise, a problem cannot be followed.

D. The physician is responsible for the information in the database and should not allow others to input this patient information.
E. Transferring laboratory data to a flow sheet increases the chance of errors.

Answer: A

Critique: The display and organization of the POMR make the logic behind clinical decisions apparent. This advantage of the POMR makes it particularly appealing for primary care. Consistent display of abnormalities is necessary, but Rakel makes it clear that a high degree of compulsion is not required of the POMR. Some recommend consistency in numbering problems, but the demands of this process may be sufficiently taxing to make it unreasonable. The physician should establish what information is in the database for all patients, but other health workers can obtain and enter the information. The transfer of laboratory data to a flow sheet is recommended in order to follow trends. Errors have not proved to be an important problem when transferring laboratory values.

Pages 1618–1620

Questions 6–12 (Matching). The POMR uses the "SOAP" note format for progress notes. Indicate the place in the progress note—subjective, objective, assessment, or plan—where each of the following items would be best entered.

A. Subjective
B. Objective
C. Assessment
D. Plan

6. Digoxin level of 1.8

7. Dizzy upon awakening

8. Nystagmus

9. Acute labyrinthitis

10. Fatigue; no energy for the last week

11. Admit to rule out deep vein thrombus

12. Cataract removed 5 years ago

Answers: 6-B, 7-A, 8-B, 9-C, 10-A, 11-D, 12-A

Critique: The "subjective" portion of the progress note includes the present complaint, symptoms, past, family, and social history. The "objective" data include physical findings, physiologic data, and special studies. The "assessment" should indicate the diagnosis or present status of the problem. The "plan" documents therapy, planned investigations to rule in or rule out diagnoses, and patient education. "Dizzy upon awakening," "fatigue," and "no energy for the last week" are subjective complaints. "Dizzy" may be subsequently used as an assessment, but it would be preferable to have it better defined (e.g., orthostatic hypotension, vertigo, disequilibrium). "Cataract removed 5 years ago" is subjective information in the past history. "Nystagmus" is an objective physical finding. The digoxin level is laboratory information and belongs in the objective section of the progress note. "Acute labyrinthitis" is a diagnostic impression and should be entered as part of the assessment. "Admit to rule out deep vein thrombus" is a specific part of a plan. Note that "rule out" is appropriate here. It is not in the assessment, and it is not a guess; rather, it is a goal.

Pages 1625, 1626

Questions 13–18 (True or False) Of the following, which items are appropriately entered into the medical record's problem list?

13. Left inguinal hernia

14. Rule out appendicitis

15. Family history of myocardial infarction

16. Hen-pecked husband

17. Violent temper

18. Nausea

Answers: 13-T, 14-F, 15-T, 16-F, 17-T, 18-T

Critique: Left inguinal hernia is a problem until it is corrected. After correction, the patient's history of hernia or surgery may be important. The physician may choose to date problems as being resolved with surgery or line them out in the record. "Rule out appendicitis" is not an appropriate entry. "Right lower quadrant pain" may be appropriate, but a guess or a goal are not problems. A family history of myocardial infarction is appropriate. It is a problem that needs to be reviewed regularly. "Hen-pecked husband" is a derogatory term that does not accurately convey medical significance or reflect on the patient's care. This type of term has no place in the physician's assessment or comments in the medical record. Notation of a violent temper should be included if it is a patient problem that the physician is addressing, or if it is a matter of safety. Although the notation may seem derogatory, and a social and potentially legal issue, the safety of the physician, staff, and consultants may be a more urgent priority. The notation should not be included if the source is a rumor of if the problem is not being addressed directly with the patient. Symptoms such as nausea are appropriate when a diagnosis has not been developed.

Pages 1617, 1618

62

Managed Health Care

Kent E. Anthony

1. The health maintenance organization (HMO) is one of the main organizational structures that delivers managed health care. Which of the following is true of the HMO.

    A. The concept, which was originally developed in Europe, was that villages would pay a physician a fixed annual stipend to meet all the medical needs of the village.

    B. The HMO assumes responsibility for all health care of the contracted population.

    C. Regardless of how much service the HMO provides, the HMO is paid only the amount contractually agreed on.

    D. If an enrollee in an HMO wants a service that the HMO physician has determined not to be indicated, the physician can perform the service and collect a fee from the patient.

    E. If the HMO denies payment for a covered service that the physician and enrollee mutually agree is desired, the physician may perform the service and bill the consenting patient.

Answer: C

Critique: HMO services are independent of utilization; however, most have stop-loss insurance, such that expenses on one enrollee above a certain level are indemnified. Mutual aid societies had their beginnings in Europe. The HMO assumes responsibility for the services explicitly stated in the contract. For example, if cosmetic surgery, dietary counseling, or smoking cessation are not included in the contract, the HMO would have no obligation to provide these services. Usual HMO contract wording clearly states that the physician may not collect from the patient for covered services. Simply determining that a service is not medically indicated, does not exclude the service from such stipulation. Most HMOs consider billing an enrollee for a covered service to be in violation of the contract. If the matter was never reported to the HMO, it might not become an issue. However, if it was discovered, it could be grounds for termination of the contract with the physician.

Page 1636

2. The staff model HMO:

    A. Uses staff to manage medical care instead of using physicians to carry out most routine services

    B. Makes contracts with community physicians for certain medical services

    C. Pays primary care physicians on a contingency basis, paying for only medical services that are determined to be appropriate and necessary

    D. Because of the relationship with physicians, is at the greatest financial risk of the managed care models

    E. May employ some physicians, pay fee-for-service to some physicians, and keep other physicians on retainer.

Answer: B

Critique: While on the surface this seems to be a strange statement, it applies to different medical specialties. The primary care and high-demand subspecialty physicians would usually be employed. Services that are rarely used would be obtained from available physicians on whatever basis the HMO could negotiate with that physician. Two examples are: (1) fee-for-service, and (2) a flat fee (retainer) plus discounted fee-for-service. The "staff model" means that the physicians are employed as staff and not that nonphysician staff manages care. Usually primary care physicians are salaried in staff model HMOs. Staff model HMOs have the most formal relationship with physicians and have the LEAST risk of the models presented.

Pages 1636, 1637

3. Staff, group, and network model HMOs all involve physicians who work together in practice. Which one of the following statements is correct regarding these types of HMOs?

    A. Physicians are direct employees in staff and group models but not in network models.

    B. The network model allows the HMO to market services throughout a service area.

C. Physicians are compensated identically in all three models; however, the method is dependent on the HMO.

D. Various sites in the network model must offer the same services as all other sites.

Answer: B

Critique: A staff model HMO directly employs physicians at practice sites. A group model HMO is a contract between an HMO and a group practice. A network model HMO is an HMO that has contracts with several group practices. Using the network model, an HMO can enter a market and, by contracting with various groups, cover a service area to which they market services. Staff models directly employ physicians. A group practice determines its financial relationship with these physicians on an internal basis—it is not a matter governed by the HMO. Services offered at a particular site are dependent on availability and on the contract with the HMO.

Pages 1636, 1637

4. Which of the following is true of the individual practice association (IPA)?

A. The majority of HMOs are IPA models.

B. If the HMO contracts with an organization of independent physicians, it may have legal problems involving restriction of trade.

C. Contracts are usually restrictive, thus the physician chooses to participate in the IPA or in private practice.

D. Capitation involves buying the capital assets of the practice of those physicians who become involved in an IPA.

Answer: A

Critique: For IPA both the terms "independent" and "individual" practice association are found in the literature. In 1992, nearly two thirds of the HMOs were IPA models. HMOs contract both directly with solo physicians and with organizations of solo physicians. If an organization of solo physicians forms specifically to keep an HMO out of their market, those physicians can face charges of restriction of trade. The physician continues to practice fee-for-service as previously. The IPA enrollees are added to the practice. Capitation is a payment structure in which a physician is paid a fixed fee for each enrollee subscribed to that practice for that month, regardless of utilization. The purchase of a physician's practice is another matter and is not part of the IPA model HMO.

Pages 1637, 1638

5. Economic credentialing is a technique used in managed health care. What does it mean?

A. All organizations that deliver medical care must credential their providers. Economic credentialing is a technique in which provider credentials are obtained easily (e.g., credentialing those with staff privileges at a certain hospital).

B. Physicians practice medicine with different levels of efficiency. Through economic credentialing, managed care organizations identify the economies by which a physician practices. The physician is invited or excluded by the organization by this information.

C. Before a managed care organization becomes involved with a physician, it is prudent to ascertain the financial risk that the physician holds. If the physician declares bankruptcy, the managed care may have obligations that it cannot honor. Economic credentialing involves credit checks of physicians.

D. Some regions of the United States are saturated with managed care organizations and would not be a good market opportunity for an expanding managed care organization. Other markets are so unfamiliar with managed care organizations that the cost of introducing managed care would be too great. However, some markets understand managed care but are not saturated. Economic credentialing distinguishes such markets.

Answer: B

Critique: Economic credentialing is a controversial matter. Measurements of efficiencies are made on the basis of a few months or years and do not reflect long-term efficiencies nor necessarily good practice of medicine. For example, a physician who was very successful in procuring kidneys for his dialysis patients would appear to be very expensive in an economic credentialing analysis. Several years of dialysis is much cheaper than a renal transplant. Long-term efficiency may be better for the renal transplant—or renal transplant patients may live longer and cost the managed care organization even more. In such case, economic credentialing would select against good practice of medicine. Another controversy of economic credentialing involves patient mix. The most skilled physicians may have obtained that skill by care of the sickest patients. The physician may deliver both the highest quality of medical care and the most cost-effective care for each patient, but because his or her patients are sicker than other physicians' patients in the community, he or she is excluded as being too expensive. Patient mix programs have been developed. Results of these programs are not automatically accepted by those physicians who are determined to be more expensive and who are not chosen on the basis of economic credentialing.

Page 1638

6. Harvey's employer selected a new medical insurance company. Harvey sat through the seminars about the different plans offered by the new insurance company. He chose the plan in which he could continue to see his own physician, whose name was not on any list, yet he would not have to pay as much for his insurance as he had been. In exchange, he would have to get second opinions before surgery and certain expensive procedures, and he would have to get preauthorization for

hospitalization or elective surgery. What type of insurance did Harvey select?

    A. Preferred provider organization (PPO)
    B. Any willing provider organization
    C. Managed indemnity
    D. HMO
    E. IPA

Answer: C

Critique: This is an indemnity insurance. Harvey's expenses will be paid to some extent. Harvey's physician is not on the list, which would exclude a PPO and an IPA. HMOs may market by their corporate name and not the physician's name, but it would be unusual for an HMO to use second opinions and preauthorizations as part of their marketing presentation. Harvey would pay less for the managed indemnity plan than he had paid for his previous indemnity insurance. "Any willing provider" is a phrase used by physician organizations resisting economic credentialing by managed care organizations. The managed care organization would be required to work with any physician who was willing to deliver care under the management structure of that organization. This is not a medical insurance option.

Pages 1637–1640

7. The PPO is another managed care structure. Which of the following could be true of an HMO but would be very unusual for a PPO?

    A. Physicians are salaried by the managed care organization.
    B. Monitor and report on a physician's utilization of services.
    C. Utilize discharge planning of hospitalized patients.
    D. Limit the patient's choice of physician.

Answer: A

Critique: HMOs may employ physicians in the staff model, but PPOs are not structured to employ physicians directly. Both HMOs and PPOs monitor physicians' use of resources. Reporting findings to respective physicians is a common management technique, allowing the physician to identify and alter unnecessary use of resources. Both HMOs and PPOs use discharge planning to identify services that can be provided outside the hospital and decrease days spent in the hospital. While HMOs restrict the choice of physician to a designated primary physician, PPOs restrict patients to a member of the panel of physicians. Use of a physician outside the designated panel will cost the patient a greater percentage of the bill or may not be covered at all.

Pages 1638–1640

8. The quality management loop is described as a dynamic process that enhances health status, prevents deterioration or injury, and promotes quality of life. Which of the following processes is NOT part of the quality management loop?

    A. Establish standards or requirements of care.
    B. Measure performance against standards of care.
    C. Compare performance to the standards and analyze to identify opportunities for improvement.
    D. Eliminate persons from the system who are not producing to standard.

Answer: D

Critique: Elimination of persons from the system who are not producing to standard is not an advisable approach under the quality management loop. Corrective action is taken, but elimination of providers is a last option. Providers who have entered into the contracting process and who have provided care under that structure are familiar with the structure. To lose them and bring in new providers will often be more expensive than helping existing providers to improve their performance. Establishing standards or requirements, measuring performance against standards, and analyzing results for opportunities for improvement are part of the quality management loop.

Pages 1644, 1645

63

Accounting Systems

Kent E. Anthony

1. Financial statements include all the following information EXCEPT:

    A. Revenues
    B. Invoices
    C. Expenses
    D. Assets
    E. Liabilities

Answer: B

Critique: Invoices are source documents for the preparation of financial statements but are not presented in the statements. An income statement reports revenues, expenses, and the difference between these—the income or loss. A balance sheet reports assets (e.g., cash, material, equipment, improvement), liabilities (e.g., loans, accounts owed), capital (e.g., owner's equity, retained earnings), and the balance of these. Assets should be equal to the total of capital and liabilities.

Pages 1648, 1649

2. Which of the following is NOT consistent with good accounting control?

    A. Reconcile transactions as often as practical, even daily if practical.
    B. Deposit all cash, checks, and credit card documents daily to minimize theft.
    C. Make unannounced spot checks of various financial processes.
    D. Separate accounting tasks among employees so that one employee can check on another employee.
    E. Keep a running account of a change fund, because it is also used for petty cash.

Answer: E

Critique: Use of the change fund for petty cash is not consistent with good accounting control. The change fund and the petty cash fund should be different. One does not take money from the change drawer and use it for petty cash. The change fund should be consistent from one day to another and should be counted daily. The petty cash fund is managed by submitting receipts, such that the total of the receipts and cash should be consistent. The other methods are all sound techniques used in maintaining accounting control.

Page 1651

3. You have just joined a new group practice. Which is an acceptable way to go about setting your fees?

    A. Obtain the relative value scale that other physicians in your community use, and apply the same geographical multiplier and other multipliers that they use.
    B. Adopt the fee schedule of the other physicians in your group.
    C. Ask your office manager to obtain a fee schedule from other physicians' offices in the area and charge your patients according to the community standard.
    D. Recognizing that Dr. A does not practice good medicine, in accord with the recommendations of the local medical society, you lower your fees for former patients of Dr. A.

Answer: B

Critique: Adoption of the same fee schedule is an appropriate practice; after all, you are in the same organization and you are not competing with the physicians in your group. As a matter of practice, by adopting the fee schedules of our community physicians whether you actually obtain a copy of their schedules or not, you are achieving fixed prices, which is illegal. Discounting fees to patients of a specific physician, regardless of altruistic motives, is clearly a restraint of trade and is illegal. The fact that a physician may practice poor medicine is not a reason to use economic measures against him. Restraint of trade in this case would be organized and illegal.

Pages 1652, 1653

4. Which one of the following basic functions of a patient accounting system is designed to detect honest errors and mistakes?

A. Posting of transactions
B. Control system operations
C. Processing insurance claims
D. Collecting delinquent accounts
E. Producing patient bills

Answer: B

Critique: All patient accounting systems, whether manual or automated, should perform several basic functions, including storage of demographic and insurance information, posting of transactions, system control operations, production of patient bills, processing of insurance claims, collection of delinquent accounts, and production of reports. Control system operations catch honest mistakes. The daily reconciliation process, in which an office assistant compares transaction totals derived from source documents with the totals on the daysheet, is one example of a system control operation.

Pages 1653–1656

5. The collection ratio measures the general effectiveness of the patient accounting system. It is calculated by:

A. Dividing total payments by gross charges
B. Dividing bad debts by gross charges
C. Subtracting bad debts from total payments, then dividing by gross charges
D. Dividing courtesies and discounts by gross charges
E. Dividing total payments by gross charges minus bad debts, courtesies, and discounts

Answer: A

Critique: The collection ratio is a percentage of the total charges collected. The numerator is a total of everything that was collected, regardless of what was billed. Gross charges are the full value of the physician's services, despite discounts, professional courtesy, and contractual discounts. Accordingly, a physician living in a university town could have very little or no bad debt yet have a low collection ratio because of extending professional courtesy to the physicians and medical students. Division of bad debts by gross charges yields a bad debt ratio. Division of courtesies and discounts by gross charges provides a courtesy and discount ratio. Division of total payments received by gross charges minus bad debts, courtesies, and discounts yields an adjusted collection ratio as a measure of the efficiency of collecting truly collectable revenues.

Page 1657

Questions 6–11 (True or False) You are setting up a new practice. When you are thinking about finding an accountant, which of the following services should you expect the accountant to perform?

6. Preparing professional tax returns

7. Paying bills

8. Preparing personal tax returns

9. Auditing the bookkeeping system

10. Advising whether to lease or purchase equipment

11. Advising the physician of changes in local market forces that may affect the practice

Answers: 6-T, 7-F, 8-T, 9-T, 10-T, 11-F

Critique: Most practices will require internal and external support for a successful business operation. An accountant or accounting firm is one such external service. Customary accounting functions include preparing professional tax returns; preparing personal tax returns (the physician's tax may best be prepared by an accountant; however, the physician should not use professional, pretax funds to pay for personal services); setting up and auditing a bookkeeping system; and advising the physician on sensible business decisions, such as whether to lease or purchase equipment. The payment of bills is usually an internal function with which the office manager or bookkeeper is charged; however, some accounting firms may offer this service. While alerting the physician to local market events may help the accountant keep a valuable client in business, it is no part of customary accounting services.

Page 1648

Questions 12–16 (True or False) The physician, as an employer, takes on several responsibilities. Which of the following examples illustrate the proper execution of these responsibilities?

12. Mary Jane, RN works 40 hours a week, 8:00 A.M. until 5:00 P.M. with an hour off sometime between noon and 2:00 P.M. It is not unusual for her to stay late, but the office is closed on Thursday afternoons. Last week, there was spring cleaning on Thursday afternoon, and Ms. Jane worked. She worked a total of 43 hours during the week. The additional 3 hours were paid in her next check.

13. Jean Marx, RN works full-time as the school nurse. You arrange with her to make home visits in the evenings and change dressings for some of your patients. You did not include her among your employees on your workers' compensation policy.

14. You and your office manager decide that the nurse will be an exempt employee. Several months later, you arrive at the office to find that it has not been opened, and patients are standing outside. There was a traffic accident that kept your receptionist and nurse from getting to work on time, but the manager lives nearby. He has been rather lax about his morning time of arrival to the office, and this tardiness has been irritating you. You dock his pay 1 hour for being late this morning but not for any previous tardiness.

15. New to practice, you submit an SS-4 and receive a federal employer identification number. You pay taxes on your employees: federal income tax, Medicare, social security, state tax, and local tax. You provide workers' compensation and unemployment compensation insurance, but you require your employees to provide their own health insurance.

16. You decide that before you settle on a practice, you will work in the hospital emergency room for 1 year. It is very economical for you. You live close by; the food in the doctor's dining room is quite good; and you can wear the hospital's scrub suits. Since you are new, you get more evening shifts and holidays. Your accountant tells you that since the hospital states that you are an independent contractor, you have to pay taxes quarterly, which you do.

Answers: 12-F, 13-T, 14-F, 15-T, 16-F

Critique: Nonexempt employees are paid time-and-a-half for hours in excess of 40 hours. The employee should have been paid for 44.5 hours in her next pay check. Ms. Marx is an independent contractor. She chooses her time, brings at least some of her tools, and does not work mainly for you. You do not need to provide her workers' compensation insurance or withhold taxes. The number of hours worked is not a basis for docking the pay of exempt employees. You have carried out the requirements of the law in becoming identified as an employer, withholding taxes, and providing insurance. It is legal for you not to provide health insurance, yet require your employees to produce proof of insurance as a condition for employment; however, your employees might not like your approach. You are not an independent contractor, and the hospital should be providing the services required for other employees. You are working full time for one employer, the hospital, which chooses your hours, location, and tools—even down to the scrubs.

Page 1650

64

Personnel and Time Management

Kent E. Anthony

1. Job descriptions are the hub of personnel management. Which one of the following statements about job descriptions is true?

   A. Prior to employing someone in a position, a job description may be no more than the physician's dreams. Only after someone has performed the work can a real job description be written.

   B. Salary review is based on performance review but is unrelated to the job description.

   C. The job description is job specific. If cross-coverage of two jobs is included, it becomes confusing and unworkable.

   D. The job description should emphasize only difficult or complex duties with a detailed description of how to accomplish the job.

   E. A well-designed job description includes primary tasks (those performed almost daily) and secondary tasks (additional tasks that are performed when needed).

Answer: E

Critique: A well-designed job description includes primary tasks, which are performed almost daily, and secondary tasks, which are additional tasks that are performed when needed. The applicant or employee needs to know what to expect on a regular basis and what he or she can be called on to perform. The job description may be refined once performance realities are indentified, but the basic tasks that need to be done can be identified before recruiting an individual for a job. Job descriptions have a role in recruiting, setting job standards, conducting performance review, and conducting salary review. The job description is job specific but includes those aspects of other jobs that are expected to be performed as cross-coverage if required. Details on how to perform any given task, regardless of the degree of difficulty, should be in the office procedures manual and not in the job description.

Page 1660

2. All the following are true of performance reviews, EXCEPT:

   A. All employees should be reviewed after the first 90 days of employment.

   B. Salary increases and other rewards may be based on the performance review.

   C. Performance review involves grading performance on specific tasks.

   D. Subjective issues, such as attitude, cannot be measured. These may be mentioned directly to the employee or ignored but should not be included in the performance review.

   E. Performance reviews should be nonconfrontational to let the employee know how he or she is performing and to establish specific goals.

Answer: D

Critique: Subjective measures should be included in the performance review. A subjective factor may become overwhelming and a reason to terminate employment. If these issues are not documented as they are recognized, then termination will be more difficult to justify in a grievance process. The initial performance evaluation should be done early in a new job. Each performance review should be specific to the job description and nonconfrontational. Salary increases and other rewards are often based on the performance review.

Pages 1660, 1661

3. Salary reviews occur 90 days after performance reviews:

   A. Across-the-board increases for all employees are recommended to keep in-fighting to a minimum.

   B. If the practice has done particularly well in a year, larger bonuses may be in order.

   C. Performance of the practice is crucial to making a decision about salary increases. Changes in salaries in the community do not necessarily have an impact on the individual practice.

D. COLA, cost-of-living policies, recognize the importance of not allowing salaries to be eroded by inflation. COLA policies are essential in order to develop employee security.

Answer: B

Critique: Bonuses can be used to reward employees in years that economic performance exceeds expectations. Note that the term "bonus" is used here, rather than salary increase. The banner year may be a blip that cannot be sustained. Salary increases are in order; however, if the blessings of the good year are incorporated into an expectation of subsequent years, the practice can find an inordinate payroll burden when performance wanes. Variation in salary increases, according to performance, is recommended. A survey of the community is important. If a physician is paying substantially less than comparable jobs pay elsewhere, there is a risk of losing good employees. A COLA policy can obligate the practice to pay salaries that it is not in a position to afford. Although cost of living should be considered in the salary increase decision process, there should not be a policy that obligates the increase to a minimum of a certain amount.

Pages 1661, 1662

4. Which of the following statements about personnel policies is correct?

A. Although an office handbook for each employee may be a nicety for large practices, posting office personnel policies is adequate for the solo practice.

B. It is wise to have policies reviewed by legal counsel.

C. A personnel policy regarding an orientation period applies only to those who are new to the field. Employees with experience elsewhere should not need to be oriented.

D. Due to the legal sensitivity of ethnic group considerations, it is advised to avoid policies involving a person's appearance.

Answer: B

Critique: Legal counsel can alert you to questionable practices reflected in the personnel policies; where policies can be enforced; and policies that may not have been considered. Counsel should also stay abreast of changes in the law. With today's print capabilities afforded by computers, it is very little trouble to generate policies and distribute them in a handbook for each employee. All employees deserve and need an orientation to learn what, when, where, why, and how to perform the job. Statements on appearance are appropriate and need not

cross ethnic lines. Intentional discrimination should not be the motivation for writing any policy.

Page 1662

5. Management of the physician's time is a key to efficient practice and to personal gratification of the practice of medicine. Which one of the following statements is true?

A. Time management means skillfully performing many tasks well; for example, being able to interweave patient care, consultant calls, pharmacy refills, patient calls, and personal business into a constant flow of practice.

B. Telephones in examination rooms may increase practice overhead but save the physician time by allowing him or her to rapidly respond to issues that could later take much time yet have minimum impact on the patient's visit.

C. Dictated notes can be time consuming but can save the physician time deciphering handwritten notes in a busy practice in which patients see different physicians.

D. Business meetings are best made in the evenings. Physicians are more likely to be in a social mood in the evenings and foster good relationships in the medical community.

E. The management of a responsible practice rests with the physician. Those who stumble into letting someone else "call the shots" lose control and slip into poor office and medical management.

Answer: C

Critique: Dictated notes are time consuming and expensive but improve the physician's speed of reviewing his or her own charts as well as those of other physicians. Other methods of achieving typed notes include check sheets, standard quick text entered by a few prompts on the computer, editing of standard notes, barcodes, and voice recognition software. Various physicians have different information-processing styles, and a group practice may do well to offer a variety of information processing tools from which to choose. Time management does involve good performance at many tasks. Telephones in examination rooms make it more tempting to interrupt the physician, often with telephone calls that should not be taken in the presence of patients. Conomikes suggests that morning meetings are preferable because they have clear time limits and should have clear-cut agendas. The physician needs to focus on the practice of medicine and should not spend inordinate amounts of time making many minor decisions. While the physician remains "captain of the ship," he or she should hire responsible and capable persons and delegate responsibility appropriately.

Pages 1662–1664

65

Computer Applications in Office Practice

Clarence A. Jernigan

1. The most common practice management use of computers is:

    A. Patient and insurance billing
    B. Appointment scheduling
    C. Quality assurance reporting
    D. Medical records management

Answer: A

Critique: Practice management software programs that automate patient and insurance billing are the most widely used software packages in medical offices. Approximately 80% of medical offices use some type of accounts receivable software. Computers have an additional advantage in that management reports such as aged accounts would be difficult to accomplish without a computer. Submitting insurance claims electronically may save paper and lead to faster reimbursements. Computers are also used for maintenance of the medical record, appointment scheduling, and quality assurance; however, they are not used as extensively in these areas as they are in management of accounts.

Page 1665

2. When considering automation and computerization of a medical practice, the physician should consider all of the following EXCEPT:

    A. Perform a careful needs assessment of the practice.
    B. Include office management software products such as billing, appointment scheduling, and patient records as the essential ingredients.
    C. Require a detailed vendor demonstration of the program and system.
    D. Select hardware and software from independent vendors to secure the most cost-effective pricing.

Answer: D

Critique: The process of selecting an office-based computer system can be difficult to accomplish for most physicians. Physicians may not be experienced in computer software and hardware and can easily be overwhelmed by aggressive vendors and suppliers. It is essential when considering the automation of an office practice for the physician to do a careful needs assessment, and he or she should include the essential components of an automated system, including patient billing, scheduling, and patient records. Educational and diagnostic support software can be added, if needed, at a later time. Physicians should research each product carefully and solicit feedback from other users. Vendors should be required to provide a careful and complete demonstration of their product. Although cost is important, low cost systems may have high cost maintenance. When possible, hardware and software should be purchased from the same vendor to ensure compatibility and excellent and timely maintenance and support. If separate vendors are used, compatibility and support should be demonstrated prior to the purchase of any components of the system.

Pages 1670, 1671

Questions 3–7 (Matching) The clinical applications of computer-based office systems are expanding almost as rapidly as the technology. Match each of the following numbered statements with the corresponding best choice of options:

    A. Expert systems
    B. Electronic reference systems
    C. Both A and B
    D. Neither A nor B

3. A system that integrates unique attributes of a patient with knowledge available in the medical literature

4. Can quickly facilitate development of a differential diagnosis

5. Provide rapid access to medical literature

6. Places less emphasis on rote memorization of an ever-increasing medical knowledge base

7. Use in a medical practice has been shown to decrease professional liability risks.

Answers: 3-A, 4-A, 5-B, 6-C, 7-D

Critique: Expert systems allow the user to integrate unique information and attributes of a patient with a vast data base of knowledge available in the world's literature. These systems can quickly help a physician to expand his or her differential diagnosis, and some systems provide suggestions or recommendations on further diagnostic tests and studies. Electronic reference systems provide a convenient way of replacing traditional reference sources, such as textbooks and journals. These products are available on traditional media as well as on CD-ROM technology. Electronic reference systems allow physicians to quickly access a wide range of reference material and to quickly search through large volumes of material to find answers to specific questions. Both expert systems and electronic reference systems de-emphasize the need for rote memorization of large amounts of knowledge. Neither system has been shown to reduce practice professional liability risks.

Pages 1667–1669

Questions 8–11 (True or False) Proponents of the computer-based patient record (CPR) claim that CPR systems have numerous advantages compared with the traditional paper record. Which of the following are reported to be advantages of CPR systems?

8. Rapid access to information at multiple sites

9. Legibility of records and organization of data

10. Improvement of quality care through computer-generated clinical reminders

11. Reduced cost for storage and record supplies

Answers: 8-T, 9-T, 10-T, 11-T

Critique: In 1991, the Institute of Medicine of the National Academy of Science published a report that advocated the adoption by the year 2000 of the CPR as the standard for all medical records in the United States. Advocates of CPR systems claim numerous advantages over traditional records. Reduced cost for storage, paper supplies, personnel, rapid access to information with multiple site availability, record legibility and data organization, and improved quality of care are all part of the advantages claimed for CPR. (*Editor's note:* The authors of the chapter cite medical literature to support only the final claim that computer-generated clinical reminders can improve the quality of care.)

Page 1666

66

Malpractice and Risk Management

Clarence A. Jernigan

1. As a result of being named in a lawsuit, physicians are LEAST likely to:

    A. Suffer physical or emotional symptoms
    B. Practice defensive medicine by ordering extra tests
    C. Stop seeing certain types of patients
    D. Stop performing certain procedures
    E. Report suffering among family members

Answer: D

Critique: Sarah Charles, MD, a psychiatrist and leading authority on the response of physicians to the malpractice crisis, reports that as a result of being named in a lawsuit, 96% of physicians suffer physical or emotional symptoms, 62% order extra tests for protection, 42% stop seeing certain types of patients, 28% stop performing certain procedures, and 50% believe that their families suffer. She concluded that malpractice litigation, the chronic character of involvement with the legal process, and the resultant stress on both sued and non-sued physicians may in the long term not serve the public interest or the quality of medicine. Excessive malpractice litigation may diminish rather than enhance the integrity and availability of medical care.

Pages 1674, 1675

2. Most malpractice suits against physicians involve:

    A. Breech of contract
    B. Product liability
    C. Claims of negligence
    D. Personal battery

Answer: C

Critique: Malpractice suits against physicians almost always involve claims of negligence. Less commonly, they can involve breech of contract, battery, product liability, or other legal theories. The plaintiff has the burden of proving, with evidence, the following four elements in

order to prevail in a malpractice case: duty, injury, negligence, and proximate cause.

Page 1675

3. In malpractice claims alleging negligence, the plaintiff has the burden to prove:

    A. Lack of informed consent
    B. Personal battery
    C. Proximate cause
    D. Breech of confidentiality

Answer: C

Critique: Most malpractice suits against physicians involve claims of negligence. The plaintiff has the burden of proving that the physician had a duty to treat the patient. This usually means that some form of a physician-patient relationship existed at the time of the alleged negligent act. The act must be shown to be at variance with what the average physician would do in a similar situation. There must be clear evidence that an injury occurred and that the act was the proximate cause of the injury. Proximate cause is often difficult to prove or disprove. In general, the plaintiff must show one of the following: (1) the injury would not have occurred "but for" the negligent act; (2) the negligent act was a "substantial factor" in the injury; or, (3) the doctrine of res ipsa loquitur ("the thing speaks for itself") is satisfied. Negligence can occur even if informed consent was obtained. Proof of personal battery is not an essential element of negligence claims.

Pages 1675, 1676

4. Which one of the following is the most common allegation against family practitioners in professional liability cases?

    A. Failure to obtain informed consent
    B. Negligent obstetric practices

C. Failure to obtain timely consultation
D. Failure to correctly diagnose a problem
E. Negligent management of fracture and other trauma

Answer: D

Critique: About one third of cases brought against family physicians involve the failure to diagnose, or diagnose in a timely manner, certain conditions. About 50% of these cases involve cancer, particularly cancer of the breast, lung, colon, or testes. Masses or significant symptoms related to these areas should be carried to diagnosis in a prompt and efficient manner. Negligent obstetric practice is the second most common allegation in suits against family physicians. Plaintiffs allege failure to obtain informed consent in about 10% of cases. Failure to obtain timely consultation, negligent management of fractures and other trauma, negligent treatment with drugs, and negligent performance of a procedure are also among the top seven allegations against family physicians.

Pages 1680, 1681

5. True statements about informed consent include all of the following EXCEPT:

A. Informed consent is best accomplished by development, with expert legal advice, of a full disclosure consent form.
B. Ten percent of malpractice cases involve informed consent as an issue.
C. Informed consent is the relationship between the patient and the physician that allows a dialogue resulting in an understanding of the relevant risks and benefits involved in a proposed treatment option and its alternatives.
D. When obtaining informed consent, the physician should empathetically share the uncertainty that lies ahead.

Answer: A

Critique: Informed consent is the relationship between the patient and the physician that allows a dialogue resulting in an understanding of the relevant risks and benefits involved in a proposed treatment option and its alternatives. When obtaining informed consent, the physician should empathetically share with the patient and other appropriate parties the uncertainty that lies ahead. Although a signed consent, acceptable to legal council, is recommended, it is not the ultimate endpoint of informed consent. Informed consent is a cause of alleged malpractice in approximately 10% of claims brought against family physicians.

Page 1681

Questions 6–10 (True or False) Truisms germane to the professional liability problems experienced in the United States health care system include the following:

6. Physicians' expectations about the professional liability system are often as unrealistic as their patients' expectations about medicine.

7. All physicians contribute equally to the professional liability crisis.

8. There is more negligence committed than is ever recognized, litigated, or compensated.

9. Increased frequency of suits and increased sizes of awards contribute to increased malpractice insurance premiums.

10. During the past decade, the annual size of malpractice awards has stabilized.

Answers: 6-T, 7-F, 8-T, 9-T, 10-F

Critique: Professional liability and medical malpractice are serious concerns for all practicing physicians. Physicians who are uninformed about the legal system often have unrealistic expectations. Similarly, patients uninformed about medical care frequently have unrealistic expectations. The United States Department of Health and Human Services, in a communication in 1987, is quoted as saying, "physician expectations about the professional liability system are often as unrealistic as their patients' expectations about medicine." There is good evidence to suggest that there is more negligence committed than is ever recognized, litigated, or compensated. The most frequently cited study is the medical insurance feasibility study. The results of this study have also been confirmed by researchers at Harvard, who showed that about only one in eight negligently injured patients ever sued, and only one in sixteen patients ever recovered damages. There is also good evidence that a few physicians contribute to a large number of lawsuits. The study from Los Angeles County showed that 0.6% of the physicians accounted for 10% of the lawsuits and were responsible for 30% of all payments. During the past decade, the annual growth in the size of malpractice awards has averaged 20 to 30% per year combined with increasing frequency. The increased size of awards has not surprisingly contributed to an increase in malpractice insurance premiums.

Pages 1673, 1674

Questions 11–16 (True or False) Health system reforms, which are directed at professional liability issues, that potentially may reduce the cost of care and improve quality of care are:

11. Capping noneconomical awards

12. Periodic, rather than lump sum, payment of awards

13. Alternate dispute resolution

14. Shifting away from enterprise liability

15. Resisting "no fault" systems of liability

16. Implementation of practice guidelines

Answers: 11-T, 12-T, 13-T, 14-F, 15-F, 16-T

Critique: Professional liability has an impact on the cost and quality of care. Obviously, any proposed health care reform should directly address this issue. Both federal and state governments have proposed a number of options to control escalating professional liability. The California MICRA provisions are popular and include placing a cap on noneconomical awards, imposing a sliding scale on attorney contingency fees, emphasizing periodic rather than lump sum payment of awards, and eliminating collateral source awards. Alternate dispute resolution, such as pretrial arbitration, has also been proposed. The Clinton administration favors an emphasis on enterprise liability, focusing on the "system" and not on the individual. No-fault systems have been successful in the automobile insurance arena and are currently in place in Virginia and Florida. Other states have advocated the use of practice guidelines to lower malpractice costs.

Page 1678

Questions 17–21 (True or False)   Effective practices of risk management in the process of clinical medicine include:

17.   Full documentation in the medical record of your disagreement with a colleague's plan of care

18.   Full disclosure of your findings and plans to the patient, patient's family, nursing staff, and colleagues involved in the patient's case

19.   Keeping legible, accurate, consistent, timely objective, and complete records

20.   Immediate acceptance of blame for poor outcomes when you feel that you have made a wrong decision

21.   Handling emergencies to the best of your ability even though you are not as well trained to deal with the problem as are colleagues who will be available later

Answers: 17-F, 18-T, 19-T, 20-F, 21-T

Critique: The reflective practitioner can reduce the risk of professional liability claims by practicing the four Cs of risk management: compassion, communication, competence, and charting. Compassion is both toward the patient and his or her colleagues. Disagreements and "jousting" have no place in the medical record; however, it is prudent to fully explain your decisions when they, justifiably, go against guidelines, recommendations, or standards of care. Full disclosure and discussion of impressions and plans with patients and other key persons promote informed choices; however, confidentiality must be maintained. Clear, legible, accurate charting is essential to reduce liability risks, especially since most claims come to light long after memories of the events are gone, clouded, or tainted. Emergencies are always a challenge, but every physician should handle an emergent situation to the best of his or her ability until a more qualified person takes over, especially if a delay in treatment is obviously going to result in an undesirable outcome.

Pages 1681, 1682